C000090584

Recent Developments *in* Gynecology *and* Obstetrics

To our parents and to our families

Recent
Developments
in # Gynecology
and # Obstetrics

Selected papers presented at the 4th World Congress of
Gynecological Endocrinology organized by the International Society
of Gynecological Endocrinology joint with the 2nd Congress of the
European Society for Gynecologic and Obstetric Investigation,
Madonna di Campiglio, Italy, February 1995.

Edited by
A. R. Genazzani, F. Petraglia, G. D'Ambrogio,
A. D. Genazzani and P. G. Artini

The Parthenon Publishing Group
International Publishers in Medicine, Science & Technology

NEW YORK   LONDON

ACKNOWLEDGEMENTS

This work has been conducted in part supported by the Italian Research Council (CNR) – targeted project 'Prevention and Control Disease Factors', subproject Maternal-Infant Disease, contract No. 95.00887.PF41

Published in the UK and Europe by
The Parthenon Publishing Group Ltd.
Casterton Hall, Carnforth,
Lancs. LA6 2LA, UK

Published in North America by
The Parthenon Publishing Group Inc.
One Blue Hill Plaza
PO Box 1564, Pearl River,
New York 10965, USA

ISBN: 1-85070-700-6

Copyright © 1996 The Parthenon Publishing Group Ltd.

No part of this publication may be reproduced, stored in a retrieval system, or transmitted in any form or by any means, electronic, mechanical, photocopying, recording or otherwise, without prior permission from the publishers.

Typeset by H&H Graphics Ltd., Blackburn, UK
Printed and bound in Great Britain by
Bookcraft (Bath) Ltd., Midsomer Norton, UK

Contents

Preface   xxi

Section 1   Gynecological Endocrinology

Regulation of LH and FSH synthesis and secretion   3
J.C. Marshall, A.C. Dalkin, D.J. Haisenleder, J.R. Kerrigan, S.E. Kirk, J.A. Aloi and M. Yasin

Autocrine/paracrine functions of activin-B, inhibin-B and follistatin in the rat anterior pituitary   5
L.M. Bilezikjian and W.W. Vale

Neurosteroids: pharmacology and possible clinical implications   9
R.H. Purdy, M.D. Brot, C.A. Dyer, L.K. Curtiss, G.F. Koob and K.T. Britton

Role of neurosteroids in the modulation of hypothalamus–pituitary–adrenal function and reproductive function in rats   11
A.R. Genazzani, F. Petraglia, Ai-Li Guo, R.E. Nappi, M.A. Palumbo, A.A. de Micheroux, V. Cela, P.G. Artini, M. Criscuolo and G.P. Trentini

Weight-loss related amenorrhoea   17
P.G. Crosignani

Analysis of pituitary hormone secretion: pulsatility and copulsatility   21
A.D. Genazzani, F. Petraglia and A. Volpe

The role of inhibin in the regulation of FSH in man: unresolved issues   27
H.G. Burger and D.M. Robertson

Thyroid hormone receptors and the reproductive tract   31
A. Pinchera and E. Macchia

Disturbed follicle selection and anovulation in polycystic ovary syndrome   35
B.C.J.M. Fauser

Role of LH in oocyte maturation   37
Z. Shoham

Intraovarian markers of follicle and oocyte development   39
B.C. Tarlatzis and H. Bili

Insulin-like growth factors and binding proteins   43
E.-M. Rutanen, F. Pekonen and T. Nyman

Insulin-like growth factors and the human ovary   47
*P.G. Artini, G. D'Ambrogio, A. Barreca, V. Cela, C. Parri, C. Battaglia and
A.R. Genazzani*

Immunosuppressive activity of human follicular fluid   53
*A. Volpe, A. Macciò, E. Turnu, G. Contu, P. Artini, N. Maxia and
A.D. Genazzani*

Puberty: the critical juncture for expression of the polycystic ovary   59
V. Insler and B. Lunenfeld

**Pathophysiology of amenorrhea: current concepts (β-thalassemia as a model
of amenorrhea)**   63
V. Markussis and G. Tolis

The pituitary–adrenal axis response to CRF in women with PCOS   67
*A. Lanzone, F. Petraglia, A.M. Fulghesu, M. Guido, F. Cucinelli, L. Soranna,
A. Caruso and S. Mancuso*

**The primate luteal paracrine system: new insights with an emphasis on
intrinsic pulsatility**   73
C. Nappi, A.R. Gargiulo and C. Di Carlo

Ovarian safety aspects of LHRH antagonists and agonists   87
C.B. Lambalk, L. Brus and J. Schoemaker

The antiprogestins – modulators of progestin and glucocorticoid function   93
I.M. Spitz and A. Robbins

The contraceptive potential of the antiprogestin mifepristone   99
I.M. Spitz and A. Robbins

Premature ovarian failure   103
C. Faiman and A.E. Mehta

Effects of aging on the female reproductive system   107
A. Pellicer, C. Simón and J. Remohi

**Progress in diagnosis and treatment of hyperandrogenism of ovarian
origin**   113
A. Milewicz

Clinical and endocrine effects of ovarian laser surgery in patients with
polycystic ovary disease 119
W.G. Rossmanith, U. Ulrich and J. Keckstein

Corticotropin releasing factor effect on the pituitary–ovary axis in the
human luteal phase 125
R. Apa, P. Villa, A.M. Fulghesu, A. Lanzone, M. Guido, V. Pavone, F. Murgia,
A. Caruso and S. Mancuso

Influences of the opioid system on hyperinsulinemia and impaired
growth hormone secretion in PCOS obese subjects 131
P. Villa, D. Valle, A.M. Fulghesu, A. Lanzone, F. Cucinelli, A. Caruso,
A.M. De Luca, A. Mancini and S. Mancuso

Correlations between bone mineral density and hormonal factors in
androgenized women 137
M. Legan and A. Kocijančič

Effect of weight loss on the pituitary response to GnRH in obese
patients 141
G. Grugni, D. Moro, A. Ardizzi, A. Minocci and F. Morabito

Steroid hormones and the human breast 147
J.H.H. Thijssen and M.A. Blankenstein

Differentiation of ambiguous genitalia 153
Q.-S. Ge, Q. Yu, F. He, L. Yeh, S. Huang and C. Gu

Cholinergic dysregulation in anorexia nervosa 157
L. De Marinis, A. Mancini, M.L. Fabrizi, G. Conte, A. Bianchi,
M. Perrelli and D. Valle

Gonadotropin pulsatility in women with premenstrual syndrome 163
S. Vujović, M. Drezgić, Z. Penezić, M. Stojanović, B.Z. Beleslin, N. Krstić and
D. Slijepčević

Headache in primary empty sella: a psychoneuroendocrinological
approach 169
A. Mancini, G. Conte, D. Valle, C. D'Amico, C. Anile, G. Maira and
L. De Marinis

Nasal spray administration of bromocriptine: a preliminary study 175
E. Cicinelli, R. Maiorino, D. Petruzzi, G. Ragno, C. Ruccia, T. Falco,
G. Matteo and L.M. Schönauer

The role of melatonin in menstrual disorders of obese adolescents during
weight loss   183
G. Grugni, G. Calò, G. Guzzaloni, E. Tonelli, C. De Medici and F. Morabito

Liver involvement in Turner's syndrome: a case of 'newborn-like'
histology   189
M. Certo, D. Valle, L. Sammartano, L. Marra, L. Rossi, G. Fadda, A. Mancini
and L. De Marinis

LHRH agonists and uterine fibroids: before hysterectomy and after
myomectomy   193
P. Galli, A. Carani, A. Colombo, R. Delli Carpini, R. Guidetti, R. Fiozzi and
D. Tavernari

Insulin-like growth factors and steroidogenesis in polycystic ovarian
syndrome   197
A. Porcelli, C. Taccani and N. Surico

PCOS and surrenalic function   203
A. Tolino, S. Ronsini, M. Pellicano, A. Petrone and C. Nappi

The side-effects of oral hormonal contraceptives   211
N. Costin, I.V. Surcel, A. Rosca and S. Parastie

Effect of medroxyprogesterone acetate on ornithine decarboxylase
activity in human endometrial tissue and in MCF7 cells   217
G. Visca, R. Bellino, M. Tessarolo and A. Lanza

Disturbances in the hypothalamic-pituitary-gonadal axis of depressed
fertile women compared to normal controls   225
B. Hartmann, W. Baischer, G. Koinig, A. Albrecht, S. Kirchengast,
J. Huber and G. Langer

Section 2   Fertility and Sterility

Clinical aspects of preimplantation diagnosis   233
P.N. Barri, A. Veiga, M. Boada, J. Santaló, F. Vidal and J. Egozcue

Usefulness of cytogenetics in preimplantation diagnosis   239
A. Veiga

Factors affecting the selection of human embryos for transfer in an
IVF–ET program   243
S.M. Walker

Implantation 245
K. El-Farra and J.G. Grudzinskas

In vitro gamete micromanipulation and intracellular ionic changes 253
L. Leybaert and H.T. Depypere

**Effect of follicular fluid on sperm motility, acrosomal reactivity and
chemotactic response** 259
*A. Revelli, P. Tacconis, M. Modotti, C. Ansaldi, M. Balerna and
M. Massobrio*

Folliculogenesis with recombinant FSH stimulation 265
F. Ubaldi, J. Smitz, A. Van Steirteghem and P. Devroey

Use of gonadotropins for assisted reproductive techniques 271
*G. De Placido, C. Carravetta, C. Alviggi, A. Mollo, C. La Rusca and
C. Cadente Colucci*

**Use of pFSH for controlled ovarian hyperstimulation in an IVF-ET
program** 277
*M. Salvatori, M.R. Sgherzi, P.G. Artini, G. Regnani, P. Traversi and
C. Battaglia*

The luteal support in stimulated cycles 281
C. Montoneri, F. Nardo and G. Zarbo

Endometriosis: impact on fertility 285
A. Caruso, G. Paradisi and A.M. Fulghesu

Superovulation and pregnancy rate in minimal and mild endometriosis 293
R. Agostini, S. Galossi, G. Pesce, A. Quinzi and G. Traficante

The surgical treatment of recurrent endometriosis 297
L. Fedele, S. Bianchi, M. Candiani, M. Busacca and M. Vignali

Atypical laparoscopic appearances of peritoneal endometriosis 301
S. Dessole, G. Ambrosini, M. Dei, A. Scapinelli and N. Vargiu

Hysteroscopy in infertile women 307
V. Benedetto, V. Palmara, M. Micalizzi, G. Zona, J. Leonardi and R. Leonardi

Reproductive outcome after hysteroscopic metroplasty 311
*N. Colacurci, A. Mollo, C. Carravetta, R. Sagliocco, T. Santoro and
G. De Placido*

Laparoscopic treatment of adnexal torsion   315
S. Dessole, P.L. Cherchi, M. Farina, G. Ambrosini and M. Dei

Idiopathic sterility and intratubaric insemination   319
R. Agostini, D.R. Ambrosio, C. Ban, M.T. Filosofi and A. Quinzi

**Psychological and clinical aspects of assisted reproduction with
donor semen**   325
G. D'Ambrogio, P.G. Artini, A.A. de Micheroux, M. Tarabusi, V. Cela,
C. Parri, C. Battaglia and A.R. Gennazzani

Psychological counselling in the infertile couple   331
P. Pezzella and L. Cersosimo

**Recurrent spontaneous abortion: epidemiology and prospective
management**   335
V. Trojano, R. Alfonso and N. Veloce

Antiphospholipid syndrome and spontaneous recurrent abortion   341
V. Benedetto, J. Leonardi, R. D'Anna, G. Zona, F.V. Ardita, A. Mancuso and
R. Leonardi

**Intrauterine auto-erotic movements: preparation to coping mechanisms
– a case report**   345
C. Battaglia, P.G. Artini, M. Salvatori, M.R. Sgherzi, P. Traversi and A. Volpe

Chronic anovulation: therapeutical strategies and clinical results   351
A.M. Mattei, P. Monti, B. Bocconcello, M. Serrani, V. Liprandi and P. Capetta

**Comparison between u-hFSH conventional protocol and a personalized
approach in controlled ovarian hyperstimulation**   357
F. Zullo, C. Di Carlo, M. Pellicano, R. De Stefano, P. Mastrantonio and
C. Nappi

**Pelvic endometriosis with histological aspects of perineural involvement:
case report**   363
A. Azzena, G. Cerri, R. Salmaso, F. Vasoin, C. Vasile and A. Ferrara

**Strange histological findings of the uterine endometriomyosis: biological
meaning**   371
S. Cianci, A. Mangiacasale and L. Milluzzo

Section 3   Menopause

Menopause and pregnancy: the woman's point of view   375
M. Boulet

**Late effects of menopausal ovarian failure: physiopathological and
clinical aspects**   385
M. Massobrio, M. Ardizzoja, M. Gallo and G. De Luigi

Urodynamic diagnosis and ultrasound findings   389
L.D. Cardozo, V. Khullar, S. Hill and A. Yip

Mammary changes during the menopausal transition   393
R. Pérez Sanz, L. Villavieja, P. de la Cueva, I. Morollón and F.R. Pérez-López

Parenteral versus oral replacement therapy with estrogens: an overview   401
A.E. Schindler

**Comparison of oral and transdermal hormone replacement therapy:
a multicenter study with a new transdermal system**   407
J. Herold, B. Sajtos, U.H. Winkler and A.E. Schindler

Estrogen–androgen hormone replacement therapy   413
M.M. Gelfand

**Effect of conjugated estrogens on skin thickness: a randomized,
double-blind, placebo-controlled study**   419
R. Maheux

**Minimizing the untoward effects of progestin in hormonal replacement
therapy**   423
A. Kauppila, T. Raudaskoski and E. Suvanto-Luukkonen

**Stimulation of prostacyclin and unaffected endothelin-1 by estradiol
provides one explanation for cardiovascular protection by estrogen
replacement therapy**   427
O. Ylikorkala

**Hemodynamic effects of hormonal replacement therapy in normal
postmenopausal women**   431
*P.L. Montaldo, M. Tronci, M.A. Fenu, C. Montaldo, P. Soi, G. Pittau,
S. Angioni and A. Volpe*

Hormones and hypertension   437
S. Palacios, C. Menendez and A.R. Jurado

Color Doppler analysis of ophthalmic and uterine arteries in
postmenopausal patients treated with hormone replacement therapy   441
*C. Battaglia, M.R. Sgherzi, P. Traversi, P.G. Artini, A.D. Genazzani and
A. Volpe*

Hemostatic variables and estrogen substitution in postmenopausal
women   447
U.H. Winkler

A new approach to postmenopausal hormonal treatment   453
N. Mercuri, P. Ardito, F. Vescio, V. Scarcella, A. Leotta, S.G. Lio and P. Vadalà

Placebo-controlled randomized trial of melbrosia pld for the treatment
of climacteric symptoms   457
M.O. Sator, D.M. Gruber, P. Frigo, W. Knogler and J.C. Huber

Kinetics of a new 17β-estradiol transdermal drug delivery system   463
U.D. Rohr, C. Nauert and A.M. Ehrly

Effect of β-estradiol therapy in menopause by transdermic means   469
E. Giannone, M.N.J. Abubakari, P. De Domenico, S. Bori and V. Lauro

Klimonorm® in postmenopausal hormonal therapy   473
P. Šuška, M. Borovský and D. Uherčík

Analysis of efficacy and the bleeding pattern during 6 months' treatment
with sequential and continuous estrogen-progestogen therapy   479
T. Moskovic and S. Runic

Occurrence of untreated climacteric and estrogen-deficient syndrome in
general medicine practice   485
E. Šuškova, P. Šuška, G. Kováč and A. Šoka

Abdominal repair of small cystocele following total hysterectomy   489
*P. Galli, P. Bellodi, R. Delli Carpini, G. Guerzoni, L. Padula,
D. Tavernnari and M.A. Vezzani*

Evaluation of ovarian activity in hysterectomized women with
conservation of the ovaries   493
E. Alba, R. Lerro, L. Corvetto, L. Nuzzo and G. Ragonesi

Feasability of reconstructive vaginal surgery according to Kelly-Kennedy
in the treatment of genital prolapse   497
A. Carbonaro, R. Cantarella, V. Aidala and S. Reitano

Medical therapy in the prevention of recurrent dysfunctional uterine bleeding   501
S. Dessole, E. Coccollone, G. Ambrosini, N. Vargiu, A. Scapinelli and
P.L. Cherchi

MAP and LHRH agonists combination in the treatment of simple endometrial hyperplasia   507
P. Galli, P. Bellodi, R. Delli Carpini, G. Guerzoni, L. Padula,
D. Tavernari and M.A. Vezzani

Hysteroscopic diagnosis in women with abnormal uterine bleeding   511
V. Benedetto, V. Palmara, G. Zona, E. Crea, M. Rigano, J. Leonardi and
M. Micalizzi

Hysterectomy in Finland   515
E.-M. Rutanen and R. Luoto

Menopausal profile: proposal of a synthetic index on menopausal state   519
G. Fiorentino, A. Celona, L. Barbaro and C. Pullè

Intrafascial vaginal hysterectomy, an alternative to traditional surgery: indications   523
S. Maffei, A. Di Gregorio, G. Sarpa, A. Re, L. Leo, A. Venuti, G. Gordini,
R. Bellino, M. Tessarolo, G. Visca, G. Osnengo, T. Wierdis and A. Lanza

Hormone replacement therapy or intact ovaries in radical surgery for cervical cancer in young women   529
S. Maffei, R. Bellino, A. Re, M. Tessarolo, L. Leo, A. Venuti, G. Sarpa,
T. Wierdis, G. Visca and A. Lanza

Section 4   Obstetric Care – Prenatal Medicine

First-trimester serum screening for Down syndrome   535
K.J. Powell and J.G. Grudzinskas

Chromosome mosaicism in prenatal diagnosis   541
S. Agosti, G. Nocera, P. Ilardi, C. Bombelli, N. Cotrozzi, F. Gramellini,
D. Coviello and L. Dalprà

Hemoglobin, glucose, α-fetoprotein and endocrine changes during normal pregnancy   547
F.R. Pérez-López, J. Hergueta, J. Robert, M.D. Abós and V. Peg

Pregnancy and diabetes   557
R. Navalesi, G. Di Cianni, L. Volpe, P. Orsini and L. Benzi

Hypertension in pregnancy and insulin-resistant syndrome 565
O. Ylikorkala

Hypoplastic left heart syndrome: implications of the prenatal diagnosis 569
P. Bogatti, G. Maso, S. Alberico, R. Pinzano and S. Guaschino

Intrauterine growth retardation and antiphospholipid antibody
syndrome 577
S. Reitano, V. Aidala, R. Platania, R. Cantarella and A. Carbonaro

Antiphospholipid antibodies and pre-eclamptic disorders 583
S. Reitano, V. Aidala, R. Cantarella and A. Carbonaro

Activin A, parturition and preterm labor 589
F. Petraglia, P. Florio, A. Gallinelli, D. De Vita, P. Scida, M. Simonelli,
C. Salvestroni, M. Lombardo and A.R. Genazzani

Neurotransmitters in the myometrium 595
N.-O. Sjöberg and M. Stjernquist

Biological changes preceding onset of labor 599
A. Skret

Endogenous oxytocin at term and preterm parturition: the intrauterine
pattern 605
A. Mauri, C. Ticconi and E. Piccione

The influence of non-clinical factors on the decision for vaginal delivery
after prior Caesarean section 609
E. Alba, R. Lerro, M. Fenocchio and G. Visca

Comparison of Ondansetron versus acupuncture to preserve
post-operative nausea and vomiting in Caesarean section: is it always
a useful preventive therapeutic intervention? 613
F. Capone, V. Cozzolino, C. D'Auria, E. Desiderio, F. Lollo, G. D'Aniello,
C. Pagano, M. Piscopo, R. Molaro, A. Castaldo, G. Lubrano and G. Vairo

Intensive care during pregnancy: our experience 619
F. Lollo, F. Capone, E. Desiderio, P. De Luca, A. Castaldo Tuccillo and
G. Vairo

Spinal block in emergency Caesarean section: our experience 625
E. Desiderio, G. Lubrano, F. Lollo, R. Molaro, M. Piscopo, M. Grieco,
C. D'Auria and G. Vairo

Incidence of ectopic pregnancy: preliminary results of a
population-based register in Lithuania   631
G. Bogdanskiene, I. Dirsaite and J.G. Grudzinskas

Blood lead levels in pregnant women: a study conducted in Pisa and
surrounding areas   637
G. Guazzelli, M.A. Celano, E. Neri, M.C. Papa, S. Masoni,
C. Salvestroni and C. De Punzio

Early transvaginal ecocardiography   643
M.A. Vezzani, R. Guidetti, A. Carani, A. Colombo, R. Fiozzi and P. Galli

Diagnostic approach to urinary incontinence in pregnancy   649
A. Carbonaro, R. Cantarella, V. Aidala and S. Reitano

Laparoscopic treatment of ectopic pregnancy   655
D. Cirillo, A. Tolino, E. Sole, A. Petrone, P. Ferrara, E. Parente,
C. Rapicano and C. Nappi

Operative hysteroscopy and pregnancies   661
V. Benedetto, V. Palmara, M. Rigano, G. Zona, F.V. Ardita, J. Leonardi and
R. Leonardi

Microalbuminuria and PIH   665
G. Menato, M. Anzivino, P. Petruzzelli, B. Masturzo, M. Massobrio and
Q. Carta

Obstetric management of PROM   671
F. Polatti, F. Perotti, C. Belloni, U. Maccarini, N. Filippa, M. Ciccarese and
A. Catinella

Section 5   Infections of the Lower Genital Tract

Sexually transmitted diseases and infertility: a global perspective   679
G. Benagiano and P. Rowe

Molecular applications in the diagnosis of sexually transmitted diseases   683
M. Comar and S. Guaschino

Cervicitis and vaginitis in elderly women diagnosed by the Papanicolaou
smear   687
V.G. Gandulfo, J.B. Silva and N.R. Pereira

Cytology in cervical screening for carcinoma and HPV infection:
which role? 693
S. Masoni, R. Parducci, G. Giovannetti, C. Salvestroni, M.C. Papa,
M.A. Celano, G. Guazzelli and C. De Punzio

HPV infections in male sexual partners 697
E. Giannone, N. Di Giulio and V. Lauro

HPV infection: cytocolpohystologic correlations in patients affected by
condylomatosis of external genitalia 701
G. Piras, F. Esposito, M.P. Bagella, L. Pinna Nossai, P. Lecca, L. Manca,
A. Scapinelli and P.L. Cherchi

Combined treatment (sytemic and topical) with α-interferon in genital
HPV infections 707
A. Azzena, G. Cerri, V. Brunetti, J. Dal Maso, C. Vasile and F. Vasoin

Section 6 Gynecological Oncology

Sex steroid receptors, LH/hCG receptor, and oncogene expression in
endometrial carcinomas 715
I. Konishi, M. Koshiyama, M. Mandai, T. Komatsu, S. Yamamoto, K. Nanbu,
S. Fujii, Ch. V. Rao and T. Mori

Tumor-associated markers of stromal origin as indicators of clinical
course of ovarian cancer 721
A. Kauppila, G. -G. Zhu, C. Tomás, U. Puistola, M. Santala, F. Stenbäck,
S. Kauppila, J. Risteli and L. Risteli

Steroid hormones and breast cancer 727
J.A. Pinotti and R. Hegg

Expression of bcl-2 and p53 in human breast cancer: relationships with
proliferative activity and clinical findings 733
M. Massobrio, L. Bianchi Malandrone, A. Demurtas, A. Durando,
O. Gaiola, M. Geuna, A. Ramella, A. Ravarino, M. Sberveglieri,
B. Torchio and G. Palestro

Endocrine management of breast cancer 739
H.P.G. Schneider

Surgical management of breast cancer 745
F.R. Pérez-López

Hormonotherapy for advanced or recurrent breast cancer   763
P. Sismondi and F. Genta

GnRH-agonists for treatment of benign and malignant breast disease   773
A.E. Schindler

Mammary and metabolic changes induced by tamoxifen   777
F.R. Pérez-López, I. Morollón, J. Hergueta and R. Pérez Sanz

Breast cancer and breast implants: can a chronic granulomatous inflammation provoked by a breast implant with rough-spongious surface produce acquired immunity against tumors? – the role of IFN-γ and TNF secreting epithelioid cells   787
I. Lyras, P. Rapti, T. Nassif, G. Cotta-Pereira and I. Pitanguy

Needle localization of clinically occult breast lesions   793
G. Ragonesi, L. Nuzzo, A. Decko, E. Alba, M. Fenocchio, L. Corvetto and S. Maffei

Intra-operative ultrasound in non-palpable mammary lesions   797
A. Di Giorgio, L. Cersosimo, P. Arnone and A. Canavese

A follicular cyst complicating tamoxifen therapy in a premenopausal breast cancer woman: a case report   803
L. Leo, A. Re, M. Tessarolo, R. Bellino, G. Gordini, A. Venuti, M. Rosso, T. Wierdis and A. Lanza

Oncogenes and ovarian cancer   807
M. Marzola, F. Morali, G. Balconi, M.G. Cantù, S. Rota and C. Mangioni

Cytokines in ovarian cancer   811
A. Gadducci, M. Ferdeghini, O. Gagetti, C. Prontera, A. Bonuccelli, V. Facchini, R. Bianchi and A.R. Genazzani

Serum CA 125 assay in the management of ovarian cancer   817
A. Gadducci, M. Ferdeghini, C. Castellani, C. Annicchiarico, A. Perutelli, V. Facchini, R. Bianchi and A.R. Genazzani

Immunoscintigraphy in ovarian cancer   821
M. Ferdeghini, A. Gadducci, G. Boni, F. Matteucci, C.R. Bellina, M. Grosso, B. Prato, V. Facchini, A.R. Genazzani and R. Bianchi

Laparoscopic treatment of serous and mucinous ovarian cystoadenomas   827
D. Cirillo, A. Tolino, G. Passannanti, E. Sole, A. Petrone, V. Graziano, P. Ferrara and C. Nappi

Laparoscopic treatment of dermoid cysts 833
D. Cirillo, A. Tolino, A. Petrone, G. Passannanti, S. Ronsini, E. Sole,
P. Ferrara and C. Nappi

Laparoscopic treatment of ovarian cysts 837
G.L. Bracco, M.E. Coccia, E. Scatena and G. Scarselli

Usefulness of presurgical staging in the prognostic evaluation of
endometrial cancer 843
P.L. Cherchi, F. Sbernardori, G. Ruiu, F. Esposito, G.B. Franco,
M.P. Bagella and A. Ambrosini

SHBG level changes after high-dose danazol in postmenopausal women
with endometrial cancer 849
A. Rigano, G. Baviera, E. Sturlese, M. Rigano and C. Pullè

Ploidy in endometrial carcinoma 855
M. Melpignano, M. Brusati, C. Merisio, L. Sansebastiano, M. Fontanesi,
A. Merialdi and E. Vadora

Hormonal pattern after high-dose danazol therapy in postmenopausal
women with endometrial cancer 863
A. Rigano, G. Baviera, E. Sturlese, M. Rigano and C. Pullè

Changes of hormone serum levels in endometrial adenocarcinoma after
progestin therapy 869
A. Re, R. Bellino, M. Rosso, M. Tessarolo, L. Leo, A. Lauricella, A. Venuti,
T. Wierdis, G. Visca and A. Lanza

Cervical cancer treated at stage I and II: evolution and surveillance 875
N. Surico and G. Ferraris

Radical hysterectomy and pelvic lymphadenectomy for cervical
cancer IB: a review of 72 cases 881
V. Vavalà, A. Monaco, M. Garizio and A. Scribanti

HPV and cervical intraepithelial neoplasia 887
G. Piras, M.P. Bagella, F. Esposito, L. Pinna Nossai, P. Lecca, M. Putzolu,
A. Scapinelli and P.L. Cherchi

Aggressive angiomyxoma of the vagina: case report and review of the
literature 891
A. Azzena, R. Salmaso, F. Vasoin, G. Cerri, M. Gardiman and T. Zen

Serous papillary ovarian carcinoma: solitary uterine polyp metatstase 897
A. Azzena, R. Salmaso, F. Vasoin, G. Cerri, S. Polonio and G. Altavilla

Relationships between proliferative activity and oncogene expression in human breast cancer   901
M. Massobrio, L. Bianchi Malandrone, A. Demurtas, A. Durando, M. Geuna, N. Ravarino, M. Sberveglieri, B. Torchio and G. Palestro

Ornithine decarboxylase activity, P21 overexpression and P53 mutation in progestin treated endometrial adenocarcinoma   905
R. Bellino, A. Venuti, L. Leo, A. Re, M. Tessarolo, S. Colombatto, L. Gubetta, S. Cappia, T. Wierdis and A. Lanza

Ovarian carcinoma metastases to the breast and axillary node: case report   915
M. Tessarolo, L. Leo, A. Re, R. Bellino, B. Ghiringhello, A. Venuti, T. Wierdis, G. Visca and A. Lanza

Author Index   921

Preface

This volume comprises some of the papers presented at the biannual joint Congress of the International Society of Gynecological Endocrinology and of the European Society of Gynecologic and Obstetric Investigation. For this reason, the chapters are concerned with reproductive endocrinology, prenatal medicine and gynecological oncology.

Several topics have been the subject of detailed discussion. The most recent advances on the role of growth factors in the regulation of reproductive function, in embryo-fetal growth, and in the pathogenesis of benign and malignant tumors of the female genital tract are presented. Considerable space is devoted to the role of the sex hormones in the modulation of mood and behaviour during reproductive life, and various aspects of gamete maturation and function, and the mechanisms of implantation are debated fully. Throughout the book, basic and clinical investigations are reported and we are confident that these proceedings reflect accurately the modern science for present and future generations of gynecologists.

SECTION 1

Gynecological Endocrinology

Regulation of LH and FSH synthesis and secretion

J.C. Marshall, A.C. Dalkin, D.J. Haisenleder, J.R. Kerrigan*, S.E. Kirk, J.A. Aloi and M. Yasin

Divisions of Endocrinology, *Departments of Internal Medicine and Pediatrics, University of Virginia Health Sciences Center, Charlottesville, VA, USA

Pituitary luteinizing hormone (LH) and follicle-stimulating hormone (FSH) consist of a common α and different ß subunits which are encoded by 3 genes. Both synthesis and secretion of LH and FSH are regulated by gonadotropin releasing hormone (GnRH). GnRH is secreted in a series of pulses which are essential to maintain protein synthesis and secretion. The amplitude and frequency of hypothalamic GnRH secretion vary in normal physiology, and are associated with differential secretion of LH and FSH. Gonadal steroids can modify GnRH secretion, and gonadotrope responses to GnRH can be modulated by both gonadal steroids and gonadal peptides such as inhibin, activin, and follistatin. Activin increases FSH ß mRNA and FSH secretion, while inhibin and follistatin reduce mRNA concentrations and serum FSH. Thus in vivo regulation of LH and FSH synthesis and secretion reflects changes in the pattern of GnRH pulse stimuli, together with the direct actions of gonadal steroids and peptides on the gonadotrope cell.

We have examined regulation of gonadotropin subunit gene expression using a GnRH deficient male and female rat models.

Physiologic regulation of gonadotropin subunit mRNAs:-

In male rats, steady state concentrations of α, LH and FSH ß mRNAs are fairly constant, whereas in females up to 3 fold changes in subunit mRNA concentrations occur during the four day estrous cycle in rats. On metestrus FSH ß mRNA is selectively increased, and on diestrus, both alpha and LH ß are transiently elevated. On proestrus, LH ß mRNA increases (3 fold) prior to the LH surge, and FSH ß mRNA increases (4 fold) during and after the LH surge. These changes reflect regulation of subunit mRNA transcription rates, particularly that on proestrus, while changes in FSH ß mRNA may also reflect alterations in plasma inhibin and in expression of pituitary follistatin.

GnRH pulse secretion varies during the estrous cycle with low amplitude slow frequency pulses on metestrus increasing in both amplitude and frequency by proestrus. A pulsatile GnRH stimulus is essential for ß subunit transcription, and GnRH appears to be the main regulator of gonadotropin subunit mRNA expression. The stability of newly transcribed FSH ß mRNA can be modulated by gonadal steroids and peptides. Estradiol and progesterone in females and testosterone in males can stabilize FSH ß mRNA. Activin also enhances FSH ß stability, while inhibin and follistatin decrease mRNA stability and reduce FSH ß mRNA. Both follistatin and inhibin subunits (components of both inhibin and activin) are present in pituitary gonadotropes. Thus the predominant regulation of gonadotropin synthesis appears to be effected by GnRH, with different patterns of GnRH pulse stimulation effecting differential expression of gonadotropin subunit mRNAs. This effect of GnRH is mediated both by direct effects on subunit transcription, and by the role of GnRH in regulating follistatin synthesis in the gonadotrope. Thus the overall regulation of subunit mRNA expression during the four day

3

estrous cycle probably reflects the combined effects of GnRH regulation of both subunit transcription and follistatin synthesis, together with the effects of gonadal steroids in regulating the stability of a newly transcribed FSH ß mRNA.

Studies in GnRH Deficient Models:-

We have used GnRH deficient rat models and have administered exogenous GnRH to study the role of GnRH pulses in subunit mRNA expression. Suppression of endogenous GnRH secretion is achieved in gonadectomized animals by continuous replacement of testosterone in males, or estradiol and progesterone in females. An alternative method is to block GnRH secretion using the α-1 adrenergic receptor blocker phenoxybenzamine (PBZ).

Studies in GnRH Deficient Male Rats:- In castrate male rats replaced with testosterone, earlier studies showed that a pulsatile GnRH stimulus is required to increase LH ß and FSH ß transcription. In subsequent studies, we examined the effects of different patterns of both GnRH pulse amplitude and frequency on subunit gene expression. All amplitudes of GnRH pulses increased α and FSH ß mRNAs by 2-3 fold. LH ß mRNA, however, was maximally expressed after 25 ng GnRH pulses (producing maximum plasma GnRH concentrations of approx 200 pg/ml). In similar studies, the 25 ng GnRH pulse dose was given at different intervals (between 8 and 480 minutes) to reproduce frequencies seen in normal physiology. Fast frequency (8 minute interval) GnRH pulses increased both α and LH ß mRNA, pulses given every 30 minutes increased all three subunits mRNA, whilst slower frequency (120 minutes or longer) pulses only increased FSH ß mRNA.

We investigated the mechanisms of this differential mRNA expression by measuring pituitary follistatin mRNA using a quantitative reverse transcriptase - polymerase chain reaction assay in RNA extracted from rat pituitaries. Initial studies showed that follistatin mRNA was regulated by GnRH, the 3 fold increase after castration being prevented by a GnRH antagonist. Measurement of pituitary follistatin mRNA after different GnRH pulse frequencies revealed that follistatin mRNA increased 3 fold after fast frequency (every 8 or 30 minute pulses), but was not increased by slower frequencies. Thus, follistatin mRNA expression was the reciprocal of FSH ß mRNA concentrations following different GnRH pulse frequencies. Thus the effects of GnRH in increasing follistatin after fast frequency stimuli, would reduce FSH ß mRNA stability and steady state FSH ß mRNA would not increase. In contrast, slow frequency GnRH pulses do not increase follistatin mRNA and FSH ß mRNA concentrations increase as a consequence of increased transcription.

Studies in GnRH Deficient Female Rats:- The alpha adrenergic antagonist PBZ was used to block endogenous GnRH secretion in ovariectomized rats. GnRH pulses were administered in the presence or absence of ovarian steroids and hypothalamic peptides. GnRH pulses given at 30 minute intervals, similar to GnRH pulse secretion during the LH surge, increased α and FSH ß mRNA (2-5 fold respectively). Similar results were observed in the presence or absence of estradiol and progesterone. Of interest, LH ß mRNA was not increased by any GnRH pulse regimen used. This suggested the possibility that other hypothalamic peptides may act in concert with GnRH on the afternoon of proestrus to rapidly increase LH ß mRNA synthesis. The peptides GnRH associated peptide (GAP), neuropeptide-Y (NP-Y), and galanin (GAL), are all increased in portal blood on proestrus afternoon and are known to enhance GnRH secretion or LH responsiveness to GnRH. Co-administration of these peptides together with GnRH however, failed to increase LH ß mRNA. This suggests that other factors, potentially of ovarian origin, are required for the rapid expression of LH ß mRNA seen on proestrus afternoon.

References

1. Marshall, J.C., Dalkin, A.C., Haisenleder, D.J., Paul, S.J., Ortolano, G.A. and Kelch, R.P. (1991). Gonadotropin releasing hormone pulses: regulators of gonadotropin synthesis and ovulatory cycles. Rec. Prog. Horm. Res. 47, 155-189
2. Kerrigan, J.R., Dalkin, A.C., Haisenleder, D.J., Yasin, M. and Marshall, J.C. (1993). Failure of gonadotropin releasing hormone (GnRH) pulses to increase LH beta mRNA in GnRH deficient female rats. Endocrinology 133, 2071-2079
3. Kirk, S.E., Dalkin, A.C., Yasin, M., Haisenleder, D.J. and, Marshall J.C. (1994). GnRH pulse frequency regulates expression of pituitary follistatin mRNA: a mechanism for differential gonadotrope function. Endocrinology 135, 876-880

Autocrine/paracrine functions of activin-B, inhibin-B and follistatin in the rat anterior pituitary

L.M. Bilezikjian and W.W. Vale

Clayton Foundation Laboratories for Peptide Biology, The Salk Institute, La Jolla, California, USA

It has become increasingly evident that the response of anterior pituitary cells to various hypothalamic and peripheral hormones is influenced by factors that are synthesized and secreted within the pituitary. The concept of autocrine/paracrine regulation of the anterior pituitary is not novel (3) and the pituitary is now established to be a site of production of a number of growth factors and bioactive peptides that may function to locally modulate pituitary function. Included in the group of local modulators are the inhibins, activins and follistatins, which have been demonstrated to exert local modulatory effects on gonadotropes and possibly on other pituitary cell types (2,1).

Activins ($\beta_A\beta_A$=activin-A, $\beta_B\beta_B$=activin-B and $\beta_A\beta_B$=activin-AB) and inhibins ($\alpha\beta_A$=inhibin-A and $\alpha\beta_B$=inhibin-B) are structurally related dimeric proteins with stimulatory and inhibitory effects on FSH secretion, respectively (7). The three subunit proteins that comprise the family of inhibin/activin proteins belong to the TGFβ superfamily of growth and differentiation factors because of their significant structural and functional similarities with members of this large family (7).

The mechanism by which activins exert their biological actions has not been fully elucidated thus far. Cross-linking experiments with [^{125}I]activin-A have revealed the presence of two major affinity-labeled complexes in most tissues examined, reflecting type I and type II receptor forms (5). The cloning of several structurally related type I and type II activin receptors has identified a novel family of receptors having an intracellular serine/threonine protein kinase domain (5). Although the exact nature of the functional interactions of the type I and the type II receptors, and the downstream substrates of their catalytic domains have not been identified, the presence of both receptor types is required for ligand binding, signal transduction and responsiveness to activins. *In situ* hybridization techniques indicate a pattern of wide-spread distribution pattern for these receptors, reminiscent of the distribution for their ligand (7,5).

In the pituitary, activins stimulate FSH secretion and FSHβ mRNA accumulation but suppress basal and GRF-stimulated GH secretion and synthesis (1). Activins also inhibit basal ACTH and PRL secretion and synthesis. In contrast to the activins, inhibins suppress FSH secretion and synthesis (7) but have little or no effect on the other pituitary cell types suggesting each pituitary cell type may express a distinct set of inhibin/activin receptor isoforms. In general, inhibins function as biological antagonists of activins (7), presumably, by either competing with activin binding to its receptor or by transducing opposing intracellular signals via specific inhibin receptors.

There is compelling evidence that gonadal inhibins function as negative feedback regulators of pituitary FSH secretion and synthesis (7). A similar endocrine function for activins, on the other hand, has not been demonstrated. Activins, unlike inhibins, may play a more important role as local autocrine/paracrine factors, given the wide-spread anatomic distribution of inhibin/activin β_A and β_B in a wide variety of tissues where their biological actions have been documented (7,2,1).

Follistatins are cysteine-rich single-chain glycoproteins that were identified in gonadal fluids based on their ability to suppress pituitary FSH secretion (4,6). Two alternatively spliced mRNA transcripts give rise to a full-length 315 amino acid protein and a carboxy-terminally truncated 288 amino acid form. Follistatin mRNA expression appears to generally coincide with that of the inhibin/activin β subunits or with activin-responsive cells, suggestive of a role for follistatins as local modulators of the actions of activins. The ability of follistatins to inhibit FSH secretion or any of the biological actions of activins is attributed to their ability to bind activins and thus biologically inactivate them.

Inhibin/activin subunits and follistatins are expressed within the pituitary, inhibin/activin α and β_B expression being restricted to gonadotropes (7,2,1). The analysis of metabolically labeled cultured rat anterior pituitary cell lysates revealed the presence of multiple forms of inhibin/activin α subunit protein but only two forms of β_B-immunoreactivity corresponding to monomeric 14-15 kDa β_B and its 90-95 kDa (or 40-45 kDa, reduced) precursor form. The expression of both α and β_B inhibin/activin subunits by gonadotropes of the rat anterior pituitary makes this tissue a likely site of production of either inhibin-B, activin-B or both. Follistatin mRNA, on the other hand, has been detected in all pituitary cell types and the protein is secreted by cultured rat anterior pituitary and bovine pituitary folliculostellate cells. Immunoreactive follistatin from rat anterior pituitary cells migrates as a broad 35-46 kDa unreduced band, characteristic of glycosylated polypeptides.

In order to evaluate if pituitary follistatin functions as a local modulator of the response of pituitary cells to activins, an antiserum directed against purified porcine follistatin was used to biologically immunoneutralize the protein. In the presence of this follistatin antiserum, the ability of activin-A to stimulate FSH secretion was significantly enhanced, confirming a functionally relevant role for locally secreted follistatin.

Evidence that activin-B is a likely local product of cultured rat of anterior pituitary cells was also obtained by the use of a monoclonal antibody directed against dimeric activin-B (7,2,1). The addition of the antibody to cultured rat anterior pituitary cells suppressed basal FSH secretion and FSHβ mRNA accumulation, suggesting that locally secreted activin-B plays an autocrine function within the anterior pituitary. The presence of locally secreted dimeric activin-B was subsequently confirmed by the analysis of secreted products of metabolically labeled rat anterior pituitary cells, *in vitro* . An N-terminally directed antiserum directed against β_B immunoprecipitated a secreted protein of 24-25 kDa (unreduced) or 14-15 kDa (reduced) apparent size. The likelihood that rat anterior pituitary cells secrete inhibin-B or a form of bioactive α is also supported by functional experiments with an immunoneutralizing antiserum to α. This α antiserum increased basal FSH secretion from cultured rat anterior pituitary cells, indicating that a biologically active inhibin-like immunoreactivity is present in these cultures.

Studies of the regulation of pituitary β_B synthesis and follistatin secretion suggested that activins and follistatins exert a reciprocal regulatory influence on each other. When cultured rat anterior pituitary cells were treated with follistatin (1 nM), the rate of β_B monomer production was stimulated by approximately 70%. A similar effect was observed upon treatment with inhibin-A (2 nM). In contrast, treatment with activin-A (1 nM) resulted in a 30% inhibition of β_B synthesis. The simultaneous addition of equimolar concentrations of activin-A and follistatin (1 nM each) produced no net change in the rate of β_B production, compared to untreated cells. Conversely, when these cells were treated with 1 nM activin-A, the secretion of follistatin was enhanced approximately 7-fold. This effect of activin-A was concentration-dependent and was completely blocked by co-treatment with inhibin-A. Inhibin-A by itself also diminished basal follistatin secretion by approximately 50%.

The rate of β_B synthesis and follistatin secretion were enhanced in response to the activation of either protein kinase A or protein kinase C by treatment with either 10 μM forskolin or 20 nM TPA, respectively. The stimulatory effect of activin on the accumulation of follistatin in the medium was also influenced by the presence of gonadal steroids. The presence of a maximal concentration of testosterone propionate diminished basal follistatin secretion to undetectable levels and attenuated the stimulatory effect of activin-A. In contrast, this steroid did not alter the rate of β_B synthesis.

The observations summarized above reveal the existence of a complex reciprocal regulatory network that modulates anterior pituitary cell functions. By influencing each other's expression and/or secretion levels, locally secreted activin-B and follistatin are proposed to exert regulatory effects on gonadotropes and other pituitary cell types.

References

1. Bilezikjian, L.M., Corrigan, A.Z., and Vale, W.W. (1994): Activin-B, inhibin-B and follistatin as autocrine/paracrine factors of the rat anterior pituitary, In: *II International Symposium on Inhibin and Inhibin-Related Proteins*, edited by J.F.a.D.R. HG Burger, Frontiers in Endocrinology, 3:81-99.
2. Bilezikjian, L.M., and Vale, W.V. (1992): Local extragonadal roles of activins, *Trends Endocrinol Metabol*, 3:218-223.
3. Denef, C. (1984): Paracrine interactions in rat anterior pituitary, *Endocrinology*, 115:495-498.
4. DePaolo, L.V., Bicsak, T.A., Erickson, G.F., Shimasaki, S., and Ling, N. (1991): Follistatin and activin: a potential intrinsic regulatory system within diverse tissues, *Proc Soc Exp Biol Med*, 198:500-512.
5. Mathews, L.S. (1994): Activin receptors and cellular signaling by the receptor serine kinase family, *Endocrine Rev*, 15:310-325.
6. Michel, U., Farnworth, P., and Findlay, J.K. (1993): Follistatins: more than follicle-stimulating hormone suppressing proteins, *Mol Cellul Endocrinol*, 91:1-11.
7. Vale, W., Hsueh, A., Rivier, C., and Yu, J. (1990): The inhibin/activin family of hormones and growth factors., In: *Handbook of Experimental Pharmacology, Vol. 95/II Peptide Growth Factors and Their Receptors II*, edited by M.B. Sporn, and A.B. Roberts, pp. 211-248. Springer-Verlag, New York.

Neurosteroids: pharmacology and possible clinical implications

R.H. Purdy, M.D. Brot**, C.A. Dyer*, L.K. Curtiss*, G.F. Koob** and K.T. Britton

Department of Psychiatry, University of California San Diego School of Medicine, San Diego and Departments of *Immunology and **Neuropharmacology, The Scripps Research Institute, La Jolla, California, USA

The term "neuroactive steroid" refers to both endogenous and synthetic steroids which rapidly alter the excitability of the central nervous system (CNS, Paul and Purdy, 1992). After parenteral administration to both experimental animals and humans, neurosteroids such as 3α-hydroxy-5α-pregnan-20-one (allopregnanolone) can produce behavioral effects within seconds to minutes through non-genomic mechanisms. This is in contrast to the effects of steroid hormones themselves, which alter endocrine and behavioral functions through their well known intracellular receptors that regulate genomic effects over longer periods of time. The term "neurosteroid", which includes allopregnanolone, was introduced in 1981 by Baulieu to designate those neuroactive steroids that are synthesized *de novo* from cholesterol in the CNS.

In the case of allopregnanolone and related steroids, there are well characterized *in vitro* binding assays which demonstrate excellent correlation between the pharmacologic and electrophysiologic interactions of these neuroactive steroids with τ-aminobutyric acid$_A$ (GABA$_A$) receptor complexes (Hawkinson *et al*, 1994). These neuroactive steroids have been demonstrated to be positive allosteric modulators of GABA$_A$ receptor complexes which potentiate chloride ion flux in neuronal membranes, resulting in the hyperpolarization of these neurons. This is demonstrated by an increase in GABA-stimulated ^{36}chloride ion uptake and GABA-activated chloride currents. Neuroactive steroids like allopregnanolone modulate the binding of radioligands that are selective for GABA$_A$ receptor complexes through their interaction with site(s) on the complex that are distinct from those for barbiturates and benzodiazepines. Comparing their concentration effectiveness, neurosteroids like allopregnanolone are about 20 times more potent than benzodiazepines and 200 times more effective than barbiturates in augmenting GABA$_A$ receptor function (Morrow *et al*, 1990). There are now believed to be multiple steroid recognition sites on individual subtypes of GABA$_A$ receptors.

Behavioral studies have demonstrated anti-conflict, hypnotic, and anti-aggressive effects of neurosteroids like allopregnanolone in rodents, as well as their anxiolytic effects using several behavioral tests. Administration of progesterone, the metabolic precursor of allopregnanolone, leads to anxiolytic activity in ovariectomized female rats that correlates with increased concentrations of allopregnanolone in serum and brain (Bitran *et al*, 1993). In a modified Geller-Seifter conflict test of anxiety, recent results in our laboratories suggested that allopregnanolone acted on $GABA_A$ receptor complexes at site(s) that were independent of the benzodiazepine binding site(s), but which can be modulated by an inverse benzodiazepine agonist. Therefore, it is apparent that allopregnanolone was capable of having a significant inhibitory effect on neuronal tone in the CNS.

In male rats exposed to brief ambient-temperature swim stress, there was a rapid (<5 min) and robust (4-20 fold) increase in the plasma and brain levels of allopregnanolone (Purdy *et al*, 1991). The brain levels (10-30 nM) were within the range of concentration which augments $GABA_A$-activated chloride currents in electrophysiological studies of $GABA_A$ receptors expressed in transformed human cells (Puia *et al*, 1990). There is no significant level of allopregnanolone in the plasma of adrenalectomized male rats before or after swim stress, but this neurosteroid is detectable in the cerebral cortex of both groups. Additionally, acute stress increases the brain level of allopregnanolone prior to its elevation in plasma. These results are consistent with some biosynthesis of allopregnanolone in the brain, however the adrenal gland appears to be the major source of allo-pregnanolone in the stressed male rat (Holzbauer *et al*, 1985; Purdy *et al*, 1991).

In non-stressed female rats, there is an estrus cycle-dependent ovarian content and ovarian secretion of allopregnanolone (Holzbauer, 1975). LH but not FSH produces a several-fold stimulation of allopregnanolone formation by the ovary (Ishikawa *et al*, 1972). Both cultured ovarian theca/interstitial and luteal cells types were shown in our laboratories to produce allopregnanolone in response to LH-stimulation. Allopregnanolone was a major product of these theca/interstitial cells, whereas it was a relatively minor product of cultured luteal cells. Moreover, theca/interstitial cell production of allopregnanolone was recently shown by Dyer *et al* (1994) to be increased 200-300% by corticosterone and dexamethasone (10-100 nM), but not by aldosterone. Therefore, it is postulated that in stressed females the secretion of adrenal glucocorticoids can lead to a significant increase in the ovarian secretion of allopregnanolone.

Progesterone is metabolized in women to both allopregnanolone and the epimeric 3α-hydroxy-5β-pregnan-20-one, termed pregnanolone, which also has comparable anxiolytic and sedative/hypnotic effects in experimental animals. After oral dosage of 1.2 g progesterone in women, the plasma levels of progesterone and its anxiolytic metabolites were measured by RIA and compared with changes in mood, cognition and motor performance (Freeman *et al*, 1993). Significant changes in fatigue, delayed verbal recall and symbol copying are found one hr after treatment in subjects where the combined plasma level of allopregnanolone and pregnanolone was >96 nM. In the third trimester of pregnancy we have found that the combined levels of allopregnanolone and pregnanolone in plasma average about 100 nM (Paul and Purdy, 1992). These results suggest that these anxiolytic steroids mediate the behavioral effects of progesterone in women.

Role of neurosteroids in the modulation of hypothalamus–pituitary–adrenal function and reproductive function in rats

A.R. Genazzani, F. Petraglia*, Ai-Li Guo**, R.E. Nappi***, M.A. Palumbo, A.A. de Micheroux, V. Cela, P.G. Artini, M. Criscuolo† and G.P. Trentini†

Department of Obstetrics andGynecology, University of Pisa, *Department of Obstetrics and Gynecology, University of Modena, Italy, **Department of Endocrinology, Peking Union Medical College, Beijing, Peoples Republic of China, ***Department of Obstetrics and Gynecology, University of Pavia, Italy and †Institute of Pathological Anatomy, University of Modena, Italy

Several data indicate that steroid hormones are synthesized in brain neurons. These steroids of central origin have been termed as "neurosteroids". Glial cells have the enzymes necessary to synthesize steroids from cholesterol [1-3]. One of the most naturally diffused steroid is 5α-pregnan-3α-ol-20-one (allopregnanolone or tetrahydroprogesterone). Many biological actions have been suggested for neurosteroids. In numerous brain areas they show a similar activity to that of steroid hormones. A neuromodulatory role for neurosteroids in the central nervous system has been proposed [4-7].

An involvement of neurosteroids on stress [8], depression and anxiety [9], and cognitive functions [10] has been demostrated. Stress and anxiety stimulate the secretory activity of hypothalamus-pituitary-adrenal (HPA) axis; allopregnanolone is a potent agonist of the $GABA_a$ receptor complex, displaying sedative-hypnotic and analgesic activity. In particular, an increased synthesis of neurosteroid has been observed in brain following acute stress [8,11,12], and thus, this steroid has been suggested to play a role in the mechanisms involved in stress response.

Central GABA receptors are known to be involved in the neuroendocrine control of HPA function. An inhibitory effect of the GABAergic pathway on adrenocorticotropic hormone (ACTH) and corticosterone secretion in rats has been observed [13-15], and it is thought to be mediated by $GABA_a$ receptors [14,15]. In order to evaluate the role of allopregnanolone in the modulation of HPA function, we investigated the effect of passive immunoneutralization of allopregnanolone on diurnal changes in corticosterone secretion and acute stress-induced corticosterone secretion in rats [16].

11

In a first protocol, four groups of male rats and three groups of female rats, all with different characteristics, were studied. Rats were injected intracerebroventricularly (i.c.v.) with antiserum to allopregnanolone or with normal rabbit serum (the latter serving as control group) before exposure to acute cold swimming stress; subsequently, rats were sacrificed before stress or 5 five minutes after stress administration. In a second protocol, a group of fertile male rats and female rats at diestrus II were injected i.c.v. with anti-allopregnanolone serum or with normal rabbit serum and then sacrificed on the following day at h. 10,00 or at h. 18,00. Truncal blood samples were collected to measure plasma corticosterone levels. An augmented release of plasma corticosterone levels was observed in prepubertal and adult fertile rats receiving passive immunoneutralization, while no significant difference in basal plasma corticosterone levels were found between passively immunoneutralized and control rats of both sexes. The same effect was observed in male castrated rats, thus excluding a possible role of gonadal steroids. In female rats the stress response of plasma corticosterone was enhanced by passive immunoneutralization of allopregnanolone in prepubertal and fertile rats throughout the estrous cycle. No difference in plasma corticosterone response to stress was found between antiserum-treated and control rats the same age of both sexes. Furthermore, we demonstrated the occurrence of diurnal changes in plasma corticosterone, with higher levels at h. 18,00, in both male and female control rats. However, subsequent administration of antiserum to allopregnanolone resulted in a significant reduction in plasma corticosterone levels at h. 18,00 in both male and female rats.

These findings suggest that neurosteroids may exert an inhibitory action on stress-activated HPA axis function, and that this effect is likely to be independent from the existence of circulating gonadal steroids in rats. Neurosteroids, presumably involved in the neuroendocrine control of changes in circadian rhythm of plasma corticosterone, may lose part of their role with the advancing age in rats. Since behavioral and neurochemical effects of neurosteroid appear to be mediated through the activation of GABA$_a$ receptor, it may be proposed that an allopregnanolone-GABA interaction occurs in response to acute stress exposure.

The evidence that estrous cycle and some sexual behavioral changes are associated to modified neurosteroid activity has suggested an impact of neurosteroids on reproductive function. Supporting this hypothesis, the suppression of basal or GnRH-stimulated FSH release in cultured rat pituitary cells from neurosteroid 3α-hydroxy-4-pregnen-20-one (3αHP) has been shown [17].

In a second study, we attempted to evaluate the possible role of neurosteroids in modulating ovulation and sexual behavior in female rats [18]. We investigated the effect of allopregnanolone or of passive immunoneutralization of brain allopregnanolone on ovulatory events. Hypothalamic and brain cortex concentrations of allopregnanolone in female rats throughout estrous cycle were evaluated. Allopregnanolone was injected intracerebroventricularly in rats on diestrus and proestrus and tests were done on estrus. The intracerebroventricular injection of allopregnanolone significantly decreased the number of oocytes collected on estrus. Antiserum to allopregnanolone was, then, centrally injected to block the activity of the endogenous neurosteroid. When administered on diestrus and proestrus or only on proestrus, the antiserum showed to be correlated with a significant increase in oocytes retrieved on estrus. In female rats injected with antiserum to allopregnanolone, sexual behavior was monitored; the lordosis intensity and the lordosis quotient resulted significantly augmented in treated rats than in controls. Finally, the possible changes of medial basal hypothalamus concentration of allopregnanolone throughout estrous cycle and at the time of ovulation were investigated. Hypothalamic extracts were eluted on high pressure liquid cromatography and allopregnanolone concentration was measured by radioimmunoassay. Brain cortex was used as control tissue. Hypothalamic allopregnanolone concentration on proestrus morning and afternoon was found significantly lower than in the remaining phases of the estrous cycle, while no significant changes were observed in brain cortex concentration of allopregnanolone.

These findings may demonstrate an inhibitory effect of centrally injected allopregnanolone on ovulation in rats, while an increased ovulatory rate and sexual behavior is obtained blocking the activity of brain allopregnanolone. The evidence of decreasing allopregnanolone concentration in hypothalamus throughout proestrus day, when ovulation occurs, supports the putative role of a neurosteroid inhibitory pathway on hypothalamus-pituitary control of ovulatory process.

Previous data have emphasized on the wide distribution of neurosteroid in various brain areas and on the functional interaction between neurosteroids and GABA receptors [11,19]. The present findings focus the attention on a specific area (medial basal hypothalamus) and on the neuroendocrine control of ovulation. An endogenous inhibitory GABAergic pathway on GnRH release has clearly been shown [20]. However, stimulatory effects on gonadotropin secretion are also seen [21]. Such stimulatory effects through the mediation of $GABA_a$ receptors have also been reported after the administration of neurosteroid 3α-hydroxy-5α-pregnan-20-one [22]. Since allopregnanolone acts as GABA receptor agonist compound, it may be hypothesized that this neurosteroid has a central site of action. However, a direct action on pituitary gonadotropin release cannot be ruled out. In fact, FSH release from cultured rat pituitary cells is decreased in presence of neurosteroid [17,23]. The substance injected in the third ventricle may diffuse to the adiacent hypothalamic areas as well as, through median eminence, may reach in part pituitary gonadotrophs. Therefore, allopregnanolone may act both on hypothalamus and on pituitary sites of action. However, the evidence that central injection of an antiserum antiallopregnanolone was able to affect the ovulatory rate supports the hypothesis of a brain more than a pituitary site of action. In the same direction are the influence on sexual behavior and the evidence of a decreasing concentration of hypothalamic allopregnanolone on proestrus.

The impact of neurosteroid on sexual behavior may be also mediated throughout an effect on GABA receptors. Indeed, GABA inhibits sexual behavior in female rats [24], with a particular evidence on lordosis behavior [25,26]. Lordosis is a steroid-dependant behavior which requires the presence of estradiol and progesterone and it is associated to ovulation in female rats. Mechanism regulating receptivity involves an interaction between ovarian steroids and GABA transmission [27].

Our data support the putative role of allopregnanolone as neuromodulator. This is also suggested by changes of hypothalamic allopregnanolone: a two-fold difference on proestrus morning reaches to five-fold lower magnitude at h. 18,00 when ovulation occurs, probably reflecting a decreasing activity of the inhibitory effect of allopregnanolone. The lack of changes in brain cortex concentration suggests that hypothalamic allopregnanolone is related to the events of ovulation. The evidence that hypothalamic concentration of allopregnanolone does not change on diestrus afternoon in part counteracts the hypothesis of a circadian change of allopregnanolone and supports the functional role of changes occurring on proestrus. The present data also suggest that different brain areas contain neurosteroids acting on different functions

In conclusion, in view of these results we hypothesize an involvement of neurosteroids, and particularly allopregnanolone, in the central mechanisms related to ovulation, probably mediating some steroid-dependant behavioral changes.

References

1. Le Goascogne C, Robel P, Gouézou M, Sananès N, Baulieu E-E, Waterman M. Neurosteroids: cytochrome P-450$_{scc}$ in rat brain. *Science* 1987; 237: 1212-5

2. Jung-Testas I, Hu ZY, Baulieu E-E, Robel P. Neurosteroids: biosynthesis of pregnenolone and progesterone in primary cultures of rat glial cells. *Endocrinology* 1989; 125: 2083-91

3. Jung-Testas I, Hu ZY, Baulieu E-E, Robel P. Steroids synthesis in rat brain cell cultures. *J Steroid Biochem* 1989; 34: 511-9

4. Paul SM, Purdy RH. Neuroactive steroids. *FASEB J* 1992; 6: 2311-22

5. Majewska MD. Neurosteroids: endogenous bimodal modulators of the GABA$_a$ receptor. Mechanism of action and physiological significance. *Prog Neurobiol* 1992; 38: 379-95

6. Mellon SH. Neurosteroids: biochemistry, modes of action, and clinical relevance. *J Clin Endocrinol Metab* 1994; 78: 1003-8

7. Robel P, Baulieu E-E. Neurosteroids: biosynthesis and function. *TEM* 1994; 5: 1-8

8. Purdy R, Morrow PH, Moore PH, Paul SM. Stress-induced elevation of GABA receptor-active 3α-hydroxysteroids in the rat brain. *Soc Neurosci Abstr* 1990; 16: 691

9. Bertholini G, Scatton B, Zivkovitz B, Lloyd KG. On the mode of antidepressant action of GABA receptors agonist and monoamine-uptake inhibitors. In: Bertholini et al., eds., GABA and Mood Disorders. New York: Raven Press, 1986: 105-12

10. Flood JF, Roberts E. Dehydroepiandrosterone sulfate improves memory in aging mice. *Brain Res* 1988; 447: 269-78

11. Corpéchot C, Young J, Calvel M, Wehrey C, Veltz JN, Touyer G, et al. Neurosteroids: 3α-hydroxy-5α-pregnan-20-one and its precursors in the brain, plasma, and steroidogenic glands of male and female rats. *Endocrinology* 1993; 133: 1003-9

12. Purdy RH, Morrow AL, Moore PH jr, Paul SM. Stress-induced elevations of γ-aminobutyric acid type A receptor-active steroids in the rat brain. *Proc Natl Acad Sci USA* 1991; 88: 4553-7

13. Racagni G, Apud JA, Cocci D, Locatelli V, Müller EE. GABAergic control of anterior pituitary hormone secretion. *Life Sci* 1982; 31: 823-38

14. Jones MT, Gillham B, Altaher ARH, Nicholson SA, Campbell EA, Walls SM, Thody A. Clinical and experimental studies on the role of GABA in the regulation of ACTH secretion: a review. *Psychoneuroendocrinology* 1984; 9: 107-23

15. Lakic N, Pericic D, Manev H. Mechanisms by which picrotoxin and a high dose diazepam elevated plasma corticosterone level. *Neuroendocrinology* 1986; 43: 331-5

16. Guo A-L, Petraglia F, Criscuolo M, Ficarra G, Nappi RE, Palumbo MA, Trentini GP, Purdy RH, Genazzani AR. Evidence for a role of neurosteroids in modulation of diurnal changes and acute stress-induced corticosterone secretion in rats. *Gynecol Endocrinol* 1995; 9: 1-7 (In press)

17. Wiebe JP, Dhanvantari S, Watson PH, Huang Y. Suppression in gonadotropes of gonadotropin-stimulated follicle stimulating hormone release by the gonadal- and neurosteroid 3α-hydroxy-4-pregnane-20-one involves cytosolic calcium. *Endocrinology* 1994; 134: 377-82

18. Genazzani AR, Palumbo MA, de Micheroux AA, Artini PG, Criscuolo M, Ficarra G, Guo A-L, Benelli A, Bertolini A, Petraglia F, Purdy RH. Evidence for a role of a neurosteroid, allopregnanolone (5α-pregnan-3α-ol-20-one), in the modulation of reproductive function in female rat. *Eur J Endocrinol* (In press)

19. Purdy RH, Morrow AL, Blinn JR, Paul SM. Synthesis, metabolism, and pharmacological activity of 3α-hydroxy-steroids wich potentiate GABA-receptors-mediate chloride ion uptake in rat cerebral cortical synaptoneurosomes. *J Med Chem* 1990; 33: 1572-81

20. Masotto C, Wisniewski G, Negro-Vilar A. Different gamma-aminobutyric acid receptor subtypes are involved in the regulation of opiate-dependent and independent luteinizing hormone-releasing hormone secretion. *Endocrinology* 1989; 125: 548-53

21. Vijayan E, McCann SM. The effects of intraventricular injection of GABA on prolactin and gonadotropin release in conscious female rats. *Brain Res* 1978; 155: 35

22. Brann DW, Putnam CD, Mahesh VB. γ-Aminobutyric acid$_A$ receptors mediate 3α-hydroxy-5α-pregnan-20-one-induced gonadotropin secretion. *Endocrinology* 1990; 126: 1854-9

23. Jussofie A. Brain area specific differences in the effects of neuroactive steroids on the GABA$_A$ receptor complexes following acute treatment with anaesthetically active steroids. *Acta Endocrinol* 1993, 129: 480-5

24. Qureshi GA, Bednar I, Forsberg G, Södersten P. GABA inhibits sexual behavior in female rats. *Neuroscience* 1988; 27: 169-74

25. McCarthy MM, Masters DB, Fiber JM, López-Colomé AM, Beyer C, Komisaruk BR, et al. GABAergic control of receptivity in the female rat. *Neuroendocrinology* 1991; 53: 473-9

26. Ågmo A, Soria P, Paredes R. GABAergic drugs and lordosis behavior in the female rat. *Horm Behav* 1989; 23: 368-80

27. Pfaff DW, Schwartz-Giblin S. Cellular mechanisms of female reproductive behaviors. In: Knobil E, Neill J, et al., eds. The Physiology of Reproduction. New York: Raven Press, 1988: 1487-1569

Weight-loss related amenorrhoea

P.G. Crosignani

1st Department of Obstetrics and Gynecology, University of Milan, Milan, Italy

---

INTRODUCTION

A moderate weight loss in the range of 10-15% of normal weight results in amenorrhoea due to hypothalamic dysfunction (1). This weight loss is equivalent to a loss of one third of body fat (2).

In addition a high proportion of well trained dancers and athletes have amenorrhoea though weight may be in the normal range, since muscle are heavy (80% water compared to 5-10% water in adipose tissue). For these subjects the psychological stress of competition may also be involved however body fat and not stress seems to be the main causative factor (3).

THE RELATIONSHIP BETWEEN BODY FAT AND MENSTRUAL CYCLE

There are at least four mechanisms by which adipose tissue may affect the menstrual cycle:

1) adipose tissue is a significant extragonadal source of oestrogen. Conversion of androgen to estrogen takes place in adipose tissue and accounts for a third of the circulating estrogen of premenopausal women (4);

2) body weight influences the direction of estrogen metabolism to more or less potent forms (5);

3) adipose tissue regulates SHBG synthesis which in turn regulates the availability of serum free estrogen (6);

4) body fat stores steroid hormones (7).

17

THE HYPOTHALAMIC DYSFUNTION

Women with this type of hypothalamic dysfunction have both quantitative and qualitative changes in the secretion of luteinizing hormone (LH), follicle-stimulating hormone (FSH), and of oestrogen:

-   LH, FSH, and oestradiol levels are low;

-   the secretion of LH and the response to gonadotrophin-releasing hormone (GnRH) are reduced in direct correlation with the amount of weight loss (1);

-   weight loss results in an age-inappropriate 24 hrs LH secretory pattern resembling that of prepubertal or early pubertal children. Weight gain restores the postmenarcheal secretory pattern (8);

-   a reduced response or absence of response to clomiphene is correlated with the degree of the loss of body weight (9).

THE CYCLE DISRUPTION

The amenorrhoea is quite probably due to an adaptative hypothalamic dysfunction preventing an unsuccesfull pregnancy outcome (10). The amenorrhoea is usually reversible with weight gain, decreased exercise on both (11).

The disruption of the cycle can be partial. Women who exercise moderately or who are regaining weight into the normal range may have an apparently normal menstrual cycle but which actually has a shortened luteal phase or is anovulatory (12).

REFERENCES

1   Vigersky, R.A., Andersen, A.E., Thompson, R.H. et al. (1977). Hypothalamic dysfunction in secondary amenorrhea associated with simple weight loss. New England Journal of Medicine **297**, 1141-5.

2. Frisch, R.E. and McArthur, J.W. (1974). Menstrual cycle: fatness as a determinant of minimum weight for height necessary for their maintenance or onset. Science **185**, 949-51.

3. Frisch, R.E., Hall, G., Aoki, T.T. et al. (1984). Metabolic, endocrine and reproductive changes of a woman channel swimmer. Metabolis **33**, 1106-11.

4   Siiteri, P.K. (1981). Extraglandular oestrogen formation and serum binding of estradiol: relatioship to cancer. J. Endocrinol. **89**, 119-29.

5. Fishman, J., Boyar, R.M. and Hellman, L. (1975). Influence of body weight on estradiol metabolism in young women. J. Clin. Endocrinol. Metab. **41**, 989-91.

6. Apter, D., Bolton, N.J., Hammond, G.L. et al. (1984). Serum sex hormone-binding globulin during puberty in girls and in different types of adolescent menstrual cycles. Acta Endocrinologica **107**, 413-9.

7. Kaku, M. (1969). Disturbance of sexual function and adipose tissue of obese females. Sanfujinka No Jissai (Tokyo) **18**, 212-8.

8. Boyar, R.M., Katz, J., Finkelstein, J.W. et al. (1974). Anorexia nervosa: immaturity of the 24-hour luteinizing hormone secretory pattern. New England Journal of Medicine **291**, 861-5.

9. Marshall, J.C. and Fraser, T.R. (1971). Amenorrhea and loss of weight. British Journal of Obstetrics and Gynaecology.

10 Van der Spuy, Z.M., Steer, P.J., McCusken, M. et al. (1988). Outcome of pregnancy in underweight women after spontaneous and induced ovulation. Br. Med. J. **296**, 962-5.

11. Frisch, R.E., von Gotz-Welbergen, A., McArthur, J.W. et al. (1981). Delayed menarche and amenorrhea of college athletes in relation to age of onset of training. Journal of the American Medical Association **246**, 1559-63.

12. Cumming D.C., Vickovic M.M., Wall S.R. et al. (1985) Defects in pulsatile LH release in normally menstruating runners. Journal of Clinical Endocrinology and Metabolism **6**, 810-2.

Analysis of pituitary hormone secretion: pulsatility and copulsatility

A.D. Genazzani, F. Petraglia and A. Volpe

Department of Physiopathology of Human Reproduction, University of Modena, Modena, Italy

Introduction

Clinical implication of hormonal pulse analysis requires the characterization of many parameters such as pulse frquency, duration and amplitude. In these last years new algorhythms for the determination of both the episodic secretion and the temporal relationship between different hormones have been created (1-3).

Physiology and pathophysiology of episodic secretion of hypophiseal hormones

Hypophiseal hormones are episodically secreted and particular attention was given to the changes that pulsatile secretion presented throughout the menstrual cycle and in some physiopathological conditions. During the menstrual cycle gonadotropins increase their frequency, together with estradiol plasma levels, while approaching ovulation (4,5). Later in the cycle, LH pulse frequency falls with the increase in amplitude of the LH secretory bursts and in progesterone plasma levels (5). Also PRL and GH have been demonstrated to change their episodic discharge all along the menstrual cycle. PRL increases its frequency while moving from follicular to the luteal phase with no changes in pulse amplitude (6) while GH increases pulse amplitude with no changes in pulse frequency (7). These data support the specific role of gonadal steroid in the modulation of pituitary hormones.

When higly sensitive immunofluorimetric assays (IFMA) endocrine characteristics of hypothalamic amenorrhea were disclosed (8, 9). Previous studies reported the absence of any detectable LH plasma concentration (10) but the use of IFMA showed that hypothalamic amenorrhea has an LH pulsatile release of higher frequency and lower amplitude than eumenorrheic women (8, 9) while FSH secretion was perfectly normal. In addition, similarly to LH, also PRL and GH secretory patterns were found significantly modified in patients affected by hypothalamic amenorrhea than in normal women (6, 7). In fact these patients showed a PRL and GH episodic release characterized by a higher pulse frequency and a reduced pulse amplitude (6, 7). Similar data were observed in hypogonadotropic men (Genazzani AD & Forti G, unpublished data). When these patients underwent to hormonal replacement therapy (HRT), both PRL and GH increased their integrated concentrations and changed the secretory characteristics, both reducing the pulse frequency and increasing the pulse amplitude (6, 7). Similar results were obtained in postmenopausal women under HRT administration (11). Indeed these data enforced the importance of the estrogen and/or the progestin milieau on the modulation of pituitary hormones since the exogenous administration of testosterone to a group of agonadal men did not modify the spontaneous PRL episodic release (12). Moreover when the specific intrinsic characteristics of several hypophiseal hormones were evaluated, that is when the instantaneous secretory rates were calculated, the duration of secretory events resulted always in the range of 22-25 minutes independently from the gonadal steroid plasma levels in young prepubertal children as well as in healthy controls of both sexes and in several physiopathological conditions (9, 12, 13).

Concomitant release of hypopheseal and gonadal hormones

The observation and characterization of an episodic pattern of release for hormones which are known to be related to, or regulated by, other hormones has led to various efforts to demonstrate concomitant pulsatile release, or more generally to characterize a temporal relationship between pulsatile secretory episodes (defined as "events") of the two hormones under study. Simple cross-correlation is no more applied to the analysis of pairs of hormone time series since is heavily influenced by circadian rhythms or trends in the hormonal concentrations. Recently new statistically validated techniques for concordance determination have been developped (2) permitting to demonstrate that LH and FSH secretory events are concomitantly released during the follicular but not during the luteal phase of the menstrual cycle (14). Indeed FSH episodic release was temporally couple to LH also in several different amenorrheic conditions (hyperandrogenic, normo and hypogonadotropic amenorrhea) and in hypoestrogenic postmenopausal women (14). On the basis of these observations, the apparent discrepancy of the lack of concomitancy between LH and FSH during the luteal phase of the menstrual cycle can be explained suggesting a negative effect exerted by progesterone on the neuroendocrine control of GnRH discharge from the hypothalamus (15) or assuming that progesterone might exert a specific negative modulation only on GnRH-induced LH secretion. During prepuberty only FSH resulted episodically released since LH is undetectable even using very sensitive IFMA When pubertal maturation takes place, LH plasma centrations increase and a secretory pattern can be described and demonstrated as synchronously coupled to FSH (16). The lack of any detectable plasma LH in prepubertal children raises the question of what drives FSH episodic release at this age. Gonadotropins are secreted synchronously in children at puberty probably because there is an increased sensitivity of the pituitary to GnRH. The hypothesis of an alternative FSH regulatory system in humans is suggested by the different FSH response to the blockade of GnRH action. The hypothesis of a GnRH-independent mechanism of FSH secretion has received support from several animal models. The administration of anti-

GnRH serum abolished LH pulsatile discharge with little effects on FSH in ewes (17). Moreover the stimulation of specific areas of the hypothalamus of rats induced the release of FSH alone, and the injection of partially purified hypothalamic extracts resulted in greater discharge of FSH compared to LH (18). When GnRH-a was administered to a group of hypoestrogenic hypergonadotropic postmenopausal women, LH pulsatile release was completely blocked and its plasma levels were almost undetectable after 21 days. On the contrary, FSH still shows an episodic discharge, even if with lower plasma concentrations (16). The temporal coupling that was observed in baseline conditions was completely cancelled by GnRH-a administration., resembling the lack of concomitancy described in prepubertal children (16). These data support that during puberty LH episodic release becomes evident after FSH and only when LH plasma concentrations are detectable, both gonadotropins resulted co-secreted probably under the positive effect of GnRH. In postmenopause GnRH-a blocked only LH secretion but not FSH, thus suggesting that FSH might have an additional stimulatory pathway that is independent of those regulating LH secretion.

The determination of the degree of concordance permitted also to establish the lagged-temporal coupling between hormones secreted by different endocrine glands. Iranmanesh et al (19) reported that within 20 minutes after β-endorphin (and ACTH) release cortisol discharge occurrs from the adrenal gland. Using a different analytical recent studies (20) reported that during the luteal phase of the menstrual cycle of healthy control and of patients suffering for premenstrual syndrome (PMS)(21), progesterone is clearly driven by LH discharge with a lagged temporal-coupling of 10-20 minutes. Indeed, the estimation of the pulsatile patterns and the degree of concordance of LH and cortisol with androstenedione permitted to verify that not all the patients with PCOS have such a disturbance only for an ovarian cause. On the basis that adrenal gland is involved in androgen secretion, 55% of a group of PCOS patients were studied and a significant synchronous release of LH with androstenedione was observed (22), thus confirming the ovarian origin of thier hyperandrogenism, while in the remaining 45% cortisol secretory patterns showed a degree of concordance androstenedione higher than LH. This last observation supported the hypothesis of the presence of an adrenal-dependent hyperandrogenism which probably starts and/or negatively affects the clinical and ovarian picture of PCOS.

In conclusion the use of specific tools to study the hormonal secretory patterns might be helpful to disclose the inner intrinsic aspects of some physiopathological conditions.

References:

1. Genazzani AD, Rodbard D. (1991). Evaluation of methods for detection of pulsatile hormone secretion: sensitivity vs. specificity. Acta Endocrinol. 124: 295-306
2. Guardabasso V, Genazzani AD, Veldhuis JD, Rodbard D. (1991). Objective assessment of concordance of secretory events in two endocrine time-series. Acta Endocrinol. 124: 208-18

3. Urban RJ, Johnson ML, Veldhuis JD. (1989). Biophysical modelling of the sensitivity and positive accuracy of detecting episodic endocrine signals. Am J Physiol 257: E88-E94

4. Filicori M, Santoro N, Merriam GR, Crowley WF. (1986). Characterization of the pattern of episodic gonadotropin secretion throughout the human menstrual cycle. J Clin Endocrinol Metab 62: 1136-44

5. Genazzani AD, Rodbard D, Forti G, Petraglia F, Baraghini GF, Genazzani AR. (1990). Estimation of instantaneous secretory rate of luteinizing hormone in women during the menstrual cycle and in men. Clin Endocrinol 32: 573-81

6. Genazzani AD, Petraglia F, Gastaldi M, Volpogni C, Surico N, Genazzani AR. (1994). Episodic release of prolactin in women with weight loss-related amenorrhea. Gynecol Endocrinol 8: 95-100

7. Genazzani AD, Petraglia F, Volpogni C, Gastaldi M, Pianazzi F, Montanini V, Genazzani AR. (1993). Modulatory role of estrogens and progestins on growth hormone episodic release in women with hypothalamic amenorrhea. Fertil Steril 60: 465-70

8. Genazzani AD, Petraglia F, Fabbri G, Monzani A, Montanini V, Genazzani AR. (1990). Evidence of luteinizing hormone secretion in hypothalamic amenorrhea associated with weight loss. Fertil Steril 54: 222-26

9. Genazzani AD, Petraglia F, Benatti R, Montanini V, Algeri I, Volpe A, Genazzani AR. (1991). Luteinizing hormone (LH) secretory burst duration is independent from LH, prolactin, or gonadal steroid plasma levels in amenorrheic women. J Clin Endocrinol Metab 72: 1220-25

10. Crowley WF, Filicori M, Spratt DI, Santoro NF. (1985). The physiology of gonadotropin-releasing hormone (GnRH) secretion in men and in women. Recent Prog Horm Res 41: 473-531

11. Mercuri N, Petraglia F, Genazzani AD, Amato F, Sgherzi MR, Maietta-Latessa A, De Leo V, Nappi C, Genazzani AR. (1993). Hormonal treatments modulate pulsatile plasma growth hormone, gonadotrophin and osteocalcin levels in postmenopausal women. Maturitas 17: 51-62

12. Genazzani AD, Petraglia F, Volpogni C, Forti G, Surico N, Genazzani AR. (1994). The duration of prolactin secretory bursts from the pituitary is independent from both prolactin and gonadal steroid plasma levels in women and in men. J Endocrinol Invest 17: 83-9

13. Genazzani AD, Petraglia F, Gastaldi M, Massolo F, Cellini M, Iori G, Surico N, Genazzani AR. (1994). Intrinsic secretory characteristics of luteinizing hormone and prolactin episodic release during pubertal development. Eur J Endocrinol 131: 80-5

14. Genazzani AD, Petraglia F, Volpogni C, D'Ambrogio G, Facchinetti F, Genazzani AR. (1993). FSH secretory pattern and degree of concordance with LH in amenorrheic, fertile and postmenopsausal women. Am J Physiol 264: E776-81

15. Genazzani AR, Petraglia F, Genazzani AD, Facchinetti F, Volpe A. (1987). Progesterone and progestins modulate β-endorphin concentrations in the hypothalamus and in the pituitary of castrated female rats. Gynecol Endocrinol 1: 61-9

16. Genazzani AD, Petraglia F, Gastaldi M, Volpogni C, Gamba O, Massolo F, Genazzani AR. (1994). Evidence suggesting an additional control mechanism regulating episodic secretion of luteinizing hormone and follicle stimulating hormone in pre-pubertal and in post-menopausal women. Hum Reprod 9: 1807-12

17. McNelly AS, Fraser HM, Baird DT. (1984). Effect of immunoneutralization of LH releasing hormone on LH, FSH and ovarian steroids in the preovulatory phase of the oestrus cycle in the ewe. Endocrinology 110: 1292-99
18. McCann SM, Mizunuma H, Samson WK, Lumpkin MD. (1983). Differential hypothalamic controlof FSH secretion: a review. Psychoneuroendocrinol 8: 299-304
19. Iranmanesh A, Lizarralde G, Johnson ML, Veldhuis JD. (1989). Circadian, ultradian and episodic release of β-endorphin in men and its temporal coupling with cortisol. J Clin Endocrinol Metab 68: 1019-26
20. Genazzani AD, Guardabasso V, Petraglia F, Genazzani AR. (1991). Specific concordance index defines the physiological lag between LH and progesterone in women during the midluteal phase of the menstrual cycle. Gynecol Endocrinol 5: 175-84
21. Facchinetti F, Genazzani AD, Martignoni E, Fioroni L, Nappi G, Genazzani AR. (1993). Neuroendocrine changes in luteal function in patients with premenstrual syndrome. J Clin Endocrinol Metab 76: 1123-27
22. Genazzani AD, Petraglia F, Pianazzi F, Volpogni C, Genazzani AR. (1993). The concomitant release of androstenedione with cortisol and luteinizing hormone pulsatile releases distinguishes adrenal from ovarian hyperandrogenism. Gynecol Endocrinol 7: 33-41

The role of inhibin in the regulation of FSH in man: unresolved issues

H.G. Burger and D.M. Robertson

Prince Henry's Institute of Medical Research, Monash Medical Centre, Clayton, Victoria, Australia

INTRODUCTION : THE INHIBIN HYPOTHESIS

The primary tenet of the inhibin hypothesis is that there is a non-steroidal endocrine regulator of FSH, inhibin, which acts as a gonadal signal to the pituitary, conveying information as to the state of spermatogenesis or follicular development. If it followed classical endocrine feedback principles, inhibin would be expected to suppress FSH, whilst FSH would be expected to stimulate gonadal production of inhibin. It should therefore be demonstrable that in states of gonadal damage or removal, circulating inhibin levels would be low or undetectable, with FSH being correspondingly elevated. In states of either autonomous inhibin over-production by the gonad, or its stimulation by exogenous trophic signals, FSH would be expected to be suppressed in the presence of elevated inhibin levels. According to this hypothesis it would be anticipated that inverse relationships or positive relationships between inhibin and FSH might be seen under various physiological circumstances, though in normal subjects, with the balance between secreted hormone and gonadal feedback product (including both peptide and steroid hormones), it may be difficult to demonstrate such a relationship (1).

FORMS OF INHIBIN IN FOLLICULAR FLUID AND BLOOD

Inhibin was first isolated from bovine follicular fluid in the 58kDa form and that isolation was rapidly followed by the recognition that a lower molecular weight form of 31kDa could also be purified from bovine and porcine follicular fluids (2) Until recently the assumption has been made that radioimmunoassays developed for inhibin would primarily measure the 31kDa form. Recent studies from this laboratory(3) have been directed to the characterisation of the range of molecular weight forms of inhibin present in human follicular fluid and in plasma/serum. In fact, inhibin both in human follicular fluid and plasma is present in a range of bioactive and bio-inactive forms, believed to originate from the differential processing of high molecular weight precursors. The 31kDa dimer consists of an approximately 20kDa α-subunit and a 15kDa ß-subunit, either ßA or ßB, giving rise to inhibin A or inhibin B respectively. In the 58kDa form, the α-subunit is N-terminally extended and a 95kDa form exists with an extended ß-subunit. A 105kDa form has a further extension of the α-subunit. Using an immunoconcentration technique with subsequent preparative polyacrylamide gel electrophoresis, a range of molecular weight forms of inhibin with varying biological and immunological activity has been identified both in follicular fluid and in serum. Male plasma pools show a similar variety of peaks of immunoactivity. The precise role of these various forms of inhibin in physiology and paraphysiology remains to be elucidated.

NEW INHIBIN ASSAYS

Because peptides related to the biologically inactive α-subunit, particularly are termed, pro-αC, are known to cross-react strongly in the heterologous Monash inhibin radio-immunoassay, it is of interest to note that several two-site immunoassays have been described which detect the biologically active αß dimer only. Several assay methods employing different antibody combinations were reported by Baly et al., (4) but the results of these assays have been difficult to interpret with no evidence of physiologically plausible fluctuations during the human menstrual cycle. More recently, Groome et al., (5) have described a new assay specific for the inhibin A dimer. Interestingly it has been found not to detect significant quantities of inhibin in male serum (6) suggesting that inhibin A may not be the physiological species in the male. This conclusion was supported by studies by Franchimont and colleagues using ELISA assays for inhibin A and inhibin B where high concentrations of inhibin B were detected in epididymal and hydrocele fluids but only very low concentrations of inhibin A (7). Thus it may be speculated that whereas the major inhibin form in the female may be inhibin A, the major species in the male may be inhibin B. This speculation will not be resolved until further developments occur with specific dimeric inhibin B assays.

INHIBIN PHYSIOLOGY

Whilst there is some evidence for a role of inhibin in the regulation of FSH in the male, much more plausible evidence exists for this role in the female for example during the menopausal transition. . Certain aspects of inhibin physiology in the female still require resolution. For example inhibin levels are inversely related to FSH during the luteal phase of the menstrual cycle and it was postulated that inhibin might have a role in the regulation of the intercycle FSH rise. However Le Nestour et al., (8) suggest that oestradiol alone is capable of providing the only necessary regulation during this transition. Observations in female rhesus monkey also support the notion that it is mainly oestradiol which is involved in FSH regulation during the luteal phase (9).

INHIBIN IN OVARIAN CANCER

Of particular recent interest is the finding of elevated inhibin levels in the serum of post-menopausal women with a variety of ovarian malignancies, particularly granulosa cell and mucinous tumours (10,11). The nature of the immunoreactivity in the circulation of such women may vary with the type of tumour, with inhibin levels generally being inverse to those of FSH in granulosa cell tumours but unrelated to FSH in those with mucinous tumours (11). Current findings using immunohistochemistry suggest that in addition to inhibin, activins are also present in ovarian tumours particularly the mucinous cystadenocarcinomas (12). The characterisation of the particular molecular species as well as the nature of the activins present in various types of ovarian malignancy may provide new insights into the biology of these tumours and even their pathogenesis.

CONCLUDING REMARKS

Overall it is clear that the feedback regulation of gonadotrophin secretion is complex and may involve inhibin and sex steroids differentially under various circumstances. A full definition of the relative roles of both feedback factors could lead to the development of new approaches to fertility regulation in both sexes.

REFERENCES

1. Burger, H.G (1993) Evidence for a negative feedback role of inhibin in follicle stimulating hormone regulation in women. *Human Reprod.* **8**, 129-132

2. Robertson, D.M., Foulds, L.M., Leversha, L., Morgan, F.J., Hearn, M.T.W., Burger, H.G., Wettenhall, R.E.H., and de Kretser, D.M. (1985) Isolation of inhibin from bovine follicular fluid. *Biochem. Biophys. Res. Commun.* **126**: 220-26

3. Robertson, D.M., Sullivan, J., Watson, M. and Cahir, N. (1994) Inhibin forms in human plasma. *J. Endocrinol.* (in press).

4. Baly, D.L., Allison, D.E., Krummen, L.A., Woodruff, T.K., Soules, M.R., Chen, S.A., Fendly, B.M., Bald, L.N., Mather, J.P. and Lucas, C. (1993). Development of a specific and sensitive two-site enzyme-linked immunosorbent assay for measurement of inhibin-A in serum. *Endocrinology,* **132**: 2099-108.

5. Groome, N.P., Illingworth, P.J., O'Brien, M., Cooke, I., Ganesan, T.S., Baird, D.T. and McNeilly, A.S. (1994) Detection of dimeric inhibin throughout the human menstrual cycle by two-site enzyme immunoassay. *Clin Endocrinol.* **40**: 717-23.

6. Lambert-Messerlian, G.M., Hall, J.E., Sluss, P.M., Taylor, A.E., Martin, K.A., Groome, N.P., Crowley Jr., W.F., and Schneyer, A.L. (1994) Relatively low levels of dimeric inhibin circulate in men and women with polycystic ovarian syndrome using a specific two-site enzyme-linked immunosorbent assay. *J. Clin. Endocrinol. Metab.* **79**: 45-50

7. Poncelet, E., and Franchimont, P. (1994) Two site enzymo-immunoassays of inhibin. In *'Inhibin and Inhibin-Related Proteins'* (Ed. H.G. Burger.) pp. 45-54. (Ares-Serono Symposia, Rome).

8. Le Nestour, E., Marraoui, J., Lahlou, N., Roger, M., de Ziegler, D. and Bouchard, P. (1993). Role of estradiol in the rise in follicle-stimulating hormone levels during the luteal-follicular transition. *J. Clin. Endocrinol. Metab.* **77**, 439-42.

9. Fraser, H.M., Smith, K.B., Lunn, S.F., Cowen, G.M., Morris, K. and McNeilly, A.S. (1992). Immunoneutralization and immunocytochemical localization of inhibin α-subunit during the mid-luteal phase in the stump-tailed macaque. *J. Endocrinol.* **133:** 341-47.

10. Lappohn, R.E., Burger, H., Bouma, J., Bangah, M., Krans, M., and de Bruijn, H. (1989) Inhibin as a marker for granulosa-cell tumors. *N. Engl. J. Med.* **321**: 790-93.

11. Healy, D.L., Burger, H.G., Mamers, P., Jobling, T., Bangah, M., Quinn, M., Grant, P., Day, A.J., Rome, R., and Campbell, J.J. (1993) Elevated serum inhibin concentrations in postmenopausal women with ovarian tumors. *N. Engl. J. Med.* **329**: 1539 - 42.

12. Gurusinghe, C.J., Healy, D.L., Jobling, T., Mamers, P., and Burger, H.G. (1995) Inhibin and activin are demonstrable by immunohistochemistry in ovarian tumor tissue. *Gynecologic Oncology* (in press)

Thyroid hormone receptors and the reproductive tract

A. Pinchera and E. Macchia

Istituto di Endocrinologia, Università di Pisa, Pisa, Italy

The effects of thyroid hormones (THs) on the female reproductive system are numerous and well-established from a clinical point of view. Both hyper- and hypothyroidism produce major gynecological disturbances. Whether these disturbances are due to a direct action of TH on the reproductive tract or to an action on the hypothalamus-pituitary axis or to an interaction with steroid metabolism mainly through modifications of circulating SHBG is uncertain. A combination of these different effects on determining the whole clinical picture is anyway likely. On the other hand, the discovery of specific THs receptors (TRs) in the female reproductive system underscores the importance of a local action of THs on reproductive tract physiology.

THs exert a wide range of actions on differentiation, development, growth and metabolism and are required for normal function of nearly all tissues. They may exert their effects at different cellular levels: the major effects result from the interaction with nuclear receptors, which are associated with chromatin, bind THs with high affinity and specificity, and regulate the transcription of target genes. Thyroxine, the primary secretory product of the thyroid gland, is relatively inactive and is converted peripherally to the active hormone, triiodothyronine (T3), by the enzyme 5'-deiodinase. TRs are members of a large superfamily of nuclear receptors, closely related to the oncogene v-erbA, which includes steroids, vitamin D and retinoic acid receptors. This superfamily shares a similar domain organization, including a central DNA binding domain, containing two zinc fingers, and a carboxy-terminal ligand-binding domain. Two distinct TR genes have been discovered, alpha and beta, located on chromosome 17 and 3, respectively. At least two alternative mRNA splice products have been described for each gene (TRalpha1 and alpha2, TR beta1 and beta2). The variant alpha2, although expressed in most tissues, is not able to bind T3 and its physiological role is still debated. In the presence of T3, the different TRs bind to specific DNA sequences, called TRE, as complexes with other related nuclear proteins, and regulate the transcription of target genes. There are both developmental and tissue-specific patterns of expression of the different TRs. TRalpha1, TRbeta1 and c-erbA alpha2 are widely expressed in different tissues, whereas TRbeta2 has been identified only in the pituitary and hypothalamus. The clinical findings in hyper- and hypothyroidism are the net result of the action of products of a variety of genes whose expression is directly or indirectly regulated by T3.

Female reproductive system and hyperthyroidism

The clinical aspects of female reproductive alterations described in hyperthyroidism should be firstly divided into those occurring in early life and adulthood. In prepubertal girls sexual maturation, as well as the onset of menses, is often delayed. After puberty, anovulation, fertility reduction, menstrual disorders (from oligomenorrhea to amenorrhea) and abortion may be present. Alterations in the metabolism of gonadal steroids are observed: a constant increase of SHBG, which leads to an increase of plasma total testosterone (T) and estradiol (E2) with a concomitant reduction of their free fractions, occurs. The latter phenomenon is partially balanced by a decrease of the metabolic clearance rates (MCR) of both hormones. Moreover, an augmented aromatization from T to E2 and androstenedione to estrone, probably related to an increased blood flow, is observed. The mean LH and FSH values are increased, but the mid-cycle LH surge may be reduced or absent. The challenge test with GnRH shows a normal pituitary LH and FSH reserve.

Female reproductive system and hypothyroidism

The reproductive tract appears to develop normally in cretins. Thus, hypothyroidism during fetal life does not appear to affect the normal development of the reproductive tract. Congenital hypothyroid patients, though, show sexual immaturity, while prepubertal girls have delayed maturation and onset of puberty. In some cases of juvenile hypothyroidism even precocious onset of menses and sellar enlargement have been described. In adults, hypothyroidism may cause diminished libido, anovulation, menometrorrhagia. This latter symptom is probably due to the fact that secretion of progesterone fails and endometrial proliferation persists, resulting in excessive and irregular menstrual bleeding. In long-standing hypothyroidism ovarian atrophy can occur. Abortion, stillbirths and prematurity are frequent in those who succeed in becoming pregnant. Hormonal data demonstrate a reduction of total E2 and T with a partial increase of the free fractions, due to a reduction of SHBG concentrations. A decrease in the MCR of androstenedione and estrone can also be observed.

TRs in female reproductive tract and their physiological implications

TRs have been demonstrated in human ovary, uterus and placenta. As far as the ovary is concerned, both alpha and beta TR isoforms were found to be expressed both in human granulosa (GC) and stromal cells (1), both at RNA and protein level, using anti-c erbA antibodies produced by our group (2). The alpha isoform is largely predominant in GC. THs, as well as insulin and cortisol, have been found to affect growth and luteinization of GC in vitro in humans and animals. Even in rabbits thyroidectomy arrests follicular develoment. THs exert maximal biological effects early in the follicular development, in agreement with the finding that the number of TRs is diminished in GC by the time the follicle is in the preovulatory phase. In vitro studies on cultured, serum free, porcine GC by Maruo and co-workers (3) show that THs act as biological amplifiers of the actions of FSH in the functional differentiation of porcine GC. The combined treatment with THs and FSH remarkably increases LH/hCG receptors and consequently P and E production, while TH alone are not able to do so. This effect is particularly manifest in GC from small follicles, but not from medium and large follicles. Moreover, since the dose/response curve of T3 used in these experiments depicts a bell-shaped curve, it appears that an optimal concentration of THs is crucial and plays a physiological role in amplifying FSH-stimulated morphological luteinization, hCG/LH receptor induction, and ovarian steroid production in immature GC. These in vitro data are consistent with the clinical observation that ovarian hypofunction is observed in conditions of both hyper and hypothyroidism, and strongly support the concept of a direct effect of THs on ovarian physiology at multiple sites. A recent paper suggests an increase of ovarian hCG/LH receptors in hypothyroid rats. This would cause a hypersensitivity to hCG leading to the formation of policystic ovaries under treatment with gonadotropins: these data need further clarification.

A direct effect of THs on the female reproductive tract is further supported by the demonstration of the existence of TRs in the rat and human uterus (4,5). In nuclear extracts of rat uterus T3 maximal binding capacity is 3-5 times lower than in liver. In immature rats the response of the uterus to estrogens is partially dependent on THs action and hypothyroidism reduces E2 action on growth and differentiation of this organ during development. On the other hand, the administration of high doses of THs causes a decline in uterine estrogen receptors both in vitro and in vivo. A direct action of T3 on the human uterus is likely since TRs have been found in both endometrium and myometrium. The precise operative effect of T3 is still unknown; however, it appears also at uterine level that an optimal concentration of THs is crucial for the physiological development and function of this organ.

The clinical effects of thyroid dysfunction in pregnancy are well known. These include an increased miscarriage rate, placenta abruption, preeclampsia and fetal damage. In this regard it is worth noting that TRs have been described in human placenta and the discovery of c-erbA beta as a THs receptor has been performed by screening a cDNA library from human placenta (6).

Open questions

As previously discussed, the clinical effects of THs on the female reproductive system depend on their interaction with nuclear TRs. Since

TRs have been cloned, considerable progress has been made in understanding the molecular basis of THs action and the mechanisms by which THs regulate the expression of their target genes. Several questions still remain open. Why are there two distinct TRs genes? Have they different functions? What is the exact tissue distribution of each receptor's isoform? How do TRs interact with other nuclear proteins and DNA-binding sites? Which genes are regulated by each TR isoform? The issue of whether, and to what extent, these questions are relevant from a clinical point of view remains to be established.

References

1. Wakim A.N., Paljug W.R., Jasnosz K.M., Alhakim N., Brown A.B., Burholt D.R.. Fertil. Steril. 62:531, 1994.

2. Macchia E., Nakai A., Jeniga A., Sakurai A., Fisfalen M.E., Gardner P., DeGroot L.J.. Endocrinology 126: 3232, 1990.

3. Maruo T., Hayashi M., Matsuo H., Yamamoto T., Okada H., Mochizuki M.. Endocrinology 121: 1233, 1987.

4. Mukku V. R., Kirkland J.L., Hardy M., Stancel G.M.. Metabolism 32: 142, 1983.

5. Kirkland J.L., Mukku V., Hardy M., Young R. Am.J. Obstet. Gynecol. 146: 380, 1983.

6. Weimberger C., Thompson C.C., Ong E.S., Lebo R., Gruol D.J., Evans R.M.. Nature 324: 641, 1986.

Disturbed follicle selection and anovulation in polycystic ovary syndrome

B.C.J.M. Fauser

Section of Reproductive Endocrinology and Fertility, Department of Obstetrics and Gynecology, Dijkzigt Academic Hospital and Erasmus University, Rotterdam, The Netherlands

Polycystic ovary syndrome (PCOS) is a frequent cause of anovulatory infertility and is characterized by polycystic transformation of ovaries together with hyperandrogenemia. Elevated androgen biosynthesis can be of ovarian or adrenal origin or both. Elevated serum luteinizing hormone (LH) levels are also involved in a proportion of patients. Although this syndrome was first described over 50 years ago by Stein and Leventhal, the exact cause underlying arrested follicle maturation in these patients is still unknown.

Based on studies performed in the early sixties measuring steroid levels in pooled follicle fluid samples it is generally believed that follicles in polycystic ovaries are atretic, due to a lack of induction of aromatase enzyme activity resulting in low intra-follicular estrogen concentrations. Much additional information has become available in recent years on regulation of follicle development under normal conditions as well as regarding follicle maturation arrest in PCOS. The primary tools used in these studies include: (1) longitudinal monitoring of follicle development using transvaginal ultrasound, (2) measurement of steroids and growth factors (in particular the insulin-like growth factor [IGF] system) in fluid obtained from individual ovarian follicles, (3) *in vitro* granulosa cell cultures, (4) classical ovarian morphology as well as immunocytochemistry and in situ hybridization, and (5) clinical observations of follicle development during gonadotropin induction of ovulation (see Table). The classical concept of disturbed FSH induction of aromatase enzyme activity in granulosa cells (by local or systemic factors) in these patients is challenged by multiple recent observations. The most crucial being that follicles can grow without the concomitant increase in estradiol (E_2) production indicating that estrogens are not mandatory follicle development. Apparently other (as yet unknown) factors drive growth of the follicle, and studies in PCOS should focus in these (growth) factors.

It seems reasonable to hypothesize that follicle development progresses normal in PCOS until a size of 6-8 mm. This is the stage where dominant follicle selection takes place under normal conditions. It appears that FSH enhance-

35

ment (auto- or paracrine upregulation by intra ovarian factors) needed for selection does not take place in PCOS.

No question that PCOS is a heterogenous syndrome, combining various etiological entities with a comparable end point. A better understanding of ovarian abnormalities in these patients may certainly help to standardize and improve classification of the disease. In this way the present confusion may be diminished and prospective therapeutic studies can be initiated in well defined patients.

Observations suggesting normal early follicle development and disturbed dominant follicle selection in PCOS

Transvaginal sonography
   dominant follicle apparent > 9 mm under normal conditions (controls)
   increased number of follicles, all < 8 mm in PCOS
Follicle fluid levels
   significant rise in E_2 only in follicles > 9 mm (control)
   follicles can grow without a concomitant rise in E_2 (control)
   E_2 levels and E_2/AD ratios same as non-dominant follicles (PCOS)
   changes in IGF binding proteins in PCOS same as control
Granulosa cell cultures
   aromatase activity only present in follicles > 6-8 mm (control)
   absent aromatase activity in PCOS
   aromatase activity can be induced in vitro in PCOS same as control
Ovarian tissue
   double the number of healthy early antral follicles
   similar changes in proteins and mRNA for the IGF system in PCOS
Gonadotropin induction of ovulation
   maximum FSH serum levels and duration of follicular phase is comparable
   to control in PCOS patients using a decremental dose regimen

---

References:

Axelrod LR, Goldzieher JW. The polycystic ovary. III. Steroid biosynthesis in normal and polycystic ovarian tissue. J Clin Endocrinol Metab 1962, 22, 431-40

Erickson GF, Hsueh AHW, Quigley ME, Rebar RW, Yen SSC. Functional studies of aromatase activity in human granulosa cells from normal and polycystic ovaries. J Clin Endocrinol Metab 1979, 49, 514-9

Fauser BCJM. Observations in favor of normal early follicle development and disturbed dominant follicle selection in PCOS. Gynecol Endocrinol 1994, 8, 75-82

Pache TD, Hop WC, de Jong FH, Leerentveld RA, van Geldorp H, vd Kamp TM, Gooren LJ, Fauser BCJM. Oestradiol, androstenedione and inhibin levels in fluid from individual follicle of normal, and polycystic ovaries, and ovaries from androgen treated female-to-male transsexuals. Clin Endocrinol (Oxf) 1992, 36, 565-71

Schoot DC, Coelingh Bennink HJT, Mannaerts BM, Lamberts SW, Bouchard P, Fauser BCJM. Human recombinant FSH induces growth of pre-ovulatory follicles without concomittant increase in androgen and estrogen biosynthesis in a woman with isolated gonadotropin deficiency. J Clin Endocrinol Metab 1992, 74, 1471-3

Role of LH in oocyte maturation

Z. Shoham

Department of Obstetrics and Gynecology, Kaplan Hospital, Rehovot 76100 Israel (affiliated to the Hebrew University, Hadassah Medical School, Jerusalem, Israel)

The onset of meiosis in mammalian oocytes occurs during prenatal life after a period of high mitotic activity. The meiotic division continues up to the diplotene stage of the first prophase and is arrested at birth. Meiotic arrest is maintained throughout infancy until the onset of puberty. In most mammalian species, the fully grown oocyte resumes meiosis a few hours before ovulation, progressing from prophase of the first meiotic division to metaphase of the second division. This process, which transforms a primary oocyte into an unfertilized egg, is generally called oocyte maturation. Resumption of meiosis is also referred to as oocyte maturation, and is induced in vivo by the preovulatory surge of pituitary LH or by exogenous hCG administration. This action of LH in the ovary is mediated by cAMP and involves activation of a cAMP-dependent protein kinase (1).

Resumption of meiosis is often roughly estimated by the visible disappearance of the nuclear envelope and also by changes in cumulus expansion. In fact, the meiotic process encompasses several events including: 1. phosphorylation of H1 and H2 histones and chromosome condensation; 2. disappearance of pores of the nuclear envelope. 3. phosphorylation and depolymerization of lamins by lamin kinase; 4. breakdown of nuclear envelope by specific proteases and kinetochore formation; 5. microtubule polymerization (assembly) by the microtubule organizing centers and anchoring at the kinetochores. Extrusion of the first polar body and formation of the second meiotic spindle are definitive proof that oocyte maturation is complete (2).

The midcycle gonadotropin surge is a major event in the dynamics of ovulation. Rapidly increasing levels of LH induce a number of key changes in both oocytes and follicular cells, which further modify the steroid and protein micro- and macroenvironment. These physiologic changes have a prominent role in the normal maturation of oocytes, the process of ovulation and subsequent fertilization and implantation. The ultimate role of the midcycle gonadotropin surge is to prepare the follicle and its cells for oocyte extrusion (ovulation), to induce resumption of meiosis in the arrested oocyte, and finally to induce the proper changes in the follicular cells to form an active corpus luteum.

37

The threshold duration for LH surge levels required to reinitiate meiosis appears to be 14-18 hours, whereas metaphase II oocytes are obtainable some 28 hours after the onset of the LH surge. The threshold amplitude of the LH surge is not known. Studies in rats have shown that only 5% of the normal LH surge amplitude is necessary for oocyte maturation, but at least 85% of peak levels is needed to activate actual ovulation (1).

During follicular growth fine projections, which emanate from the innermost layer of the cumulus, traverse the zona pelucida and contact the oocyte surface. These regions of membrane specialization are thought to contain the channels that allow intracellular communication. Communication between the cumulus and the oocyte has been demonstrated in the form of ionic coupling and transfer of small molecules. Shortly before ovulation, the physical integrity of the cumulus-oocyte complex is disrupted and communication between the cumulus and oocyte is terminated. At the same time, the oocyte is released from meiotic arrest (3).

The effect of LH, or rather its biologic substitute hCG, on communication in the cumulus-oocyte complex was initially reported by Gilula and her colleagues. These investigators demonstrated that following hCG administration, coupling in the cumulus-oocyte complex is terminated. In a later study it was shown that follicle enclosed oocytes induced to mature in vitro by LH, are uncoupled from the cumulus cells (4).

In a study done by Dekel et al. (4) it was found that interruption of communication between the cumulus and the oocyte leads to relief of meiotic arrest. It was also found that in the rat ovary (3), uncoupling occurs prior to oocyte maturation. This might lead to resumption of meiosis by decreasing the flow of a meiosis-inhibiting factor to the oocyte. As cAMP is known to directly inhibit oocyte maturation, and as this nucleotide can apparently move from the cumulus cells to the oocyte, it could serve as the physiological inhibitory factor of oocyte maturation. The fact that a reduction in intra-oocyte levels of cAMP is associated with resumption of meiosis is consistent with this idea.

In general the mechanism of LH action upon the ovary starts with the binding to a specific LH receptor on the theca and/or the granulosa cell, followed by a rapid stimulation of adenylate cyclase activity. Stimulation of adenylate cyclase results in elevated levels of cAMP which then interact with the regulatory subunit of protein kinase, resulting in production or activation of appropriate enzymes.

It has also been demonstrated in several species that granulosa cells from small and immature follicles lack LH receptors and are incapable of responding to LH stimulation with increased cAMP production. However, as these follicles mature and reach the antral stages, these cells gradually acquire the capacity to bind LH and the ability to synthesize cAMP. Indeed, mature granulosa cells have the capacity for initiating the mechanism leading to follicle rupture, stimulating luteal P secretion, promoting the expansion of the cumulus oophorus and its detachment from the granulosa layer of the follicle and activation of morphological luteinization in response to stimulation by LH.

38

Intraovarian markers of follicle and oocyte development

B.C. Tarlatzis and H. Bili

1st Department of Obstetrics and Gynecology, Aristotle University of Thessaloniki and IVF Center "Geniki Kliniki", Thessaloniki, Greece

INTRODUCTION

Follicular fluid (FF) is the microenvironment that surrounds the oocyte and influences its development and maturation. The main constituents of the FF are steroids and various proteins which can be affected by the stimulation protocol chosen to induce preovulatory follicles.

A   Steroids

In general, steroid levels in FF seem to correlate with successful IVF outcome. Thus, previous studies have shown that FF estradiol (E_2), progesterone (P) or P/E_2 ratio are correlated with subsequent oocyte fertilization, embryo development, implantation and the achievement of pregnancy (1).

Furthermore, some authors found higher P follicular levels in patients treated with GnRH analogues (GnRHa) and HMG than in patients treated with clomiphene citrate (CC) and HMG. On the other hand, others using the same protocols, found no differences in FF steroid levels. Similarly, in a recent study (2) we did not observe any significant differences in FF E_2, P and testosterone (T) levels between women treated either with HMG or GnRHa/HMG. We also found that the mean concentrations of these hormones were higher in follicles with oocytes of intermediate maturity (Fig. 1, 2) (2).

FOL. FLUID E2 VS OOCYTE MATURITY

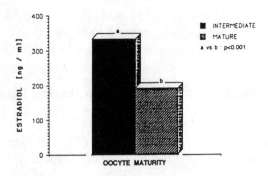

Figure 1 Follicular fluid estradiol (E_2) levels versus oocyte maturity (Adapted from Tarlatzis et al [2])

FOL. FLUID PROG. VS OOCYTE MATURITY

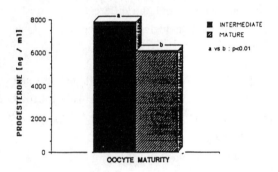

Figure 2 Follicular fluid progesterone (P) levels versus oocyte maturity (Adapted from Tarlatzis et al [2])

B´ Proteins

Proteins in the FF, e.g. cytokines, renin-angiotensin, inhibin and insulin-like growth factors seem to have specific actions and may play a significant role in ovarian physiology. The presence of cytokines and especially of interleukin (IL)-1, IL-2, IL-6 and tumor necrosis factor α (TNFα) in FF has been confirmed by several studies (3), in women stimulated either with CC/HMG or GnRHa/HMG without reporting any significant differences. The effect of IL-1 and TNFα on follicular steroidogenesis and prostaglandin production is similar, since both induce progesterone production and the synthesis of prostaglandins by human granulosa cells. We have previously demonstrated a correlation between FF IL-1α and TNFα with leukotriene B_4 (LTB_4), supporting the notion that IL-1α and TNFα are involved in the synthesis of LTB_4 (4).

Studies from our group (5) as well as from others (6) have shown the presence of the renin-angiotensin system (RAS) in human FF. RAS components are present in FF from both unstimulated and HMG-stimulated cycles (7) and are found in higher concentrations in FF than in plasma. RAS has been implicated in ovarian angiogenesis and was correlated with oocyte maturity and the achievement of pregnancy after IVF/ET (8).

CONCLUSIONS

Despite the growing amount of data concerning the relationship of FF markers with follicle and oocyte development, the results are still conflicting. These discrepancies are possibly due to the difficulties in assessing accurately the actual status of ovum maturity and the different stimulation protocols used as well as to the different methodologies that have been adopted by the various investigators.

REFERENCES

1. Tarlatzis, B. C. (1992). Oocyte collection and quality. Assist. Reprod. Rev., 2, 16-22

2. Tarlatzis, B.C., Pazaitou, K., Bili, H., Bontis, J., Papadimas, J., Lagos, S., Spanos, E., Mantalenakis, S. (1993). Growth hormone, oestradiol, progesterone, and testosterone concentrations in follicular fluid after ovarian stimulation with various regimes for assisted reproduction. Hum. Reprod., 8, 1612-1616

3. Barak, V., Mordel, N., Holzer, H., Zajicek, G., Treves, A.J., Laufer, N. (1992). The correlation of interleukin-1 and tumour necrosis factor to oestradiol, progesterone and testosterone levels in periovulatory follicular fluid of in vitro fertilization patients. Hum. Reprod., 7, 462-464

4. Bili, H., Tarlatzis, B. C., Daniilidis, M., Fleva, A., Bontis, J., Tourkantonis, A., Mantalenakis, S. (1994). Cytokines and leukotriene B_4 levels in human perioculatory follicular fluid and in preimplantation embryo culture media. Hum. Reprod., 9 (Suppl. 4), 11

5. Tarlatzis, B. C., Lightman, A., Rzasa, P. J., Culler, M. D., Fernandez, L. A., Caride, V. J., Negro-Vilar, A. F., DeCherney, A. H., Naftolin, F. (1987). The renin-angiotensin system in the human ovary. Serono Symposia Publications, 35, 57-63

6. Pampfer, S., Van Krieken, L., Loumaye, E., DeHertogh, R., Thomas, K. (1989). Inhibin and renin in follicular fluids of patients with one or two ovaries stimulated with GnRH agonist and gonadotropins. Hum. Reprod., 4, 396-402

7. Lightman, A., Tarlatzis, B., Rzasa, P., Culler, M. D., Caride, V. J., Negro-Vilar, A. F., Lenuard, D., DeCherney, A. H., Naftolin, F. (1987). The ovarian renin-angiotensin system: Renin-like activity and angiotensin II/III immunoreactivity in gonadotrophin-stimulated and unstimulated human follicular fluid. Am. J. Obst. Gynecol., 156, 808-816

8. Itzkovitz, J., Rubattu, S., Rosenwaks, Z., Liu, H. C., Sealey, J. E. (1991). Relationship of follicular fluid prorenin to oocyte maturation, steroid levels and outcome of in vitro fertilization. J. Clin. Endocrinol. Metab., 72, 165-171

Insulin-like growth factors and binding proteins

E.-M. Rutanen, F. Pekonen* and T. Nyman*

Department of Obstetrics and Gynecology, Helsinki University Central Hospital and *Minerva Institute for Medical Research, Helsinki, Finland

Endometrial homeostasis is primarily controlled by ovarian steroid hormones. Changes in ovarian hormone secretion as well as treatment with exogenous hormones are reflected in endometrial morphology and function. Current interest in research on the endometrium has been focused on the mechanisms by which the actions of ovarian steroid hormones are mediated and/or modulated in different endometrial cell types. Evidence is emerging that the insulin-like growth factor (IGF) system, including IGF-I and IGF-II, receptors and binding proteins, is involved in the autocrine/paracrine regulatory process of the endometrium. Therefore, understanding the nature of endometrial IGF system and its physiologcal significance is a fundamental goal of endometrial research today. This communication surveys major findings on the search for endometrial IGF system and also addresses the clinical implications of these observations.

The messenger ribonucleic acids (mRNAs) for both IGF-I and IGF-II have been identified in human endometrium throughout the menstrual cycle. Studies of the hormonal regulation of endometrial IGF gene expression have revealed that IGF-I, but not clearly IGF-II, is stimulated by estrogen (Giudice L,1994). High level of IGF-I mRNA is expressed in late proliferative phase endometrium, suggesting that IGF-I mediates the proliferative effect of estrogen. The IGF-II mRNA level has been found to be higher in late secretory endometrium and early pregnanct decidua, suggesting that IGF-II may have a role in endometrial differentiation process. By in situ hybridization studies, IGF-I mRNA was localized mainly to the stromal cells (Ghahary and Murphy, 1990).

The mRNAs for IGF-I and IGF-II receptors as well as functional receptors are also expressed in human endometrium. Studies with cycling endometrium have demonstrated that both type I and type II IGF receptor mRNAs are more abundantly expressed in the secretory phase and during early pregnancy than in proliferative phase. No data on the hormonal regulation of IGF receptor mRNAs in human endometrium are availble.

Under physiological conditions, the IGFs in body fluids and tissues are bound to specific binding proteins (IGFBP). So far six distinct IGFBP cDNAs have been cloned and characterized. In contrast to ubiquitous IGFs, IGFBPs are more tissue specific, and their regulation, and presumably also function, vary in different organs. The best characterized IGFBP is IGFBP-1, which is a major secretory protein in human endometrium (see review, Rutanen, 1992). IGFBP-1 mRNA expression as well as protein secretion are induced by progesterone and inhibited by insulin. IGFBP-1 is produced by predecidualized/decidualized endometrial stromal cells which appear in late secretory phase- and pregnant endometrium. IGFBP-1 mRNA expression and protein secretion are greatly enhanced during pregnancy as compared to late secretory phase of the normal menstrual cycle. IGFBP-1 inhibits the receptor binding and biological action of IGF-I in human endometrium and in cultured trophoblast cells, suggesting a role as a local inhibitory regulator of IGF action in the endometrium and placental trophoblast. Thus, one of the mechanisms how progesterone counteracts estrogen effects may occur through the function of IGFBP-1.

In contrast to IGFBP-1 mRNA which is expressed in late secretory phase endometrium only, the mRNAs encoding IGFBP-2, -3, -4, -5 and -6 are expressed in the endometrium throughout the menstrual cycle. IGFBP-2 and IGFBP-3 production by cultured endometrial stromal cells was reported to be stimulated by progestin, suggesting hormonal regulation in the endometrium. Using ligand blotting and quantitative RT-PCR, we have been unable to show significant cyclic variation in the expression of these binding proteins or their mRNAs in endometrial tissue samples obtained at various phases of the menstrual cycle. In contrast, a clear cyclic variation was found in IGFBP-6 mRNA levels in the same endometrial samples (Rutanen et al. 1994). The IGFBP-6 mRNA levels are higher in late secretory to early proliferative phase than around the mid-cycle. What is the factor suppressing IGFBP-6 expression in the endometrium during periovulatory period, remains to be studied. Gonadotropins, which have been shown to inhibit the IGFBP-6 expression in ovarian granulosa cells, are possible candidates.

Talavera and coworkers (1990) have shown that the number of ^{125}I-IGF-I binding sites in membranes obtained from endometrial carcinoma was significantly higher when compared to normal endometrium, suggesting that IGF-I may play an important role in the growth of endometrial carcinoma. We compared the IGFBP mRNA expression in well differentiated endometrial adenocarcinoma to that in cycling endometrium. The most striking difference between normal endometrium and endometrial carcinoma tissue was the lack of IGFBP-1 mRNA in all endometrial tissues (Rutanen et al., 1994). IGFBP-6 mRNA level in endometrial cancer tissues was comparable to that in periovulatory endometrium. IGFBP-2, -4 and -5 mRNA expression in endometrial cancer did not differ from that in cycling endometrium. Endometrial carcinoma, which is known as an estrogen dependent neoplasia, most commonly occurs in postmenopausal women who have no ovarian function. However, IGFs and their receptors are expressed in postmenopausal endometrium as well and may thus have proliferation stimulating action even in the absence of estrogen. In such occassion, suppressed expression of IGFBP-1 might allow IGF action to continue, leading finally to uncontrolled cell proliferation and development of cancer. Interestingly, conditions known to increase the risk of endometrial cancer, such as postmenopausal age, anovulation, obesity, hypertension and type II diabetes, are all characterized either by hyperinsulinemia or absence of progesterone i.e. states in which endometrial IGFBP-1 production is decreased or absent, and therefore, the bioavailability and functional activity of IGF-I increased. These data suggest the lack of IGFBP-1 may be one of the molecular mechanisms associating endometrial cancer with its risk factors.

A levonorgstrel-releasing intrauterine device (LNG-IUD) was introduced for contraceptive purpose in late 1970'. The morphological changes induced by LNG-IUD, including epithelial atrophy and stromal decidualization, are well characterized, but relatively little is known about the effects of LNG-IUD in endometrial biochemistry. By using immunohistochemistry, we have shown that decidualized stromal cells in the endometrium exposed to LNG-IUD secrete IGFBP-1 so long as the IUD is in situ (Pekonen et al., 1992). The IGFBP-1 mRNA level and protein concentration in LNG-IUD endometrium are as high as those in early pregnancy decidua. Epithelial atrophy associated with stromal decidualization in LNG-exposed endometrium supports the hypothesis that IGFBP-1 is a paracrine factor of stromal origin inhibiting epithelial growth. In contrast to IGFBP-1, the IGF-I mRNA levels are significantly lower in endometrium exposed to intrauterine LNG than in cycling endometrium. Taken together, the above data suggest that LNG-IUD effectively suppresses IGF-I action in the endometrium and may thus be beneficial in protecting endometrium from hyperplasia and carcinoma during hormone replacement therapy, in which it has recently been used.

In summary, cyclic changes in the expression of various components of endometrial IGF system during normal menstrual cycle, and alterations induced by hormone therapy, implie that this growth factor system may be important in endometrial physiology and pathophysiology.

REFERENCES:

Ghahary A and Murphy LJ: In situ localization of the sites of synthesis and action of insulin-like growth factor-1 in the rat uterus. Mol Endocrinol. 1990;4:191-195.

Giudice LC: Growth factors and growth modulators in human uterine endometrium: their potential relevance to reproductive medicine. Fertil Steril 1994;61:1-17.

Pekonen et al.: Intrauterine progestin induces continuous insulin-like growth factor-binding protein-1 production in the human endometrium. J Clin Endocrinol Metab 1992;75:660-664.

Rutanen E-M: Insulin-like growth factor binding protein-1. Seminars in Reprod Endocrinol 1992;10:154-163.

Rutanen et al.: Suppressed expression of insulin-like growth factor binding protein-1 mRNA in the endometrium: a molecular mechanism associating endometrial cancer with its risk factors. Int J Cancer 1994;59:307-312.

Talavera et al.: Insulin-like growth factor receptors in normal and neoplastic human endometrium. Cancer Res 1990;50:3019-3024.

Insulin-like growth factors and the human ovary

P.G. Artini, G. D'Ambrogio, A. Barreca*, V. Cela, C. Parri, C. Battaglia** and A.R. Genazzani

Departments of Obstetrics and Gynecology, University of Pisa and **University of Modena, and *Department of Endocrinology, University of Genoa, Italy

The primary endocrine regulators of gonadal differentiation and function are the pituitary follicle-stimulating hormone (FSH) and luteinizing hormone (LH). Recently, however, experimental data have shown that differentiation of gonadal cells is also modulated by several factors through a paracrine and/or autocrine mechanism. In particular, some growth factors, initially evaluated for their ability to stimulate ovarian cell proliferation, have been shown to be capable of inducing, directly or by regulating gonadotrophin activity, some differentiated functions in the follicular cells (1). They also seem to be involved in the mechanisms which underline the selection and dominance of the ovulatory follicle.

The insulin-like growth factor system (IGFs) are a family of peptides which are synthesized by several tissue and cell lines and circulate almost exclusively bound to specific carrier proteins IGF-binding proteins (IGFBPs), in the form of high molecular weight complex. It has recently been hypothesized that IGFBPs may have a role in regulating the local action of the IGFs in the ovary. Particularly in rat, it has been demonstrated that both IGFs and their specific binding proteins are synthesized in the ovary (2-4). The fact that, using the in situ hybridization technique, the mRNA for IGFBP-2, IGFBP-3 and IGFBP-4 have been localized to the interstitial cells corpora lutea and atretic granulosa cells (GC) of the rat, hints a different regulation for each of these IGFBPs, which may have a role as autocrine or paracrine factors in regulating the local actions of the IGFs in the ovary (5).

47

Experimental data (6) have indicated that IGF-I can act via paracrine or autocrine mechanisms in human ovary. Indeed, the synthesis of IGF-I and the presence of its specific receptors have been demonstrated in the follicular cells which appear to be sensitive to the action of IGF-I in a dose-dependent fashion (7). The production in the rat ovary has been further confirmed by the presence of high levels of IGF-I mRNA in the granulosa cells, notably in the granulosa cells of developing follicles. Ovarian IGF-I synthesis appears to be dependent on growth hormone (GH) (8,9), gonadotropins and estradiol (10), epidermal growth factor (EGF) and transforming growth factor-α (TGF-α) (11).

In the last few years, the concept of the IGFs as modulators of other hormonal actions has been expanded with the demonstration that, besides the effect of gonadotropin, particularly FSH, on ovarian and testicular tissues, IGF-I is also able to amplify the effects of TSH on thyroid cells (12,13). Some of the well-known actions of GH on the gonads could also be mediated by IGF-I.

GH therapy infact increases the ovarian response to gonadotropin in women presenting with ovaries that are relatively resistant to conventional gonadotropin therapy (14-15). As it is not completely certain whether GH modulates the actions of FSH on granulosa cells directly or via IGF-I production, we studied the effect of GH on steroid release by human granulosa cells (16) and also the production of the IGFBPs and the role of IGFBP-3 in the regulation of ovarian cell responsiveness to IGFs and FSH.

To this purpose after follicular aspiration, 1×10^6 granulosa cells of patients affected with unexplained infertility or male factor infertility were cultured in serum-free conditions. The superovulation for in vitro fertilization-embryo transfer was induced by treatment with gonadotropins or GH in association with gonadotropins.

The effects of the different in vivo treatments were evaluated in the conditioned medium obtained after the first 24 h of incubation; granulosa cells of patients treated with GH/gonadotropin therapy released higher amounts of estradiol and progesterone into the medium than did granulosa cells of patients treated with gonadotropins alone.

When the in vivo GH-induced release of steroid due to the in vivo treatment was exhausted, cells were subjected to increasing concentrations of GH in the presence or absence of 200 nmol anti-IGF Sm 1.2 monoclonal antibody (MoAb) or the antitype I receptor α IR3 MoAb.

The results showed that GH stimulates estradiol production in a dose-dependent fashion, and the presence of the MoAbs drastically reduces the GH effect. These data demonstrate that the established stimulatory effect of GH on ovarian function is dependent not only on the increased levels of circulating IGF-I, but also on a direct effect of GH on granulosa cells, which seems to be mediated, at least partially by the autocrine action of IGF, particularly IGF-II. Infact, chromatographic analysis of medium conditioned by human granulosa cells revealed that these cells clearly produce IGF-II and IGFBP and only small amounts of IGF-I. Since GH appears to be able to increase the in vitro effect of both IGF-I and IGF-II, we can hypothesize a sensitization of the granulosa cells to the IGF-II produced by the cells themselves, acting through the IGF-I receptor.

Moreover, we have investigated the effect of increasing concentrations of recombinant deglycosylated and partially glycosylated IGFBP-3 on basal and stimulated estradiol release by human granulosa cells in vitro. About 1×10^6 granulosa cells were picked-up and subsequently submitted to 0,2,4,8 nmol of IGFBP-3 for 48h, in presence or absence of IGF-I, and Des-(1-3)-IGF-I, a truncated analogue of human IGF-I with markedly reduced binding ability to IGFBPs and FSH (5-20mU/ml). The results demonstrate that human granulosa cells release IGFBP-1 -2 and -3 into the medium conditioned and FSH is able to inhibit this release, while GH is clearly inhibitory on IGFBP-1 and stimulatory on IGFBP-3. Both IGF-I and anti Des-(1-3)-IGF-I, significantly (p<0.001) stimulate estradiol production by human granulosa cells in culture medium in a fashion comparable to that of FSH in the dose range used; the addition of IGF-I to FSH resulted in a more than additive effect. IGFBP-3 alone was ineffective at 2 nmol but inhibitory at 4 and 8 nmol probably by inhibiting the action of the IGF-II produced by the cultured cells.

Preincubatory 2h at room temperature with IGFBP-3, to allow the formation of the IGF-I-BP complex, significantly reduced the stimulatory effect of FSH alone or in combination with IGF-I but not that of Des-(1-3)-IGF-I on estradiol production by human granulosa cells.

These data show that:

1) the IGF peptide is less active when bound to IGFBP-3;

2) as IGFBP-3 does not affect the potency of Des-(1-3)-IGF-I, its inhibitory action is exerted upstream by the membrane receptor binding;

3) as the action of IGFBP-3 is exerted by binding the IGF peptide, its inhibitory effect on FSH points out the role of the autocrine IGF-II in potentiating the FSH action on human granulosa cells.

In conclusion, the data demonstrate that the stimulatory effect of IGF peptides on ovarian function can be modulated by the presence of their specific binding proteins. IGFs and IGFBPs in the ovary are important modulators of gonadotropin actions, so together they contribute to normal growth and maturation of ovarian follicles.

References

1. Giordano, G, Barreca, A and Minuto, F (1992). Growth factors in the ovary. J. *Endocrinol Invest*, 15, 689-707.

2. Mondschein, JS, Etherton, TD, Hammond, JM (1990). Production of insulin-like growth factor binding proteins (IGFBPs) by porcine granulosa cells: identification of the IGFBP-2 and -3 and regulatio by hormones and growth factors. *Endocrinology*, 127 (4), 2298-306.

3. Ricciarelli, E, Hernandez, ER, Tedeschi, C, Botero, LF, Kokia, E, Rohan, RM, Rosenfeld RG, Albiston AL, Herington, AC, Adashi, EY (1992). Rat ovarian insulin-like growth factors binding protein-3: a growth hormone-dipendent theca intestitial cell-derived antigonadotropin. *Endocrinology*, 130 (5), 3092-4.

4. Erickson, GE, Nakatani, A, Ling, N, Shimasaki, S (1992). Cyclic changes in insulin like growth factor protein-4 messanger ribonucleic acid in the rat ovary. *Endocrinology*, 130 (2), 625-36.

5. Nakatani, A, Shimasaki, S, Erickson, GE, Ling, N, (1991). Tissue-specific expression of four insuline-like growth factors binding proteins (1,2,3 and 4) in the rat ovary. *Endocrinology*, 129 (3), 1521-9.

6. Adashi, EY, Resnick, CE, D'Ercole, AJ, Svoboda, ME, and Van Wyk, JJ (1985). Insuline -like growth factors as intraovarian regulators of granulosa cells growth and function. *Endocrine Reviews*, 6, 400-20.

7. Artini, PG, Battaglia, C, D'Ambrogio, G, Barreca, A, Droghini, F, Volpe, A and Genazzani, AR (1994). Relationship between human oocyte maturity, fertilization and follicular fluid growth factors. *Human Reproduction* 9, 902-906.

8. Davoren, GB, Hsueh, AJW (1986). Growth hormone increases ovarian levels of immunoreactive somatomedin-C/insulin-like growth factor-I in vivo. *Endocrinology*, 118, 888-890.

9. Hsu, CJ, Hammond, JM (1987). Concomitant effects of growth hormone on secretion of insulin-like growth factor-I and progesterone by cultured porcine granulosa cells. *Endocrinology*, 121, 1343-48.

10. Hsu, CJ, Hammond, JM (1987). Gonadotropin and estradiol stimulate immunoreactive insulin-like growth factor-I by porcine granulosa cells in vitro. *Endocrinology*, 120, 198-207.

11. Mondschein, JS, , Hammond, JM (1988). Growth factors regulate immunoreactive insulin-like growth factor-I by porcine granulosa cells in vitro. *Endocrinology*, 123, 463-468.

12. Minuto,F, Barreca, A, Del Monte, P, Cariola, G, Torre, CG, Giordano, G, (1989). Immunoreactive Insulin-like growth factor-I and IGF-I binding protein content in human thyroid tissue. *J Clin Endocrinol Metab*, 8,621-626.

13. Smith, P, Wynford-Thomas, D, Stringer, MJ, Williams, ED (1986). Growth factor control of rat thyroid follicular cells proliferation. *Endocrinology*, 119, 1439-45.

14. Volpe, A, Coukos, G, Barreca, A, Artini PG, Minuto, F, Giordano, G and Genazzani, AR (1989). Ovarian response to combined growth hormone-gonadotropin treatment in patients resistant to induction of superovulation. *Gynecol. Endocrinol.*, 3, 125-33.

15. Homburg, R, Eshel, A, Abdalla, HI, Jacobs, HS (1988). Growth hormones facilitates ovulatio induction by gonadotropins. *Clin Endocrinol (Oxf)*, 29,113-117.

16.Barreca A, Artini PG, Del Monte P, Ponzani P, Pasquini P, Cariola G, Volpe A, Genazzani AR, Giordano G and Minuto F (1993). In vivo and in vitro effect of growth hormon on estradiol secretion by human granulosa cells. *J Clin Endocrinol Metab*, 77 (1),61-67.

Immunosuppressive activity of human follicular fluid

A. Volpe, A. Macciò*, E. Turnu*, G. Contu*, P. Artini**, N. Maxia and A.D. Genazzani

Physiopathology of Human Reproduction, University of Modena, *Department of Obstetrics and Gynecology, University of Cagliary and **Department of Obstetrics and Gynecology, University of Pisa, Italy

INTRODUCTION

Recent studies have shown that follicular fluids (FFs) obtained from gonadotropin-stimulated ovaries of women (1) and mares (2) exert a marked immunosuppressive effect. In addition, media from cultured granulosa cells exert a specific immunosuppressive effect (3) thus suggesting that FF contains substances which are able to negatively affect the immunologic response. Immunosuppression might be induced by several substances such as estrogens (4), progesterone (5) and prostaglandins (6) through the specific mediate activation of lymphokine production. Other studies demonstrated the presence these lymphokine, such as interleukin (IL) -1 (7) IL-2, and the soluble IL-2 receptor (8) in human FF.

To better understand the role of the immunosuppressive activity of the FF, it is to remember that IL-1 is released from activated macrophages which are essential in the control of the cellulomediate immunoresponse (9). IL-1 stimulates T lymphocytes and induces both a higher production of IL-2 from CD4+ T lymphocites and the expression of IL-2 receptor on the lymphocites (10). IL-2 acts on T lymphocites by autocrine and paracrine mechanisms through the specific IL-2 receptor which is expressed on the membranes of the lymphocites after the antigenic activation and then is released as a soluble form in the serum (11). To evaluate the mechanism of these immunosuppressive activity of the FF, we studied how the FF was able to modulate and/or modify the blastic response of peripheral blood mononuclear cells (PBMCs) of women undergoing GIFT program. Blastic response was stimulated by the use of phytohemoagglutinin (PHA) and it can be compared with the antigenic activation of cellulo-mediated immunity (12). Since it induces the release of IL-1 from the macrophages, IL-2 from CD4+ helper lymphocites and the expression of IL-2 receptor on lymphocites, we evaluated all these parameters on PHA-stimulated PBMC.

MATERIALS and METHODS

The experimental protocol was carried out on the follicular fluids from 15 women (25-35 years of age) undergoing gonadotropin stimulation for GIFT. All subjects were stimulated with purified FSH (Metrodin; Serono, Rome, Italy) starting on the 2nd day of the menstrual cycle and follicules were aspirated (through a laparoscopic guide) 36 hours after the administration of 10,000 IU of hCG (Profasi; Serono). Only two FFs for each patient were selected for a total of 30 FFs according to the fact that E_2 and P plasma levels were above 40 and 1 ng/ml, respectively. FFs were centrifuged at 500 g for 10 minutes to remove all cellular components.

A sample from peripheral blood was taken from each patient and then mononuclear cells were separated by Ficoll-Hypache density gradient from heparinized peripheral blood and were washed three times in Hank's solution. The cells were then kept in RPMI 1640 medium at the appropriate concentration.

Experiments were carried out using fluorescein isothiocyanate-coniugated monoclonal antibodies anti-CD3 (OKT3), anti-CD4 (OKT4), anti-CD8 (OKT8), anti-CD16 (OKNK), anti-CD11b (OKTM1) and anti-CD36 (OKTM5) (Ortho Pharmaceutical, Raritan, NJ, USA).

PERIPHERAL BLOOD MONONUCLEAR CELL PROLIFERATIVE RESPONSE TO PHA, FHA PLUS RECOMBINANT IL-2, AND RECOMBINANT IL-2 ALONE

The response of PBMC to PHA, PHA plus recombinant IL-2, and recombinant IL-2 alone was evaluated using flat-bottomed microliter 96-microwell plates, triplicates cultures of 1.5×10^5/well cells were performed in 200 μl RPMI 1640 supplemented with 10% autologous serum 2 nmol glutamine, 10 μg gentamicine; or 1 μg of PHA plus 20 IU of recombinant IL-2; or 20 IU of recombinant IL-2 alone. 40 μl per well of FFs was added into the appropriate wells. Controls were rapresented by cultures without the addition of FF. Cultures were incubated at 37° C in a 5% CO_2 atmosphere for 72 hours. Fourteen hours before harvesting, 1μCi/well of ^{3}H-thymidine (^{3}H-Tdr) were added. The blastic response was evaluated counting the ^{3}H-Tdr incorporated by the cells.

IL-1α, IL-2 AND GONADAL STEROIDS ASSAYS

Citokines were assayed in supernatant cultures from PHA-stimulated PBMC (at 24 hours), both in the presence and in the absence of FF, as above described. The assay was performed with a sandwich ELISA test (Immunotech SA, Marseille, France). The adsorbance at 405 nm was measured with a spectrofotometer (Unidata, Rome , Italy). Estradiol and progesterone were determined using commercially available RIA.

DETECTION OF FLOW CYTOMETRY OF MEMBRANE-BOUND IL-2 RECEPTOR P55 CHAIN (CD25) ON PHA-STIMULATED PBMC.

After stimulation with PHA and the following IL-2 release by T cells, a variable percentage of T lymphocytes undergoes to blastic transformation, as they express the receptor for IL-2. For this study the cells at the concentration of 1.5×10^6 / ml were incubated with PHA (10 µg/ml) and autologous FF (20%) for 72 hours at 37°C in a 5% CO_2 atmosphere. Lymphocytes coltures without FF with 30% autologous serum were used as controls. Then the cells were washed twice in Hank's solution and resuspended at a concentration of 2×10^6 /ml in RPMI 1640 solution. 100 µl of this cellular suspension was treated with 5 µl of fluorescein isothiocianate-coniugated monoclonal antibody anti-CD25, incubated for 15 minutes at 4°C, washed once with Hank's solution resuspended in 400 µl of RPMI 1640 solution, and tested for CD25 expression using flow cytofluorometry.

Results were expressed as mean±SEM and as a percentage of ^{3}H-Tdr suppression incorporation by PBMC in cultures with FF compared with those without FF, according to the formula:

$$\% \text{ suppression} = [1-(\text{cpm in culture with FF})/(\text{cpm in control cultures})] \times 100$$

RESULTS

Our data show that the lymphocyte blastic response to PHA was suppressed by the addition of FF.In fact the incorporation ^{3}H-Tdr was significantly lower in presence of FF than without FF. The presence of FF reduced also the blastic response to recombinant IL-2 alone, to PHA plus recombinat IL-2.

In the presence of FF the percentage of CD25 expression on PHA-stimulated PBMC was significantly lower than in controls.

In addition, the levels of IL-1α and IL-2 in culture medium of PHA-stimulated PBMC without FF were higher than those found in culture medium of PHA-stimulated PBMC with FF.

DISCUSSION

The high failure rate of embryo preimplantation in humans is still not clear and several reports suggested that this may depend from a prevalence of the maternal immune defense over the immunosuppressive defense of the embryo. In fact human embryos produce a soluble factor that reduces lymphocyte proliferation (13) and recently a major role was given to the inhibitory role of FF. FF was demonstrated to inhibit lymphocite blastic response through the stimulation of suppressor T cells and an important modulatory role is played by progesterone (1).

The present study confirms the findings that preovulatory human FF contains one or more factors which act(s) as immunosuppressor. In fact our data demonstrate that FF inhibit the production of IL-1 or IL-2, as well as of IL-2 receptor expression or negatively modulated the IL-2 interaction with its receptor. The presence of the FF in culture medium significantly inhibited ^{3}H-Tdr uptake and incorporation in PBMC. Moreover, the fact that the addition of recombinat IL-2 to culture medium did not completely reverse this inhibition induced by FF, let us infer that more than one mechanism is involved in this action. We have to keep in mind that many substances, such as estradiol, progesterone and prostaglandins E_2, contained in the FF may play an immunosuppressive effect (5, 6, 14,15).

In conclusion our data show that preovulatory follicles of gonadotropin-stimulated ovaries inhibit the immune system by means the reduction of IL-1 or IL-2 production, as well as of IL-2 receptor expression. These observations might disclose the important role of FF as immunosuppressive factor to positively accomplish the oocyte fertilization and/or implantation.

REFERENCES

1. Castilla JA, Molina R, Lopez-Nevot MA, Vergara F, Garrido F, Herruzo AJ. (1990). Immunosuppressive properties of human follicular fluid. Fertil Steril 53: 271-5.
2. Watson ED, Zanecosky HG. (1990). Immunosupressive properties of follicular fluid from preovulatory horse follicles. J Reprod Fertil 89: 627-32.
3. Armstrong DT,Cahaouat G, Guiciard A, Cetard L, Andreu G, Denver L. (1989). Lack of correlation of immunosupressive activity secreted by human in vitro fertilization (IVG) ova with successful pregnancy. J In Vitro Fert Embryo Transf 6: 15-20.
4. Macciò A, Mantovani G, Serri FG, Mauri A, Andria G, Arangino S, et al. (1990). In vitro estrogen-induced inhibition of PHA-stimulated proliferation of peripheral blood lymphocytes:reversal by recombinant interleukin 2 and oxytocin. J Immunol Res 2: 90-4.
5. Low BG, Hansen PJ. (1988). Action of steroids and prostaglandins secreted by the placenta and uterus of the cow and ewe on lymphocyte proliferation in vitro. Am J Reprod Immunol Mycrobiol 17: 71-5.
6. Chouaib A, Welte K, Mertelsmann R, Dupon B. (1985). Prostaglandin E2 acts at two distinct pathawys of T lymfocyte activation:inhibition of interleukin 2 production and down-regulation of transferrin receptor expression. J Immunol 135: 1172-9.
7. Khan SA, Schmidt K, Hallin P, Di Pauli R, De Geyter CH, Nieschlag E. (1988). Human testis cytosol and ovarian follicular fluid contain high amounts of interleukin-1-like factor(s). Mol Cell Endocrinol 58: 221-30.
8. Barak V, Mordel N, Zajicek G, Kalichman I, Treves AJ, Laufen N. (1992). The correlation between interleukin 2 and soluble interleukin 2 receptors to oestradiol, progesterone and testosterone levels in periovulatory follicles of in-vitro fertilization patients. Hum Reprod 7: 926-9
9. Dinarello CA. (1989). Interleukin-1 and its biologically related cytokines. Adv Immunol 44: 153-205.
10. Dinarello CA. (1988). Biology of interleukin-1. FASEB J 2: 108-12.
11. Nelson DL, Rubin LA, Kurman CC, Fritz ME, Boutin S. (1986). An analysis of the cellular requirements for the production of soluble interleukin-2 receptors in vitro. J Clin Immunol 6: 114-20.

12. Ruscetti FW, Gallo RC. (1981). Human T lymphocyte growth factor: regulation of growth and function of T lymphocytes. Blood 57: 379-94.

13. Daya S, Clark DA. (1988). Identification of two species of supressive factor of differing molecular weight released by in vitro fertilized human oocytes.Fertil Steril 49: 360-3.

14. Fujisaki S, Kawano K, Haruyama Y,Mori N. (1985). Synergistic effect of progesterone and prostaglandin E modulation of the mitogenic response of human peripheral lymphocytes. J Reprod Immunol 7: 15-26.

15. Vercammen C, Ceuppens JL. (1987). Prostaglandin E inhibits human T-cell proliferation after cross-linking of CD3-Ti complex by directly affecting T cell at an early step of the activation process. Cell Immunol 104: 24-36.

Puberty: the critical juncture for expression of the polycystic ovary

V. Insler and B. Lunenfeld*

Department of Obstetrics and Gynecology, Kaplan Hospital, Rehovot, Israel, affiliated to the Hebrew University Hadassah Medical School, Jerusalem, Israel and *Department of Life Sciences, Bar-Ilan University, Ramat-Gan, Israel

Our hypothesis is that polycystic ovarian disease (PCOD) is a multifactorial disease in which the full clinical expression is the result of a synergistic pathological action of several different systems, or the effect triggered by one factor and eliciting an abnormal response of other systems.

The physiological basis of normal follicular development is briefly summarized in order to provide better understanding of processes leading to PCOD.

Puberty is a crucial juncture in the development (and function) of different body systems in general and the reproductive complex in particular. The changes in adrenal function, GnRH pulsatility, gonadotropin levels and ratios, ovarian size and response to stimulation taking place during the peripubertal period are examined with regard to their possible impact on development of PCOD. It is logical to assume that all parts of the complicated reproductive system which are finally developing during the peripubertal period are particularly fragile instable and prone to extraneous influences at this time juncture.

Hence, it is a reasonable inference that, whatever the underlying pathology, the final expression of PCOD is manifested during the peri- or post-pubertal period. Clinical reports supporting this hypothesis are briefly scrutinized.

The peripubertal period is characterized by at least three features congruous to development of PCO: the ovarian volume is enlarging dramatically, the GnRH pulsatility pattern is yet prone to modifications, and the FSH:LH ratio is slanted towards the latter. If one accepts the assumption that PCOD is a multifactorial disease it seems to be salient that it will reach full expression if either the type of stimulation or the ovarian response are excessive, incorrect or ill-balanced during the formative stages of reproductive system, i.e. during puberty.

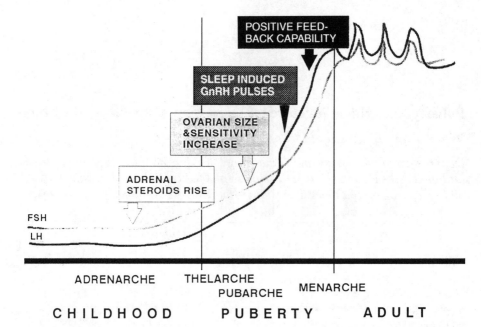

FSH

LH

ADRENARCHE   THELARCHE
              PUBARCHE   MENARCHE

C H I L D H O O D   **P U B E R T Y**   **A D U L T**

<u>Fig. 1.</u> Main events of the peripubertal period. The first important signal is a significant increase in adrenal androgens appearing concomitant with adrenarche. Sometimes later the ovaries increase in size and their sensitivity to gonadotropins is enhanced. During this period, or a little later, hypothalamic GnRH secretion acquires a pulsatile character resulting in intermittent (pulsatile) stimulation of ovaries which is essential for their proper response. The development of reproductive system is finalized when the hypothalamic-pituitary complex acquires the capability to respond to positive feedback signals, thus enabling the midcycle LH surge.

1. Urdl, W. Polycystic ovarian disease:endocrinological parametres with special reference to growth hormone and somatomedin-C. *Arch Gynecol Obstet* 243:13-36, 1988.
2. Insler, V. and Lunenfeld, B. Polycystic ovarian disease: a challenge and controversy. *Gynecol.Endorinol.* 4:51-69, 1990.
3. Insler, V., Shoham, Z., Barash, A., et al. Polycystic ovaries in non-obese and obese patients: possible pathophysiological mechanism based on new interpretation of facts and findings. *Hum. Reprod.* 8:379-384, 1993.
4. Bridges, NA, Cooke, A, Healy, MJR, Hindmarsh, PC, Brook, ChGD Standards for ovarian volume in childhood and puberty. *Fertil Steril* 60:456-460, 1993.
5. Beitins, IZ, Padmanabhan, V and Urban, RJ Serum bioactive follicle-stimulating hormone concentrations from puberty to adulthood: a cross-sectional study. *J Clin Endocrinol Metab* 71:1022, 1990.

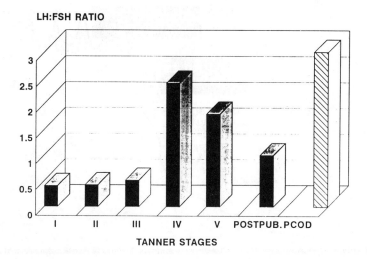

Fig. 2. Bioactive LH:FSH ratio during peripubertal period. Based on data reported by Reiter et al (1982) and Beitins et al (1990) and in patients with PCOD on own material.

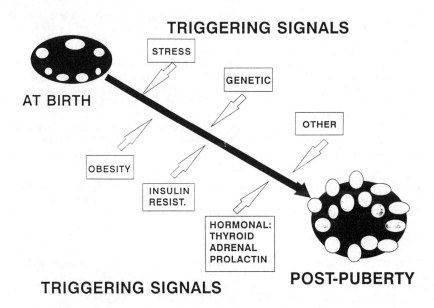

Fig. 3. Different signals promoting expression of PCOD. Girls with apparently normal sonographic picture of ovaries at birth and during childhood may develop PCOD later in life if exposed during the pubertal period to triggering effects such as obesity, stress, hyperinsulinemia etc.

Pathophysiology of amenorrhea: current concepts (β-thalassemia as a model of amenorrhea)

V. Markussis and G. Tolis

Department of Endocrinology, Hippokration Hospital, Athens, Greece

Beta-Thalassaemia is a hereditary haemolytic anaemia which is more prevalent in the Mediterranean countries. Patients are currently managed by overtransfusion (to keep Hgb > 10 mg %) and chelation with sc desferrioxamine. Despite regular chelation, iron deposition ensues and is manifested by cardiomyopathy, hepatic cirrhosis, hyperpigmentation and multiple endocrinopathies; the most common manifestation being hypogonadotrophic hypogonadism.

Transfusional haemosiderosis, as in the case of thalassaemia, is a useful model to study amenorrhoea. With improvement in the treatment of these patients, almost half of them enter puberty normally (1). However, a considerable proportion of female patients present with primary (30.1 %) or secondary (26.5 %) amenorrhoea. The timing of destruction of pituitary gonadotrophs is important to judge entry into puberty. Pathologic reports support the idea of selective pituitary siderosis, with no iron deposition in the hypothalamus (2). Similar findings were documented in patients with primary haemochromatosis (3). The gonads appear atrophic with cystic appearance and minimal siderosis. Once iron is deposited in the pituitary, gonadotrophs cannot recover their function, despite intense chelation. This is not necessarily the case with other endocrine glands (e.g. thyroid, pancreas etc.). The increased sensitivity of pituitary gonadotrophs to iron deposition may be explained by the finding that these cells selectively express the transferrin receptor (3,4).

The GnRH pulsatility pattern has been studied in thalassaemic patients (5). An increasing number of female patients is presenting with amenorrhoea, with almost all of them becoming amenorrheoic within 10 years from menarche. Even during the period of normal cyclic menstruation, there is evidence of reduced spontaneous and induced gonadotrophin secretion. This is consistent with subtle damage to the hypothalamic GnRH pulse generator, although pituitary gonadotrophs appeared more severely affected. LH pulse defects (reduced number, low amplitude, combined defects, etc) progressively deteriorate over time, and patients become apulsatile, despite continuing chelation. In another study (6), three years of intense chelation failed to restore FSH/LH responsiveness to GnRH, even when a six-month pulsatile GnRH therapy was aditionally introduced. The decreased gonadotrophin reserve was less marked in patients with delayed puberty, in comparison with those with primary amenorrhoea (7).

This situation is best described as sexual maturational arrest. The site of this abnormality has again been located in the pituitary, with autopsy data supporting conclusions from GnRH administration (8). Indeed, in this study, there was no gonadotrophin response to acute or chronic GnRH stimulation. The same happened after prior priming with GnRH, HCG and oestrogens. This implies not only a diminished pituitary gonadotrophin reserve, but also an absent positive oestrogen feedback. However, there was adequate gonadal steroid response to exogenous HMG, showing that gonads of patients with thalassaemia major retain the ability to secrete sex steroids in a normal fashion, after appropriate stimulation.

Basal prolactin levels and responses to stimuli like TRH or metoclopramide are suboptimal in female thalassaemic patients (9). Oestradiol valerate administration restored the impaired prolactin response to TRH, but not to metoclopramide. Thus, impaired prolactin dynamics are caused by hypoestrogenaemia rather than by iron infiltration in the pituitary. Alternatively, it may represent some alteration in the dopamine tone.

Another factor that may be operative in the pathophysiology of amenorrhoea in this group of patients, is the stress caused by their chronic disease state. Since hypothalamic CRF/β-endorphin and dopamine function as modulators of the secretory activity GnRH neurons, activation of the CRH/opioidergic system may significantly affect the LH pulse frequency (10). We can speculate that CRH modifies the supra-chiasmatic nucleus / locus ceruleus interactions, leading to altered norepinephrine / GnRH release dynamics and, hence, to impaired pituitary gonadotrophin secretion. Moreover, hypercortisolaemia, *per se*, may adversely affect the hypothalamic-pituitary-ovarian axis in normal women (11). There is preliminary data for increased cortisol production rates in a thalassaemic patient population.

At present, early chelation treatment appears to be the best option to offer thalassaemic patients a normal sexual maturation (12). If, however, amenorrhoea ensues, patients should be offered hormone replacement treatment, with adequate uterine response and cyclic menstruation in most cases. In conclusion, thalassaemia appears as a model of amenorrhoea caused mainly by pituitary iron overload. Possible further input by complex neuroendocrine aberrations cannot be excluded.

<u>References</u>

1. Vullo, C., De Sanctis, V., Katz, M., Wonke, B., Hoffbrand, A. V., Bagni, B., Torresani, T., Tolis, G., Masiero, M., Di Palma, A., *et al.* (1990). Endocrine abnormalities in thalassemia. *Ann. N.Y. Acad. Sci.*, **612**, 293-10.

2. Sonacul, D. (1995). Endocrine pathology in thalassemia. In Ando-Brancatti (eds.) *Endocrine Disorders in Thalassemia*, pp. 75-80. (Heidelberg: Springer-Verlag)

3. Atkin, S. L., Burnett, H. E., White, M. C., Lombard, M. (1993). Human gonadotrophin-secreting pituitary adenomas express the transferrin receptor *in vitro*. *J. Endocrinol.*, **139** (Suppl.), 121.

4. Bergeron, C., Kovacs, K. (1978). Pituitary siderosis. *Am. J. Pathol.*, **93**, 295-306.

5. Chatterjee, R., Katz, M., Cox, T. F., Porter, J. B. (1993). Prospective study of the hypothalamic-pituitary axis in thalassemic patients who developed secondary amenorrhoea. *Clin. Endocrinol.*, **39**, 287-296.

6.   Wang, C., Tso S. C., Todd, D. (1989). Hypogonadotrophic
      hypogonadism in severe β-thalassemia. Effect of chelation and
      pulsatile GnRH Therapy. *JCEM*, **68**, 511-6.

7.   De Sanctis, V., Vullo, C., Katz, M., Wonke, B., Tanas, R., Bagni, B.
      (1988). Gonadal Function in patients with β-thalassemia major. *J.
      Clin. Pathol.*, **41**, 133-37.

8.   Kletzky, O. A., Costin, G., Marps, R. P., Bernstein, G., March, C. M.,
      Mishell, D. R. (1979). Gonadotropin insufficiency in patients with
      thalassemia major. *JCEM*, **48**, 901-905.

9.   Spitz, I. M., Landau, H., Gross, V., Trestian, S., Palti, Z.,
      Rachmilewitz, E. (1982).Prolactin responsiveness to TRH and
      metoclopramide in thalassemia. *Clin. Endocrinol.*, **16**, 275-82,

10,   Berga, S. L., Mortola J. F., Girton, L., Suh, B., Laughlin, G., Pham, P.,
      Yen, S. S. C. (1989). Neuroendocrine aberrations in women with
      functional hypothalamic amenorrhea. *JCEM*, **68**, 301.

11,   Saketos, M., Sharma, N., Santoro, N. F. (1993). Suppression of the
      hypothalamic-pituitary-ovarian axis in normal women by glucocorticoids.
      Biol. Reprod., **49**, 1270-6.

12.   Bronspiegel-Weintrob, N., Olivieri, N. F., Tyler, B., Andrews, D. F.,
      Freedman, M.H., Holland, F. J. (1990). Effect of age at the   start of iron
      chelation therapy on gonadal function in β-thalassemia major. *NEJM*, **323**,
      713-19.

The pituitary–adrenal axis response to CRF in women with PCOS

A. Lanzone*, F. Petraglia, A.M. Fulghesu, M. Guido, F. Cucinelli, L. Soranna, A. Caruso and S. Mancuso

Department of Obstetrics and Gynecology, Catholic University of Sacred Heart and *OASI Institute of Research, Troina, Italy

Introduction

It is well known that polycystic ovarian syndrome is characterized by multifactorial pathogenic events (1): several authors have concentrated their attention on the possible role played by the hypothalamus-pituitary-adrenal axis in the ethiology of this syndrome. Often, patients with Cushing's syndrome or with androgen-secreting tumors develop PCOS, in association, (2) as well as women suffering from congenital adrenal hyperplasia (3) develop the PCOS. Furthermore, in some cases, PCOS can represent the final stage of an excessive adrenarche or of a chronic exposure to stressing events. Nevertheless, there are in literature many studies that analyse the presence of adrenal alteration in patients suffering from PCOS (5,10). The knowledge on the role played by corticotropic hormone in the reproductive disfunctions correlated to the stress (4) is more recent; it is known that CRF is implicated in the alteration of gonadotrophin secretion by pituitary (11); furthermore, other Authors valued the possible relation between HPA axis and amenorrhoea, thus suggesting a potential role of HPA in the onset of important stressing events with a possible loss of weight which may cause desorders in the reproductive sphere.(12) In view of this evidence, we wanted to value the dynamics of HPA in the PCOS analyzing the ACTH and cortisol production in response to a test to CRF.

Subjects and Methods

We studied 8 women (17-32 years) suffering from PCOS whereas fifteen normoovulatory patients have been studied as a control group (C). The Syndrome has been diagnosed by clinical findings, endocryne data (high to high normal plasma levels LH associated with low to low normal FSH levels), echographic and laparoscopic visualization of bilaterally normal or enlarged ovaries with multiple small cysts (diameter ranging from 6 to 8 mm). Congenital enzymatic defects of adrenal gland are excluded according to New and coll. criteria (13). In the early follicular phase (3°-5° day) of a spontaneous or progestin-induced menstrual cycle, every patient has been subjected to a clinical study. At 8.00 a.m. every patient was injected intravenously 1µg/Kg of human CRF (INALCO, Milan); blood samples have been collected basally (time 0) and 15, 30 ,60 and 90 minutes after the stimulus. At time 0 plasma levels of prolactin (PRL), 17-beta-oestradiol (E2), androstenedione, testosterone, dehydroepiandrosterone sulphate (DHEAS), 17-hydroxy progesterone, LH, FSH have been assayed, whereas ACTH and cortisol have been assayed in every blood sample: Body weight was calculated as a percentage in comparison to the ideal body weight (IBW) according to Lorentz's criteria (14). All results have been expressed as a mean ± SD of the absolute values. ACTH and cortisol response to CRF has also been expressed as an area under the curve (AUC) calculated by the trapezoidal rule. The increment area (AUC) has been calculated after the basal area of hormonal concentration (AUCb) had been subtracted.

Results and Conclusion

The two groups of studied patients, are similar, in terms of age and weight (25 ± 4 vs 28 ± 6; IBW 125 ± 40 vs 105 ± 25 in PCOS subjects and in controlling groups respectively), while PCOS patients have shown significantly higher plasma levels of LH, A and T (P< 0,05) in respect to control subjects.

In PCOS patients, ACTH basal levels are higher, though not significantly; nevertheless, after administring CRF, ACTH levels result by far higher in PCOS than in the controlling groups (fig 1). In fact, it results that after CRF stimulus in PCOS patients both ACTH and the percentage increase are significantly higher than those in controls (fig 2). Response in terms of cortisol has also been estimated. cortisol basal levels are slightly higher, though not significantly, in controls. In control groups, after CRF administration, cortisol basal levels increase at time 15 and 30 while starting from time 60 concentrations are lower than those found at time 0. In the group of PCOS patients, cortisol increase after CRF remains constant during the whole test with a percentage increment at time 30, 60, 90 significantly higher than that found in controls; the highest peak of cortisol concentration has been obtained between 30 and 60 after stimulus with CRF.

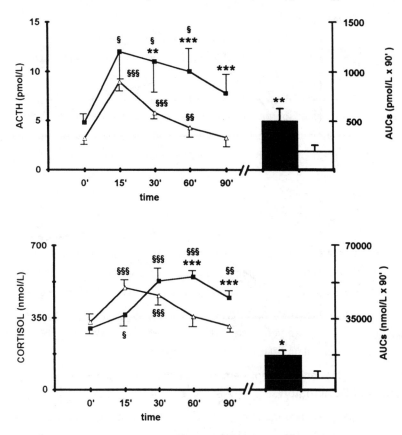

Figure 1: ACTH and Cortisol plasma levels and AUC in response to CRF stimulus in PCOS patients (■—■; ■) and controls (△—△;□).

Thus, it results that AUC values in terms of cortisol are significantly higher in PCOS than in control patients (P < 0,001). Data from this study clearly demonstrate that starting from similar ACTH and cortisol basal levels, PCOS patients show a significantly higher response to CRF as for both hormones studied and besides in PCOS patients this response remains high during the whole test while in controls ACTH and cortisol plasma levels have a decrement similar to basal levels. These results seem to enhance the hypothesis that PCOS patients present a hyperfunction of HPA axis; this phenomenon may be secondary to an increased pituitary sensitivity to CRF that unfolds in a hypersecretion of ACTH. Moreover, it's interesting to note how the percentage increase both of ACTH and cortisol is similar to the control group as for AUCs values; this may suggest that in PCOS patients an increased activity of HPA axis occurs, perhaps this in partly due to central origins. Since the reproductive and endocryne pattern in PCOS seems to be similar to that of the excessive

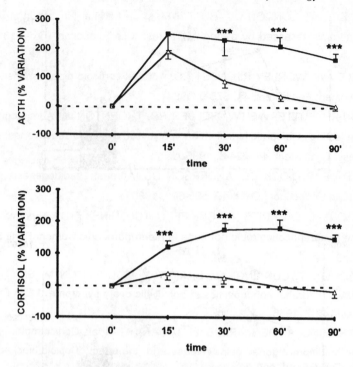

Figure 2: ACTH and Cortisol percent variation with respect to basal values in response to stimulus with CRF in PCOS patients (■—■;■) and controls (Δ—Δ;❑).

adrenarche, partly depending on chronic stressing events, it is, thus, possible to hypothesize that HPA axis alterations are implicated in the patho-physiological events leading to the irreversibility of the Syndrome. Anyway, in order to clarify this interesting hypothesis further exhaustive studies on the subject are needed.

References

1) YEN SSC. Polycystic ovary syndrome. Clin Endocrinol; 12: 177-208, 1980

2) KASE N, KONWALD J, PERLOFF W, SOFFER LL. In vitro production of androgens by a virilizing adrenal adenoma and associated polycystic ovaries. Acta Endocrinol (Copenh); 44: 15-19,1963

3)HORROCKS PM, FRANKS S, HOCKLEY AD, HOCKLEY AD, ROLFE EB, VAN NOORDEN S, LONDON DR. An ACTH secreting pituitary tumor arising in a patient with congenital adrenal hyperplasia. Clin Endocrinol (Oxf); 17: 457-68, 1982

4) LAATIKAAINEN TJ. Corticotropin-releasing hormone and opioid peptides in reproduction and stress. Annals of Medicine; 23:489-95,1991

5) KANDEEL FR, LONDON DR, BUTT WR, et al. Adrenal function in subgroup of PCO syndrome assessed by a long ACTH test. Clin Endocrinol (Oxf) 13: 601-12, 1980

6) MEIKLE AW, WORLEY RJ, WEST CD. Adrenal corticoid hiperresponsiveness in hirsute women. Fertil Steril; 41: 575-9, 1984

7) COBIN RH, FUTTERWEITW, FIELDER RP, THORNTON JL. Adrenocorticotropic hormone testing in idiopatic hirsutism and polycystic ovarian disease: a test of limited usefulness. Fertil Steril; 44: 224-6, 1985

8) CHILD DF, BU'LOCK DE, ANDERSON DC. Adrenal steroidogenesis in hirsute women. Clin Endocrinol (Oxf); 12: 595-601, 1980

9) GIBSON M, LACKRITS R, SCHIFF I, TULCHINSKY D. Abnormal adrenal response to adrenocoticotropic hormone in hiperandrogenic women. Fertil Steril; 33: 43-8, 1980

10) LOUGHLIN T, CUNNINGHAM S, MOORE M, CULLITON M, SMYTH PPA, McKENNA TJ. adrenal abnormalities in polycystic ovary syndrome. J Clin Endocrinol Metab; 62: 142-7, 1986

11) BARBARINO A, DE MARINIS L, TOFANI A, et al. Corticotropin releasing hormone inhibition of gonadropins release and the effect of opioid blockade. J Clin Endocrinol Metab; 68: 523-28,1989

12) BILLER BM, FEDEROFF HJ, KOENIG JI, KLIBANSKI A. Abnormal cortisol secretion and responses to Corticotropin-releasing hormone in women with hiptalamic amenorrhea. J Clin Endocrinol Metab; 70: 311-17, 1990

13) NEW MI, LORENZEN F, LERNER AJ, et al. Genotyping steroid 21-hidroxilase deficency: hormonal reference data. J Clin Endocrinol and Metabol; 57: 320-6, 1983

14) LORENTZ FH. Ein never costitutios index. Klin Wonchenschr; 8: 348-54, 1929

The primate luteal paracrine system: new insights with an emphasis on intrinsic pulsatility

C. Nappi, A.R. Gargiulo* and C. Di Carlo

Department of Obstetrics and Gynecology, University of Naples "Federico II" Medical School, Italy and *Department of Obstetrics, Gynecology and Reproductive Sciences, University of Texas Medical School at Houston, Texas, USA

The importance of intercellular communication among different cell types in a dynamic organ such as the corpus luteum (CL) is a well-established concept supported by experimental evidence accumulated over the past decade (1). However, pituitary luteinizing hormone (LH) is clearly the central drive that controls and maintains luteal function from ovulation to its demise, as showed by some classic in vivo and in vitro studies (2-8).

Administration of a GnRH antagonist alone consistently reduced progesterone (P) secretion and the life span of the CL (4-6) in the human and primate female: an effect which could be avoided by coadministration of human menopausal gonadotropins (7). When LH is immunoneutralized in macaque monkeys, plasma progesterone levels decline promptly and luteolysis ensues (3). In a similar fashion biologically inactive hCG (obtained by deglycosylation) inhibits luteal function in vitro (2).

Studies on the temporal relationship between pituitary LH and luteal steroids secretion further support the pivotal

73

role of this gonadotropin. Indeed, a few studies report a consistent correlation between episodes of LH and P secretion in women, with release of P always occurring after an LH pulse. Backstrom et al. were the first to suggest an increase in estradiol (E2) and P secretion from the human corpus luteum in response to an LH pulse, using criteria of obvious overlapping of visually detected peaks (9). More recent studies employing standardized pulse-detecting algorhythms showed a significant cross-correlation between the episodic release of pituitary LH and P secretion in the mid- and late luteal phases, during which serum LH increases occurred with or were followed closely by increases in serum P (10, 11). Parallel observations in the primate confirm the above chronobiological relationships (12, 13). In particular, a one to one relationship was seen between LH pulses and secretory episodes of P release in the rhesus monkey, (13). However, other studies show that in women, discrete pulses of serum P can occur four times more frequently as those of bioactive LH (14) and can be observed even without antecedent LH pulses (15-17).

Some of the inconclusive results reported by earlier studies may be ascribed to the fact that luteal LH receptor binding characteristics vary throughout the cycle (with maximal binding during mid-luteal phase), which makes the timing of the sampling a fundamental variable (18, 19). However, even when profiles of steroid hormone secretion and LH secretory patterns are compared at the mid-luteal phase of the cycle (when one should expect the best correlation based on optimal binding) two distinct populations of steroid pulses are described: large amplitude pulses, preceded by an LH pulse, and small amplitude pulses, associated with periods of relative pituitary LH quiescence (20).

Overall, the incomplete cross-correlation between luteal and pituitary secretion suggests some degree of autonomy of luteal steroidogenesis in the woman and nonhuman primates. Similarly, in the cow and sheep, analysis of the relationship between the pulses of LH and P and the persistence of episodic P secretion after LH suppression with GnRH antagonist supports partial intra ovarian control of CL secretion of P (21-23). Measurements of LH and P in both the ovarian and the systemic blood of the ewe showed two different cycles of P pulses, one similar to that of the LH pulses, and the other independent of LH (21). More recently, a study employing superfusion of small slices of bovine CL showed that P is secreted episodically in vitro, in complete absence of gonadotropin drive for observation periods of 3-5 hours (24). Finally, with the use of in vitro microdialysis on the baboon CL, pulsatile secretion of P over an extended period of 24 hours in absence of LH was demonstrated, suggesting for the first time the presence of an intra luteal oscillator or pulse generator for P secretion in the early, mid and late luteal phases in the primate (25).

Microdialysis is a technique based on the use of an artificial capillary vessel, widely employed in neurochemical research and more recently in endocrinological studies (26-29), in this instance, the probe was housed within the CL. With microdialysis as carried out in our studies, the concentration of all solutes in the two solutions, namely the intercellular fluid and the dialysis fluid flowing through the microdialysis probe containing the permeable membrane, will constantly tend toward equilibrium (30). Thus, P measured from the sample microdialysis reflects the P secreted into the intercellular fluid by the surrounding cells. This technique allows for preservation of intact tissue architecture and continuous sampling from the intercellular space, without distortion of intercellular volumes (31, 32). The closed loop system of the microdialysis technique employed maintains the integrity of the CL with minimal trauma. Therefore, microdialysis provides a very suitable and useful approach for investigating cell-to-cell interactions and paracrine systems within the CL. Superfusion studies, such as the one reported with bovine CL (24), although still preserving the gross parenchymal architecture, entail that the tissue be sliced and/or minced, which is likely to cause the release of mediators that can potentially affect the regulatory mechanisms of steroid secretion. The pulse frequency of P secretion over a 24 hour period by the baboon CL is less than that obtained with perifused slices of bovine CL observed for a smaller window of time, and varies with the age of the CL, suggesting that an autochtone oscillator synchronizes luteal P secretion once the CL is completely formed. The pulse frequency is not random, as attested to by the bell-shaped distribution of the pulses when plotted against the ranges of interpulse intervals, with the maximum number of puls es having a pulse frequency of 21-40 minutes. The presence of an intra luteal P oscillator is further strengthened by nonrandom distribution of the pulses. Although the data do not show statistical significance in this respect, there appears to be a trend toward a decrease in pulse frequency of autonomous P secretion by the primate CL as it reaches the late luteal phase or the end of the normal life-span of the CL of the menstrual cycle. What causes this episodic release of steroids in the absence of neuroendocrine stimuli, and which luteal cell population is primarily responsible for it is not yet understood.

In the ovine CL, there are two clearly different cell types: large and small (33). Both have LH receptors, however it appears that LH stimulates P release only from the small luteal cells (34, 35), whereas the large luteal cells secrete greater amounts of P than the small cells and contribute to most of the P secreted by the CL under basal conditions (36). Thus, the autonomous oscillatory secretion of P by the sheep CL is likely to depend on the large luteal cells. The ovine CL displays a particularly high level of local autonomy, as suppression of gonadotropin pulsatility in vivo with GnRH antagonist treatment has no significant effect on the life span or secretory activity of the gland (22).

We have previously described a two-cell model for the primate corpus luteum, which is based on histochemical and functional, rather then morphological, differentiation between two different types of luteal cells (37) It is, therefore, tempting to hypothesize that a similar source is responsible for the episodic secretion in the primate CL.

Although the site or source of the pulsatile P secretion may be predominantly the large luteal cells, the mechanisms responsible for the oscillatory secretion may be partially, if not exclusively, autocrine, regulated by P itself. The demonstration of progesterone receptors in primate luteal cells (38) suggests that this steroid may also act as a local regulator, inhibiting its own release via an ultra-short autocrine feedback in the corpus luteum and therefore functioning as an important component of the proposed intra luteal oscillator.

Recent data indicate another fundamental role of progesterone in controlling the number of luteal cells that ultimately develop within a corpus luteum (39). Such control appears to be exerted at two levels: by inhibiting granulosa cell EGF-induced mitosis and by influencing the rate of granulosa cell luteinization. The observation that the progesterone antagonist mifepristone attenuates such anti-mitotic effects of progesterone suggests that these are mediated through specific receptors, which have been identified on human granulosa cells (40). Progesterone exposure increases the percentage of granulosa cells and decreases the percentage of large luteal cells, suggesting an auto-regulatory mechanism by which luteinization is prevented when a critical threshold level of progesterone is reached. In rats, ovarian 3ß-hydroxysteroid dehydrogenase activity is increased in a dose-dependent manner by P, which also reverses the inhibitory effect of mifepristone when coadministered (41). RU 486 not only decreased CG-stimulated P production by rat CL through a decrease in 3ß-hydroxysteroid dehydrogenase, but also simultaneously increased 20V-hydroxysteroid dehydrogenase activity (42). In the above mentioned study with superfusion of slices of bovine CL, P pulse frequencies and amplitudes are suppressed by inhibition of intracellular calcium with calcium channel blockers, and enhanced by inhibition of local prostaglandin production with indomethacin (24). Wether these mechanisms are operational or function to the same extent in the primate CL and when examined with microdialysis, which delivers and allows exchange of molecules in a controlled and compartmentalized manner into an intact CL compared with the open perfusion method with tissue slices, remains to be examined.

In conclusion, a new level of luteal chronobiology seems to unravel as a promising avenue of investigation. The corpus luteum, a peripheral and temporary gland, seems to have an internal biochemical mechanism responsible for autonomous maintenance of an intrinsically pulsatile hormonal release, similar to the one described for the isolated human hypophysis in vitro (43). The clinical implications of such a concept are difficult to foresee at this early stage of research.

REFERENCES

1) Nappi, C., Gargiulo, A.R. (1994) The human luteal paracrine system: current concepts. J. Endocrinol. Invest. 17, 825-36.

2) Stouffer, R.L., (1990) Corpus luteum function anD dysfunction. Clin. Obstet. Gynecol. 33, 668-89.

3) Groff, T.R., Raj, H.G., Tolbert, L.M., Willis, D.L. (1984) Effects of neutralization of luteinizing hormone on corpus luteum function and cyclicity in macaca fascicularis. J. Clin. Endocrinol. Metab. 59, 1054-7.

4) Hamberger, L., Hahlin, M., Hillensjo, T., Johanson, C., Sjogren, A. (1988) Luteotropic and luteolytic factors regulating human corpus luteum function. Ann. N.Y. Acad. Sci. 541, 485-97.

5) Mais, V., Kazer, R.R., Cetel, N.S., Rivier, J., Vale, W., Yen, S.S.C. (1987) The dependency of folliculogenesis and corpus luteum function on pulsatile gonadotropin secretion in cycling women using a gonadotropin-releasing hormone antagonist as a probe. J. Clin. Endocrinol. Metab. 62, 1250-5.

6) Fraser, H.M., Abbott, M., Laird, N.C., McNeilly, A.S., Nestor Jr., J.J., Vickery, B.H. (1986) Effects of a LH-releasing hormone antagonist on the secretion of LH, FSH, Prolactin and ovarian steroids at different stages of the luteal phase in the stumptailed macaque (Macaca arctoides). J. Endocrinol. 111, 83-90.

7) Fraser, H.M., Nestor Jr., J.J., Vickery, B.H. (1987) Suppression of luteal function by a luteinizing hormone-releasing hormone antagonist during the early luteal phase in the stumped-tailed macaque monkey and effects of subsequent administration of a human chorionic gonadotropin. Endocrinology. 121, 612-8.

8) McLachlan, R.I., Cohen, N.L., Vale, W. (1989) The importance of luteinizing hormone in the control of inhibin and progesterone secretion by the human corpus luteum. J. Clin. Endocrinol. Metab. 68, 1078-85.

9) Backstrom, C.T., McNeilly, A.S., Leask, R.M., Baird, D.T. (1982) Pulsatile secretion of LH, FSH, Prolactin, oestradiol and progesterone during the human menstrual cycle. Clin. Endocrinol. 17, 29-42.

10) Filicori, M., Buttler, J.P., Crowley Jr., W.F. (1984) Neuroendocrine regulation of the corpus luteum in the human – evidence for pulsatile progesterone secretion. J. Clin. Invest. 73, 1638-47.

11) Veldhuis, J.D., Christiansen, E., Evans, W.S., Kolp, L.A., Rogol, A.D., Johnson, M.L. (1988) Physiological profiles of episodic progesterone release during the mid-luteal phase of the human menstrual cycle: analysis of circadian and ultradian rhythms, discrete pulse properties and correlations with simultaneous luteinizing hormone release. J. Clin. Endocrinol. Metab. 66, 414-21.

12) Zeleznik, A.J., Hutchinson, J. (1987) Luteotrophic actions of LH on the macaque corpus luteum. In Stouffer, R.L. (ed.) The primate ovary, pp. 163-74. (New York: Plenum Publishing).

13) Ellinwood, W.E., Norman, R.L., Spies, H.G. (1984) Changing frequency of pulsatile luteinizing hormone and progesterone secretion during the luteal phase of the menstrual cycle of rhesus monkeys. Biol. Rep. 31, 714-22.

14) Beitins, I.Z., Dufau, M.L. (1986) Pulsatile secretion of progesterone from the human corpus luteum: poor correlation with bioactive LH pulses. Acta Endocrinol. (Copenh). 111, 553-7.

15) Soules, M.R., Clifton, D.K., Steiner, G.R., Cohen, N.L.. Bremner, W.J. (1988) The corpus luteum: determinants of

progesterone secretion in the normal menstrual cycle. Obstet. Gynecol. 71, 659-66.

16) Rossmanith, W.G., Laughlin, G.A., Mortola, J.F., Johnson, M.L., Veldhuis, J.D., Yen, S.S.C. (1990) Pulsatile cosecretion of estradiol and progesterone by the midluteal phase corpus luteum. Temporal link to luteinizing hormone pulses. J. Clin. Endocrinol. Metab. 70, 990-5.

17) Healy, D.L., Schenken, R.S., Lynch, A., Williams, R.F., Hodgen, G.D. (1984) Pulsatile progesterone secretion: its relevance to clinical evaluation of corpus luteum function. Fertil. Steril. 41, 114-21.

18) McNeilly, A.S., Kerin, J., Swanston, I.A., Bramley, T.A., Baird, D.T. (1980) Changes in the binding of human chorionic gonadotropin/luteinizing hormone, follicle stimulating hormone and prolactin to human corpora lutea during the menstrual cycle and pregnancy. J. Endocrinol. 87, 315-25.

19) Vega, M., Devoto, L., Navarro, V., Castro, O., Kohen, P. (1987) In vitro net progesterone production by human corpora lutea: effects of human chorionic gonadotropin, dibutyryl adenosine 3',5'- monophosphate, cholera toxin, and forskolin. J. Clin. Endocrinol. Metab. 65, 747-53.

20) Rossmanith, W.G., Laughlin, G.A., Mortola, J.F., Yen, S.S.C. (1990) Secretory dynamics of oestradiol (E2) and progesterone (P4) during periods of relative pituitary LH quiescence in the midluteal phase of the menstrual cycle. Clin. Endocrinol. 32, 13-23.

21) Baird, D.T., Swanston, J., Scaramuzzi, R.J. (1976) Pulsatile release of LH and secretion of ovarian steroids in sheep during the luteal phase of the estrous cycle. Endocrinology 98, 1490-6.

22) McNeilly, A.S., Crow, W.J., Fraser, H.M. (1992) Suppression of pulsatile luteinizing hormone secretion by gonadotropin-releasing hormone antagonist does not affect episodic progesterone secretion or corpus luteun function in ewes. J. Reprod. Fertil. 96, 865-74.

23) Hixcn., J.E., Pijanowski, G.J., Weston, P.G., Shanks, R.D., Wagner, W.C. (1983) Evidence for an oscillator other than luteinizing hormone controlling the secretion of progesterone in cattle. Biol. Reprod. 29, 1155-62.

24) Rossmanith, W.G., Schick, M., Benz, R., Lauritzen, C. (1991) Autonomous progesterone secretion from the bovine corpus luteum in vitro. Acta Endocrinol. (Copehn) 124, 179-87.

25) Khan-Dawood, F.S., Gargiulo A.R., Dawood, M.Y. (1994) Baboon corpus luteum: autonomous pulsatile progesterone secretion and evidence for an intraluteal oscillator demonstrated by in vitro microretrodialysis. J. Clin. Endocrinol. Metab. 79, 1790-6.

26) Khan-Dawood, F.S., Gargiulo, A.R., Dawood, M.Y. (1994) In vitro microdialysis of the ovine corpus luteum of pregnancy: effects of insulin-like growth factor on progesterone secretion. Biol. Rep. 51, 1299-306.

27) Jarry, H., Einspanier, A., Kanngieber, L., et al. (1990) Release and effects of oxytocin on estradiol and progesterone secretion in porcine corpora lutea as measured by an in vitro microdialysis system. Endocrinology. 126, 2350-60.

28) Einspanier, A., Jarry, H., Pitzel, L., Holtz, W., Wuttke, W. (1991). Determination of secretion rates of estradiol, progesterone, oxytocin, and angiotensin II from tertiary follicles and freshly formed corpora lutea in freely moving sows. Endocrinology 129, 3403-9.

29) Miyamoto, A., Schams, D. (1991) Oxyticin stimulates progesterone release from microdialyzed bovine corpus luteum in vitro. Biol. Rep. 44, 1163-70.

30) Benveniste, H., Huttemeier, PC. (1990) Microdialysis - Theory and application. Prog. Neurobiol. 35, 195-215.

31) Ungerstedt, U., Pycock, C. (1974) Functional correlates of dopamine neurotransmission. Bull Schweiz Akad Wiss. 1278, 1-13.

32) Benveniste, H. (1989) Brain microdialysis. J. Neurochem. 52, 1667-79.

33) Fitz, T.A., Mayan, M.H., Sawyer, H.R., Niswender, G.D. (1982) Characterization of two stroidogenic cell types in the ovine corpus luteum. Biol. Reprod. 27, 703-11.

34) Rao, C.V., Estergreen, V.L., Carman, F.R., Moss, G.E. (1979) Receptors for gonadotropin and prostaglandin F2V in

bovine corpora lutea of early, mid and late luteal phase. Acta Endocrinol. (Copehn). 91, 113-24.

35) Rodgers, R.J., O'Shea, J.D., Bruce, N.W. (1984) Morphometric analysis of the cellular composition of the ovine corpus luteum. J. Anat. 138, 757-69.

36) Wiltbank, M., Diskin, M.G., Niswender, G.D. (1991) Differential actions of second messenger systems in the corpus luteum. J. Reprod. Fertil. 43 (Suppl), 65-75.

37) Dawood, M.Y., Gargiulo, A.R., Nappi, C., Montemagno, U. (1992) Progesterone secretion by the human corpus luteum: mechanisms of control. In: Genazzani A.R. and Petraglia F. Hormones in Gynecological Endocrinology. Carnforth, U.K.: Parthenon Publishing Group, UK, 52, 547-65.

38) Hild-Petitom, S.A., Stouffer, R.L., Brenner, R.M. (1988) Immunocytochemical localization of estradiol and progesterone receptors in the monkey ovary throughout the menstrual cycle. Endocrinology. 123, 2896-905.

39) Chaffkin, L.M., Luciano, A.A., Peluso, J.J. (1993) The role of progesterone in regulating human granulosa cell proliferation and differentiation in vitro. J. Clin. Endocrinol. Metab. 76, 796-800.

40) Greenberg, L.H., Stouffer, R.L., Brenner, R.M., Molskness, T.A., Hild-Petito, S.A., Yu, Q. (1990) Are human luteinizing granulosa cells a site of action for progesterone and relaxin? Fertil Steril 53, 46-53.

41) Tanaka, N., Iwamasa, J., Matzura, K., Okamura, H. (1993) Effects of progesterone and anti-progesterone RU 486 on ovarian 3ß-hydroxysteroid dehydrogenase activity during ovulation in the gonadotropin-primed immature rat. J. Reprod. Fertil. 97, 167-72.

42) Kawano, T., Okamura, H., Tajima, C., Fukuma, K., Katabuchi H. (1988) Effects of RU 486 on luteal function in the early pregnant rat. J. Reprod. Fertil. 83, 279-85.

43) Gambacciani, M., Liu, J.H., Swartz, W.H., Tueros, V.S., Yen, S.S.C., Rasmussen, D.D. (1987) Intrinsic pulsatility of luteinizing hormone release from the human pituitary in vitro. Neuroendocrinology 45, 402-8.

Ovarian safety aspects of LHRH antagonists and agonists

C.B. Lambalk, L. Brus and J. Schoemaker

Institute of Endocrinology, Reproduction and Metabolism, Division of Reproductive Endocrinology, Department of Obstetrics and Gynecology, Free University Hospital, Amsterdam, The Netherlands

INTRODUCTION

Some years ago the use of LHRH agonists was introduced in in vitro fertilization (IVF) programs in order to prevent the preovulatory spontaneous luteinizing hormone (LH) surge by means of desensitizing the pituitary[1]. In the near future LHRH antagonists may become introduced for this purpose. Their mechanism of action is via direct blockade of the pituitary LHRH receptor. This presentation will shortly review the safety aspect of this application in light of possible direct effects of LHRH analogs on the ovaries. For the purpose of understanding these effects some attention will be adressed to the issue of ovarian LHRH receptors.

LHRH RECEPTORS IN THE PRIMATE OVARY?

The direct effects of LHRH agonists and antagonists observed on rat ovarian tissue suggest receptor mediated action. Indeed in the rat ovary high affinity LHRH receptors have been demonstrated[2]. Specific binding of LHRH agonist was observed in rat granulosacell, and theca interna and externa, and in the corpus luteum by means of autoradiography[3]. Conflicting data exist on the presence of LHRH receptors in primate ovarian tissue. Recently, LHRH agonist binding sites with high affinity have been localized with autoradiography in the granulosa of a single preovulatory follicle in one human ovary among negative observations in the ovaries of 5 other subjects[4]. No other high affinity pituitary type LHRH receptors have been identified in human or non-human primate ovarian tissue[5]. Bramley and coworkers demonstrated low affinity LHRH binding sites present in human midluteal corpus luteum.[6] Recently, Kakar and collegues demonstrated, by means of PCR (polymerase chain reaction) technique, the presence of cDNA coding for the human LHRH receptor in human ovarian tissue[7]. Others have not been able to confirm this by means of in situ hibrydization until sofar(Eidne et al. Personal Communication). In our own laboratory we have not been able to demonstrate specific binding of a radiolabeled LHRH antagonist and agonist in human preovulatory follicles while clear specific binding with the same analogues was present in rat ovarian tissue (unpublished data).

DIRECT EFFECTS OF LHRH AGONISTS IN THE PRIMATE OVARY

In the human some experiments have been conducted on the biological action of LHRH agonists on the ovary and the results appear to be contradictory. One study showed an effect of LHRH on follicle stimulated hormone (FSH) and LH stimulated granulosacell progesterone accumulation in vitro from cells harvested in the mid to late follicular phase[8]. In contrast, another report demonstrated no effect on FSH stimulated aromatase activity and progesterone accumulation from cells obtained in the early to mid follicular phase[9]. Similar observations were made by Dodson et al.[10]. It should be mentioned that LHRH agonist treated patients have luteinized granulosacells with a significantly higher Proliferative Index associated with lower Mullerian Inhibiting Substance levels in the follicular fluid[11]. This indicates a possible indirect pathway of the mode of action of LHRH and its agonists. FSH induced progesterone production by granulosa-lutein cells from preovulatory follicles, aspirated after hCG administration in in vitro fertilization patients, was also inhibited by the LHRH agonist Buserelin[12]. On the other hand an increase of progesterone and a decline of estradiol and LH binding has been observed under unstimulated conditions[12,13].

DIRECT EFFECTS OF LHRH ANTAGONISTS IN THE PRIMATE OVARY

Some data indicate that LHRH may act directly on the human ovary. Tureck et al. noted an inhibitory effect of a LHRH agonist on progesterone production of cultered human granulosacells[8]. A LHRH antagonist could prevent the inhibitory action of LHRH agonist on FSH stimulated progesterone production suggesting LHRH receptor mediated effects. On the other hand others were not able to demonstrate an inhibitory effect of LHRH agonist on human granulosacell-culture FSH-dependent steroidogenic function[9]. Similar observations were made on cultured luteal cells[14]. In the non-human primate it was shown that inhibition of FSH stimulated steroid and cyclic AMP production of cultured marmoset granulosacells can be achieved by both LHRH agonist and antagonist[15]. If both drugs were given together, even a synergistic effect could be observed. The latter observation indicate that a mechanism is involved that is not LHRH receptor specific.

CONCLUSION

Rat gonadal tissue does contain LHRH receptors and LHRH influence seems to be receptor mediated. LHRH antagonists have shown to exert direct effects on rat gonadal tissue which are compatible with receptor binding, while in primate and human ovarian tissue LHRH antagonistic effects do not seem to be LHRH receptor mediated. Untill now no clear evidence exists that high affinity LHRH receptors are present in primate and human ovarian tissue, although, uncertainty still exists on this issue. With the possible introduction of a new drug that will be given during the follicular phase of the cycle it seems appropriate to further explore possible overt direct ovarian effects of LHRH antagonists prior to their large scale application in Assisted Reproduction.

REFERENCES

1. Porter R.N., Smith W., Craft I.L. and et al (1984).Induction of ovulation for in-vitro fertilisation using buserelin and gonadotropins. *Lancet.*,**2**,-1284-1285

2. Clayton R.N., Harwood J.P. and Catt K.J. (1979).GnRH analogue binds to luteal cells and inhibits progesterone production. *Nature*,**282**,90

3. Seguin C., Pelletier G., Dube D. and Labrie F. (1982).Distribution of luteinizing hormone-releasing hormone receptors in the rat ovary. *Regul. Pept.*,**4**,183-190

4. Latouche J., Crumeyrolle Arias M., Jordan D., Kopp N., Augendre Ferrante B., Cedard L. and Haour F. (1989).GnRH receptors in human granulosa cells: Anatomical localization and characterization by autoradiographic study. *Endocrinology.*,**125**,1739-1741

5. Clayton R.N. and Huhtaniemi I.T. (1982).Absence of gonadotropin-releasing hormone receptors in human gonadal tissue. *Nature*,**299**,56-59

6. Bramley T.A., Stirling D., Swanston I.A. and et al (1987).Specific binding sites for gonadotrophin-releasing hormone, LH/chorionic gonadotrophin, low-density lipoprotein, prolactin and FSH in homogenates of human corpus luteum. II: Concentrations throughout the luteal phase of menstrual cycle and early pregnancy. *J. Endocrinol.*,**113**,317-327

7. Kakar S.S., Musgrove L.C., Devor D.C., Sellers J.C. and Neill J.D. (1992).Cloning, sequencing, and expression of human gonadotropin releasing hormone (GnRH) receptor. *Biochem. Biophys. Res. Commun.*,**189**,289-295

8. Tureck R.W., Mastroianni L.J., Blasco L. and Strauss J.F.I.I.I. (1982).Inhibition of human granulosa cell progesterone secretion by a gonadotropin-releasing hormone agonist. *J. Clin. Endocrinol. Metab.*,**54**,-1078-1080

9. Casper R.F., Erickson G.F., Rebar R.W. and Yen S.S.C. (1982).The effect of luteinizing hormone-releasing factor and its agonist on cultured human granulosa cells. *Fertil. Steril.*,**37**,406-409

10. Dodson W.C., Myers T., Morton P.C. and Conn P.M. (1988).Leuprolide acetate: Serum and follicular fluid concentrations and effects on human fertilization, embryo growth, and granulosa-lutein cell progesterone accumulation in vitro. *Fertil. Steril.*,**50**,612-617

11. Seifer D.B., Charland C., Berlinsky D., Penzias A.S., Haning R.V.J., Naftolin F. and Barker B.E. (1993).Proliferative index of human luteinized granulosa cells varies as a function of ovarian reserve. *Am. J. Obstet. Gynecol.*,**169**,1531-1535

12. Parinaud J., Beaur A., Bourreau E., Vieitez G. and Pontonnier G. (1988) Effect of a luteinizing hormone-releasing hormone agonist (Buserelin) on steroidogenesis of cultured human preovulatory granulosa cell. *Fertil. Steril.*,**50**,597-602

13.   Guerrero H.E., Stein P., Asch R.H., de Fried E.P. and Tesone M. (1-993).Effect of a gonadotropin-releasing hormone agonist on luteinizing hormone receptors and steroidogenesis in ovarian cells. *Fertil Steril.*,**59**,803-808

14.   Casper R.F., Erickson G.F. and Yen S.S.C. (1984).Studies on the effect of gonadotropin-releasing hormone and its agonist on human luteal steroidogenesis in vitro. *Fertil. Steril.*,**42**,39-43

15.   Wickings E.J., Eidne K.A., Dixson A.F. and Hillier S.G. (1990).Gonadotropin-releasing hormone analogs inhibit primate granulosa cell steroidogenesis via a mechanism distinct from that in the rat. *Biol. Reprod.*,**43**,30-5-311

The antiprogestins – modulators of progestin and glucocorticoid function

I.M. Spitz and A. Robbins

Center for Biomedical Research, The Population Council, New York, USA

INTRODUCTION

Following the discovery of the progesterone receptor, it was recognized that a progesterone receptor antagonist i.e. an agent which will inhibit the action of progesterone would open many therapeutic possibilities for female reproductive health. In 1981, Philibert, Deraedt and Teutsch announced the discovery of RU 38486, a glucocorticoid antagonist with antiprogestin properties. RU 38486 was subsequently abbreviated to RU 486 and is now known by its generic name mifepristone. It was the first antiprogestin to be developed. This synthetic steroid binds strongly to both progesterone and glucocorticoid receptors and minimally to the androgen receptor. It failed to bind estrogen or mineralocorticord receptors. Further biological tests in animals showed that mifepristone behaved as a potent progestin and glucocorticoid antagonist(1).

Mifepristone is a derivative of the progestin norethindrone and possesses an additional 4-(dimethylamino) phenyl side chain at the 11β position and a 1-propynyl chain at the 17α position(2,3).

Since the original report of mifepristone, over 400 additional antiprogestins have been synthesized and several are undergoing preliminary clinical evaluation. The 2-dimensional structure of onapristone (ZK 98299) is similar to those of mifepristone. However, it has a different molecular shape due to configurational inversions at the C13 and C17 positions(2,3).

CLINICAL EFFECTS

A. Medical Abortion

In 1982, Herrmann et al, published the first report describing the successful termination of pregnancy with mifepristone in 9 out of 11 subjects(4). Numerous studies have been conducted over the last decade using different regimens with total doses ranging from 140 to 700 mg administered over 1-7 days. In all these studies, the success rate in women with pregnancy duration of 7 weeks or less usually ranges from 64 to 85%(3,5).

This low response rate is attributed to an inadequate prostaglandin effect. An increase in prostaglandin action is critical for the initiation of the abortive process. In pregnancy, prostaglandins are low and uterine contractibility is suppressed. During spontaneous abortion and labor there is an increase of prostaglandin production. In *in vitro* conditions, antiprogestins induce an increase in prostaglandin production with a significant decrease in prostaglandin metabolism(6). When the use of mifepristone is followed within 36 to 48 hours by a prostaglandin, the abortion rate exceeds 95% in women whose pregnancy duration is less than 49 days(3).

The initial prostaglandin used in conjunction with mifepristone belonged to the PGE_2 series and it was administered by injection. However this specific preparation, which is known as sulpostrone, was associated with cardiovascular complications in approximately 1 in 20,000 subjects and its use was subsequently withdrawn(3). Currently prostaglandins of the PGE_1 series are used. These include the vaginal pessary preparation known as gemeprost and an orally administered prostaglandin, misoprostol(7). The use of mifepristone followed 36 to 48 hours later by either misoprostol or gemeprost has now been approved for the medical termination of pregnancy of up to 49 days duration in France and China and 63 days duration in the United Kingdom and Sweden.

B. Other Gynecological Uses

Another major action of antiprogestins is to promote dilation of the uterine cervix(3,5). As a consequence, mifepristone has been found to be useful in the preparation of women for first and second trimester vacuum aspiration. It is usually administered 24-48 hours prior to surgical abortion and it is as effective as prostaglandins which are currently used. Moreover, mifepristone has significantly fewer side effects. Because of its effect on the uterine cervix, mifepristone has also been used for the induction of labor following intra-uterine fetal death. Indeed, mifepristone has been registered in France for these indications. Another proposed use of mifepristone is to induce labor at the end of normal pregnancy. However, since this agent may cross into the fetal circulation, further studies are required to establish its safety(3,5).

In view of its antiestrogenic activity, mifepristone may be used in the treatment of estrogen dependent gynecological disorders such as uterine myoma or endometriosis(8). Preliminary studies have shown that both these conditions may improve following mifepristone administration. However, further clinical trials need to be conducted. Another potential use of mifepristone is in contraception. This subject is reviewed elsewhere in these proceedings (Spitz, I.M. and Robbins, A.).

C. Treatment of Tumors

In view of its unusual progesterone agonist and antagonistic activity, the effect of this agent has also been evaluated in hormone dependent tumors. In several *in vitro* studies with human breast cancer cells in culture, mifepristone demonstrated an antiproliferative effect with both progestin agonistic and antagonistic activities. In view of the multiple and varied effects of mifepristone on tumor cells *in vitro*, the action of this agent must be explored on breast cancer and other tumors *in vivo*. There have been two preliminary published trials on the use of mifepristone in advanced carcinoma of the breast. The results were not conclusive(9,10). To establish where antiprogestins might form a treatment modality in the endocrine treatment of human breast cancer, long term comparative studies are required.

Another tumor which may be amenable to antiprogestin administration is meningioma which is a benign brain tumor. Most meningiomas are devoid of estrogen receptors but contain significant concentrations of progesterone receptors. Mifepristone has been used in the treatment of patients with unresectable meningioma. In one study comprising 14 subjects, there was objective and subjective improvement is 5 subjects(11). Further trials need to be conducted to determine the efficacy of this treatment. In this regard there are other carcinomas which possess steroid receptors and antiprogestins may have a potential role in their treatment.

D. Antiglucocorticoid Action

All antiprogestins possess antiglucocorticoid activity although this varies from compound to compound. Mifepristone may be used to treat patients with adrenal overactivity known as Cushing's syndrome due to inoperable tumors(3). On the basis of studies in animals, other applications for the antiglucorticoid effects of antiprogestins have been suggested. These include the local application of eye drops containing mifepristone in order to lower intraoccular pressure in patients with glaucoma and oral administration of the drug to prevent the progression of viral diseases in humans. It has also been suggested that this compound could be used to prevent steroid-induced muscle atrophy. All these and other potential applications must be evaluated in the clinic(3).

SIDE EFFECTS

Few women who receive single doses of mifepristone to interrupt pregnancy have side effects. When such effects do occur, they include heavy bleeding, nausea, vomiting, abdominal pain and fatigue. It is often difficult to dissociate many of these symptoms from those that result from normal pregnancy and spontaneous abortion. Prolonged high dose administration of mifepristone is associated with anorexia, nausea and vomiting. Other side effects include slight weight loss and skin rashes(3,5).

Because a few women do not abort and continue with their pregnancies following the administration of mifepristone, it is important to determine whether antiprogestins have teratogenic effects. None have been observed in monkeys, mice, or rats. There are isolated case reports of normal pregnancies and offspring when women have taken mifepristone alone or in combination with prostaglandin have not aborted and elected to continue their pregnancies(3,5). None the less, at the current state of knowledge, women who do not abort following administration of mifepristone and prostaglandins should be warned about possible teratogenic effects and offered surgical abortion.

CONCLUSIONS

It has been estimated that world wide approximately 55 million pregnancies are terminated by abortions each year. When abortion is performed in less than ideal situations, there is significant maternal mortality and morbidity, including infections and uterine perforation. The availability of a safe and effective method of medical abortion would thus have a marked impact on maternal health throughout the world.

It must be stressed that medical induced abortion is only one indication for this new group of compounds. Antiprogestins are among the most interesting therapeutic compounds developed over the past two decades and they may also be used for the treatment of patients with hormone dependent tumors, gynecological disorders and for contraception. In view of their antiglucocorticoid properties, these agents may also be used to treat Cushing's syndrome, a condition characterized by an excess of glucocorticoids and other situations where a decrease in glucocorticoid action is desired.

REFERENCES

1. Ulmann, A., Teutsch, G., and Philibert, D. (1990). RU 486. *Sci. Amer.*, **262**,42-48

2. Beier, H.M. and Spitz (eds.), I.M. (1994). Progesterone antagonistic in Reproductive Medicine and Oncology. *Human Reprod.*, **9 (Suppl.1)**

3. Spitz, I.M. and Bardin, C.W. (1993). Clinical pharmacology of RU 486 - An antiprogestin and antiglucocorticoid. *Contraception*, **48**,403-444

4. Herrman, W., Wyss, A., Riondel, A., Philibert, D., Teutsch, G., Sakiz, E., and Baulieu, E.E. (1982). Effect d' un-steroide anti-progesterone chez la femme: Interuption du cycle metruelet de la grossesse au debut. *C.R. Acad. Sci. Paris*, **294**,933-938

5. Spitz, I.M. and Bardin, C.W. (1993). Mifepristone (RU 486) - A modulator of progestin and glucocorticoid action. *N. Engl. J. Med.*, **329**,404-412

6. Cheng, L., Kelly, R.W., Thong, K.J., Hume, R., and Baird, D.T. (1993). The effects of mifepristone (RU486) on prostaglandin dehydrogenase in decidual and chorionic tissue in early pregnancy. *Human Reprod.*, **8**,705-709

7. Peyron, R., Aubeny, E., Targosz, V., Silvestre, L., Renault, M., Elkik, F., Leclerc, P., Ulmann, A., and Baulieu, E.-E. (1993). Early termination of pregnancy with mifepristone (RU 486) and the orally active prostaglandin misoprostol. *New Engl. J. Med.*, **328**,1509-1513

8. Kettel, L.M., Murphy, A.A., Morales, A.J., and Yen, S.S.C. (1994). Clinical efficacy of the antiprogesterone RU486 in the treatment of endometriosis and uterine fibroids. *Human Reprod.*, **9 (Suppl. 1)**,116-120

9. Romieu, G., Maudelande, T., Ullman, A., Pujol, H., Grenier, J., Cavalie, G., Khalaf, S., and Rochefort, H. (1987). The antiprogestin RU 486 in advanced breast cancer: Preliminary clinical trial. *Bull. Cancer*, **74**,455-461

10. Klijn, J.G.M., deJong, F.G., Bakker, G.H., Lamberts, S.W.J., Rodenburg, C.J., and Alexieva-Figusch, J. (1989). Antiprogestins, a new form of endocrine therapy for human breast cancer. *Cancer Res.*, **49**,2851-2856

11. Grunberg, S.M., Weiss, M.H., Spitz, I.M., Ahmadi, J., Sadun, A., Russell, C.A., Lucci, L., and Stevenson, L.L. (1991). Treatment of unresectable meningioma with the antiprogesterone agent mifepristone. *J. Neurosurg.*, **74**,861-866

The contraceptive potential of the antiprogestin mifepristone

I.M. Spitz and A. Robbins

Center for Biomedical Research, The Population Council, New York, USA

INTRODUCTION

Mifepristone (RU486) is a potent progesterone and glucocorticoid antagonist. Since progesterone is critical for the initiation and maintenance of pregnancy, the major clinical application of antiprogestins is in the interruption of early pregnancy. In women with amenorrhea of less than seven weeks, the incidence of termination of pregnancy is over 95% when mifepristone (600 mg) is followed within 36 to 48 hours by the administration of a prostaglandin by the oral (misoprostol) or vaginal (gemeprost) route (1).

Progesterone also has other important actions. Together with estradiol it facilitates the luteinizing hormone (LH) surge. It also transforms the endometrium from a proliterative to a secretory state and maintains endometrial integrity. Thus, antiprogestins may have contraceptive potential by virtue of i) inhibition of the LH surge delaying ovulation, ii) prevention of endometrial transformation, and iii) shedding of the endometrium and induction of menstrual bleeding.

FOLLICULAR PHASE ADMINISTRATION

Mid and late follicular phase mifepristone administration in doses ranging from 25 to 100 mg for three days or longer blocks follicular development and delays the LH surge and ovulation by approximately 12 days (1). Thereafter follicular growth resumes or a new follicle is recruited. To inhibit ovulation, either continuous or intermittent mifepristone regimens have been employed. In monkeys, oral mifepristone [25mg] once

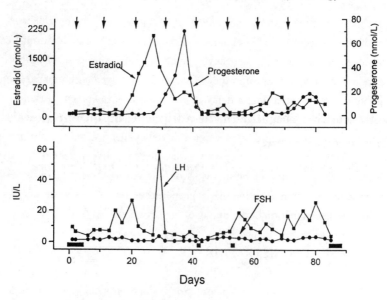

Figure 1   Responses of serum estradiol and progesterone (upper panel) and LH and FSH (lower panel) to mifepristone administered in a dose of 50 mg for 3 consecutive days every 10 days. This is indicated by the arrows. Bleeding episodes are shown as rectangles in the lower panel.

weekly for 1 month successfully inhibited ovulation (2). However once weekly administration of 10 mg or 50 mg to normal women and even administration of 50mg a day for three days repeated every 10 days for three consecutive months (Fig. 1) did not consistently inhibit the LH surge and corpus luteum function (3). In contrast to inter-mittent mifepristone administration, the continuous administration of daily doses of 2 to 10 mg for one month did block ovulation (4,5). However, under these circumstances there is suppression of serum progesterone with normal estradiol levels. This raises the possibility of unopposed estrogen action on the endometrium. Intermittent progestins have been administered in an attempt to obviate any unopposed estrogen effect on the endometrium. However with exogenous progestins, an LH surge is frequently induced (6). Since antiprogestins do not reliably inhibit ovulation and may adversely effect the endometrium, this method is unlikely to have contraceptive potential.

DELAY IN ENDOMETRIAL TRANSFORMATION

A daily 1 mg dose of mifepristone for one month did not interfere with bleeding patterns or hormonal profiles of ovulation. However this dose did produce morphological changes in the endometrium which indicates that the endometrium is markedly sensitive to mifepristone (5). In another study, a single of mifepristone (10 mg) given 5 and 8 days after the LH surge also did not alter the menstrual cycle or hormone patterns. However there was disturbance of endometrial maturation with reduced stromal edema and delayed glandular secretion and development (7). A single dose of mifepristone (200 mg) administered 48 hours after the LH surge also did not alter hormonal events of the cycle but was associated with a delay in endometrial development already evident after twelve hours, becoming more pronounced after 36 and 72 hours (8). Administration of this regimen to 21 unprotected women in 169 cycles resulted in only one pregnancy (9). This indicates that mifepristone has contraceptive potential by altering endometrial function without inhibiting ovulation. However at this stage of its development, the schedule of administration that appears most effective is not practical since it requires precise determination of the timing of the LH surge.

LUTEAL PHASE ADMINISTRATION

When administered in the late luteal phase, mifepristone promotes endometrial sloughing and vaginal bleeding. Attempts have been made to utilize this property of antiprogestins to develop a contraceptive based on antiprogestin given each month at the end of the cycle. This would be administered independently of whether the woman is pregnant or not. However this strategy is not efficacious as a contraceptive since up to 20% of proven pregnancies are not interrupted and the menstrual bleeding pattern is frequently disrupted (1,3).

POSTCOITAL ADMINISTRATION

Antiprogestins are very promising postcoital agents. Mifepristone administered within 72 hours of unprotective intercourse is as effective and safe a postcoital contraceptive as is high dose estrogen-progesterone administration. Moreover it has fewer untoward side effects although the menstrual bleeding patterns may be disturbed. (10) The mechanism for its effectiveness as a postcoital agent depends on the time of the cycle when it is administered. Inhibition of ovulation, delay in endometrial development or endometrial sloughing may be operating.

CONCLUSION

In conclusion, at the current stage of development of antiprogestins as potential contraceptives, it would appear that they are best used as post-coital agents within 3 days of unprotected intercourse. They also probably have contraceptive potential in view of their ability to disrupt endometrial maturation. However, further studies are required in unprotected women to determine the utility of this method. Ovulation inhibition and once monthly administration do not appear likely as contraceptive possibilities.

REFERENCES

1. Spitz, I.M. and Bardin, C.W. (1993). Mifepristone (RU 486) - A modulator of progestin and glucocorticoid action. *N. Engl. J. Med.*, **329**,404-412

2. Danforth, D.R., Dubois, C., Ulmann, A., Baulieu, E.E., and Hodgen, G.D. (1989). Contraceptive potential of RU 486 by ovulation inhibition. III. preliminary observations on once weekly oral administration. *Contraception*, **40**,195-200

3. Spitz, I.M., Croxatto, H.B., Lähteenmäki, P., Heikinheimo, O., and Bardin, C.W. (1994). Effect of mifepristone on inhibition of ovulation and induction of luteolysis. *Human Reprod.*, **9 (Suppl. 1)**,69-76

4. Ledger, W.L., Sweeting, V.M., Hillier, H., and Baird, D.T. (1992). Inhibition of ovulation by low-dose mifepristone (RU 486). *Human Reprod.*, **7**,6

5. Croxatto, H.B., Salvatierra, A.M., Croxatto, H.D., and Fuentealba, A. (1993). Effects of continuous treatment with low dose mifepristone throughout one menstrual cycle. *Human Reprod.*, **8**,201-207

6. Kekkonen, R., Alfthan, H., Haukkamaa, M., Heikinheimo, O., Luukkainen, T., and Lähteenmäki, P. (1990). Interference with ovulation by sequential treatment with the antiprogesterone RU 486 and synthetic progestin. *Fertil. Steril.*, **53**,747-750

7. Greene, K.E., Kettel, L.M., and Yen, S.S.-C. (1992). Interrruption of endometrial maturation without hormonal changes by an antiprogesterone during the first half of luteal phase of the menstrual cycle: a contraceptive potential. *Fertil. Steril.*, **58**,338-343

8. Swahn, M.L., Bygdeman, M., Cekan, S., Xing, S., Masironi, B., and Johannisson, E. (1990). The effect of RU 486 administered during the early luteal phase on bleeding pattern, hormonal parameters and endometrium. *Human Reprod.*, **5**,402-408

9. Gemzell-Danielsson, K., Swahn, M.-L., Svalander, P., and Bygdeman, M. (1993). Early luteal phase treatment with mifepristone (RU 486) for fertility regulation. *Human Reprod.*, **8**,870-873

10. Glasier, A., Thong, K.J., Dewar, M., Mackie, M., and Baird, D.T. (1992). Mifepristone (RU 486) compared with high-dose estrogen and progestogen for emergnecy postcoital contraception. *N. Engl. J. Med.*, **327**,1041-1044

Premature ovarian failure

C. Faiman and A.E. Mehta

Department of Endocrinology, The Cleveland Clinic Foundation, Cleveland, Ohio, USA

INTRODUCTION

Is premature ovarian failure a homogeneous entity? What is the definition of premature? Does failure imply irreversibility? How can it be treated? These are the major questions facing us today. There is growing evidence in the literature which indicates that premature ovarian failure is multifactorial and encompasses a spectrum of clinical presentations ranging from permanent hypergonadotropic amenorrhea to the apparent presence of a prematurely early perimenopausal state, to a condition waxing and waning from normogonadotropic menstrual cycles to hypergonadotropic amenorrhea.

THE NORMAL MENOPAUSE

The mean age at menopause in North America is 52 years and appears to be unrelated to the age of menarche, parity, ethnic extraction, nutrition or environmental factors. Menopause, due to ovarian failure and the virtual absence of primordial follicles in the ovary, is characterized by low estradiol levels, amenorrhea, and sustained elevation of gonadotropin levels. The final cessation of menses may be preceded by two to ten years of progressively irregular cycles with prolonged intermenstrual intervals.[1] During this time, gonadotropins, particularly FSH, may be variably elevated but estradiol levels are usually normal; ovulation is sporadic and hot flashes are a common accompaniment.

Studies indicate a correlation between the size of the residual follicular stock and the preservation of more normal menstrual function at this stage.[2] Although the primary cause of cessation of menstrual function is no doubt due to the disappearance of ovarian follicles, the nature of pituitary-ovarian interrelationships and a change in the ovarian milieu may help to explain the apparent gonadotropin resistance and relative infertility at this stage.[3]

For example, diminished ovarian inhibin production may have a cascade effect, in which the resultant hypersecretion of FSH leads to down-regulation of gonadotropin receptors and the development of a "resistant" state. Such a series of events has been postulated for both the aging primate ovary as well as for ovulation-induced cycles in older women.

PREMATURE MENOPAUSE

Since less than 2% of women reach the menopause prior to age 40, this is the currently accepted cut off for the definition of prematurity. The etiology of POF is outlined in Table 1. Classification based upon the presence or absence of follicles on an ovarian biopsy (at a particular time point) may be overly simplistic since factors which govern the number of endowed ova, the rate of follicular atresia, the changes in ovarian steroid and peptide hormone production and the intra-ovarian milieu as a function of age, remain poorly understood. Two categories will be discussed further - autoimmune oophoritis and idiopathic premature ovarian failure since these typify our inability to categorize the etiology with any degree of certainty.

AUTOIMMUNE OOPHORITIS

Circulating antibodies against some ovarian component (including gonadotropin receptors) defines the condition of autoimmune oophoritis in patients presenting with primary or secondary hypoestrogenic, hypergonadotropic amenorrhea and the biopsy-proven presence of ovarian follicles. It occurs in between 15-40% of such individuals.[4] Follicular lymphocytic infiltration, often transient, may also be found in ovarian biopsy specimens particularly during the early evolution of the condition.

TABLE 1: ETIOLOGICAL CLASSIFICATION OF PREMATURE OVARIAN FAILURE

1) CHROMOSOMAL:
    - X Linked: Turner syndrome and variants
                   Familial long arm X deletion
                   Triple X syndrome
    - Autosomal: Trisomy 13
                   Trisomy 18

2) ENZYMATIC DEFECTS:
    - 17 *a*-hydroxylase deficiency
    - Galactosemia

3) GONADOTROPIN APPARATUS DEFECTS:
    - Abnormal gonadotropin molecules
    - Abnormal gonadotropin receptors

4) INFECTION
    - Tuberculosis
    - Mumps
    - Others

5) IATROGENIC
    - Surgery
    - Chemotherapy
    - Irradiation

6) VASCULAR
    - Torsion/hemorrhage

7) IMMUNOLOGIC
    - Deficiency   - Ataxia Telangiectasia
                    - DiGeorge's Syndrome
    - Autoimmune   - "Oophoritis"

8) IDIOPATHIC
    - With follicles   - Resistant ovary syndrome
    - Afollicular

Variables such as the type of antigen used, assay technic, and the time of testing in relationship to disease onset appear to be of critical importance in the detection of this disorder. This concept should not seem surprising in light of identical issues which apply to the prototypic autoimmune glandular disease Hashimoto's thyroiditis.[5] In this condition, the antibody mix is heterogenous (organ damaging, anti-enzyme, thyroglobulin, growth promoting, TSH receptor agonist, TSH receptor blocking, etc.), not fixed in proportion with time, the response varying with the antibody mix and the state of the thyroid gland at a particular time so that transient or permanent hypofunction (or even hyperfunction) may occur, and the antibodies may disappear after organ death.

The coexistence of autoimmune premature ovarian failure in patients with Addison's disease may be as frequent as 25% and may relate to the presence of antibodies directed against common steroidogenic enzymes shared by the two organs.[6] The association of premature ovarian failure with hypothyroidism is less frequent but more so than is the general population. As with type 1 diabetes mellitus and Hashimoto's thyroiditis, there is an HLA-DR3 association with autoimmune oophoritis.[7]

IDIOPATHIC PREMATURE OVARIAN FAILURE AND THE RESISTANT OVARY SYNDROME

A significant proportion of women with premature ovarian failure, in whom circulating autoantibodies are either not detected or not looked for, and no other cause has been identified, are defined as having idiopathic premature ovarian failure. If ovarian follicles are present the term resistant ovary syndrome has been used to define the condition.[8] The presence or absence of follicles in patients presenting with premature ovarian failure is pivotal not only for establishing a diagnosis but also in delineating therapeutic options.

INVESTIGATION OF PREMATURE OVARIAN FAILURE

History and physical examination may help to establish the diagnosis. Documentation requires the presence of hypoestrogenemic hypergonadotropism especially on more than one occasion. A karyotype is mandatory in primary amenorrhea and can be of help in secondary amenorrhea as well. Searching for antibodies may be helpful and, if positive, opens up a number of therapeutic options. However, testing is not available generally and the procedures have not been standardized. Establishing the presence or absence of primordial follicles in the ovary is crucial. The gold standard has been a full thickness biopsy of the ovary to look for primordial follicles. The major disadvantage of such biopsies is the fact that the results are qualitative and presume appropriate representation in the specimen obtained. Moreover, the ensuing potential risk of adhesions and mechanical infertility is added to the already existing infertile state.

Thus, it would seem to be crucial to devise a non-invasive method for investigation. The endovaginal ultrasonographic technic permits detailed visualization of the ovaries and seemed to be a novel way to view ovaries in individuals with premature ovarian failure.[9] Whereas primordial follicles are far too small to be visualized, small cysts of about 2-3 mm diameter can be detected. Our contention has been that the visualization of such small cystic structures within the ovary indicates the presence of primordial follicles.

In a group of postmenopausal women in their 50's, we detected no follicles, whereas in women whose ovaries were rendered "quiescent" by oral contraceptives, numerous follicles were visualized. In the group with premature ovarian failure, two distinct subgroups were identified -one with and one without follicles. In those in whom follicles were visualized, the number of follicles per ovary was significantly smaller than in the oral contraceptive controls. While we did not correlate our findings on ultrasound with ovarian biopsies, or attempt to stimulate individuals with follicles to see if they could be induced to ovulate under supraphysiologic gonadotropin stimulation, we feel that focusing our attempts to induce ovulation in such individuals with primordial follicles may be more likely to succeed and prove of cost benefit. Indeed, such studies are currently underway although preliminary results are not encouraging.[10]

THERAPY OF PREMATURE OVARIAN FAILURE

The impetus to find methods to treat premature ovarian failure has been obtunded or lost in the 1990's by the availability of successful egg donation, *in vitro* fertilization and embryo transfer programs. However, in those individuals desiring biological offspring, the whole question of our ability to better differentiate the heterogenous group of POF patients is crucial if successful and presumably less costly treatment programs are to evolve. The group with no primordial follicles, if clearly defined, are really untreatable except by donor I.V.F. techniques. The group with immunologic abnormalities and discernible primordial follicles might benefit from such therapies as high dose glucocorticoids and/or plasmapheresis. Others might benefit from megadoses of exogenous gonadotropins or short-term down-regulation by estrogen. Estrogens might also act by ameliorating the autoimmune process. Such regimens have been variably reported to yield successful pregnancies.[11] A more recent approach has been the "down-regulation" by gonadotropin releasing hormone agonists followed by attempts at ovulation induction with exogenous gonadotropins.[12]

Overall, the success with therapeutic intervention has been remarkably small and most schools of thought feel that such attempts are exercises in futility.[13] The easy, safe and highly successful egg donation/IVF programs have therefore mainly replaced all such endeavors.

PREVENTION OF PREMATURE OVARIAN FAILURE

It is difficult to prevent that which cannot be influenced (idiopathic, genetic) or which is detectable only after it occurs. To the extent that some conditions clearly predispose to premature ovarian failure, attempts have been made to prevent the process. Theoretically, the institution of a galactose-free diet during pregnancy might prevent premature ovarian failure in fetuses at risk for galactosemia; such diets are not of primary value in protecting the ovaries when instituted early in neonatal life or infancy, even though some of the other clinical manifestations are favorably influenced.[14]

Shielding the ovaries may help during abdominal irradiation. On theoretic grounds, the deleterious effects on follicles of either irradiation or chemotherapy might be ameliorated by down-regulation using GnRH analogues. There are no long-term, large-scale definitive studies regarding efficacy; indeed, a few reports with small numbers of patients indicate that this technic may not be protective.[15]

CONCLUSION

Premature ovarian failure remains an enigma. The etiology in most cases is unexplained. Although it fortunately affects a small percentage of women, it is a devastating psychological, emotional and physical insult to women desirous of fertility. Accurate diagnosis is crucial and attempts to further develop and define non-invasive techniques are worthwhile.

The major challenges are: (1) to develop and define accurate and reproducible non-invasive diagnostic technics; (2) to identify and treat those patients, who have follicles capable of responding, with selected therapeutic modalities.

105

BIBLIOGRAPHY

1. Reyes FI, Winter JSD, Faiman C: Pituitary-ovarian relationships preceding the menopause. I. A cross-sectional study of serum follicle-stimulating hormone, luteinizing hormone, prolactin, estradiol and progesterone levels. Amer. J. Obstet. Gynecol. 129:557-564, 1977.

2. Richardson SJ, Senikas V, Nelson JP: Follicular depletion during the menopausal transition: Evidence for accelerated loss and ultimate exhaustion. J. Clin. Endocrinol. Metab. 65:1231-1237, 1987.

3. Jewelewicz R, Schwartz M: Premature ovarian failure. Bull. N.Y. Acad. Med. 62:219-236, 1986.

4. Coulam CB: Premature gonadal failure. Fertil. Steril. 38:645-655, 1982.

5. Weetman AP, McGregor AM: Autoimmune thyroid disease: Further developments in our understanding. Endocrine Rev. 15:788-829, 1994.

6. Cohen I, Speroff L: Premature ovarian failure: Update. Obstet. Gynecol. Survey. 46:156-162, 1991.

7. Walfish PG, Gottesman IS, Shewchuk AB, *et al.*: Association of premature ovarian failure with HLA antigens. Tissue Antigens 21:168, 1983.

8. Vaitukaitis JL: In, "Case records of the Massachusetts General Hospital." N. Engl. J. Med. 315:1336-1343, 1986.

9. Mehta AE, Matwijiw I, Lyons EA, Faiman C: Noninvasive diagnosis of resistant ovary syndrome by ultrasonography. Fertil. Steril. 57:56-61, 1992.

10. Taylor AE, Mulder J, Adams J, Fuh V, Martin K, Crowley WF, Jr: Estrogen therapy does not increase spontaneous ovarian activity in women with premature ovarian failure. Abstract #839. Endocrine Soc. 76th Annual Meeting. June 1994, Anaheim, CA.

11. Check JH, Nowroozi K, Chase JS, et al: Ovulation induction and pregnancies in 100 consecutive women with hypergonadotropic amenorrhea. Fertil. Steril. 53:811-816, 1990.

12. Surrey ES, Cedars MI: The effect of gonadotropin suppression on the induction of ovulation in premature ovarian failure patients. Fertil. Steril. 52:36-41, 1989.

13. Rebar RW, Cedars MI: Hypergonadotropic forms of amenorrhea in young women. Endocrinol. Metab. Clinics N.A. 21:173-191, 1992.

14. Holton JB, Leonard JV: Clouds still gathering over galactosemia. Lancet 344:1242-1243, 1994.

15. Kreuser ED, Klingmüller D, Thiel E: The role of LHRH-analogues in protecting gonadal functions during chemotherapy and irradiation. Eur. Urol. 23:157-164, 1993.

Effects of aging on the female reproductive system

A. Pellicer, C. Simón and J. Remohi

Instituto Valenciano de Infertilidad, and Department of Pediatrics, Obstetrics and Gynecology, Valencia University School of Medicine, Valencia, Spain

Introduction

The current trend toward delayed childbearing has increased our interest in the changes produced in the physiology of the human reproductive system with age. There is an evident decline in fecundity with age, clearly observed in populations in which contraception has not been employed (1). In such circumstances, fecundity decreases as well as infertility increases with age, suggesting that either the uterus, the ovary, or both are responsible for this impairment of fertility with age.

When the ovary is individually analysed, the oocyte as well as the granulosa cells forming the follicle must be separated. There is little doubt that the quality of the egg is affected by age. Studies performed in unfertilized human oocytes showed a significant increase in chromosome abnormalities in women > 35 (2). Similarly, recent studies employing fluorescence in situ hybridization in human preimplantation embryos have shown that aneuploidy is more frequent in women > 40 than in younger patients (3), suggesting that the quality of the oocyte and the resulting embryo in women >40 may be one of the mechanisms involved in the decline of fecundity with age.

The effect of age on granulosa cells is a matter of discussion. High serum FSH levels have been detected with age being most probably the consequence of variations in ovarian physiology that affect the secretory pattern of the gonadotrope. Specifically, observations made comparing natural (4,5) and stimulated cycles (6) in young and older women have shown decreased serum inhibin levels in the latter group, suggesting that this induces elevated FSH secretion. It is unknown, however, whether this decline in ovarian inhibin production is due to a reduction in the number of follicles in the failing ovary or to an impairment of the maximum ability of each granulosa cell to produce inhibin. Similarly, the impact of age on the steroidogenesis ability of human granulosa cells remain to be determined. Clinical studies have shown decreased midcycle and luteal phase estradiol (E_2) levels in aged women in natural (7) and stimulated cycles (8). However, other observations (5) have found similar peak E_2 levels in the preovulatory phase of the IVF-ET cycle when young and older women are compared.

Aging of the uterus is a more controversial subject. Ovum donation may prove a good in vivo model to search for an answer because many variables influence the end result which is pregnancy, while manipulation of the artificial cycle and selection of donors may help for correction of such differences in order to test appropriate hypotheses. While some authors have observed decreased pregnancy rates in women >40 years as compared to younger patients (9-11), others have not found such differences (12-16). Thus, although the model seems to be valid, some controversy still exists as to whether the uterus ages with the ovary.

Because of the physiological and clinical implications of these matters, we have been interested in the fundamental questions regarding aging of the female reproductive system. Two sets of clinical studies were designed to address the effects on the granulosa cells (17) and the uterus (Cano et al, in Press), respectively. This report summarizes both contributions.

The effect of aging on granulosa cell function

Thirty-three patients participating in our IVF-ET programme were divided into two groups according to age: patients in group 1 (n=15) were 32.0 ± 0.7 years old, while the mean age in group 2 (n=18) was 40.3 ± 0.3. Pituitary desensitization and multiple follicular development were employed in all cases.

All visible follicles in women included in the present study were harvested by US-guided vaginal aspiration. Oocytes were identified under the dissecting microscope and isolated for further insemination and culture. The remaining follicular contents were centrifuged at 1,500 rpm for 10 minutes and the supernatants decanted. Cells from all follicles in each woman were combined, washed twice in 2 mL Ham F-10 medium supplemented with 20 % FCS and centrifuged at 1,500 rpm for 10 minutes. Subsequently, cells were layered onto 5 mL 50% Percoll columns and centrifuged at 500 rpm for 30 minutes to pellet red cells. A purified granulosa- luteal cell preparation was aspirated from the interface, washed, resuspended, and counted in a hemocytometer. Viability in all cases was > 95%, as assessed by trypan blue staining. All cell cultures were performed in triplicates at a density of 20,000 cells/ well in tissue culture dishes. Cells were incubated in 1 ml M-199 supplemented with 10% FCS, 2 mM L- Glutamine in a 5% CO_2 in air atmosphere at 37° C. Cultures were maintained up to 4 days, and medium changed every 2 days. Culture medium progesterone was measured using commercially avalilable RIA kits. Accumulation of immunoreactive α-inhibin production by the cells cultured in vitro was measured using an immunoenzymetric assay.

Immunoreactive α-inhibin accumulation in culture medium after 48 and 96 hours incubation in basal conditions was significantly higher in younger than in older patients ($P < 0.01$). No stimulation of immunoreactive α-inhibin secretion was detected after 96 hours. The results of progesterone accumulation in culture medium after 48 and 96 hours in both groups of cells showed a significantly ($P < 0.05$) higher ability to produce progesterone in younger patients as compared to older women after 48 as well as 96 hours.

This study showed for the first time that the decline in immunoreactive α-inhibin production by human granulosa- luteal cells seems to be the consequence of a reduction in the maximum ability of the granulosa cell to produce the peptide. This mechanism does not necessarily exclude the possibility that a reduction in the number of follicles in the failing ovary may contribue to the lower serum levels of inhibin detected.

The effect of aging on the uterus

In this study, recipients of different ages received oocytes from the same source and quality so as to test the receptivity of their uteri, since we know that implantation in ovum donation is influenced by the source of the oocytes (18). The quality of the oocytes can be corrected when oocytes from the same cohort of follicles are randomly distributed between women <40 and >40 years undergoing ovum donation. This approach has been recently employed by Navot et al (15), who found similar pregnancy rates between younger and older patients, concluding that uterine aging is not an important factor in determining the success of oocyte donation. From this study it can be inferred that waning oocyte quality rather than reduced uterine receptivity is responsible for the age-related decline in female fertility potential in natural life and assisted reproduction.

Further evidence, however, reveals that the uterus may be affected by age. Meldrum (13) showed that a decrease in ongoing/delivered pregnancy rates in older patients may be corrected by increasing the dose of exogenous progesterone administered to the recipient. From this study it can be concluded that the uterus may be affected by age, although progesterone may correct the defect. In keeping with this concept, it is of enormous interest to assure an adequate action of progesterone on the endometrium in women entering an ovum donation programme.

Thus, we addressed the issue of uterine aging in a study in which progesterone administration was adjusted in order to obtain an appropriate transformation of the endometrium, and oocyte quality was corrected. Fourty-five cycles of oocyte donation were performed in 9 fertile women subjected to tubal sterilization, who voluntarily decided to donate oocytes, and 36 women undergoing IVF who had a high response to gonadotropins and voluntarily donated part of their oocytes for our anonymous oocyte donation programme. They were stimulated for oocyte retrieval, and always

Table 1: Influence of age in the results of oocyte donation. Oocyte quality corrected by study design.

	<40 years	>40 years
Cycles	45	45
Age	33.5+0.4a	43.7+0.5
Oocytes donated	7.8+0.3	7.6+0.3
Oocytes fertilized	5.4+0.2	5.3+0.2
Embryos transferred	4.2+0.1	4.4+0.1
Pregnancies(%)	21/45(46.6)	25/45(55.5)
Implantation(%)	33/193(17.1)	34/200(17.0)
Abortion(%)	1/21(4.7)b	12/25(48.0)

a $P<0.01$
b $P<0.05$

donated oocytes to two different recipients: one <40 years and another >40 years of age. The ovarian stimulation protocol and general IVF procedure have been described above.

Recipients were 76 women undergoing 90 cycles of oocyte donation because of low response to follicular stimulation in previous IVF cycles and menopause. They were matched by age. The protocol of ovum donation for recipients has been previously described (18). Pregnant patients were followed every two weeks by ultrasound scans and serum determinations of E2, progesterone and ß-hCG, until exogenous medication was withdrawn. Blood samples were measured using commercially available kits. Estradiol and ß-hCG were analysed by an immonoenzymatic assay. Progesterone was measured by RIA.

The comparison of the transfer cycles in the recipients aged <40 and >40 years, when oocytes came from the same cohort of follicles showed no difference between groups in the period of time women waited on unopposed estradiol valerate replacement prior to embryo transfer (Table 1). Similarly, the number of oocytes donated, the total number of embryos replaced as well as the proportion of good quality embryos transferred, were not different between groups. As a result, pregnancy and implantation rates were similar between groups. However, miscarriage was significantly ($P<0.05$) increased in the group of recipients >40 as compared to younger patients. Miscarriage occurred on week 10 in one patient included in the group<40, while 12 abortions were present in the group >40; five were observed at week 7, 5 at week 8, and 2 at week 17.

There was a significant ($P<0.05$) increase in serum E2 levels on pregnancy week 8 as compared to week 6 in the group of women <40. A significant ($P<0.05$) rise in serum E2 in the group of single pregnancies >40 was detected on week 10 as compared to week 8 in the group of women <40.

Navot et al (15) found no difference between groups of recipients when the source of the donated oocytes was controlled by study design, but, our results did show a significant increase in abortion rates in the older group, suggesting the existence of a reproductive failure at the uterine level. We followed our patients during the first trimester of pregnancy, and analysed those data to find an explanation for an increased miscarriage rate in women > 40. Initially, known causes of miscarriage such as immunological problems and uterine malformations were ruled out by the data available.

Serum levels of E2 were analysed in single ongoing pregnancies in order to find the moment of the luteoplacental shift in these cases, a concept raised by Csapo et al (19) who showed that it takes place around pregnancy weeks 7 to 8. The term luteoplacental shift is inappropriate in these medically/surgically/naturally agonadal patients, but it is of interest because it shows the ability of the placenta to secrete steroids, which in turn is a direct evidence that the fetoplacental unit has been turned on. For estrogen formation by the placenta to occur, precursors must reach it from both the fetal and the maternal compartments whereas placental progesterone formation is accomplished in large part from circulating maternal cholesterol. Thus, the activation of the fetoplacental unit and secretion of steroids is fully dependent of a normal development of the maternal site of the placenta, with a complete vascular network which provides the substrate for steroid synthesis. Unfortunately, we did not learn much from the analysis of progesterone secretion.

A intra-group comparison of serum E2 levels in single pregnancies showed that the luteoplacental shift is produced between weeks 6 to 8 in women <40, whereas patients >40 had the shift later (weeks 8 to 10). These data are in agreement with Devroey et al (20) who observed a shift in E2 production by pregnancy week 7. These findings suggest that the mechanism(s) responsible for the normal functioning of the fetoplacental unit is retarded in older patients. Since, a normal delivery of substrate seems to be of crucial importance, it is tempting to speculate that an abnormal vascularization of the pregnant uterus in older women may be responsible for this delay. Likewise, we found an increased incidence of abortions in the group of older women, 10 out of 12 of whom occurred at weeks 7 to 8 of pregnancy, just when the placenta started to be autonomous. Thus, it seems reasonable to suggest that an increase in miscarriage rates in older women might be related to the ability for vascularization in older pregnant uteri.

In conclussion, we have conducted a series of studies in order to test the changes induced by age in the female reproductive system. The first series of experiments, based in in vitro studies described herein, but also in vivo measurements of steroids and inhibin (17), showed that the quality of the follicles in older patients is seriously impaired, in parallel to the changes observed in the quality of the oocytes (2) and embryos (3). In addition, we have also tested the effect of senescence of the ability of the uterus to sustain a pregnancy to term, observing that abortion is significantly increased in older patients, and suggesting a deficient uterine vasculature as the primary cause of this clinical observation. Thus, we believe that age affects the entire reproductive system and these observations should be taken into account in order to advice properly our patients.

References

1- Menken J, Trussell J, Larsen U (1986). Age and Infertility. Science **233**:1389-1394.

2- Plachot M, Veiga A, Montagut J, de Grouchy J, Calderón G, Lepretre S, Junca AM, Santaló J, Carles E, Mandelbaum J, Barri P, Degoy J, Cohen J, Egozcue J, Sabatier JC, Salat-Baroux J (1988). Are clinical and biological IVF parameters correlated with chromosomal disorders in early life: a multicentric study. Hum Reprod **3**: 627-635.

3- Grifo J, Rosenwaks Z, Cohen J, Munné S (1994). Implantation failure of morphologically normal embryos is due largely to aneuploidy. Abstract book of the 50th Annual Meeting American Fertility Society, San Antonio, November 5-10, p.S2

4- Buckler HM, Evans CA, Mamtora H, Burger HG, Anderson DC (1991). Gonadotropin, steroid, and inhibin levels in women with incipient ovarian failure during anovulatory and ovulatory rebound cycles. J Clin Endocrinol Metab **72**: 116-124.

5- Lenton EA, de Kretser DM, Woodward AJ, Robertson DM (1991). Inhibin concentrations throughout the menstrual cycles of normal, infertile, and older women compared with those during spontaneous conception cycles. J Clin Endocrinol Metab **73**: 1180- 1190.

6- Hughes EG, Robertson DM, Handelsman DJ, Hayward S, Healy DL, de Kretser DM (1990). Inhibin and estradiol responses to ovarian hyperstimulation: Effects of age and predictive value for in vitro fertilization outcome. J Clin Endocrinol Metab **70**: 358-364.

7- Sherman BM, Korenman SG (1975). Hormonal characteristics of the human menstrual cycle throughout reproductive life. J Clin Invest **55**: 699- 706.

8- Jacobs SL, Metzger DA, Dodson WC, Haney AF (1990). Effect of age on response to human menopausal gonadotropin stimulation. J Clin Endocrinol Metab **71**: 1525-1530.

9- Flamigni C, Borini A, Iolini F, Bianchi L, Serrao L (1993). Oocyte donation: comparison between recipients from different age groups. Hum Reprod **8**:2088-2092.

10- Abdalla HI, Baber R, Kirkland A, Leonard T, Power M, Studd JWW (1990). A report on 100 cycles of oocyte donation; factors affecting the outcome. Hum Reprod **5**:1018-1022.

11- Yaron Y, Botchan A, Amit A, Kogosowski A, Yovel I, Lessing JB (1993). Endometrial receptivity: the age-related decline in pregnancy rates and the effect of ovarian function. Fertil Steril **60**:314-318.

12- Rotsztejn DA, Asch RH (1991). Effect of aging on assisted reproductive technologies (ART): experience from egg donation. Sem Reprod Endocrinol 9:272-279.

13- Meldrum DR (1993). Female reproductive aging-ovarian and uterine factors. Fertil Steril 59:1-5.

14- Check JH, Askari HA, Fisher Ch, Vanaman L (1994). The use of a shared donor oocyte program to evaluate the effect of uterine senescence. Fertil Steril 61:252-256.

15- Navot D, Drews MR, Bergh PA, Guzman I, Karstaedt A, Scott RT, Garrisi GJ, Hofmann GE (1994). Age-related decline in female fertility is not due to diminished capacity of the uterus to sustain embryo implantation. Fertil Steril 61:97-101.

16- Balmaceda JP, Bernardini L, Ciuffardi I, Felix C, Ord T, Sueldo CE, Asch RH (1994). Oocyte donation in humans: a model to study the effect of age on embryo implantation rate. Hum Reprod 9:2160-2163.

17- Pellicer A, Marí M, De los Santos MJ, Simón C, Remohí J, Tarín JJ (1994). Effects of aging on the human ovary: the secretion of immunoreactive α-inhibin and progesterone. Fertil Steril 61:663-668.

18- Remohí J, Vidal A, Pellicer A (1993). Oocyte donation in low responders to a conventional stimulation for in vitro fertilization. Fertil Steril 59:1208-1215.

19- Csapo AI, Pulkinnen KO, Wiest WG (1973). Effects of luteectomy and progesterone replacement therapy in early pregnant patients. Am J Obstet Gynecol 115:759-765.

20- Devroey P, Camus M, Palermo G, Smitz J, Van Waesbergue L, Wisanto A, Wijbo I, Van Steirteghem AC (1990). Placental production of estradiol and progesterone after oocyte donation in patients with primary ovarian failure. Am J Obstet Gynecol 162:66-70.

Progress in diagnosis and treatment of hyperandrogenism of ovarian origin

A. Milewicz

Department of Endocrinology, Medical Academy ul. Pasteura 4, Wroclaw, Poland

INTRODUCTION

A detailed history concerning the chronological development of symptoms and signs is critical in establishing the direction of evaluation for the diagnosis.Hyperandrogenemia should be considered in an adolescent with hirsutism, menstrual irregularity or obesity.
Hirsutism may or may not be progressive,but other signs of virilization usually reflect the presence of an androgen-producing tumor or ovarian hyperthecosis. The time course of development of the androgenic signs is of great importance: a recent rapid onset of androgenization requires urgent and special diagnostic methods for distinguishing the PCOS from other more serious causes of androgen excess.

DIAGNOSIS

As laboratory screening for hyperandrogenemia I recommend measurements of blood levels of free testosterone,androstenedione (A-dione) and DHEA-S, LH, FSH, PRL and TSH. Plasma testosterone level in the male range (over 350 ng/dl) indicated a virilizing tumors, however cases of adrenal tumor with normal plasma DHEA-S were also presented (1).
Rosenfield proposed maximal diagnostic information from limited sampling on the basis of low-dose dexametasone suppression test (2). Dex, was given in a low dose of 1,0 mg/m2 daily in divided doses orally for 5 days. the

113

pattern of response of plasma free testosterone, DHEA-S
and cortisol segreates patients diagnostically. Normal
suppresion of androgens is for testosterone less than 8
pg/ml, for DHEAS 70um/dl and for cortisol 3ug/dl. After 4
days dex.,subnormal suppresion of plasma free
testosterone points toward PCOS (if both DHEAS and
cortisol suppress normally), tumor (if only cortisol
suppresses normally), or Cushing's syndrome (if cortisol
does not supress normally). PCOS is present in the vast
majority of patients with subnormal suppression. An
elevated serum LH level may be a useful corroborative
test; however elevation of LH is not specific for PCOS.
Pelvic ultrasound examination may also be supportive of
the diagnosis, but the sensitivity and specificity are
relatively low. Serum 17-OHP level 24 hour after the
injection above 224 ng/dl in response to a 100 ug
s.c.test dose of the GnRH agonist Nafarelin seems
promising as specific test for PCOS. Normal suppression
of hyperandrogenemia is an indication for ACTH testing. A
rise in 17-OHP to over 1200 ng/dl 60 min after i.v. inj.
of 250 ug Cosyntropin is then diagnostic for virilizing
congenital adrenal hyperplasia (2,3).
In suspcted cases for virilizing tumor,immediate work-up
and treatment are mandatory. Magnetic resonance imaging
(MRI), computed tomography (CT) and ultrasonography may
be helpful in localizing tumor.
Retrograde venous catheterisation to determine the site
adrenal versus ovary) and the side (left or right) of
hormonal excess has been utilized extensively prior to
surgical removal.
Recently, scan with (6-beta-131 I)
iodomethylnorcholesterol (NP 59) has been successful in
establishing the precise location of the tumor
preoperatively (4). Stimulation and suppression tests in
different combinations may be misleading because a wide
range of responses for both ovarian and adrenal tumors
have been observed (1,5).

MEDICAL TREATMENT

Hyperandrogenism in women is still an important
therapeutic problem.Except for ovarian tumor (surgical
removal of the tumor is suggested), other cases of
hyperandrogenism can have endocrine therapy.Weight
reduction is indicated for obese hyperandrogenic
patients. This is sometimes successful in reversing
hyperandrogenemia and menstrual disorders (1,2,5).

Therapeutic intervention in the treatment of the clinical signs of hyperandrogenism (acne and/or hirsutism) may be directed at the source of androgens at the level of their target tissue. The treatment of functional ovarian hyperandrogenism (that is, PCOS and hyperthecosis) depens on the symptoms. Cyclic progestin administration is the method of choice for initiating treatment of menstrual irregularities. Medroxyprogesterone acetate, 10 mg at bedtime daily for 5 days, is prescribed, commencing at intervals of 3 weeks to 2 months (1,2).

The only indication for the use of estrogen/progestin contraceptive pills or recently transdermally (ST 1435) in the management of isolated menstrual irregularity is recommended in those patients with dysfunctional uterine bleeding that cannot be controlled with progestin alone (6).

The maximal effect of pharmacologic agents takes 9 to 12 months because of the long growth cycles of hair follicles. Cosmetic measurements are necessary concomitantly. Combination estrogen/progestin therapy will lower free T levels by reducing serum gonadotropin levels, increasing SHBG levels, and modestly decreasing DHEAS levels. This can be expected to arrest hirsutism but not to lead to substantial improvement (1,2,5,6).Severe hyperandrogenism and hirsutism can be improved by treatment with antiandrogens. This class of hormone antagonist inhibits the binding of androgens to the androgen receptor (1,2). Agents in this category include cyproterone acetate without or with ethylinestradiol (Diane), spironolactone, and most recently, flutamide.

Cyproterone acetate in a 50 mg dose for the first 10 day of 21 days course of estrogen is quite effective and has limited adverse effects (1,2,5).Spironolactone is clinically antiandrogenic and progestational in doses of 50 to 100 mg/24 h. Simultaneous administration of cyclic estrogen/progestin is indicated. This prevents pseudohermafroditismus in the fetus if the mother should become pregnant. It also ensures regular menstrual cycles (1,2,7). Flutamide is a potent nonsteroidal selective antiandrogen that is currently under investigation. Many reports suggest 250 mg daily as a sufficient dose, in combination with an estrogen-progestin without complications (1,2,5).

Recent studies show that GnRh agonists are potent suppressors of ovarian androgen biosynthesis even in the face of severe hyperandrogenism (e.g.hyperinsulinemia, hyperthecosis). GnRh-agonists in the inhibition of

ovarian androgen steroidogenesis, mostly were
administered in single dose i.m. leuprolide depot 3.75 mg
every 28 days. Literature shows that GnRh-A-nist
utilization in hirsutism therapy can reduce A-dione of
50-70%,T of 43-70%, free T of 62-67% and Ferriman-Gallwey
score objectively decrease of 43-65%.

Usually GnRh-A treatment does not last more than 6 month
because of osterporosis risk, consequence of
hypoestrogenism. This time limit, though is temptative,
as hyperandrogenic patients have a thicker trabecular
bone mass (1,2,8). Many authors use GnRh-A in association
with estrogen/progestin combination in order to avoid
osteoporosis risk, to increase therapeutical efficacy and
to enable cyclic deprivation bleeding (1,8).

Ketoconazole has been proposed as a new therapeutic drug
in the non-tumor hyperandrogenism treatment, providing
its selective inhibitory effect on ovarian and adrenal
steroidogenesis (9,10). Serum T and hair growth rate
declined in patients while on 600 to 1000 mg nizoral
daily.

Diani at al. published very successful results of studies
with Finasteride, a steroid 5-alfa-reductase inhibitor
(11). This diminishes the activity of 5-alfa
reductase enzyme and reduces DHT production.

In conclusion, the treatment of functional ovarian
hyperandrogenism , depends on the clinical symptoms and
contrindication.

REFERENCES

1. Yen, S.C.C. (1991).Chronic anovulation caused by
peripheral endocrine disorders. IN Yen, S.C.C. and Jaffe,
R.B.(eds.) *Reproductive endocrinology.*pp. 631-689
(Saunders, W.B. Company , Philadelphia, London, Toronto,
Montreal, Sydney, Tokyo)

2. Rosenfield, R.L. (1990). Hyperandrogenism in
peripubertal girls. *Ped.Clin.Nort.Am.* 37.6:1333-1358

3. Milewicz, A. (1988). 21-deoxycortisol in endocrine
disorders . In.Genazzani, A.R., Petraglia, F., Volpe, A.,
Faccinetti (eds) *Recent Research on Gynecological
Endocriology.* pp.571-576 (The Parthenon Publishing
Goup,Lancs. New Jersey)

4. Mountz,J.M., Gross, M.D., Shapiro, B., Barkan, A.L.
and Woodbury, M.C. (1988). Scintigraphic localisation of
ovarian dysfunction. *J.Nucl.Med.* 29.10,1644-1650

5.Leidenberger, F.A.(1992). Klinische Endokrinologie fur
Frauenarzte. pp.262-263. (Springer-Verlag)

6. Laurikka-Routti, M., Haukkamaa, M.,Lahteenmaki, P. (1992). Suppression of ovarian function with the transdermally given synthetic progestin ST 1435. *Fertil.a.Steril.* 58,4,680-684

7. Milewicz, A., Silber, D.and Kirschner, M.(1983). Therapeutic effects of spironolactone in polycystic ovary syndrome. *Obstet.a.Gynecology.* 61,4,429-432

8. Adashi, E.Y. (1990).Potential utility of gonadotropin-releasing hormone agonits in the management of ovarian hyperandrogenism. *Fertil.a.Steril.* 53,5:765-779

9. Pepper, G., Brenner, S.H. and Gbrilove, J.L. (1990).Ketocenazole use in the treatment of ovarian hyperandrogenism. *Fertil.a.Steril.* 54,3,438-444

10. Manusharova, R.A. (1992). The effect of nizoral on the function of the hypothalamo-hypophyseal-ovarian system in virilism. Vrach-Delo. 8,89-91

11. Diani, A.R., Mulholland, M.J., Shull, K.L., Kubicek, M.F., Johnson, G.A., Schostarez, H.J., Breunden, M.N. and Buhl, A.E. (1992). Hair growth effects of oral administration of finasteride, a steroid 5-alfa-reductase inhibitor, alone and in combination with topical minoxidil in the balding stumptail macaque. *J.Clin.Endocrinol.Metab.* 74,2,345-349.

Clinical and endocrine effects of ovarian laser surgery in patients with polycystic ovary disease

W.G. Rossmanith, U. Ulrich and J. Keckstein

Department of Obstetrics and Gynecology, University of Ulm, Ulm, Germany

OBJECTIVE

Only a few years after the first description of the syndrome of polycystic ovaries (PCO), bilateral ovarian wedge resection was propagated as a surgical method for the treatment of the infertility of PCO patients (1). Until recently, this surgical approach was still in general use, as this type of ovarian surgery induces profound local and systemic endocrinological changes (2). It allows the majority of PCO patients treated in this way to spontaneously ovulate. Alternatively, if spontaneous ovulations do not occur, ovarian surgery can markedly reduce the risks associated with ovarian stimulation regimens (3,4). However, the high efficacy of this surgical procedure is hampered by the general risks of a laparotomy and in particular, by peri-ovarian or peri-tubal adhesions frequently encountered after ovarian wedge resection (5). Therefore, alternative approaches have been utilized, involving minimal invasive surgery via laparoscopy. It was hoped that the operative and post-operative risks of bilateral ovarian surgery in PCO patients could be minimized and thus, with no loss of effectiveness surgery of polycystic ovaries could still be considered an alternative treatment modality in PCO patients wishing to conceive. Various means such as laparoscopic ovarian electrocautery (6), bilateral ovarian laser incisions (7) oder wedge-like laser vaporization of the ovarian surfaces together with excision of atretic cysts (8,9) have all been successfully employed.

In the present study, a cohort of PCO patients with infertility were treated by laparoscopic bilateral ovarian laser coagulation. The outcome was assessed by establishing clinical and endocrinological parameters before and after laser surgery. The results have been compared with those reported for conventional ovarian wedge resections (10).

METHODOLOGY

52 patients with the clinical and endocrinological characteristics of PCO syndrome (11) were enrolled in this investigation. In particular, all patients were anovulatory and presented with menstrual cycle disturbances (oligo- or amenorrhea); most women had facial or abdominal hirsutism and were obese (81 %). Polycystic ovaries were found on ultrasound examination in all women, characterized by an abnormally large volume, multiple small cysts, thickened ovarian capsules and enlarged ovarian stroma (12). Endocrinologically, hyperandrogenemia was confirmed by increases in both total and free testosterone (T) and androstenedione (AD); additionally, an elevated LH/FSH ratio attributed to a selective LH release together with an exaggerated gonadotropin secretion GnRH stimulation was observed in all women (13). All PCO patients desired pregnancy, but had not ovulated in response to administration of clomiphene citrate (up to 100 mg daily) or of HMG (up to 150 IE daily).

Laparoscopic bilateral ovarian surgery was performed in all PCO patients, using the Nd:YAK laser (n=11) with 40-70 watts or the CO_2 laser (n=41) with 15-25 watts in non-contact modes (8,9). During this procedure, the ovarian surfaces were coagulated and thinned in a wedge-like fashion and atretic cysts were drained in both ovaries. Furthermore, the adjacent androgen producing stroma was partly destroyed (Figure 1). Multiple laser vaporizations were applied to the ovarian surfaces so that the ovaries appeared like "golfballs" at the end of the procedure. For prevention of adhesions, a meticulous hemostasis was carried out and Ringer´s lactate was left as artificial ascites.

Clinical parameters (menstrual cycles, ovulations, hirsutism) were assessed before laparoscopic laser surgery and compared with those found after surgery. In addition, endocrinological profiles were established conventional raidoimmunoassays (13) before surgery, when the patients were oligo- or amenorrheic, and again after resumption of menses 4 to 6 weeks after surgery .

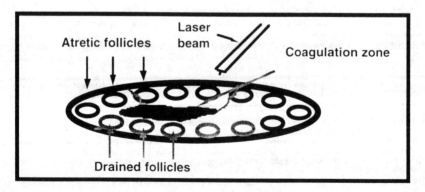

Figure 1 Schematic presentation of laparoscopic laser coagulation of polycystic ovaries.

RESULTS

The laser procedure was not complicated by any untoward side-effects. All PCO patients recovered uneventfully and were discharged on the second post-operative day. While all women were anovulatory before surgery, 89 % of these women had regular menstrual cycles within 3 months after ovarian laser treatment. 62 % had spontaneous ovulations, while a further 21% ovulated successfully with clomiphene citrate or HMG (Table 1). Within a year after surgery, 38 % of the treated patients conceived with singleton pregnancies, of 23 % of these pregnancies were delivered at term. Hirsute changes were not affected by ovarian laser surgery (Table 1).

Table 1   Clinical (given in percent) and endocrinological parameters before and after laparoscopic ovarian surgery in 52 patients with PCO syndrome. Gonadotropin secretory profiles were established in 11 patients before and after surgery (mean ± SE). * $p<0.05$, $p<0.01$ vs values before surgery.

	Before surgery	After surgery
Cliniscal characteristics		
Menstrual cycle disturbances	52 (100 %)	6 (11 %) *
Spontaneous ovulations	0 (0 %)	32 (62 %) *
Induced ovulations	0 (0 %)	11 (21 %) *
Pregnancies within a year	0 (0 %)	20 (38 %) *
Hirsutism (moderate to severe)	38 (73 %)	36 (69 %)
Periovarian adhesions (14 patients)	0 (0 %)	2 (14 %)
Endocrinological findings		
LH mean secretion (IU/L)	14.7 ± 1.1	8.2 ± 1.2 *
LH pulse frequencies (pulses / 8 h)	4.5 ± 0.5	4.4 ± 0.4
LH pulse amplitudes (IU/L)	3.6 ± 0.4	2.9 ± 0.3 **
FSH mean secretion (IU/L)	5.9 ± 0.5	7.8 ± 0.6 *
LH / FSH	2.5 ± 0.2	1.1 ± 0.2 **
GnRH stimulated LH secretion (IU/Lxmin)	$12.6 \pm 3.1 \times 10^3$	$5.8 \pm 2.1 \times 10^3$*
GnRH stimulated FSH secretion (IU/Lxmin)	$4.1 \pm 0.5 \times 10^3$	$3.8 \pm 0.5 \times 10^3$
Testosterone T (mmol/L)	2.9 ± 0.3	1.6 ± 0.2 *
Androstenedione AD (nmol/L)	9.6 ± 0.6	6.5 ± 0.5 *
Dehydroepiandrosterone DHEAS (µmol/L)	6.2 ± 0.9	5.5 ± 1.0
Estrone E_1 (pmol/L)	267 ± 33	122 ± 20 *
Estradiol E_2 (pmol/L)	282 ± 60	138 ± 38 *

Endocrinological evaluation revealed increased serum levels of androgens (T,AD, DHEAS) before surgery (Table 1). Serum values were decreased (p<0.05) by laser surgery to the range of normally cycling women. As for serum concentrations of estrone (E_1) and estradiol (E_2), they were significantly (p<0.05) reduced post-operatively. While high LH pulse amplitudes and frequencies prevailed before surgery, they were found to be markedly attenuated (p<0.05) after surgery. In contrast, FSH secretion increased (p<0.01) after surgery; therefore, the LH/FSH ratio initially found to be elevated declined (p<0.01). GnRH-stimulated gonadotropin release was attenuated (p<0.01) post-operatively (Table 1).

The clinical and endocrinological changes induced by ovarian laser surgery persisted for a maximum of two years; thereafter, all patients had relapsed into anovulation. It is important to note that weeks before resumption of chronic anovulation, serum levels of androgens began to rise in a similar range to that seen pre-operatively. In 14 patients, re-laparoscopy was scheduled for the control of the status and for re-treatment. In 2 patients, minimal periovarian adhesions were noted, the other 12 patients did not present any at all. The ovaries found at re-laparoscopies were characterized by a scarring of the ovarian surfaces, characteristically observed after ovulations; however, the ovarian sizes did not differ noticeably from the pre-operative volumes (Table 1).

DISCUSSION AND CONCLUSIONS

The results of our study suggest that laparoscopic bilateral ovarian laser surgery produces profound clinical and endocrine changes in patients with PCO syndrome. Following surgery, the majority of patients resume regular ovulations, clearly increasing the chance of conception. Ovarian laser surgery proves to be clinically at least as effective as bilateral ovarian wedge by laparotomy (10), but additionally shows a major advantage over the conventional approach in the drastic reduction of peri-ovarian and peri-tubal adhesions. By contrast, a rate of adhesion formation of up to 100 % has been reported for the classical wedge resection by laparotomy (5). The atraumatic laser application in a non-contact mode, as well as a skilful hemostasis, provide the basic premise for the prophylaxis of adhesions (8,9). In addition, reduced peri- and post-operative risks and a shorter time of hospitalization argue in favour of the minimal invasive approach.

In our investigation, serum levels of androgens and estrogens were decreased in response to ovarian laser surgery; they were then found comparable with values of women with normal menstrual cycles (13). Reduced ovarian androgen synthesis may be responsible for this, resulting from the surgical destruction of androgen-producing stroma. Furthermore, changes in the follicular micro-environment after drainage and spilling of atretic cysts with high androgen contents may play a role (13). Increased ovarian blood flow in sequence of healing processes after ovarian coagulations may also be an important part in this process. Following ovarian surgery, changes in the central nervous control of gonadal function were observed, leading to profound changes in gonadotropin secretion in our investigation. The LH secretion initially found inappropriately high in relation to FSH release (14) was attenuated, thus preventing an excessive ovarian androgenesis. These effects are likely to originate from changes in the negative feedback control by serum androgens on the central regulatory units of the hypothalamus and pituitary (3). The reduction in circulating serum androgens presumably disrupts the pathophysiological vicious cycle, which continuously perpetuates itself by an inadequate gonadotropin secretion followed by hyperandrogenemia, which in turn sensitizes the anterior pituitary (3,4).

The results of the current study demonstrate that the clinical and endocrinological effects of laparoscopic ovarian surgery are transient. Similar to classical ovarian wedge resection (3,10) and to other laparoscopic means of ovarian surgery (6-9), the effects of laser surgery do not persist for a longer period than two years. Laparoscopic laser surgery represents temporary relief for patients with the PCO syndrome, permitting them to ovulate and conceive within a limited time-frame. As is the case for the mechanisms subserving the effects of ovarian laser surgery, the reasons for this delayed relapse into chronic anovulation still remain to be explored. Presumably the identical pathogenetical changes present before surgery are still operative in the ovary, ultimately leading to anovulation and menstrual cycle disturbances as a consequence of hyperandrogenemia. Increased stroma proliferation, capsular thickening or follicular atresia by virtue of ovarian incompetence to convert an androgenic into an estrogen-dominated micro-milieu should also be considered (3,4). Alternatively, the recurrence of aberrations in the gonadotropin secretion may also be relevant, since laser surgery fails to influence the abnormal neurotransmitter control of gonadotropin release (15). This possibly results in a resumption of inappropriately high LH secretion with subsequent stimulation of ovarian androgen synthesis. At any rate, relapse into a state of chronic hyperandrogenemic anovulation supports the notion that laparoscopic bilateral ovarian coagulation in PCO patients represents merely a transient symptomatic rather than causal relief.

Collectively, we conclude from the current observations that ovarian laser surgery by laparoscopy is an effective mean for the treatment of infertility in PCO patients. It renders such women able to ovulate spontaneously or in response to stimulation regimens. Unfortunately, the effects of this surgical approach are transient and time-limited. Further, other accompanying symptoms of a chronic hyperandrogenemia, such as hirsutism, are not noticeably affected. Therefore, ovarian laser surgery by laparoscopy should only be recommended for patients with the PCO syndrome who actually wish to conceive in the immediate future.

REFERENCES

1. Stein, I.F. and Cohen, M.R. (1939). Surgical treatment of bilateral polycystic ovaries - amenorrhea and sterility. *Am. J. Obstet. Gynecol.* **29**, 465-78

2. Katz, M., Car, P.J., Cohen, B.M. and Millar, R.P. (1978). Hormonal effects of wedge resection of polycystic ovaries. *Obstet. Gynecol.* **51**, 437-44

3. Yen, S.S.C. (1980). The polycystic ovary syndrome. *Clin. Endocrinol.* **12**, 177-208

4. Franks, S. (1989). Polycystic ovary syndrome: a changing perspective. *Clin. Endocrinol.* **31**, 87-120

5. Buttram, V.J. and Vaquero, C. (1975). Post-ovarian wedge resection adhesive disease. *Fertil. Steril.* **26**, 874-6

6. Gjonnaess, H. and Norman, N. (1987). Endocrine effects of the ovarian electro-cautery in patients with polycystic ovarian disease. *Brit J. Obstet. Gynecol.* **94**, 779-83

7. Huber, J., Hosmann, J. and Spona, J. (1989). Laser incision by endoscopy of the polycystic ovary. *Geburtsh. Frauenheilk.* **49**, 37-40

8. Keckstein, J., Börchers, K., Wolf, A., Rossmanith, W. and Steiner, R. (1989). Is laparoscopic laser surgery an alternative treatment for polycystic ovarian disease? In: Donnez, J. (ed.). *Laser operative laparoscopy and hysteroscopy*, pp. 95-110. (Leuven, Nauwelaerts Printing).

9. Keckstein, G., Rossmanith, W., Spatzier, K., Schneider, V., Börchers, K. and Steiner, R. (1990). The effect of laparoscopic treatment of polycystic ovarian disease by CO_2 laser or Nd:YAG laser. *Surg. Endosc.* **4**, 103-7

10. Szilagyi, A., Rossmanith, W.G., Csermely, T. and Csaba, I. (1990). Changes in circulating hormonal levels after ovarian wedge resection in patients with polycystic ovary syndrome. *Arch Gynecol. Obstet.* **248**, 31-5

11. Goldzieher, J.W. and Green, J.A. (1962). The polycystic ovary. I. Clinical and histological features. *J. Clin. Endocrinol. Metab.* **22**, 325-38

12. Adams, J., Polson, D.W. and Franks, S. (1986). Prevalence of polycystic ovaries in women with anovulation and idiopathic hirsutism. *Brit Med. J.* **293**, 355-9

13. Rossmanith, W.G., Keckstein, J., Spatzier, K. and Lauritzen, C. (1991). The impact of ovarian laser surgery on the gonadotrophin secretion in women with polycystic ovarian disease. *Clin. Endocrinol.* **34**, 223-30

14. Rebar, R., Judd, H.L., Yen, S.S.C., Rakoff, J., Vandenberg, G. and Naftolin, F. (1976). Characterization of the inappropriate gonadotropin secretion in polycystic ovary syndrome. *J. Clin. Invest.* **57**, 1320-9

15. Szilagyi, A., Hole, R., Keckstein, J. and Rossmanith, W.G. (1993). Effects of ovarian surgery on the dopaminergic and opioidergic control of gonadotropin and prolactin secretion in women with polycystic ovarian disease. *Gynecol. Endocrinol.* **7**, 159-66

Corticotropin releasing factor effect on the pituitary–ovary axis in the human luteal phase

R. Apa, P. Villa, A.M. Fulghesu, A. Lanzone*, M. Guido, V. Pavone, F. Murgia, A. Caruso and S. Mancuso

Department of Obstetrics and Gynecology, Catholic University School of Medicine, Rome and *OASI Institute for Research, Troina, Italy

Introduction

In animals hypotalamic corticotropin-releasing factor (CRF) is known to negatively affect the reproductive function by suppressing the GnRH release into the hypophisial-portal circulation (1). It is unclear wheter CRF plays a similar role in attenuating LH pulsatility in humans. Gonadotropin levels were unaltered after intravenous (IV) bolus administration of ovine CRF in normal men (3) and after IV administration of human CRF (hCRF) in agonadal women (4). In cycling women a 3-hour infusion of hCRF was reported to induce a naloxone-reversible inhibition of LH and FSH release during the midluteal phase of the menstrual cycle (5). In previous studies we demonstrated that the corpus luteum (CL) is able to increase its Progesterone (P) production after a bolus of GnRH via increase of gonadotropin discharge (7).
The aim of the study was: a) to clarify the effect of CRF on gonadotropin release b) to evaluate the hypophysial response, in terms of gonadotropins release, to a GnRH test during a CRF infusion c) to investigate a possible direct effect of CRF on the steroidogenesis of corpus luteum since a periferal effect of this peptide on both animals and human has been recently demonstrated (8,9).

Subjects and methods

Five normally cycling women, aged 23-38 yr, were recruited for this study. All patients were within 20% of the ideal body weigth and in their mid luteal phase (MLP) (day 6-7 of the luteal phase). Each women had an hystory of regular menstrual cycle and none had evidence of endocrinopathies.
Two consecutive GnRH test were performed in each patients in two days of their mid luteal phase so that each women was control of her-self. The first day all patients underwent a GnRH test; for two hour samples blood were collected every 10 min, then 25 microg. of GnRH (Relisorm- Serono- Rome- Italy) were acutely injected and blood samples were collected at 0, +15, +30, +60, +90, +120 min after the GnRH bolus. The

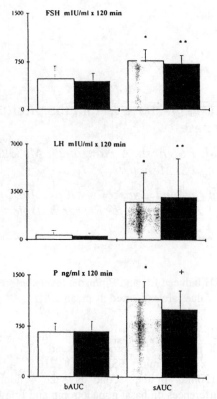

Fig. 1: Basal (bAUC) and GnRH stimulated (sAUC) LH, FSH, P secretory area before (□) and during (■) the CRF infusion. § P<0.01 vs bAUC before CRF infusion * P<0.01 vs bAUC during CRF infusion + P<0.05 vs bAUC during CRF infusion

following day, after two blood samples at -30 min and 0, a 4-hour human CRF infusion (hCRF, Novabiochem, Switzerland) (100 microg./h) was started. The blood samples were collected every 10 min for two hours, at this time a GnRH test was performed with the same modalities of the day before.

Serum levels of LH, FSH, Cortisol, and P were assayed in duplicate using RIA kits (Radim-Rome-Italy). Intra- and inter assay coefficients of variation were <8% and 15% respectively for P, 3.6% and 6% respectively for cortisol. Results were expressed as integrated secretory area (AUC) for 120 min measured before (bAUC) and after (sAUC) the GnRH injection and calculated by the trapezoidal rule. Statistical analysis was performed by the Wilcoxon rank sum test and signed rank test for the unpaired and paired comparisons between two means.

Results

The lenght of luteal phase has been normal in all studied patients.

Fig. 1 shows the AUC of LH, FSH, and P exibithed by the studied patients in their first day of examination before and after the GnRH test. The bAUC were: LH 328.7±299.5 mUI/ml x 120 min; FSH 486±201 mUI/ml x 120 min; P 665.7±181.5 x 120 min.

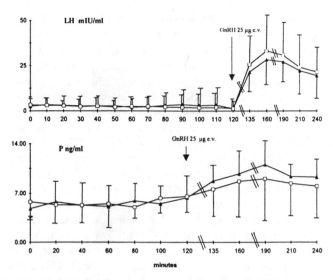

Fig. 2 : Basal and GnRH induced LH and P plasma levels before (▲) and during (□) the CRF infusion. Values are expressed as mean ± SD

The GnRH bolus significantly increased the gonadotropin secretion which in turn determined a significant increase of P production and infact the sAUC were: LH 2732±1131.2 mUI/ml x 120 min; FSH 736.4±216.8 mUI/ml x120min; P 1149.4±113.8 ng/ml x120min. In the second day, the 4 hours of CRF infusion produced no apparent differences on basal gonadotropin and P levels. Infact as shown in Fig. 1 the bAUC of LH, FSH and P determined after 2 hours of CRF infusion were superimposable to those observed the day before in the same period of observation; similarly the response to the GnRH test was not affected by the CRF infusion since the sAUC of gonadotropins and P observed after the GnRH bolus were not significantly different from those observed the day before. In Fig. 2 are illustred the means±SD of LH and P absolute values of the five women during all the studied points in the two days of test. Again neiter the basal gonadotropin and P values nor their response to the GnRH test were modified by the CRF treatment. Moreover during the CRF infusion ther was a significant increase in the cortisol plasma levels when compared to basal values.

Discussion

Considerable attention has recently been focused on CRF modulation of reproductive function . In animals CRF has been shown to impair the reproductive axis by reducing circulating levels of LH through the attenuation of the frequency of pulsatile GnRH secretion and the suppression of the electrophysiological activity of the GnRH pulse generator (1, 10, 11). The CRF action on GnRH neuronal activity appears to be mediated by endogenous opioids since its effect is reversible by the naloxone administration (2, 12). In human the CRF effect on the reproductive function is much less definied. In our study the IV infusion of CRF performed in normally cicling women in their MLP produced, as expected, a significant increase of cortisol plasma levels. On the contrary, during CRF treatment no modification of both basal and GnRH-stimulated LH and FSH levels, was seen. The lack of an inhibitory effect of CRF on basal gonadotropin levels that we observed differs from the data of Barbarino et al (5). Infact this author demonstrated that a 3-hour of IV CRF infusion (100 nanogrammi/h), performed in the same our conditions, induced a significant inhibition of gonadotropin release and that this CRF negative effect was probably mediated by the the opiods since the administration of naloxone prevented the inhibition. Our data are in agrement with those of Fischer (6) who reported no basal gonadotropin inhibition after a prolonged (8 hours) IV infusion of CRF at high doses (5 nanogrammi/Kg) in either premenopausal or postmenopausal women. Similarly Thomas failed to demonstrate any gonadotropin inhibition by CRF in agonadal women (4). The contrasting results obtained in human can be probably explained by the different protocols used as well as by the unrecognized differences existing in patient populations. Furthermore, we believe that the peripheral administration of CRF in all human studies so far conducted, does not allow the simulation of a real intracerebroventricular increase of CRF. This technical difficulty can induce different experimental situations and therefore different findings. Recently CRF and its receptor have been find in several peripheral tissues, including the ovary and the testes. Furthermore the presence of immunoreactive CRF has been detected in normal and polycystic human as well as rat ovaries (14-13). Based on these informations regarding a local involvement of this peptide in the ovarian phisiology we assayed, during the CRF infusion, the P to evaluate if CRF could affect the corpus luteum steroidogenesis directly through its own receptors or indirectly through a reduction of the LH levels. As already reported the LH levels were not altered by CRF and similarly also the hypothesis of a direct negative effect of CRF on P production, at least for the studied period, was excluded since basal levels determined during the CRF treatment were not reduced. In conclusion in our study the CRF wasfound to be uneffective on both hypotalamic and pituitary activity. Furthermore, we first demonstrated a lack of CRF effect also peripherically on corpus luteum steroidogenesis. However our study provides data only about responses to a brief exposure to CRF. Therefore, the role of CRF in human stress-associated reproductive dysfunctions, characterized by chronic high levels of the neuropeptide, remains at the moment completely unknown.

Refereces

1. Petraglia, F., Sutton, S., Vale, W., Plotsky, P.(1987) Corticotropin- releasing factor decreases plasma luteinizing hormone levels in femal rats by inhibiting gonadotropin-releasing hormone release into hypophyseal-portal circulation. *Endocrinology*, **120**,1083-1088
2. Gindoff, P.R., Ferin, M.(1987). Endogenous opiod peptides modulate the effect of corticotropin-releasing factor on gonadotropin release in the primate. *Endocrinology*, **121**, 837-842
3. Orth, D.N., Jackson, R.V., Decherney, G.S., DeBold, C.R., Alexander, A.N., Island, D.P.(1983). Effect of synthetic ovine corticotropin-releasing factor. *J.Clin. Invest.*, **71**,587-595

4.   Thomas, M.A., Rebar, R.W., Labarbera, A.R., Pennington, F.J., Liu, J.H. (1991). Dose-response effects of exogenous pulsatile human corticotropin-releasing hormone on adrenocorticotropin, cortisol and gonadotropin concentrations in agonadal women. *J.Clin. Endocrinol:Metab.*, **72**, 1249-1254

5.   Barbarino, A., De Marinis, L., Tofani, A., Della Casa, S.,D' Amico, C., Mancini, A., Corsello, S.M., Sciuto, R., Barin, A. (1989). Corticotropin-releasing hormone inhibition of gonadotropin release and the effect of opiod blockade. *J. Clin. Endocrinol. Metab.*,**68**, 523-528

6.   Fisher, U.G., Wood, S.H., Bruhn, J., Rosef, S.J., Mortola, J., Rivier, J.E., Yen, S.S.C. (1992). Effect of human corticotropin-releasing hormone on gonadotropin secretion in cycling and postmenopausal women. *Fertil. Steril.*, **58**, 1108-1112

7.   Lanzone, A., Fulghesu, A.M., Di Simone, N., Apa, R.,Guida, C., Caruso, S., Mancuso, S (1989). Effect of human chorionic gonadotropin administration on pituitary luteal respons to gonadotropin-releasing hormone. *Horm. Res.*, **32**, 203-207

8.   Calogero, A.E., Burrello, N., Papale, L., Palumbo, M., Cianci, A., Sanfilippo, S., D' Agata, R. (1993). Corticotropin-releasing hormone inhibits estrogen productionfrom rat granulosa and human granulosa cells in vitro. *J. Endocrinol. Invest.*, **16** (suppl), p.5

9.   Ulisse, S., Fabbri, A., Dufau, M.L. (1989). Corticotropin-releasing factor receptors and actions in rat Leyding cells. *J.Biol. Chem.*, **264**, 2156-2163.

10. Gambacciani, M., Yen, S.S.C., Rasmussen, D.D. (1986) GnRH release from the mediobasal hypothalamus: in vitro inhibition by corticotropin-releasing factor. *Neuroendocrinology*, **43**, 533-536

11. Williams, C.L., Nishihara, M., Thalabard, J.C., Grosser, P. M., Hotchkiss, J., Knobil, C. (1990). Corticotropin-releasing hormone and gonadotropin-releasing hormone pulse generator activity in the rhesus monkey. *Neuroendocrinology*, **52** ,133-137

12. Petraglia, F., Vale, W., Rivier, C. (1986). Opiods act centrally to modulate stress-induced decrease in luteinizing hormone in the rat. *Endocrinology*, **119**, 2445-2450

13. Mastorakos, G., Webster, E.L., Friedman, T.C., Chrousos, G.P. (1993). Immunoreactive corticotropin releasing hormone and its binding sites in the rat ovary. *J.Clin. Invest.*, **92**, 961-968

14. Vryonidou, A., Mastorakos, G., Scope, C.D., Kattis, D. , Chousos, G.P., Phenecos, C. (1993). Presence of immunoreactive corticotropin releasing hormone in normal and polycystic human ovaries. *J. Endocrinol. Invest.*, **16** (suppl), p.195

Influences of the opioid system on hyperinsulinemia and impaired growth hormone secretion in PCOS obese subjects

P. Villa, D. Valle*, A.M. Fulghesu, A. Lanzone**, F. Cucinelli, A. Caruso, A.M. De Luca***, A. Mancini**** and S. Mancuso

Departments of Obstetrics and Gynecology, *Internal Medicine II, **OASI Institute Troina, ***SERT RM12 and ****Institute of Endocrinology, Catholic University School of Medicine, Rome, Italy

INTRODUCTION

PCOS (polycystic ovary syndrome) is characterized by chronic anovulation, elevated serum androgen levels, and an elevated incidence of obesity and hyperinsulinism. Recent data (1, 2) indicate that an altered opiod tone could be involved in the mechanisms leading to hyperinsulinemia and insulin resistance in women with PCOS. On the other hand, patients affected by essential obesity (EO) show frequently hyperinsulinemia and hyperβ-endorphinemia. Moreover, it has been reported that EO and PCOS are associated with an altered GH secretion (3, 4, 5, 6). Conflicting reports exist about the basal GH secretion in PCOS(5, 6, 7). More recently a reduction in GH response to provocative stimuli was found. Lee et al. (8) suggested a reduction in GH response to L-DOPA test, and Lanzone et al. (9) demonstrated a decreased GH response to GHRH test in the obese and hyperinsulinemic PCOS patients. However obesity is associated with an altered control of GH secretion and previous works have investigated the opiod involvement in anterior pituitary hormone secretion (10). Secretory control of GH by the pituitary somatotroph cells is performed by two specific neurohormones, the GHRH which has stimulatory action and the somatostatin which has inhibitory effect. Therefore, other neurotrasmitters such as dopamine and opiods can affect the release of GH. Since insulin and GH may reciprocally influence their secretion and the opioid system may have a role in the pathogenesis of hyperinsulinemia and of reduced growth hormone secretion both in PCOS and EO patients, we explore the involvement of neuroendocrine mechanisms in these disorders by the use of an opiate antagonist.

SUBJECTS AND METHODS

We studied seven PCOS patients (**group 1**) and six women with EO (**group 2**). All women were in good health and took no medications known to affect glucose metabolism or gonadal function. PCOS was diagnosed by the presence of clinical findings, echographic data and elevated androgen plasma levels or at the upper limit of the normal range. A normal LH/FSH ratio was not considered an exclusion criterion. All diagnosises were confirmed by laparoscopy. EO was definined when the BMI exceeded 30 Kg/m^2, in the absence of other endocrinopathies. All patients showed a BMI > 30 Kg/m^2 (ranging from 31.2 to 40.8 -group 1- and from 32.7 to 39.3 -group 2-). The mean age of group 1 patients was 26.2 $\pm$ 5.1 yr; the mean age of group 2 patients was 27.6 $\pm$ 4.4 yr. All subjects exhibited normal indexes of hepatic or renal function. In follicular phase, all patients underwent an OGTT (75 g p.o.) and, on following day, a GHRH-test (1 µG/Kg i.v.). The two tests were performed before and after a thirty days naltrexone (NTX) treatment (50 mg/day). All tests were performed at 8:00 a.m. after an overnight fasting, in randomized order. Blood samples were collected for insulin at 0, 30, 60, 90, 120 minutes from the glucose load, and for GH at -15, 0, 15, 30, 60, 90 minutes from the peptide administration. Insulin and GH plasma levels were expressed as Areas Under the Curves (AUC) and calculated by trapezoidal rule. Statistical comparison between the tests in the same group was performed employing the Wilcoxon rank-sum test; intergroup analysis was performed by the Mann-Whitney U-test (we assumed p < 0.06 as significant value). GH and insulin values were determined by RIA method, using kits by Ares Serono Diagnostics, Milan Italy.

RESULTS

GH AUC (AUC-GH)

The fig. 1 shows the GH response to GHRH before and after NTX treatment. The basal AUC-GH of the group 1 did not differ from group 2. After NTX treatment PCOS patients showed a trend toward a lower response of GH to GHRH; otherwise patients with EO presented an enhanced response.

Insulin AUC (AUC-I)

The fig. 2 shows the insulin response to OGTT before and after NTX treatment. In Group 1 basal AUC-I did not significantly differ when compared to group 2 (vs). Opioid antagonist administration reduced significantly AUC-I in the group 1 (17973 $\pm$ 4332 vs 9692 $\pm$ 6086 µIU/ml; p < 0.06) but failed to modify AUC-I in the group 2 (11626 $\pm$ 5366 vs 9117 $\pm$ 2456 µIU/ml).

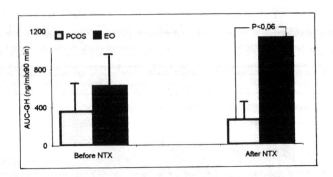

Fig. 1 (see text for details)

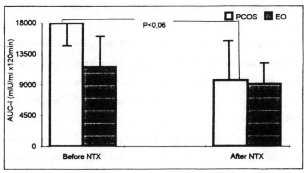

Fig. 2 (see text for details)

DISCUSSION

It is possible to suggest that hyperinsulinism rather than obesity is related to the glucoregulatory action of endogenous opiates. Patients with EO show frequently hyperinsulinemia and hyper-ß-endorphinemia. Several studies have shown that endogenous opioids are involved in complex metabolic alterations of obesity:

a) ß-endorphin (ß-end) plasma levels are increased in obese subjects (11);

b) this increase is not corrected by weight loss (12);

c) in obesity there is an increased sensitivity of pancreas to ß-end (13);

ß-end, in obese patients, increases after glucose load but not after the ingestion of a carbohydrate rich meal. The ß-end increase after glucose load is not observed in normal subjects (14). The hyperendorphinemia is not corrected by weight loss suggesting a control of peptide not related to body weight per se (12). ß-end has been also found in human pancreas (15). Contrasting data are reported about the employ of an opiate receptor blocker, naloxone (NAL). In human studies NAL has been used in different doses. In one study, Mason and Haber (16) demonstrated in NIDDM obese subjects a 50% of decrease in insulin response to OGTT during NAL infusion (0.8 mg i.v. as a bolus followed by 0.1 mg/i.v./min). Vettor et al. (17) showed that NAL reduced the plasma insulin response to oral glucose load in obese subjects but not in lean controls. Our previous work (18) showed that insulin secretion is unaffected by NAL infusion (bolus of 1.6 mg/i.v., followed by a continuous infusion of 2 mg/i.v./hr for two hours) performed after a standard meal, despite a slight but not significant increase, both in NIDDM subjects and in non-diabetic obese subjects. Therefore, opioid peptides are involved in the control of appetite, as documented by experimental data both in animals and humans (19); the use of a receptor antagonist (naltrexone NTX) has been proposed for the treatment of human obesity, to improve the compliance of obese subjects to dietary treatment (20).

In PCOS patients it was hypothesized that:

a) brain opiods may be either decreased or unaltered (21, 22)

b) the circulating levels of ß-end seems to be altered in PCOS and in irsute women and ß-end levels are directly correlated to the body weight (12).

Givens et al. (23) demonstrated that NAL infusion produced a partial reduction of hyperinsulinemia, without altering glucose levels, in hyperandrogenic and hyperinsulinemic obese PCOS patients. We found that the effectiveness of Nal infusion on reducing the insulinemic response to OGTT was related to the hyperinsulinemic status (1). In fact the opiod-antagonist treatment was able to reduce the insulinemic response in hyperinsulinemic group, wheras it had no effect in normoinsulinemic subjects with PCOS or in controls. The degree of such reduction was greater after the chronic treatment with NTX (2).

In agreement with our previous data the present findings show that opiods system is mainly involved in the regulation of insulin secretion in PCOS obese patients. After the NTX treatment we observed the significant reduction of AUC-I in group 1. Moreover the chronic opiod antagonist treatment does not affect the insulinemic response to glucose load in EO patients. In fact after the chronic treatment the AUC-I value in the group 2 does not significantly differ from basal AUC-I. Moreover, it is well known that EO and PCOS are associated to a GH reduced secretory response to provocative stimulus. Recent data suggested the existence of a relationship between GH secretion and gonadal function (24, 25, 26). Lanzone et al. demonstrated that GH response to GHRH is blunted in PCOS patients, among these patients the obese and hyperinsulinemic subjects exhibited a markedly decreased response of GH to GHRH (9). It has been reported that in EO a NAL infusion restores the normal food-induced GH inhibition (10). Obesity is associated with an altered control of GH secretion, since obese subjects exhibit an impaired GH response to a variety of stimulation tests as GHRH (3). A partial restoration of GH responsiveness after weight loss has been described (27). We have previously observed that food ingestion has an inhibitory effect on GH respone to GHRH in normal subjects, but not in obese patients (4).

Previous works have investigated the opioid involvement in anterior pituitary hormone secretion in obesity (8). We observed that a standard meal is capable to produce an increase of GHRH-induced GH-release, which is blocked by a NAL infusion. This datum further underlines the relationship between metabolic fuels and opioid tone. We observed that GH was not blocked by food ingestion and that this paradoxical GHRH-induced GH response was reverted by NAL infusion (10). Our data show the involvement of endogenous opioids in the GH secretion in EO even if there is no significant difference in AUC-GH between before- and after-NTX treatment. However NTX is able to induce a significant intergroup difference (fig. 2), suggesting an enhanced sensitivity to the antagonist in EO, or an highest opiod tone that is not reversible by the employed dose of NTX. Otherwise, the data confirm the role of the opioid system in the regulation of the exaggerated insulin secretion in PCOS subjects and our previous data about the failure of the opiate antagonists to modify the insulin secretion in the human EO. Our data suggest a significant difference in the opioid system function in the PCOS and EO subjects and need further observations to explain the complex correlation between central and peripheral opioids effects.

REFERENCES

1. Lanzone, A., Fulghesu, A. M., Fortini, A., Cutillo, G., Cucinelli, F., Di Simone, N., Caruso, A., Mancuso, S. (1991). Effect of opiate receptor blockade on the insulin response to oral glucose load in polycystic ovarian disease. Human Reproduction, 6 (8): 1043-49.

2. Fulghesu, A.M., Lanzone, A., Cucinelli, F., Caruso, A., Mancuso, S.(1993) Long term Naltrexone treatment reduces the exaggerated insulin secretion in patients with polycystic ovary disease. Obstet. Gynecol. 82,2; 191-196

3. Williams,T., Berelowitz, M., Joffe, S.N., Thorner, M.O., Rivier, J., Vale, W. and Frohman, L. (1984) Impaired growth hormone responses to growth hormone-releasing factor in obesity. New Engl. J. Med. 311, 1403-07.

4. De Marinis, L., Folli, G., D'Amico, C., Mancini, A., Sambo, P., Tofani, A., Oradei, A. and Barbarino, A. (1988) Differential effects of feeding on the ultradian variation of the growth hormone response to GH-releasing hormone in normal subjects and patients with obesity and anorexia nervosa. J. Clin. Endocrinol. Metab. 66, 598-604.

5. Urdl, W. (1988) Polycystic Ovarian Desease: Endocrinological parameters with specific reference to growth hormone and somatomedia-C. Arch. Gynecol. Obstet. 243, 13-36.

6. Kazer, R.R., Unterman,T.G. and Glick,R.P. (1990) An abnormality of the growth hormone/insulin-like growth factor-I axis in women with polycystic ovary syndrome. J. Clin. Endocrinol. Metab. 71, 958-62.

7. Lanzone,A., Fulghesu,A.M., Pappalardo,S., Proto,A., Le Donne,M., Andreani,C.L., Muscatello,R., Caruso, S., Mancuso,S.(1990) Growth hormone and somatomedin-C secretion in patients with polycystic ovarian disease. Ginecol. Obstet. Inv. 29, 149-153.

8. Lee,E.J., Park,K.H., Lee,B.S., Song,C.H., Lee,H.C., Huh,K.B. (1993) Growth hormone response to L-dopa and pyridostigmine in women with polycystic ovarian syndrome. Fertil. Steril. 60, 53-57.

9. Lanzone, A., Villa, P., Fulghesu, A.M., Pavone, V., Caruso, A., Mancuso, S. The growth hormone response to growth hormone releasing hormone is blunted in polycystic ovary syndrome: relation with obesity and hyperinsulinism. Human Reproduction (in press)

10. De Marinis, L., Mancini, A., Folli, G., D'Amico, C., Corsello, S.M., Sciuto, R., Tofani, A., Sambo, P., Barbarino, A. (1989). Naloxone inhibition of postprandial growth hormone releasing hormone-induced growth hormone release in obesity. Neuroendocrinology, 50, 529-532.

11. Givens, J.R., Wiedemann, E., Andersen, R.N., Kitabchi, A.E. (1980). ß-endorphin and ß-lipotropin plasma levels in hirsute women: correlation with body weight. J. Clin. Endocrinol. Metab., 50, 975-976.

12. Giugliano, D., Lefebvre, P.J. (1991). A role of Beta- endorphin in the pathogenesis of human obesity? Horm. Metab. Res., 23, 251-256.

13. Dubois, M., Pickar, D., Cohen, M.R., Roth, Y.F., Macnamara, T., Bynney jr, W.E. (1981). Surgical stress in humans is accompanied by an increase in plasma beta-endorphin immunoreactivity. Life Sci., 29, 1249-1254.

14. Scavo, D., Facchinetti, F., Barletta, C., Petraglia, F., Buzzetti, R., Monaco, M., Giovannini, C., Genazzani, A.R. (1987). Plasma beta-endorphin in response to oral glucose tolerance test in obese patients. Horm. Metab. Res., 19, 204-207.

15. Bruni, J., Watkins, W. and Yen S.S.C. (1979). B-endorphin in the human pancreas. J. Clin. Endocrinol. Metab., 49, 649- 651.

16. Mason, J.S., Haber, D. (1982). Endogenous opiates modulate insulin secretion in flushing non-insulin-dependent diabetics. J. Clin. Endocrinol. Metab., 54, 693-697.

17. Vettor, R., Martini, C., Manno, M., Cestaro, S., Federspil, G., Sicolo, N. (1985). Effects of naloxone-induced opiate receptors blockade on insulin secretion in obesity. Horm. Metab. Res., 17, 374-375.

18. De Marinis, L., Mancini, A., De Luca, A.M., Fiumara, C., Zuppi, P., Sammartano, L. and Valle D. (1993) Naloxone effects on post-prandial glucose, insulin and C-peptide levels in obese subjects.Diab. Res. 23, 83-91.

19. Morley, J.E., Levine, A.S., Gosnell, B.A., Billington, C.J. (1984) Which opioid receptor mechanism modulates feeding? Appetite 5:61

20. Sternbach, H.A., Annitto, W., Pottash, A.L.C., Gold, M.S. (1982): Anorectic effects of naltrexone in man. Lancet 1:388-89

21. Wortsman, J., Weherberg, W.B., Govin, J. R., Allen, J.P. (1984) Elevated levels of plasma beta-endorphin and gamma 3-melanocyte stimulating hormone in the polycystic ovary syndrome. Obstet. Gynecol 63; 630-634

22. Cumming, D.C., Reid R.L., Quigley, M.E., Rebar, R.W., Yen, S.S.C.(1984) Evidence for decreased endogenous dopamine and opiod inhibitory influences on LH secretion in polycystic ovary syndrome. Clin. Endocrinol. 20, 643-648

23. Givens JH, Kortz BR, Kitabchi AE, Tittle JB, Karas TG, Mirchell JA, Howes JF (1987) Reduction of hyperinsulinemia and insulin resistence by opiate receptor blockade. Endocrinol Metab 64, 377-382.

24. Homburg,R., West,C., Torresani,T., Jacobs,H.S. (1990) Cotreatment with human growth hormone and gonadotropins for induction of ovulation: a controlled clinical trial. Fertil. Steril.53 254-260.

25. Jacobs,H.S. (1992) Growth hormone and ovulation: is there an indication for treatment of infertile women with growth hormone? Horm. Res. 38, 14-21.

26. Katz,E., Ricciarelli,E., Adashi,E.Y. (1993) The potential relevance of growth hormone to femal reproductive physiology and pathophiysiology. Fertil.Steril. 59, 8-34.

27. Jung, R. (1984) Endocrinological aspects of obesity. In: Clinics in Endocrinology and metabolism (W.P.T. James, ed.) vol. 13, Obesity 597-612, Sauders, Philadelphia.

Correlations between bone mineral density and hormonal factors in androgenized women

M. Legan and A. Kocijančič

Department of Endocrinology and Metabolism, University Medical Centre, Ljubljana, Slovenia

PURPOSE OF THE STUDY

Women with functional hyperandrogenism have higher bone mineral density (BMD) than controls (1,2).

We proposed that special hormonal status of androgenized women explains gaining higher BMD in the case of eumenorrhea, as well as preventing bone loss in the case of hypoestrogenemia (3). Hormones that are elevated in women with androgen excess - and in the same time potencially anabolic for bone -are androgens and insulin (4,5).

Special expectations in this study we put on insulin. Mostly because the expected correlations between serum androgen levels and BMD in premenopausal androgenized women have not been found (2).

Insulin affects bone indirectly (stimulates renal 1- alpha hydroxilase activity, enhances active calcium absorption in duodenum in animal models) (6) and directly (increases replication and function of osteoblasts, in vitro studies) (7). In vivo studies on diabetics type I showed that the lack of insulin is connected with lower BMD (8,9). Studying diabetics type II gave conflicting results, probably for the sake of the special insulin dynamics in diabetes mellitus type II.

DESIGN OF THE STUDY:

To examine the impact of hormonal status on BMD of premenopausal androgenized women we designed a prospective study of 26 women with functional hyperandrogenism. The including criteria were:
- age between 18 and 35 yrs
- ideal body weight (within 20%)
- signs and symptoms of androgenisation (hirsutism, Ferriman-Galwey index >8, and/or acne and/or androgenic alopecia)
- elevated at least one of three serum androgens
- no medical pretreatment of hyperandrogenism
- no contraceptive pill
- otherwise excellent health.

After the informed consent of participants, the inicial interwiev was obtained with special emphassis on calcium containing food consumption and physical activity. Fasting blood specimen was taken in the early follicular phase of menstrual cycle (between 1-st and 8-th day) in eumenorrhoeic and oligomenorrhoeic women, and in casual fasting state in amenorrhoeic women. We determined serum concentrations of:

- free testosterone (FT)
- androstendione (A)
- DHEAS
- estradiol (E2)
- insulin (IRI)
- blood glucose
- IGF - 1
- IGFBP - 3

Blood glucose and rutine biochemistry of the blood was also measured.
We measured BMD of lumbar spine (L2-4) by dual photon absorptiometry method.

RESULTS OF THE STUDY:

Table 1. Clinical data of participants

age (yrs)	23.5 (4.3)
menarchal age (yrs)	10.2 (4.9)
weight (kg)	62.1 (11.1)
BMI (kg/m²)	22.14 (3.82)

Values are the mean (+/- SD)

Table 2. Bone mineral density and hormonal measurements of participants

BMD (g/cm²)	1.075 (0.084)
FT (pmol/l)	9.6 (5.8)
A (nmol/l)	7.9 (4.9)
DHEAS (μmol/l)	8.5 (3.7)
E2 (nmol/l)	0.26 (0.15)
IRI (mE/l)	8.9 (4.3)
IGF-1 (μg/l)	312 (165)
IGFBP-3 (mol/E)	3.86 (0.82)

Table 3. Bivariate correlations between BMD and hormonal parameters

	BMD
FT	r= -0.26 p= 0.10
A	r= 0.20 p= 0.16
DHEAS	r= -0.27 p= 0.12
E2	r= 0.63 **p= 0.001**
IRI	r= 0.18 p= 0.19
IGF-1	r= -0.01 p= 0.47
IGFBP-3	r= -0.11 p= 0.33

Table 4. Multiple regression analyse in the context of multivariate canonical analyse.

	BMD
FT	b= -0.49 p= 0.082
A	b= -0.07 p= 0.68
DHEAS	b= -0.52 **p= 0.010**
E2	b= 0.49 **p= 0.013**
IRI	b= 0.68 **p= 0.008**
IGFBP-3	b= 0.15 p= 0.278

In simple regression analyses (Table 3) only E2 shows significant positive correlation with BMD. In the context of multivariate canonical analyses, the multiple regression analyse (which involves FT, A, E2, DHEAS, IRI and IGFBP-3 in correlation with BMD) discovered strong and significant role of IRI on BMD (Table 4). Important stays the correlation of E2 with BMD, whereas DHEAS is in negative correlation with BMD (Table 4).

CONCLUSIONS OF THE STUDY:

There is an important positive correlation between the level of serum insulin and BMD in androgenized premenopausal women. Androgens show no significant positive correlation with BMD.

REFERENCES:

1. Di Carlo, C., Shoham, Z., MacDougall, J., Patel, A., Hall, HL. and Jacobs, HS. (1992). Polycystic ovaries as a relative protective factor for bone mineral loss in young women with amenorrhoea. Fertil. Steril., 57, 314-9.

2. Preželj, J. and Kocijančič, A. (1993). Bone mineral density in hyperandrogenic amenorrhoea. Calcif. Tissue. Int., 52, 422-4.

3. Dixon, JE., Rodin, A., Murby, B., Chapan, MG. and Fogelman, I. (1989). Bone mass in hirsute women with androgen excess. Clin. Endocrinol., 30, 271-7.

4. Barbieri, RL., Smith, S. and Ryan, KJ. (1988). The role of hyperinsulinemia in the pathogenisis of ovarian hyperandrogenism. fertil. Steril., 50, 197-212.

5. Dunaif, A., Segal, KR., Futterwiet, W. and Dorjansky, A. (1989). Profound peripheral insulin resistance, independent of obesity, in PCOS. Diabetes, 38, 1165-74.

6. Bouillon, R. (1991). Diabetic bone disease. Calcif. Tissue. Int., 45, 155-60.

7. Kream, BE., Smith, MD., Canalis, E. and Raisz, LG. (1985). Characterization of the effect of insulin on collagen synthesis in fetal rat bone. Endocrinology, 116, 296-301.

8. Rosenbloom, AL., Lezotte, DC., Weber, FT., Gudat, J., Heller, DR., Weber, ML., Klein, S. and Kennedy, BB. (1977). Diminution of bone mass in childhood diabetes. Diabetes, 26, 1052-5.

9. Levin, ME., Boisseau, VC., and Avioli, LV. (1976). Effects of diabetes mellitus on bone mass in juvenile and adult-onset diabetes. N. Engl. J. Med., 294, 241-5.

Effect of weight loss on the pituitary response to GnRH in obese patients

G. Grugni, D. Moro, A. Ardizzi, A. Minocci and F. Morabito

Italian Auxological Centre of Piancavallo – IRCCS, Milan, Italy

INTRODUCTION

Undernutrition associated with weight loss has been reported to cause alterations in the reproductive function both in the experimental (1-2) and human model. Calorie deprivation may determine in the healthy man a reduction in testosterone secretion (3) that may even develop into impotency (4); similarly dietetic restriction in normal weight women often determines dysfunctional uterine bleeding and inadequacy of the luteal phase (5) besides leading to specific disorders of menstrual cycle rhythm (6) and rapid weight loss often leads to amenorrhea (7). It is also known that an absence of menstrual flow is characteristic of situations in which there is an extreme weight reduction such as in anorexia nervosa (8).

When obese subjects undergo calorie restriction, changes in the hypothalamic-pituitary -gonadal axis function may be observed at least in men (9), particularly during short-term fasting (10). On the contrary, in women with moderate obesity it does not appear that serum gonadotropin (Gn) levels vary during a brief period of complete fasting (11), even if in such conditions it has been seen there is a clear increase in their urinary excretion (12).

On the basis of these observations this study examines the effects of more prolonged dietetic restrictions on spontaneous and stimulated Gn secretion in a group of young female subjects with essential obesity.

PATIENTS AND METHODS

Eight female subjects were studied. The patients were admitted to our Centre for obesity of high degree (Table 1). A complete medical work-up was carried out to confirm the condition of essential obesity, such as study of thyroid and suprarenal glands function.

Table 1 Subjects characteristics and response to the diet. BMI: Body Mass Index (Kg/m2); (A) before and (B) after diet. *p<0.001 vs basal conditions.

Subject no.	Age (yrs.)	BMI (A)	BMI (B)
1	17.9	42	38.5
2	17.2	33.5	30.5
3	16.3	40.3	31.4
4	14.6	42	37.4
5	17.3	33.8	31.1
6	16.6	38.3	34.7
7	17.6	41.6	37.1
8	14.9	42.5	37.6
mean	16.6	39.3	34.8*
± SE	0.4	1.3	1.1

All the patients had regular menstrual cycles (mean 28 days) and none had taken hormone treatment for at least 12 months preceding the study.

During hospitalization the patients were given a Very Low Calorie Diet (VLCD: 600 KCal = 2,512 kJ/day; protein g 48 (30.6%), lipids g 20.7 (29%) and carbohydrate g 62.1 (39.4%)) for a total period of 60 days and without any type of pharmacological treatment. None of the women participated in a strenous exercise program (<8 hours aerobic exercise /week).

In all subjects the GnRH test was performed both in basal conditions and at the end of the dietary restriction period (100 mcg iv at time 0') with venous blood samples taken at times 0, 15, 30, 60, 90 and 120 minutes for the determination of LH, FSH and at time 0' also of 17-beta-estradiol (E2). In both occasions the stimulation tests were performed during the follicular phase of the cycle.

Individual and parental informed consent was obtained from all the subjects; the entire study protocol was approved by the local Ethical Committee. Serum LH and FSH concentrations were determined by IRMA techniques, using commercially available kits (IRMA-mat, Byk-Sangtec Diagnostica, Dietzenbach, Germany); E2 levels were measured by RIA kits, provided by Medical Systems, Genova, Italy.

All data were expressed as mean+SE. The LH and FSH response to GnRH was evaluated as area under the curve (AUC: mU/ml/h), using the trapezoidal method. The statistical analysis was performed by appling the Student's t test for paired data; values of p less than 0.05 were considered significant.

RESULTS

Hypocaloric dietetic treatment determined a significant weight reduction (Table 1). In six subjects weight loss determined the onset of menstrual disorders (oligomenorrhea)

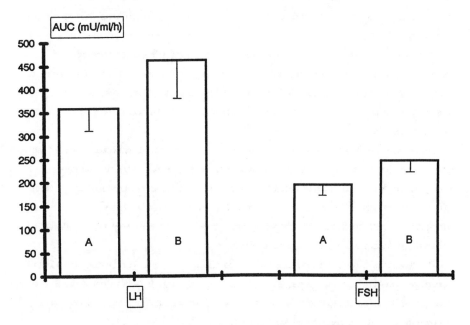

Figure 1 Gn responses to GnRH before (A) and after (B) weight loss.

whereas in the remaining two patients there was no change in menstrual cycles.

The analysis of Gn response to GnRH did not show any difference between results obtained before (A) and after (B) weight loss: LH AUC = 359+52 (A) vs 462+77 (B): p=0.2; FSH AUC = 193+12 (A) vs 245+30 (B): p=0.1 (Figure 1). Similarly we did not find any variation in the basal levels of LH (4.1+1.1 (A) vs 3.8+0.9 (B) mU/ml: p=0.7), FSH (4.4+ 0.7 (A) vs 4.9+0.6 (B) mU/ml: p=0.6) and E2 (43+5 (A) vs 51+8 (B) pg/ml: p=0.7).

DISCUSSION

In this study the effects of dietary restrictions prolonged over 60 days on Gn basal and stimulated levels were evaluated in a group of young normally menstruating women. Weight reduction determined the onset of menstrual irregularities in 75% of our patients.Though this result does not support what observed in young healthy women after short-term fasting (13), it does confirm the results of normal weight women after six weeks of dietary treatment (14).

The analysis of the effects of calorie restriction on Gn secretory pattern in normal subjects gives contrasting results: in women besides the absence of any modification in LH and FSH serum levels after both short-term (13, 15) and long-term fasting (14), a reduction of LH pulse frequency, especially during waking hours (16), and an increased

Gn responsiveness to GnRH (15) were observed. In men instead a brief period of fasting may determine a significant decrease both in LH and FSH concentrations and LH pulse frequency (17).

As concerns Gn behaviour in obese subjects after calorie restriction, it has been seen that in males short-term fasting determines an alteration of Gn responsiveness to GnRH with a reduction in basal LH (10) and FSH (18) levels. When instead dietary restriction is more prolonged, no change has been seen in the spontaneous and stimulated levels of Gn (19).

These data are in accordance with those referred to obese postmenopausal women, fasted for 10 days for weight reduction, in whom weight loss does not determine changes in the Gn serum concentration both in basal condition (12) and after stimulation with GnRH (6). These results are similar to those obtained in our group of obese patients which suggests a certain integrity of the Gn secreting axis after prolonged calorie restriction also in the period of fertility.

It thus seems possible to conclude that the onset of alterations in the reproductive sphere of juvenile obesity consequent to a decrease of food intake is not so much due to changes in Gn secretory pattern as to selective involvement of supra-hypothalamic components of the neuroendocrine system (20).

REFERENCES

(1) Knuth, U.A., Friesen, H.G. (1983). Starvation induced anoestrus: effect of chronic food restriction on body weight, its influence on oestrus cycle and gonadotrophin secretion in rats. Acta Endocrinol. 5Copenh.) 104, 402-9.

(2) Cameron, J.L., Nosbisch, C. (1991). Suppression of pulsatile Luteinizing Hormone and testosterone secretion during short term food restriction in the adult male Rhesus monkey (Macaca mulatta). Endocrinology 128, 1532-40.

(3) Rojdmark, S. (1987). Influence of short-term fasting on the pituitary-testicular axis in normal men. Horm. Res. 25, 140-6.

(4) Smith, S.R., Chhetri, M.K., Johanson, A.J., Radfari, N., Migeon, C.J. (1975). The pituitary-gonadal axis in men with protein-calorie malnutrition.J. Clin. Endocrinol. Metab. 41, 60-9.

(5) McArthur, J.W., Beitins, I.Z., Bullen, B.A. (1984). Motility, nutrition and reproduction: recent clues to an ancient relationship. In Givens, J.R. (ed.): The Hypothalamus, pp. 71-8. (Chicago: Year Book)

(6) Kapen, S., Sternthal, E., Braverman, L. (1981). A "pubertal" 24-hour luteinizing hormone (LH) secretory pattern following weight loss in the absence of anorexia nervosa. Psychosom. Med. 43, 177-82.

(7) Vigersky, R.A., Andersen, A.E., Thompson, R.H., Loriaux, D.L. (1977). Hypothalamic

dysfunction in secondary amenorrhea associated with simple weight loss. N. Engl. J. Med. 297, 1141–4.

(8) Garfinkel, P.E., Garner, D.M. (1982). Anorexia Nervosa, pp. 58–99. (New York: Brunner/Mazel)

(9) Strain, G.W., Zumoff, B., Miller, L.K., Rossner, W., Levit, C., Kalin, M., Hershcopf, R.J., Rosenfeld, R.S. (1988). Effect of massive weight loss on hypothalamic-pituitary-gonadal function in obese men. J. Clin. Endocrinol. Metab. 66, 1019–23.

(10) Rojdmark, S., Asplund, A., Rossner, S. (1989). Pituitary-testicular axis in obese men during short-term fasting. Acta Endocrinol. (Copenh.) 121, 727–32.

(11) Beitins, I.Z., Barkan, A., Klibanski, A., Kyung, N., Reppert, S.M., Badger, T.M., Veldhuis, J., McArthur, J.W. (1985). Hormonal responses to short term fasting in postmenopausal women. J. Clin. Endocrinol. Metab. 60, 1120–6.

(12) Beitins, I.Z., Shah, A., O'Loughlin, K., Johnson, L., Ostrea, T.R., Van Wart, J., McArthur, J.W. (1980). The effects of fasting on serum and urinary gonadotropins in obese postmenopausal women. J. Clin. Endocrinol. Metab. 51, 26–34.

(13) Soules, M.R., Merriggiola, M.C., Steiner, R.A., Clifton, D.K., Tolvola, B., Bremert, W.J. (1994). Short-term fasting in normal women: absence of effects on gonadotrophin secretion and the menstrual cycle. Clin. Endocrinol. 40, 725–31.

(14) Pirke, K.M., Schweiger, U., Lemmel, W., Krieg, J.C., Berger, M. (1985). The influence of dieting on the menstrual cycle of healthy young women. J. Clin. Endocrinol. Metab. 60, 1174–9.

(15) Rojdmark, S. (1987). Increased gonadotropin responsiveness to Gonadotropin-Releasing Hormone during fasting in normal subjects. Metabolism 36, 21–6.

(16) Loucks, A.B., Heath, E.M. (1994). Dietary restriction reduces luteinizing hormone (LH) pulse frequency during waking hours and increases LH pulse amplitude during sleep in young menstruating women. J. Clin. Endocrinol. Metab. 78, 910–5.

(17) Cameron, J.L., Weltzin, T.E., McConaha, C., Helmreich, D.L., Kaye, W.H. (1991). Slowing of pulsatile luteinizing hormone secretion in men after forty-eight hours of fasting. J. Clin. Endocrinol. Metab. 73, 35–41.

(18) Klibanski, A., Beitins, I.Z., Badger, T., Little, R., McArthur, J. (1981). Reproductive function during fasting in men. J. Clin. Endocrinol. Metab. 53, 258–63.

(19) Hoffer, L.J., Beitins, I.Z., Kyung, N., Bistrian, B. (1986). Effects of severe dietary restriction on male reproductive hormones. J. Clin. Endocrinol. Metab. 62, 288–92.

(20) Berga, S.L., Mortola, J.F., Girton, L., Suh, B., Laughlin, G., Pham, P., Yen, S.S.C. (1989). Neuroendocrine aberrations in women with functional hypothalamic amenorrhea. J. Clin. Endocrinol. Metab. 68, 301–8.

Steroid hormones and the human breast

J.H.H. Thijssen and M.A. Blankenstein

Department of Endocrinology, Academisch Ziekenhuis, Utrecht, The Netherlands

INTRODUCTION

Long-term effects of exogenous hormones on the human breast and especially the effects on the occurence of malignant tumours have attracted much attention since the large scale use of oral contraceptives and hormone replacement therapy. Because the aetiology of breast cancer is rather complex, more information of the physiological role of steroids in the development and maintenance of breast tissues is required in order to more meaningful discuss the possible (lack? of) effects of exogenous steroids.

Epidemiological studies have been able to identify risk factors for breast cancer and additional studies have indicated a number of possible mechanisms how steroids can exert their effects on the incidence of clinically detectable tumours. In the following article, aspects related to normal and malignant growth of the breast will be discussed.

STEROIDS AND THE DEVELOPMENT OF THE HUMAN BREAST

The first signs of growth of the breasts are observed at the beginning of pubertal maturation in girls, related to the start of ovarian secretion of oestrogens. Close analysis of the hormonal data reveals that oestrogen levels may not be the only determinant factor in normal development, the presence of glucocorticosteroids, gonadotrophins and/or GnRH may also be required for adequate development (1).

The female sex hormones induce growth activity in the glandular epithelial cells, the surrounding collagenous connective tissue, and the accumulation of fatty tissue in the breast. Then the growth ceases and additional steroids are unable to induce further increases in the total size of the breasts. Examination of the glandular tissue shows that the distal, free end of each mammary duct has developed into new branches and the terminal ducts into alveolar buds, equivalent to terminal end buds in the rat (2). Lobule formation occurs within one or two years after the first menstrual period. At this stage, after menarche but before first pregnancy, the human breast has not matured completely, the influence of a pregnancy is necessary for a full differentation. After birth many cells regress. Later in life involution of tissues in the breast occurs. The variation in the growth rates is reflected in the thymidine labelling index.

It recently was concluded that oestrogens appear to be important in priming the breast cells for other factors to be effective (3). The difficulty of extrapolating results from animal models for studies on the human breast was noted, however, as in women the breasts have a unique and complex structure, different from that in rodents (3).

AETIOLOGY OF HUMAN BREAST CANCER

The age-specific incidence of breast cancer shows large variations between populations in different countries (4), it is highest in women living in western countries; nutritional and reproductive factors are involved. Oestrogens play a role in the pathogenesis of breast cancer but they are not considered to be carcinogenic *per se*. It is likely that they act mainly as promotors of tumour growth after malignant transformation, during the promotion and/or the progression phases.

A recent unifying hypothesis (5) describes the known risk factors in one pathogenetic framework, indicated by the formation of "pre-cancerous" lesions. Early menarche and tall body height are related to the formation of such lesions, with an increased carcinogenic potential. Early age at first pregnancy leads to a reduction in the formation of "pre-cancerous" lesions by the terminal differentiation of mammary gland epithelium during pregnancy. The "pre-cancerous" lesions may be promoted to clinical breast cancer in subsequent years under the influence of a number of factors, among which oestrogens appear to play a major role (5). In postmenopausal women the oestrogenic effects of obesity possibly act as growth-enhancers of oestrogen-responsive tumors; the incidence of oestrogen receptor (ER) positive tumours is higher in western than in non-western countries (6) and higher in tumours from obese women than in those from lean women (7) within western populations.

Because oestrogens have to be taken up by cells, interest focusses on factors responsible for the accumulation of oestrogens in mammary tissues. High intratissue concentrations of oestradiol, independent of the menopausal status of women, have been found; they do not reflect plasma levels. Local factors must be involved in the intratissue accumulation, especially in postmenopausal women.

LOCAL PRODUCTION OF OESTROGENS IN THE BREAST

It seems likely that a large part of the intratissue oestradiol is derived from *in situ* biosynthesis; especially the role of local aromatase got much attention (8,9,10). The activity of the enzymes will be reflected in the concentrations of androgens and oestrogens in the tissue. The signicantly lower concentration of 4-androstenedione in tumours is in agreement with the fact that the aromatase uses 4-androstenedione as its main substrate *in vivo*, the product being oestrone. Secondary to the formation of oestrone, conversion to oestradiol must take place as especially in malignant tissues oestradiol is more abundant than oestrone. This secondary conversion is catalyzed by the enzyme 17ß-hydroxysteroid dehydrogenase (17-OHSD). The local production of oestradiol seems to play an important role of clinically manifest breast tumours in postmenopausal women.

EXOGENOUS STEROIDS AND BREAST CANCER

The maintenance of oestradiol levels in tumors would imply that exogenous steroids would not influence the intratissue levels to a large extent and thus would not influence the growth promotion of premalignant lesions or existing small tumors. This might account for the very small breast tumour-stimulating effects of hormone replacement therapy in postmenopausal women (11). Whereas the protection of the endometrium against malignant transformation by progestins is clear, no agreement exists as to their effects on the human breast. For the endometrium the protective influence is thought to be, at least partly, due the stimulation of the 17-OHSD, resulting in an inactivation of oestradiol. In the breast an opposite picture emerges: oestradiol is at much higher levels than oestrone. Future studies will have to clarify some of these points.

CONCLUSIONS

It is not possible to understand how all factors, that have an influence on the occurrence of abnormal growth in the human breast, exert their effects. The background of the large variation in the incidence rates between different populations needs more attention as westernization of many non-western societies will lead to increases in the incidence of breast cancer. Additionally, the effects of changes in life-style in the western world during the last decades, the accompanying decreases in age at menarche, and the increases in body height and thus in weight are fascinating but again remain as yet unexplained. It seems logical to focuss on nutritional compo-nents (12) that can be interesting because of their possible infuence on hormonal effects in breast tissues. Large changes have taken place in the nutritional habits and thus identification of the responsible components in such interactions will not be an easy task (13).

In the preceeding pages the possibility of local hormone synthesis in the human breast has been described. The conclusion has been reached that this local process is relevant for the promotion of premalignant breast

lesions and that the independent synthesis of local hormones has consequences for the effects of exogenous hormone administration. Especially in
postmenopausal hormone replacement therapy, local hormone synthesis
could be an important factor that could account for the almost negligible
effect of the exogenous hormones on breast cancer risk. Also in this
respect, the influence of nutritional components on the local processes
should be considered, as relatively little information is available regarding
this aspect.

REFERENCES

1. Laron, Z., Kauli, R. and Pertzelan, A. (1989). Clinical evidence on the role
    of oestrogens in the development of the breasts. *Proc. Royal Soc. Edin-
    burgh*, **95B**, 13-22
2. Russo, J., Gusterson, B.A., Rogers, A.E., Russo, I.H., Wellings, S.R, and
    van Zwieten, M.J. (1990). Biology of disease: comparitive study of human
    and rat mammary tumorigenesis. *Lab. Invest.*, **64**, 244-78
3. Anderson, T.J. and Battersby, S. (1989). The involvement of oestrogen in
    the development and function of the normal breast: histological evidence.
    Proc. Royal Soc. Edinburgh, **95B**, 23-32
4. Parkin, D.M. (1989). Cancers of the breast, endometrium and ovary: geo-
    graphic correlations. *Eur.J.Cancer Clin.Oncol.*, **25**, 1917-25
5. De Waard, F. and Trichopoulos, D. (1988). A unifying concept of the
    aetiology of breast cancer. *Int.J.Cancer*, **41**, 666-9
6. Nomura, Y., Kobayashi, S., Takatani, O., Sugano, H., Matsumoto, K. and
    McGuire, W.L. (1977). Estrogen receptor and endocrine responsiveness in
    Japanese versus American breast cancer patients. *Cancer Res.*, **37**, 106-10
7. De Waard, F., Poortman, J. and Collette, H.J.A. (1981). Relationship of
    weight to the promotion of breast cancer after menopause. *Nutrition
    Cancer*, **2**, 237-40
8. O'Neill, J.S., Elton, R.A. and Miller, W.R. (1988). Aromatase activity in
    adipose tissue from breast quadrants: a link with tumour site. *Brit. Med.J.*,
    296, 741-3
9. Thijssen, J.H.H., Daroszewski, J., Milewicz, A. and Blankenstein, M.A.
    (1993). Local aromatase activity in human breast tissues. *J.Steroid Bio-
    chem.Molec.Biol.*, **44**, 577-82
10. Bulun, S.E., Mahendroo, M.S., Price, T., Aitken, J. and Simpson, E.R.
    (1993). A link between breast cancer and local estrogen biosynthesis
    suggested by quantification of breast adipose tissue aro-matase cytochrome
    P450 transcripts by competitive PCR. *J.Clin.Endocrin.Metab.*, **77**, 1622-8
11. Staffa, J.A., Newschaffer, C.J., Jones, J.K. and Miller, V. (1992). Progest-
    ins and breast cancer: an epidemiological review. *Fert. Steril.*, **57**, 473-91
12. Adlercreutz, H., Mousavi, Y. and Hockerstedt, K. (1992). Diet and breast
    cancer. *Acta Oncol.*, **31**, 175-181
13. Marshall, E. (1993). Search for a killer: focus shifts from fat to hormones.
    Science, **259**, 618-621

Differentiation of ambiguous genitalia

Q.-S. Ge, Q. Yu, F. He, L. Yeh*, S. Huang* and C. Gu

Division of Reproductive Endocrinology and Infertility, Department of Obstetrics and Gynecology, Peking Union Medical College Hospital and *Department of Medical Genetics, Institute of Basic Medical Sciences, Chinese Academy of Medical Sciences, Beijing, Peoples Republic of China

Assessment of sex in cases with ambiguous genitalia is of extreme importance to the patient and the family to avoid psychic trauma. Genital ambiguity is the result of either excess or insufficiency of androgen. When one is familiar with the genesis of genital differentiation, it will not be difficult to understand the different variations of genital ambiguity. Clinically ambiguity showed a wide spectrum from slight enlargement of clitoris to that of full male type of genitalia. The degree of ambiguity depends upon the amount and duration of androgenic effect during different stages of fetal life. After birth, excess androgen only stimulate enlargement of the clitoris.

Within a period of 17 years, 417 cases of disorders of sexual differentiation were encounterd in our endocrine clinic. They were classified into 3 main groups: abnormalities of chromosome, dysgenesis of gonad, and disorders of sex hormone (Table 1). Among the 417 cases, 91 (21.8%) cases in 6 type of disorders, showed genital ambiguity (Table 2). In congenital adrenal hyperplasia, maternal intake of androgen, incomplete androgen insensitivity syndrome and testicular regression, all cases showed genital ambiguity; while in XO/XY gonadal dysgenesis and true hermaphrodites, not all cases showed genital ambiguity.

Special features in the history such as similar diseases

153

Table 1. Classification of disorders of sexual differentiation

Disorders		Total	%
Abnormalities of chromosome		175	42.0
Turner's syndrome	157		
XO/XY gonadal dysgenesis	10		
Super-female	6		
True hermaphrodite	1		
Klinefelter's syndrome	1		
Dysgenesis of gonad		137	32.8
XX pure gonadal dysgenesis	111		
XY pure gonadal dysgenesis	16		
True hermaphrodite	9		
Testicular regression	1		
Disorders of sex hormone		105	25.2
Androgen excess			
Congenital adrenal hyperplasia	52		
Exogenous androgen	1		
Androgen deficiency	12		
Androgen insensitivity syndrome	40		
Total		417	100.0

Table 2. Disorders of sexual differentiation
with ambiguous genitalia

Disorders	Case no.		%
	Total	Ambiguous	
XO/XY gonadal dysgenesis	10	6	6.6
True hermaphrodite	10	5	5.5
Testicular regression	1	1	1.1
Congenital adrenal hyperplasia	52	52	57.1
Maternal intake of androgen	1	1	1.1
Incomplete androgen insensitivity syndrome	26	26	28.6
Total	100	91	100.0

in the family or consanguineous marriage will help in the diagnosis of those with hereditary causes, such as congenital adrenal hyperplasia and androgen insensitivity syndrome. Positive maternal history of using androgens during early pregnancy, will help in the differentiation of the cause of ambiguity. During routine physical examination, height and secondary sex characteristics are of diagnostic importance. Low height is diagnostic for Turner's syndrome. Presence or absence of secondary sex characters will indicate presence or absence of sex steroids. Karyotype examination will clarify those with XX, XY or mosaic sex chromosome. Degree of clitorial enlargement and perineal fusion will indicate the time and degree of virilization during patient's fetal life. Determinations of androgen and corticoid hormones will be of diagnostic importance in androgen excess or deficiency. SRY is now referred to as the most possible gene for testicular determinig factor. In 3 true hermaphrodites with karyotype of 46,XX all showed presence of SRY gene using the polymerase chain reaction technique, showing the cause of testicular development in these patients.

All cases with Y chromosome or doubtful cases, laparoscopy and/or laparotomy were performed to have a direct view of the gonads. To our surprise, in one case with karyotype 45,X/46,XY preoperatively diagnosed as mixed gonadal dysgenesis, after laparotomy and histological examination, both gonads were ovaries and one even showed presence of primordial follicles. Some of the XX males, upon laparotomy were found to be true hermaphrodites. Laparoscopy and/or laparotomy had helped us clear up some of the puzzling cases. This has now become one of the routine examinations and also in the early removal of tumors. Among 55 cases operated, 8 showed presence of tumor.

As far as marriage is concerned, when the perineum is not very tight, they all can have satisfactory sexual relationships. Those with tight vaginal orifice need perineoplasty. With the development of medically assisted procreation, there will be more chances of having offsprings. From our series, some may still have normal pregnancies and children. 11 patients with congenital adrenal hyperplasia were married, 7 had successful pregnancies and 5 delivered normal babies. True hermaphrodites also had successful pregnancies and normal children. One of the incomplete androgen insensitivity syndrome after correction of hypospadias was married and had a daughter.

Patients with ambiguous genitalia should be investigated and given proper advices as to future marriages and possibilities of pregnancies. Help them to live as much as a normal individual.

KEYWORDS: Ambiguous genitalia; Androgen; Karyotype;
Laparoscopy and/or laparotomy

REFERENCES

1. Dewhurst, S.J. (1981) Integrated Obstetrics and Gynecology for Postgraduates, 3rd edn. pp. 37-48. (Oxford:Blackwell Scientific Publications)

2. Emans, S.J.H. and Goldstein, D.P. (1990) Pediatric and Adolescent Gynecology, 3rd edn. pp. 47-66. (Boston:Little, Brown and Company)

3. McPhaul, M.J., Marcelli, M., Tilley, W.D., Griffin, J.E. and Wilson, J.D. (1991) Androgen resistance caused by mutations in the androgen receptor gene. FASEB J 5,2910-2915

Cholinergic dysregulation in anorexia nervosa

L. De Marinis, A. Mancini, M.L. Fabrizi, G. Conte, A. Bianchi, M. Perrelli and D. Valle*

Institute of Endocrinology and *Department of Internal Medicine II, The Catholic University School of Medicine, Rome, Italy

INTRODUCTION

Anorexia Nervosa (AN) is a psychogenic disturbance of eating behaviour, leading to an extreme starvation, in which a large number of endocrine dysfunctions has been described (1). The GH-IGF1 axis has shown to be widely involved: in fact, high basal levels of GH, usually associated with lower IGF1 values, have been described. Moreover, an altered control of GH secretion, probably related to a hypothalamic dysfunction, has been demonstrated in such a condition (2, 3, 4, 5).

Among the neuroendocrine pathways controlling the GH secretion the role of the cholinergic system has been widely investigated in psychogenic disturbances (6); in AN, a cholinergic dysfunction has been suggested by the observation of the lacking effect of pirenzepine, a cholinergic receptor antagonist, in blunting the GHRH-induced GH release (7, 8). Data by Muller et al have also shown the lack of the effect of a cholinergic agonist (pyridostigmine) on the GH response to GHRH (9).

In order to clarify the role of the cholinergic pathway on the altered GH secretion in AN, we have tested the effect of a cholinergic stimulation on basal levels of GH and on the GHRH-induced GH release in a group of anorectic women. Two drugs, acting at different anatomical levels, were employed: pyridostigmine (PYR), inhibitor of acetylcholinesterase, and oxiracetam (OX), which directly stimulates the central cholinergic neurones (10). The study was performed at 1.00 p.m., since, in our experience, at this time the somatotroph cells exhibit the maximum sensitivity to the modulation exerted by the neurohormones and by the metabolic fuels (3).

MATERIALS AND METHODS

24 anorectic women, aged 15-24 yr., were studied. AN was diagnosed according to DSM IV criteria. All patients were in a stabilised phase of their illness, when their weight was stable and they were eating their customary diet. No one of them was taking medications which could interfere with pituitary secretion. The patients had their usual breakfast at 8.00 a.m., and ate nothing thereafter until after the tests; at 1.00 p.m. (time 0), in a quite room, normal saline was infused into an arm vein through a 19-gauge needle; blood samples were collected through this needle at times 0, 30, 45, 60, 90 and 120 min.

The following tests were performed:

a) PYR-test: PYR (Mestinon, Roche) was administered at time 0 (60 mg p.o.). Blood samples were collected as above indicated.

b) OX-test: OX (Neuromet, Smithlike) was administered at time 0 (400 mg p.o.). Blood samples were collected as above indicated.

c) GHRH-test: GHRH 1-29 (Geref, Serono) was injected i.v. at time 30, as a bolus (50 μg) and blood samples were collected at the times indicated.

d) PYR + GHRH-test: PYR was administered at time 0 and GHRH at time +30, at the same doses and in the same way. Blood samples were collected as above indicated.

e) OX + GHRH-test: OX was administered at time 0 and GHRH at time +30, at the same doses and in the same way. Blood samples were collected as above indicated.

The different tests, when in the same subject, were performed at least 3 days from each other.

Blood samples were centrifuged within two hours and plasma for GH determination was frozen at -20° C until assayed. GH was measured by specific RIA kits, supplied by Radim (Pomezia-Rome, Italy). The sensitivity of the method was 0.5 ng/ml. Intra- and inter-assay coefficients of variation were, respectively, 5.0-6.5% and 6.7-8.9%. The normal range (in adult subjects) was 0.2-10 ng/ml. All samples from each test were measured in the same assay.

Statistical evaluation: basal and peak values in each test were compared by Student's t-test for paired data. One-way analysis of variance (ANOVA) and Student-Newman-Keuls post hoc test were employed for comparing the peak values in the different tests. Results are given as mean $\pm$ SEM.

RESULTS

The response of GH to the administration of OX and PYR alone is reported in fig 1. The peak response occurred between 30 and 90' after the administration of the drug. Both cholinergic agonists induced a slight increment of GH levels.

Fig 2 shows the response of GH to the administration of GHRH, PYR + GHRH and OX + GHRH. Both cholinergic agonists induced a significant increment in the peak response of GH, although the response was more elevated after the administration of PYR.

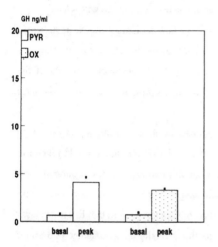

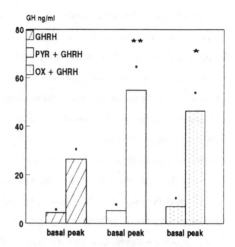

Fig 1: Mean ± SEM GH response to the administration of PYR and OX in AN patients. Basal and peak values are shown.

Fig 2: Mean ± SEM GH response to the administration of GHRH, PYR+GHRH and OX+GHRH in AN patients. Basal and peak values are shown. *p<0.05 and **p<0.01 vs GHRH alone.

DISCUSSION

The cholinergic control of GH secretion is thought to be exerted through the mediation of somatostatin (11). In normal subjects, the augmenting effect of the cholinergic agonists on the basal levels of GH and on the GHRH-induced GH release is therefore due to a inhibition of a somatostatinergic tone.

We have tested the effect of two different cholinergic drugs on basal and GHRH-stimulated GH levels in AN:

PYR is an inhibitor of acetylcholinesterase and acts through an enhancement of the endogenous cholinergic activity.

OX is a 2-pirrolidinone derivative which, despite a gabaergic structure, has shown a cholinergic activity in the central nervous system in animal models, which is due to a direct stimulation of cholinergic neurones. This drug easily crosses the blood-brain barrier and enhances the high affinity choline uptake in the hyppocampus (12, 10, 13). In humans, OX has shown an increasing effect on basal GH levels in normal subjects and on the response of GH to L-dopa in normal and obese subjects (14, 15, 16).

In our study performed in AN patients tested at noon in a chronic phase of the illness, both drugs have shown an slight increasing effect on basal GH levels and a significant increment on the GHRH-induced GH release, which is more evident in the tests performed with PYR.

These data seem to indicate that the cholinergic control of GH is blunted in AN, as indicated by the slight response to the administration of PYR or OX alone, which, in normal subjects, are both able to increase basal GH levels (14, 17). However, a substantial integrity of the cholinergic-somatostatinergic neurotransmission in chronic AN has been shown by the tests performed with PYR+GHRH and OX+GHRH.

It is interesting to compare our data with those reported by Muller et al (9): in fact, they showed the lack of the effect of the cholinergic agonist on the GHRH-induced GH release in acute AN. The different phase of the illness could explain this datum: in fact, our patients were tested in a stabilised phase of the illness, when their weight was stable and they were eating their customary diet. A different cholinergic modulation of GH secretion in the different phases of AN could be therefore suggested. According to this hypothesis, a different pattern of response of GH to GHRH after a cholinergic receptor blockade has been demonstrated by Rolla et al (8) in the acute vs the recovery phase of AN. It is also interesting to underline that the personality and the affective pattern of AN patients can influence the cholinergic control of GH in AN patients (18).

In conclusion, the variations of the nutritional status in the various phases of AN can interfere with the GH dynamics. A careful evaluation of the patients' status and of the phase of the illness is therefore recommended before hormonal evaluations in AN.

REFERENCES

1. Brown, G.M., Garfinkel, P.E., Jeuniewic, M., Moldofsky, H., Stancer, H.C. (1977): Endocrine profiles in anorexia nervosa. In Vigersky RA (ed) Anorexia Nervosa, New York: Raven Press, pp 123-135.

2. Maeda, K., Kato, Y., Yamaguchi, K. (1976): Growth hormone release following thyrotropin releasing hormone injection into patients with anorexia nervosa. Acta Endocrinol (Copenh) 81:1.

3. De Marinis, L., Folli, G., D'Amico, C. (1988): Differential effects of feeding on the ultradian variation of the growth hormone (GH) response to GH-releasing hormone in

normal subjects and patients with obesity and anorexia nervosa. J Clin Endocrinol Metab 66:598-604.

4. De Marinis, L., Mancini, A., Zuppi, P. (1994): Opioid dysregulation in anorexia nervosa: naloxone effects on preprandial and postprandial growth hormone response to growth hormone-releasing hormone. Metabolism 43:140-143.

5. Rolla, M., Andreoni, A., Belliti, D., Federghini, M., Ferrannini, E. (1990): Failure of glucose infusion to suppress the exaggerated GH response to GHRH in patients with anorexia nervosa. Biol Psychiatry 27:215-222.

6. O'Keane, V., O'Flinn, K., Lucey, J.V., Dinan, T.G. (1992): Pyridostigmine-induced growth hormone responses in healthy and depressed subjects: evidence for cholinergic supersensitivity in depression. Psychol Med 22:55-60.

7. Tamai, H., Komaki, G., Matsubayashi, S. (1990). Effect of cholinergic muscarinic receptor blockade on human growth hormone (GH) - releasing hormone (1-44) induced GH secretion in anorexia nervosa. J Clin Endocrinol Metab 70:738-741.

8. Rolla, M., Andreoni, A., Belliti, D., Cristofani, R., Federghini, M. and Muller, E.E. (1991): Blockade of cholinergic muscarinic receptor by pirenzepine and GHRH-induced GH secretion in the acute and recovery phase of anorexia nervosa and atypical eating disorders. Biol Psychiatry 29:1079-1091.

9. Muller, E.E., Locatelli, V., Cocchi, D. (1991): Aspects of growth hormone secretion in GH hypersecretory states. In Faglia G, Beck Peccoz P, Ambrosi B, Travaglini P, Spada A (eds) Pituitary Adenomas, New York: Excerpta Medica, pp 29-38.

10. Mochizuki, D., Sugiyama, S., Shinoda, Y. (1992): Biochemical studies of oxiracetam (CT-848) on cholinergic neurons. Nippon Yakurigaku Zasshi 99: 27-35.

11. Locatelli, V., Torsello, A., Redaelli, M., Ghigo, E., Massara, F. and Muller, E.E. (1986): Cholinergic agonists and antagonists drugs modulate the growth hormone response to growth hormone releasing hormone in the rat: evidence for mediation by somatostatin. J Endocrinol 111:271-278.

12. Pedata, F., Moroni, F., Pepeu, G. (1984): Effect of nootropic agents on brain cholinergic mechanisms. Collegium Internationale Neuro-psychopармacologicum - 14th CINP congress, Firenze.

13. Raiteri, M., Costa, R., Marchi, M. (1992): Effects of oxiracetam on neurotransmitter release from rat hippocampus slices and synaptosomes. Neurosci Lett 145:109-113

14. Mancini, A., De Marinis, L., Fiumara, C. (1988): The role of acethylcholine in the in the regulation of growth hormone secretion: growth hormone response to oxiracetam and L-

dopa in obese subjects. In: Proc. of the I Int Congress "Anorexia, Bulimia and Obesity eating disorders", pp 267-272.

15. De Marinis, L., Mancini, A., Zuppi, P. (1991): Cholinergic control of post-prandial growth hormone secretion in obese children: comparison between direct and indirect cholinergic drugs. In Cavallo L, Job JC, New MI (eds) Growth disorders: the state of art, New York: Raven Press, pp 283-286.

16. De Marinis, L., Mancini, A., Fiumara, C. (1993): Cholinergic modulation of GH secretion in obesity: comparison between direct and indirect stimuli. In Ferrari E, Brambilla F, Solerte SB (eds), Advances in the Biosciences - Vol 90: Primary and Secondary Eating Disorders, Oxford: Pergamon Press, pp 297-300.

17. De Marinis, L., Mancini, A., Zuppi, P. (1992): Influence of Pyridostigmine on the growth hormone (GH) response to GH-releasing hormone pre- and postprandially in normal and obese subjects. J Clin Endocrinol Metab 74:1253-1257.

18. Mancini, A., De Marinis, L., Fabrizi M.L. (1993): Correlation of Growth Hormone dynamics and personality or affective patterns in anorexia nervosa: preliminary data. In: "Advances in Diagnosis and Treatment of Anorexia, Bulimia and Obesity", (M. Cuzzolaro, G. Caputo, V. Guidetti, G. Ripa di Meana Eds), 415-419, Promo Leader Service, Firenze.

Gonadotropin pulsatility in women with premenstrual syndrome

S. Vujović, M. Drezgić, Z. Penezić, M. Stojanović, B.Z. Beleslin, N. Krstić and D. Slijepčević

Institute of Endocrinology, Diabetes and Diseases of Metabolism, KCS, Belgrade, Yugoslavia

ABSTRACT

In order to investigate gonadotropin pulse characteristics in women with premenstrual syndrome we have formed two groups. PMS group: diagnosis was confirmed according to modified Moos's menstrual distress questionnaire. CONTROL group: healthy women without PMS. All of them had regular cycles. Blood samples for FSH, LH, prolactin, estradiol and progesterone were obtained on 7th and 24th day. Pulsatility of FSH and LH was determined on 24th day. All hormones were detected by RIA. Statistic analysis was done by Wilcoxon Mann Whitney test. In the luteal phase estradiol, progesteron and prolactin levels were significantly higher in PMS group than in control. Number and frequency of LH pulses were the same in follicular and luteal phase in PMS group. In luteal phase there were increased number and frequency of LH pulses, compared to controls. Complex interplay of high E_2/Pg ratio, neuropeptides and catecholamines result in increased number and frequency of LH pulses in luteal phase of PMS group.

INTRODUCTION

Premenstrual syndrome is a set of symptoms and signs occuring either abruptly or gradually 2-14 days prior to menstruation and dissapear or become tolerable at the onset of menstration (1-3).The most common physical symptoms are abdominal distension,painfull breasts and acne;and phychical are irritability,anxiety and sudden changes of mood.Among numerous etiological hypothesis (hormones, neuropeptides, neurotransmitters, prostaglandins etc.) very possible one is relative progesterone deficiency and disturbance between estradiol and progesterone prior to menstruation in PMS.

Relationship between LH pulsatile activity and steroid hormone millieu is well known (4,5). Gonadotropin pulse characteristics depends on hypothalamus pacemaker for episodic gonadotropin release,autonomous rhythmic secretion from the pituitary (6), steroid hormones, opioids etc.

The aim of this study was to investigate gonadotropin pulse characteristics in women with PMS in the follicular and luteal phase and compare them with controls.

MATERIALS AND METHODS

Subjects

There were 23 women in PMS group, 28.5 ±4.2 y. old, BMI 22.8 ±2.3 kg/m^2.The diagnosis was confirmed according to Modified Moos menstrual questionnaire. Control group consisted of 18 women without PMS,26.0 ±3.4 y.old,BMI 23.2 ±2.8 kg/m^2.All of them had regular ovulatory cycles and were free of diseases and medications. Blood samples for follicular stimulating hormone (FSH),luteinizing hormone (LH),prolactin (PRL), estradiol (E$_2$) and progesterone (Pg) were obtained on 7th and 24th day of the cycle.On 24th day an indwelling heparin-lock cannula was inserted into a forearm vien 30 min prior to the start of FSH and LH sampling,6 h on 15 min intervals.

Hormone assays

Serum levels of FSH,LH and Pg were determined by comercial RIA kit (INEP Zemun, Yugoslavia), with intra- and interassay coefficients: FSH 6.34% and 10.73%, LH 4.99% and 15.98%, Pg 10.55% and 7.9%. PRL and E$_2$ were measured with comercial RIA (Delfia, Wallac Oy),with intra- and interassay coefficients: PRL 2.0% and 5.7%;and 10% and 9.7% for E$_2$.

Statistic analysis

Statistic analysis was done with Wilcoxon Mann Whitney test. Results were expresed as mean (± SD). Pulse characteristics were analysed by Pulsar Peak Identification Algorithm.

RESULTS

In luteal phase (24th day), FSH,LH and PRL levels and E_2/Pg ratio were significantly higher in PMS group (Tab.1).

Table 1 Plasma hormone concentrations (mean ±SD) of PMS and control group on 24th day of the menstrual cycle

	PMS	CONTROLS	p
FSH (IU/L)	5.0 ±2.3	4.6 ±1.9	<0.05*
LH (IU/L)	4.8 ±2.4	3.5 ±1.6	<0.05*
PRL (mIU/L)	446.4 ±223.8	210.0 ±112.0	<0.05*
E_2 (nmol/L)	346.2 ±245.2	190.0 ±86.0	<0.05*
Pg (nmol/L)	3.2 ±1.6	32.6 ±13.4	<0.05*
E2/Pg	108.1 ±23.2	5.8 ±2.3	<0.05*

* Wilcoxon Mann Whitney test

Maximal progesterone value in PMS group was 9 days prior to menstruation,while in control was 6 days prior.According to our previous PMS study (7),progesterone rise from ovulation to 19th day,than sharply falls down low on 24th day (Fig.1).

Table 2 Pulsatile characteristics of LH in PMS and control group on 24th day of menstrual cycle

	PMS	CONTROLS	p
No of peaks	5 ± 2	1 ± 1	<0.05*
Amplitude (IU/L)	0.95 ±0.38	0.45 ±0.24	<0.05*
Peak lenght (min)	45.0 ±22.1	15.0 ±9.0	<0.05*
Frequency (1/s)	0.0139 ±0.053	0.0028±0.001	<0.05*
Inter-peak (min)	71.25 ±22.7	0.0	<0.05*

* Wilcoxon Mann Whitney test

LH pulse characteristics of both groups in luteal phase are shown on Tab.2 and Fig.2. Pulse frequency and amplitude were significantly higher in PMS group than in controls. There were no significant diferences in pulsatility of LH

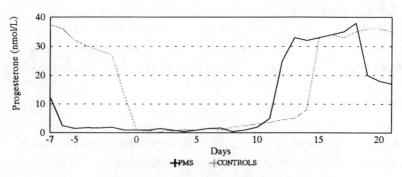

Fig.1. Progesterone levels during the cycle in PMS & control group.

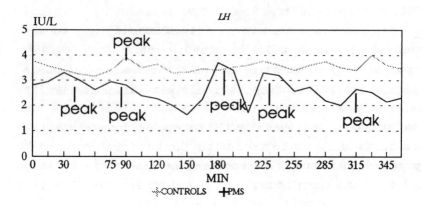

Fig.2. Pulsatility of LH in the luteal phase in PMS & control group.

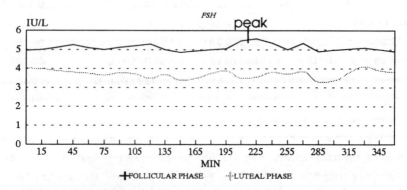

Fig.3. Pulsatility of FSH in follicular & luteal phase in PMS group.

and FSH between follicular and luteal phase in PMS group (Fig.3).

DISCUSSION

Women with PMS have very dynamic daily variations of hormone levels. Our previous study indicated higher FSH level in PMS group than in control prior to menstruation and higher FSH and LH in the follicular phase in PMS group. Such a hormonal milieu plays an important role in earlier separation of the dominant follicle and earlier ovulation in PMS group (12th day). Progesterone rise until 19th day (or 9 days prior to menstruation) and then rapidly falls down (on 24th day plasma level is 3.2 nmol/L). Hyperestrogenemia on the same day, is possibly due to higher FSH level. E_2/Pg ratio is high. In that particular time symptoms become severe. Similar results were shown by Rubinow et al.,1989 (8).

LH pulsatility is changing during the cycle. In the period of low estradiol exposure,as in follicular phase of the cycle,LH pulses are of high frequency and low amplitude (9). Soules et al.,(10) found that inter-peak interval in that period is 64 min, while in our patients is 60 min. In the luteal phase of control group there is decline in LH pulse frequency, but amplitude is high. Progesterone,acting sinergistically with estrogens exerts negative feedback on the hypothalamus during the luteal phase, thus limiting GnRH pulsatility and slowing down LH pulse frequency possibly via an opioid mechanism. Filicori et al.(11), found LH pulses of low amplitudes interimposed between those of larger amplitude and that low amplitudes could represent autonomous secretory activity of the pituitary.

In our PMS group on 24th day there were high E_2/Pg ratio and relative progesterone deficiency.That could be one of the reasons for high frequency of LH pulses.The feedback by ovarian steroids differentially modulates both the release of hypothalamic GnRH, pituitary sensitivity and character of ultradian and circadian LH pulse patterns. ß-endorphine, met-enkephalin and dynorphin are gonadal steroid dependent and they have influences on GnRH pulse generator as well. GnRH neurons possess intrinsic pulsatility regulated by aminergic input with neuropeptides acting either in concert with aminergic system, or by modulating it. Endogenous catecholamines, such as dopamine, inhibit pulsatile LH release, and they are possibly low on 24th day of the cycle in PMS group.

Complex interplay of high E2/Pg ratio, neuropeptides and catecholamines result in increased number and frequency of LH pulses in the luteal phase in PMS group.

REFERENCES

1. Bäckstörm, T. (1983). The relationship between mood change and hormonal levels during the menstrual cycles in women with premenstrual syndrome and normal volounteers. *Psychosom.Med.*, **45**, 503-512

2. O'Brien, P.M. (1985). The premenstrual syndrome. *J.Reprod.Med.*, **30**, 113-6.

3. Slijepčević, D. (1993). Pulsatilnost gonadotropina. In Slijepčević, D. *Reproduktivna endokrinologija*, pp.156-180. (Beograd, Naučna knjiga)

4. Rossmanith, W.G., Laughlin, G.A., Mortola, J.F. and Yen, S.S.C. (1990). Secretory dynamics of estradiol (E2) and progesterone (Pg) during periods of relative pituitary LH quiescence in the midluteal phase of the menstrual cycle. *Clin Endocrinol.*, **32**, 23-32

5. Schweiger, U., Tuschl, R., Broocks, A. and Pirke, K.M. (1990). Gonadotropin secretion in the second half of the menstrual cycle: comparasion of women with normal cycles, luteal phase deffects and disturbed follicular development. *Clin.Endocrinol.*, **32**, 33-39

6. Rossmanith, W.G., Gambacciani, M. (1994). Autonomous gonadotropin release from the human pituitary in vitro and factors influencing this secretion. *Gynecol.Endocrinol.*, **8**, 265-275.

7. Vujović, S. (1991). Pulsatilnost gonadotropina u žena sa PMS. In Vujović, S. *Ultrasonografske i funkcione karakteristike žena sa predmenstruacionim sindromom.*, pp 165-190. (Beograd, BIGZ)

8. Rubinow, D.R., Smith, P.J. (1989). Models for development and expresion of symptoms in premenstrual syndrome. *Psych.Clin North.Am.*, **12**, 53-68

9. Rossmanith, W.G. (1993). Ultradian and circadian patterns in LH secretion during reproductive life in women. *Hum.Reprod.*, **8**, 77-83

10. Soules, M., (1987), Corpus luteum insufficiency induced by rapid gonadotropin releasing hormone induced gonadotropin secretion pattern in the follicular phase. *J.Clin.Endocrinol.Metab.*, **65**, 457-464

11. Filicori, M., Santoro, N., Merriam, G.R, Crowley, W.F. (1986). Characterization of the physiological pattern of episodic gonadotropin secretion trought the human menstrual cycle. *J.Clin.Endocrinol.Metab.*, **62**, 1136-1144

Headache in primary empty sella: a psychoneuroendocrinological approach

A. Mancini, G. Conte, D. Valle**, C. D'Amico, C. Anile*, G. Maira*** and L. De Marinis

Institutes of Endocrinology and *Neurosurgery, **Department of Internal Medicine II, Catholic University of Rome and ***Department of Neurosurgery, University of Perugia, Italy

INTRODUCTION

Empty Sella Syndrome (ESS) is a clinical picture due to a herniation of the subarachnoidal space into the sella turcica in subjects who have not received neurosurgical interventions or radiotherapy on the pituitary gland (Primary Empty Sella, PES). It is due to a chronic or intermittent (benign) intracranial hypertension and causes a progressive compression of the pituitary stalk, leading to an impairment of pituitary secretion (1, 2). It is usually found in young, hypertensive women, often associated with overweight or obesity, and causes headache, hirsutism, irregular menses (up to amenorroea), galactorroea and, in a few cases, rinoliquorroea. Due to these symptoms, ESS and PES are often casual findings in the differential diagnosis of pituitary adenomas (3-5).

The endocrine picture of PES shows an altered control of prolactin secretion, with normal as well as high basal levels. In a few cases a panhypopituitarism or a selective impairment of pituitary function (regarding the gonadotropin, the adrenal and/or the thyroid axes) has been described (6-8).

Previous studies of ours have investigated the neuroendocrine alterations involved in this syndrome and leading to the altered secretion of gonadotropins, prolactin and growth hormone. The dopaminergic system, the endogenous opioids and the serotoninergic tone have demonstrated to be involved, possibly through a reciprocal, complex interaction (9-11).

We have now focused our attention on the symptom headache, which is commonly present in ESS, and is often the only symptom appearing in these patients. In some cases it persists even after a liquoral shunt in hypertensive subjects. This parameter has been compared with the main psycho-endocrinological elements and with the evaluation of intracranial pressure (ICP).

MATERIALS AND METHODS

30 female subjects, aged 30-54 ys, underwent this study after informed consent. They came to our observation because of the symptoms of headache (73%), oligo-amenorroea (22%), overweight (56%), hypertrichosis (26%). Eight of them showed amenorroea and the evaluation of basal FSH, LH and $17\beta E_2$ confirmed the post-menopausal status. The diagnosis of PES, suspected on the clinical and hormonal picture and on the basis of skull X-Ray, was confirmed in all subjects through a high performance CT scan or MRI. All patients underwent a standard GnRH-test (Relisorm L-100, Serono, 100 μg i.v., blood samples collection at times 0, 15, 30, 60 and 120 min.). The test, in the premenopausal patients, was performed in the follicular phase of the menstrual cycle, as assessed through the determination of $17\beta E_2$ levels. An increment of 50-200% for FSH and of 200-400% for LH after GnRH administration was considered normal. 13 subjects underwent the evaluation of diurnal ICP in basal conditions and after hypertonic infusion, as previously described (7). As previously reported, normal values of mean ICP, in an awake, relaxed patients with normal respiration are lower than 15 mmHg; an increase in ICP during REM sleep or during a lumbar infusion test is abnormal when higher than 25 mmHg. We also performed other tests of pituitary function and reserve: PRL and TSH after metoclopramide (10 mg p.o.), basal determination of plasma T_3, T_4, cortisol and $17\beta E_2$. FSH and LH were measured through specific radioimmunoassay kits, supplied by Ares-Serono Diagnostica (Milan, Italy); PRL, TSH, T_3, T_4, cortisol, $17\beta E_2$ were assayed by RIA as previously described (8).

Statistical evaluation was performed employing one-way ANOVA for comparing peak responses among groups of patients.

RESULTS

The patients were classified in two groups on the basis of the symptom "headache": group A: patients with headache (n = 22); group B: patients without headache (n = 8). There was no clear correlation between ICP and the symptom "headache". In fact, among the 13 patients tested, showed increased ICP values in basal condition and/or after infusion test: 5 of them belonged to group A and 3 to group B. Similarly, patients with normal ICP were present in both groups (4 in group A and 1 in group B). The gonadotropin response to GnRH allowed to furtherly distinguish group A patients as follows:

170

group 1A (n = 12): patients with an exaggerated response of FSH and LH to GnRH;

group 2A (n = 10): patients with a normal response of FSH and LH to GnRH.

A normal gonadotropin responsiveness to GnRH administration was observed in all patients of group B. They also showed other symptoms, such as weakness and lipotimic episodes, more often than group A patients.

Statistical evaluation showed a significant difference between group 1A and group B (p < 0.01) and between group 1A and group 1B (p<0.001) when considering the percentage of increment of LH after GnRH administration (peak value, fig 1).

Moreover, among the 10 patients of group 2A, who showed headache without a gonadotropin hyperresponsiveness, 6 were postmenopausal (mean LH = 41.6, mean FSH = 67.2); in two other subjects ICP determination showed a hypertensive PES. Other pituitary hormones, T_3, T_4, cortisol and $17\beta E_2$ levels are reported in table I.

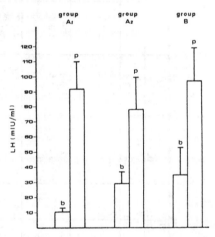

Fig 1. Mean ± SEM basal level and peak response of LH after GnRH administration in the three groups of patients (see text for groups description).

DISCUSSION

PES is a clinical picture in which the symptom of headache is quite common (73% in our casuistry). Although the term is derived from post-mortem studies, a pathophysiological finding can explain the genesis of this anatomic abnormality in vivo: a chronic or intermittent elevated ICP can explain the intrasellar herniation of the arachnoid (1, 2, 12). A clear correlation of elevated ICP and endocrine abnormalities, particularly the altered PRL circadian rhythm, has been demonstrated (7, 8). However, it is difficult to explain the mechanism underlying this relationship: in fact, the stalk compression is only one of the possible explanations. The coexistence of a pituitary (micro)adenoma or of autoimmune

TABLE I. Mean (± SEM) plasma hormone levels in 30 patients affected by ES, with (group A) or without (group B) headache (see text for further group division).
° post-menopausal subjects
* follicular phase
z after metoclopramide (10 mg p.o.)
y after GnRH (100 µg i.v.)

	PRL (basal)	PRL (peak)[z]	TSH (basal)	TSH (peak)[z]	T_3	T_4	cortisol	$17\beta E_2$	FSH (basal)	FSH (peak)[y]
group A1 (n=12)	12.9 ±2.7	139.4 ±14.8	1.7 ±0.2	2.3 ±0.4	93.8 ±3.9	8.0 ±0.4	121.1 ±9.7	41.4 ±13.7	10.0 ±1.2	22.6 ±2.9
group A2 (n=10)	12.4 ±2.7	112.9 ±18.7	1.7 ±0.2	2.3 ±0.4	108.9 ±11.6	8.1 ±0.3	153.1 ±20.6	89.3 ±44.7 12.7° ±1.4	7.9 ±2.5 70.2° ±14.5	11.5 ±2.5 90.8° ±17.3
group B (n=8)	14.2 ±3.7	149.1 ±21.7	1.7 ±0.3	2.3 ±0.4	105.4 ±5.8	8.4 ±0.8	140.5 ±10.2	56.3 ±21.9 11.5° ±0.5	10.8 ±1.5 63.8° ±5.5	16.1 ±1.2 106.6° ±13.9
normal range	5-25 (ng/ml)		0.5-5 (µU/ml)		60-180 (ng/dl)	4-11 (pg/dl)	75-210 (ng/ml)	20-70* 10-30° (pg/ml)	5-15* 40-130° (mIU/ml)	

mechanisms have been considered (4, 13, 14). The endocrine dynamics, particularly the altered prolactin secretion, suggest a dysregulation of the neurotransmitter control of the gland (15). From this hypothesis, PES can be considered a useful model to investigate the central mechanism of regulation of pituitary secretion (11).

In this paper we have considered the symptom headache, which is often a pre-diagnostic finding in these patients.

We have observed a normal gonadotropin responsiveness in patients without this symptom (group B). The hyperresponsiveness of FSH and LH appears only in a group of cephalalgic subjects (group 1A). The analysis of group 2A, however, allows to hypothesise that menopause or elevated basal ICP can contribute to mask this response. A common neuroendocrine abnormality could therefore underlie the increased gonadotropin reserve and the symptom headache. Moreover, the gonadotropin dynamic could be considered a useful marker for the classification of PES patients.

A suggestive hypothesis, which requires further experimental confirmations, regards a possible serotoninergic dysregulation which could explain both headache and gonadotropin hyperresponsiveness in PES. In a previous study (16) we observed a restoration of a normal PRL circadian rhythm in PES patients after the administration of L-Triptophane, precursor of serotonine. Therefore, the hypothesis of a neuroendocrine genesis of the altered hormonal secretion in PES and a possible correlation with the clinical picture should be worth considering for further investigations.

REFERENCES

1. Neelon, F.A., Goree, J.A., Lebowitz, H.E.: The Primary Empty Sella: clinical and radiographic characteristics and endocrine function. Medicine 52 (1973) 73-92.

2. Kaye, A.H. Tress, B.M., Brownbill, D, King, J: Intracranial pressure in patients with the empty sella syndrome without benign intracranial hypertension. J. Neurol. Neurosurg. Psychiat. 45 (1982) 209-216.

3. Brismar, K: Prolactin secretion in the empty sella syndrome, in prolactinomas and in acromegaly. Acta Med. Scand. 209 (1981) 397-405.

4. Kleinberg, D.L., Noel, G.L., and Franz, A.G.: Galactorrhoea: a study of 235 cases, including 48 with pituitary tumors. N. Engl. J. Med. 296(11) (1977) 589-600.

5. Malerkey, W.B., Goodenow, T.J., Lanese, R.R.: Diurnal variation of prolactin secretion differentiates pituitary tumors from the primary empty sella syndrome. Am. J. Med. 69 (1980) 886-890.

6. Brisinai, K., and Efendic, S: Pituitary function in the empty sella syndrome. Neuroendocrinology 32 (1981) 70-77.

7. Maira, G., Anile, C., Cioni, B., Menini, E., Mancini, A., De Marinis, L., and Barbarino A.: Relationships between intracranial pressure and diurnal prolactin secretion in primary empty sella. Neuroendocrinology 38 (1984) 102-107.

8. Barbarino, A., De Marinis, L., Mancini, A., D'Amico, C., Sambo, P., Passeri, M., Anile, C., and Maira, G.: Prolactin dynamics in normoprolactinemic primary empty sella: correlation with intracranial pressure. Hormone Res. 27 (1987) 141-151.

9. Grossman, A., Moult, P.J.A., McIntyre, H., Evans, J., Silverstone, T., Rees, L.H., and Besser, G.M.: Opiate mediation of amenorroea in hyperprolactinaemia and in weight-loss related amenorroea. Clin. Endocrinol. 17 (1982) 379-388.

10. Mancini, A., Fiumara, C., Fabrizi, M.L., Colosimo Jr, C., D'Amico, C., Conte, G., and De Marinis, L.: The primary empty sella: relationship between gonadotropin dynamics and dopaminergic tone. Experimental and Clinical Endocrinology (Life Sci. Adv.), Trivandrum (India) 11 (1992) 209-213.

11. Mancini, A., Conte, G., Fiumara, C., Fabrizi, M.L., Iacona, T., Zuppi, P.,Colosimo, C. and De Marinis, L.: Opioid-dopaminergic interactions in primary empty sella. Exp. Clin. Endocrinol. 101 (1993) 277-282.

12. Weisberg, L.A., Housepian, E.M., Saur, D.P.: Empty sella syndrome as complication of benign intracranial hypertension. J. Neurosurg. 43 (1975) 177-180.

13. Bierre, P., Gyldensted, C., Riishede, J., Lindholm, J.: The empty sella and pituitary adenomas. A theory on the causal relationship. Acta Neurol. Scand. 66 (1982) 82-92.

14. De Marinis, L., Mancini, A., Minnielli, S., Masala, R., Anile, C., Maira, G., Barbarino, A.: Evaluation of dopaminergic tone in hyperprolactinemia. III. Thyroid-Stimulating Hormone response to Metoclopramide in differential diagnosis and postoperative follow-up of prolactinoma patients. Metabolism 34 (1985) 917-922.

15. Delitala, G., Devilla, L., Arata, L.: Opiate receptor and anterior pituitary hormone secretion in man. Effect of Naloxone infusion. Acta Endocrinol. 97 (1981) 150-156.

16. De Marinis, L., Mancini, A., Fiumara, C., Conte, G., Fabrizi, M.L., Iacona, T. and Sammartano, L.: Nocturnal prolactin increase in primary empty sella: role of serotonin. In: Genazzani, A.R., D'Ambrogio G. and Artini P.G. (eds). Current investigations in Gynecology and Obstetrics, pp 117-122, The Parthenon Publishing Groups, Carnforth, UK, 1993.

Nasal spray administration of bromocriptine: a preliminary study

E. Cicinelli, R. Maiorino, D. Petruzzi, G. Ragno*, C. Ruccia, T. Falco, G. Matteo and L.M. Schönauer

Cattedra di Ginecologia ed Ostetricia and *Dipartimento Farmaco-Chimico, University of Bari, Italy

INTRODUCTION

Bromocriptine mesylate (BCP) is the most commonly used compound in the treatment of hyperprolactinemia. Nausea and vomiting are recognized as common side-effects particularly at the initiation of the oral BCP assumption (1, 2). Gastro-intestinal side-effects can determine in some cases heavy discomfort to the patients so that they are estimated to cause at least 10% of patient to discontinue treatment (3). Therefore, alternative administration routes for BCP have been investigated with the aim to minimize the undesired side-effects and improve compliance. Both intramuscular and vaginal routes have shown to be therapeutically effective and free of significant gastro-intestinal disturbances (3,4). A new promising administration route for drugs subject to intestinal and liver first-pass metabolism after oral dosing is the nasal mucosa. Nasal route has been largely investigated in animals and humans for administering both proteic and steroidal molecules; among steroid hormones, progesterone when nasally administered to menopausal women showed a bioavailability comparable to that of the intramuscular route (5). Moreover, nasal route allows BCP not only to reach systemic circulation avoiding first-pass intestinal and liver metabolism but also, by considering the close anatomical relationships between the olfactory nasal mucosa and the brain, it could offer a direct delivery of the drug to hypothalamic areas (Fig. 1).

The aim of this preliminary study was to investigate the effectiveness of nasal route for administering BCP in physiologically hyperprolactemic women in the early days of puerperium.

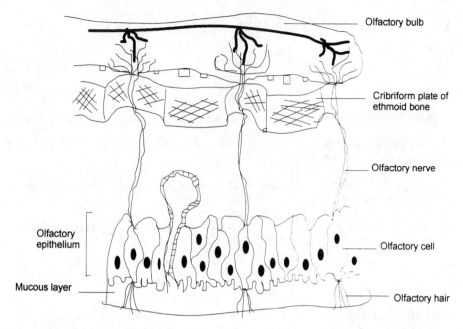

Fig. 1 Schematic representation of anatomical relatioships between nasal olphactory mucosa and brain through the lamina cribrosa of the ethmoyd bone.

MATERIALS AND METHODS

Six women in 3rd-5th day of puerperium after spontaneous delivery were enrolled in the study previous their informed consent. All of the women had asked of interrumpting breats feading because of psychological reasons.

Bromocriptine was dissolved in isopropyl alcohol 10 ml, propylene glycol 20 ml, water 30 ml at a final BCP concentration of 1.67 mg/ml. The solution was intranasally sprayed in single administration by an appropriate dispenser. The administered dose was 0.25 ml per nostril corresponding to 0.8 mg of BGP. All the administrations were given by the same doctor, with the patients in a sitting position and their head up.

Extensive blood pressure measurements during the experiment were performed; the occurrence of nausea, vomiting, dizziness, unpleasant taste and endonasal burning was also monitored.

Three blood samples were drawn after inserting a cannula in the antecubital vein at 45, 30 and 15 minutes before the administration and after the following times: 15, 30, 45, 60, 120, 180, 240, 300, 420 and 480 minutes. Serum was separated by centrifugation and stored at -20 C until analyzed.

SERUM LEVELS OF PRL

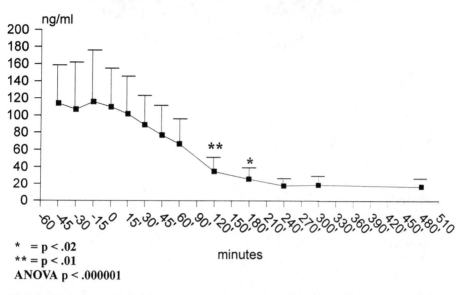

* = p < .02
** = p < .01
ANOVA p < .000001

Fig. 2 The time course of serum PRL levels before and after the nasal BCP administration. Data are mean ± SD.

Serum were assayed by RIA by using a commercial kit (Prolactin SR1, Ares Serono, Milan, Italy). The sensitivity of the assay was 0.5 ng/ml. Intra-assay and interassay variability was < 15%.

Statistical analysis was performed by ANOVA and Student t-test. A level of P < .05 was considered statistically significant.

RESULTS

The time course of serum PRL levels (mean ± SD) before and after administration is shown in Fig. 2. The side-effects referred by the patients are listed in Table 1.

After the administration serum levels of PRL decreased dramatically in all of the women. The reduction of mean serum levels was significant between the 1st and 2nd hour (P < .01) and between the 2nd and 3rd hour (P < .02). Anova analysis of PRL serum levels observed in the same subjects at different times showed a statistically significant difference (F = 8.70, dfD = 40, P < .000001). Four hours after the administration mean serum levels of PRL resulted in the normal range (< 20 ng/ml); at the 8th hour the PRL levels were still normal.

Table 1 Side-effects referred by the patients after the nasal BCP administration.

NASAL SPRAY BCP
SIDE EFFECTS

Patients Initials	A.L.	T.R.	A.F.	C.R.	E.C.	N.N.
Nausea	+	-	-	-	-	-
Vomiting	-	-	-	-	-	-
Hypotension	-	-	-	-	-	-
Dizziness	-	-	-	-	-	-
Unplesant taste	+	+	++	+	-	-
Endonasal burning	+	++	+	+	+	+

Grading:
+ = light
+ + = mild
+ + + = strong

No one patient complained of dizziness and hypotension; one patient had a light nausea and four patients (67%) referred mild or slight endonasal burning and unpleasant taste that disappeared in a few minutes.

DISCUSSION

Bromocriptine, when orally administered, is promptly metabolized in the liver and only a little fraction (3-4%) reaches the systemic circulation unchanged (6,7). Gastro-intestinal disturbances are the most frequent undesired side-effects of the oral therapy with BCP; although these symptoms are though to reflect BCP action at the central nervous system level, they have been also related to the local concentration of the dopamine agonist in the stomach and gut when taken orally. Experiences with long-acting depot form of Parlodel by injections have demonstrated that even if the serum levels of BCP reached by this way are higher with respect to those following oral intake the number of side-effects is significantly lower (8). Therefore, investigations on new administration route allowing th avoidance the intestinal passage have raised up. Bromocriptine, intravaginally administered, resulted effective in the treatment of symptomatic PRL-producing pituitary macroadenoma in a patient in whom protracted nausea and vomiting precluded the oral administration of the drug (9). Jasonni and coworkers have demonstrated the effectiveness of the vaginal route in both hyperprolactemic patients and puerperal women (3); they referred the occurrence of vaginal burning as single side-effect. However, vaginal route, in our opinion, has two further limits consisting in the discomfort due to the possible vaginal discharge and in the limited acceptance by many women.

Nasal route has been demonstrated to be useful for sistemic administration of drugs. From a pharmacokinetic point of view, the nasal mucosa possesses suitable characteristics such as a wide mucosa surface (>150 cm^2), the presence of microvillous structures, a reach vascularization, the possibility to avoid the intestinal and liver first-pass metabolism and probably the chance of a direct access to the brain. Indeed, on the basis of the observation that nasally administered β-endorfine was more effective in elevating serum prolactin levels in monkeys than equal doses administered intravenously, it has been suggested that nasal dosing could increase delivery to the brain (10). In particular, nasal administration may provide access to brain through areas unprotected by the blood-brain barrier (11,12); the mechanisms of this direct pathway have been speculated to consist in the passage through the intracellular spaces (13) or in pinocytotic processes inside the olfactory neurous (11-14).

The mean serum levels of PRL started to drop a few minutes after the administration and they halved within one hour; the greatest reduction, that was statistically significant, occurred in the second hour from the administration. Mean serum levels reached normal range (< 20 ng/ml) four hours after the administration and lasted until the last blood sampling at 480 minutes; unfortunately, the study design did not allow us to determine the overall duration of the effect because the sampling was discontinued after 8 hours.

It must be stresses that the total nasally administered dose (0.8 mg) is about one third of that normally used by mouth (2.5 mg).

Although the number of patients was very limited, encouraging results were obtained also about undesired side-effects. No one complained of gastro-intestinal effect or sistemic reactions; in four out six women only a mild or light endonasal burning and unpleasant taste were referred.

Considering the small number of patients, we cannot draw definitive conclusions; however, our results suggest that nasal route could be an effective and probably safe administration route for BCF especially in cases of oral BCP intolerance and demonstrate the opportunity for further investigation on nasal administration of BCP.

REFERENCES

1. Thorner MO, Fluckinger E, Calne DB (1980). Bromocriptine. A clinical and pharmacological review. New York, Raven Press, p 42, 143.

2. Cuellar FG (1980). Bromocriptine mesylate (Parlodel) in the management of amenorrhea-galactorrhea associated with hyperprolactinemia. Obstet Gynecol, 55, 278-84.

3. Jasonni VM, Raffelli R, De March A, Frank G, Flamigni C (1991). Vaginal bromocriptine in hyperprolactinemic patients and puerperal women. Acta Obstet Gynecol Scand, 70, 493-5.

4 Katz E, Weiss BE, Hassell A, Schran HF, Adashi EY (1991). Increased circulating levels of bromocriptine after vaginal compared with oral administration. Fertil Steril 55, 882-4.

5. Cicinelli E, Savino F, Cagnazzo I, Scorcia P (1993). Comparative study of progesterone plasma levels after nasal spray and intramuscolar administration of natural progesterone in menopausal. Gynecol Obstet Invest, 35, 172-174.

6. Aellig WH, Nuesch E (1977). Comparative pharmacokinetic investigations with tritium-labeled ergot alkaloids after oral and intravenous administration in man. Int J Clin Pharmacol Res 15, 106-12.

7. Schran HF, Bhuta SI, Scwarz HJ, Thorner MO (1980). The pharmacokinetics of bromocriptine in man. In Ergot Compounds Brain Function: Neuroendocrine and Neuropsychiatric Aspects, Edited by M Goldstein, DB Calne, A Lieberman, MO Thorner. New York, Raven Press, 125-39.

8. Rolland R (1990). On Parlodel^R LAR and optimal treatment of hyperprolactinemia. In RJ Pepperel: New Aspects of dopamine agonist therapy in menstrual cycle disorders and infertility. The Parthenon Publishing Group ed, Casterton Hall, Carnforth, Lancs UK, 33-46.

9. Katz E, Schran HF, Adashi EY (1989). Successful treatment of a prolactin-producing pituitary macroadenoma with intravaginal bromocriptine mesylate: a novel approach to intolerance of oral therapy. Obstet Gynecol 73, 517-20.

10. Jagannadha RA, Moudal NR, Li CH (1986). beta-Endorphin: intranasal administration increases the serum prolactin level in monkeys. Int J Pept Protein Res 28, 546-8.

11. Gopinath PG, Gopinath RD, Anad Kumar TC (1978). Target site of intranasally sprayed substances and their transport across the nasal mucosa: a new insight into intranasal route of drug delivery. Curr Ther Res 23, 596-607.

12. Balin BJ, Broadwell RD, Salcman M, el-Kalliny M (1986). Avenues for entry peripherally administered protein to the central nervous system in mouse, rat, and squirrel monkeys. J Comp Neurol 251, 260-80.

13. Faraj JA, Hussain AA, Aramaki Y, Iseki K, Kagoshima M, Dittert LW (1990). Mechanism of nasal absorption of drugs. III: nasal absorption of leucine enkephalin. J Pharm Sci 79, 698-702.

14. Hussain MA, Rakestraw D, Rowe S, Aungst B (1990). Nasal administration of a cognition enhancer provides improved bioavailability but not enhanced brain delivery. J Pharm Sci 79, 771-2.

The role of melatonin in menstrual disorders of obese adolescents during weight loss

G. Grugni, G. Calò, G. Guzzaloni, E. Tonelli, C. De Medici and F. Morabito

Italian Auxological Centre of Piancavallo – IRCCS, Milan, Italy

INTRODUCTION

Though the first reports concerning the role of the pineal gland date back a century or so ago, only in the last years it has been demonstrated how the gland exercises its influence on the endocrine system (1-2), particularly on those mechanisms responsible for determining onset of puberty (3), and on the immune system (4-5) as well as in a number of psychiatric disorders (6-7). Amongst the latter are found the eating disorders that include anorexia nervosa and bulimia nervosa, diseases in which an abnormal secretion of melatonin (aMT), the most important hormone secreted by the epiphyseal gland (8-9) has been observed. With regard to this, it is well known that variations in calorie intake determine changes in nocturnal aMT secretion also in healthy normal weight subjects (10), so confirming the presence of a relationship of body weight to aMT. In this context studies on the light/darkness rhythm of the pineal gland hormone in obese subjects have showed contrasting results since both a normal (11) and altered (12) diurnal aMT circadian pattern have been reported. However, when obese subjects undergo short-term complete fasting, changes in aMT nocturnal secretory pattern can be seen, probably secondary to hypoglycæmia that develops in this condition (13). It is also known that in these patients the calorie restrictions can alone determine, besides positive effects following weight loss, also alterations of reproductive function with significant abnormalities both in gonadotropin (Gn) secretion (14) as in their urinary excretion (15); altered menstrual cycles may also appear similarly to what observed in normal weight women undergoing calorie deprivation (16), with consequent weight loss.

Since aMT has an inhibitory effect on reproductive function (17-18), this study examines the aMT secretory pattern in a group of obese female subjects in whom after protracted calorie restriction oligomenorrhea was observed, with the aim to demonstrate a possible relationship between aMT and menstrual disorders.

PATIENTS AND METHODS

Ten female subjects with severe obesity (Table 1) were included in the study. A complete medical work-up was carried out to confirm the condition of essential obesity, such as the endocrinological evaluation of thyroid, pancreatic and suprarenal glands. In all cases menarche had taken place at least two years before and all subjects had regular cycles at the beginning of the study (mean 30 days). During hospitalization subjects were given a Very Low Calorie Diet (VLCD: 600 KCal = 2,512 kJ/day; protein g 48 = 30.6%, lipids g 20.7 = 29% and carbohydrate g 62.1 = 39.4%) for 45 days, without any pharmacological treatment that could interfere with this regimen.

Besides assaying basal values for LH, FSH and 17-beta-estradiol (E2), in all subjects the aMT circadian pattern was evaluated in basal conditions as well as after dietary restriction, by means of venous blood samples drawn at 1 pm, 5 pm, 9 pm, 1 am, 5 am and 9 am. During the darkness hours, the blood was sampled under a dim red light to minimize any influence on aMT synthesis (19); all the examinations were performed during the winter period.

Individual and parental informed consent was obtained from all the subjects; the entire study protocol was approved by the local Ethical Committee.

Serum levels of aMT were determined, after extractions with dyethylether, by means of a double antibody RIA using commercially available kits (Bioscience Product, The Netherlands). Coefficients of intra- and inter-assay variation were 3% and 8% respectively. All data were expressed as mean+SE.

aMT circadian rhythm was evaluated as area under the curve (AUC: pg/ml/h), using the trapezoidal method, and as a mean of the values obtained at the various times. The statistical analysis was performed using Student's t test for paired data; values of p less than 0.05 were considered significant.

Table 1 Clinical characteristics of the study group. BMI: Body Mass Index (Kg/m2); (A) before and (B) after diet. *p<0.001 vs basal conditions.

subjects (no.)	10
mean age (yrs.)	15.7
mean menarcheal age (yrs.)	13
BMI (A)	38.8+1.1
BMI (B)	34.4+1.0*

RESULTS

Hypocaloric dietetic treatment determined considerable weight loss (Table 1) and in all patients this was accompanied by oligomenorrhea (mean 36 days). The analysis of variations in aMT secretory pattern expressed as AUC, after weight reduction, revealed a significant increase in serum levels of pineal gland hormone with respect to basal levels: 845+52 vs 690+50 (p<0.05). The analysis of aMT mean concentrations taken at 4 hour intervals, showed the physiological light/darkness rhythm of the hormone, characterized by the peak of nocturnal secretion both at the beginning and the end of the study (Figure 1). However, after weight reduction aMT values were higher at all times with significant differences for samples taken at 1 am (83+6 vs 63+8 pg/ml), 5 am (66.5+5 vs 51.4+6 pg/ml) and 9 am (19+1 vs 15+1 pg/ml). As concerns the values of Gn and E2, there was no change between values at the beginning (A) and end (B)of the study: LH: 3.6+0.9 (A) vs 4.5+1.7 (B) mU/ml:p=0.6. FSH:4.6+0.7 (A) vs 4.7+0.6 (B) mU/ml: p=0.6; E2: 47+7 (A) vs 61+8 (B) pg/ml: p=0.1 .

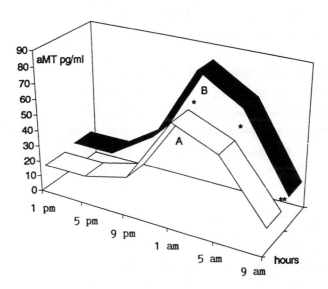

Figure 1 aMT circadian rhythm before (A) and after (B) weight loss. *p<0.01; **p<0.05.

DISCUSSION

In normal weight conditions calorie restriction determines an increase in serum aMT levels in the experimental model (20), whereas in man an inhibitory effect has been seen on epiphyseal secretory pattern (21). In this study a reduction in calorie intake in a group of subjects with severe obesity was accompanied by a significant increase in aMT epiphyseal secretion, similarly to what seen in post menopausal age women (22). In particular an increase was seen in the serum pineal gland hormone levels in samples taken during the night and early morning hours. The increase in aMT blood levels might be due to changes determined by weight reduction on the autonomic nervous system: in fact, it is well known that the condition of obesity is accompanied by an imbalance of the ortho/parasympathetic system (23) following hypertonia of the parasympathetic system and reduced activity of the orthosympathetic system. Because the main neurotransmitter involved in the regulation of epiphyseal function is noradrenalin (24), it derives that changes in orthosympathetic activity, as take place in obese subjects on weight reduction regimens, may determine an increase in noradrenergic tone at the level of the pineal beta receptors with a consequent increase in pineal gland secretion and thus in serum aMT levels.

Another possible explanation might concern the role of the pineal gland on body adaptation to stress (25). Among these are the drastic reduction in calorie intake over a brief period (21), as well as a more moderate dietary restriction over a longer period (26).

The increase in aMT levels is accompanied by the onset of menstrual irregularities in all subjects examined, without changes in Gn and E2 levels confirming what seen after exogenous administration of pineal gland hormone (27). Since aMT can determine an inhibitory effect on normal gonadic function (28), our results suggest that variations in its levels may have a role in determining the menstrual disorders seen. The mechanism involved in this effect remain to be explained considering the absence of important variations of Gn secretory axis in the patients of this study.

REFERENCES

(1) Piovesan, A., Terzolo, M., Revelli, A., Guidetti, D., Puligheddu, B., Codegone, A., Ali, A., Cassoni, P., Massobrio, M., Angeli, A. (1993). Sex related effects of exogenous melatonin on the pulsatile secretion of prolactin, TSH and LH in healthy human subjects. In Touitou, Y., Arendt, J., Pevet, P. (eds.): Melatonin and the Pineal Gland, pp. 355-8. (Amsterdam: Excerpta Medica)

(2) Waldhauser, F., Lieberman, H.R., Lynch, H.J., Waldhauser, M., Herkner, K., Frisch, H., Vierhapper, H., Waldhausl, W., Schemper, M., Wurtman, R.J., Crowley, W.F. (1987). A pharmacological dose of melatonin increase PRL levels in males without altering

tone of GH, LH, FSH, TSH, testosterone or cortisol. Neuroendocrinology 46,125–30.

(3) Cardinali, D.P., Vacas, M.I. (1984). Pineal gland, photoperiodic responses, and puberty. J. Endocrinol. Invest. 7,157–65.

(4) Maestroni, G.J.M., Conti, A., Pierpaoli, W. (1988). The immunoregolatory role of melatonin. In Gupta, D., Attanasio, A., Reiter, R.J. (eds.): Brain Research Promotion, pp. 133–43. (London–Tubingen)

(5) Maestroni, G.J.M., Conti, A., Pierpaoli, W. (1987). Role of the pineal gland in immunity. Clin. Exp. Immunol. 68, 384–92.

(6) Monteleone, P., Catapano, F., Maj, M., Kemali, D., Reiter, R.J. (1993). Circadian melatonin rhythm in patients with paranoid schizophrenia and obsessive-compulsive disorder. In Touitou, Y., Arendt, J., Pevet, P. (eds.): Melatonin and the Pineal Gland, pp. 363–6. (Amsterdam: Excerpta Medica)

(7) Rosenthal, M.E., Sack, D.A., Jacobsen, F.M., James, S.P., Parry, B.L., Arendt, J., Tamarkin, L., Wehr, T.A. (1986). The role of melatonin in seasonal affective disorder (SAD) and phototherapy. In Wurtman, R.J., Waldhauser, F. (eds.): Melatonin in Humans, pp. 233–42. (Amsterdam: Elsevier)

(8) Tortosa, F., Puig-Domingo, M., Peinado, M.A., Oriola, J., Webb, S.M., De Leiva, A. (1989). Enhanced circadian rhythm of melatonin in anorexia nervosa. Acta Endocrinol. (Copenh.) 120, 574–8.

(9) Kennedy, S.H. (1994). Melatonin disturbances in anorexia nervosa and bulimia nervosa. Int. J. Eat. Dis. 16, 257–65.

(10) Arendt, J., Hampton, S., English, J., Kwasowski, P., Marks, V. (1982). 24-hour profiles of melatonin, cortisol, insulin, C-peptide and GIP following a meal and subsequent fasting. Clin. Endocrinol. 16, 89–95.

(11) Rojdmark, S., Berg, A., Rossner, S., Wetterberg, L. (1991). Nocturnal melatonin secretion in thyroid disease and in obesity. Clin. Endocrinol. 35, 61–5.

(12) Ferrari, E., Foppa, S., Bossolo, P.A., Comis, S., Esposti, G., Licini, V., Fraschini F., Brambilla, F. (1989). Melatonin and pituitary-gonadal function in disorders of eating behaviour. J. Pineal Res. 7, 115–24.

(13) Rojdmark, S., Rossner, S., Wetterberg, L. (1992). Effect of short-term fasting on nocturnal melatonin secretion in obesity. Metabolism 41, 1106–9.

(14) Hoffer, L.J., Beitins, I.Z., Kyung, N., Bistrian, B. (1986). Effects of severe dietary restriction on male reproductive hormones. J. Clin. Endocrinol. Metab. 62, 288–92.

(15) Beitins, I.Z., Shah, A., O'Loughlin, K., Johnson, L., Ostrea, T.R., Van Wart, J., Mc Arthur, J.W. (1980). The effects of fasting on serum and urinary gonadotropins in obese postmenopausal women. J. Clin. Endocrinol. Metab. 51, 26–34.

(16) Kapen, S., Sternthal, E., Braverman, L. (1981). A "pubertal" 24-hour luteinizing

hormone (LH) secretory pattern following weight loss in the absence of anorexia nervosa. Psychosom. Med. 43, 177–82.

(17) Berga, S.L., Mortola, J.F., Yen, S.S.C. (1988).Amplification of nocturnal melatonin secretion in women with functional hypothalamic amenorrhea. J. Clin. Endocrinol. Metab. 66, 242–4.

(18) Kauppila, A., Kivela, A., Pakarinen, A., Vakkuri, O. (1987). Inverse seasonal relationship between melatonin and ovarian activity in humans in a region with a strong seasonal contrast in luminosity. J. Clin. Endocrinol. Metab. 65, 823–8.

(19) Reiter, R.J. (1988). The Pineal Gland. In De Groot, L.J. (ed.): Endocrinology, pp. 240–53. (Philadelphia: Saunders Company)

(20) Chik, C.L., Ho, A.K., Brown, G.M. (1987). Effect of food restriction on 24-h serum and pineal melatonin content in male rats. Acta Endocrinol. (Copenh.) 115, 507–13.

(21) Rojdmark, S., Wetterberg, L. (1989). Short-term fasting inhibits the nocturnal melatonin secretion in healthy men. Clin. Endocrinol. 30, 451–7.

(22) Beitins, I.Z., Barkan, A., Klibanski, A., Kyung, N., Reppert, S.M., Badger, T.M., Veldhuis, J., McArthur, J.W. (1985). Hormonal response to short term fasting in postmenopausal women. J. Clin. Endocrinol. Metab. 60, 1120–6.

(23) Jeanrenaud, B., Rohner-Jeanrenaud, F., Ionescu, E., Bobbioni, E., Niijima,A. (1986). Dysfunction of the central nervous system in VMH-lesioned and genetically obese rats. Excerpta Med. Internat. Congr. Series 700, 225–31.

(24) Arendt, J. (1988). Melatonin, a review. J. Clin. Endocrinol. Metab. 69, 205–29.

(25) Vaughan, G.M., McDonald, S.D., Jordan, R.M., Allen, J.P., Bell, R., Stevens, E.A. (1979). Melatonin, pituitary function and stress in humans.Psychoneuroendocrinology 4, 351–62.

(26) Anderson, I.M., Gartside, S.E., Cowen, P.J. (1990). The effect of moderate weight loss on overnight melatonin secretion. British J. Psych. 156, 875–7.

(27) Terzolo, M., Revelli, A., Guidetti, D., Piovesan, A., Cassoni, P., Paccotti, P., Angeli, A., Massobrio, M. (1993). Evening administration of melatonin enhances the pulsatile secretion of prolactin but not of LH and TSH in normally cycling women. Clin. Endocrinol. 39, 185–91.

(28) Brzezinski, A., Seibel, M.M., Lynch, H.J., Deng, M.H., Wurtman, R.J. (1987). The circadian rhythm of plasma melatonin during the normal menstrual cycle and in amenorrheic women. J. Clin. Endocrinol. Metab. 66, 891–5.

Liver involvement in Turner's syndrome: a case of 'newborn-like' histology

M. Certo, D. Valle, L. Sammartano*, L. Marra**, L. Rossi, G. Fadda***, A. Mancini* and L. De Marinis*

Department of Internal Medicine II, *Institute of Endocrinology, **Department of Internal Medicine I and ***Department of Pathology, Catholic University, Rome, Italy

---

INTRODUCTION.

Turner's Syndrome (TS) is genetic disorder occurring in 1:2500 female newborns (1). It is determined by defects of the chromosome X (absence, mosaicism, deletions, translocations). The first observation was reported by Henry H. Turner (2). He described a 16 years old female, showing short stature, pterigium colli, absence of sexual secondary findings and cubitus valgus. He hypothesised that the ovarian failure was secondary to a hypophiseal disease.

Since then on, several studies have been performed in order to investigate the systemic involvement observed in the syndrome. Skeletal abnormalities, hypostaturalism, cardiovascular gastrointestinal, endocrine diseases and others, are very common in this syndrome.

In this report we suggest that the liver involvement could contribute, close to the hypophiseal factor, to the short stature, since the absence of the response to the recombinant hGH therapy.

CASE REPORT

A 24 years old female affected by TS was admitted to our Medical Centre for a persistent alteration of hepatic function indexes, found during periodical controls. She showed the typical features of the syndrome and assumed steroid replacement therapy by transdermal root since 8 years (25 µg twice weekly). Above all she had assumed

189

recombinant hGH therapy for six months until one month before (0.5 IU/Kg/week s.c.).

The abdominal examination did not reveal liver or spleen enlargement.

An ecotomography showed no appreciable alterations of the liver and a slight splenomegaly.

HAV, HBV and HCV markers were found negative. ALT, AST and γ-GT were found at 2-3 folds over the normal range.

Autoantibodies (ANA, ASMA and antimitochondrial) were absent.

IGF-I plasma values were found low during and after the therapy (160 and 143 ng/ml respectively; normal values in our laboratory: 170-330 ng/ml)

Bone Mass Densitometry revealed a severe osteopenia (bone mass density less than 50 % of normal).

Liver biopsy showed cytoplasmatic regressive aspects and focal nuclear glycogenosis (fig.1); the hepatocytes were disposed as glandular acins with rare portal spaces (fig. 2).These findings were similar to those in other two cases described in literature and named "newborn-like arrangement" (3, 4).

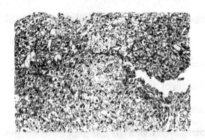

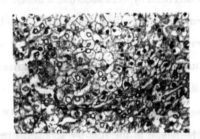

Fig.1 Liver biopsy shows cytoplasmatic regressive aspects and focal nuclear glycogenosis (40X).

Fig.2 The photo shows a detail (100X) of the fig.1. The hepatocytes are disposed as glandular acins with rare portal spaces. These findings have been named "newborn-like arrangement".

DISCUSSION

Previous works have investigated the pituitary involvement in the genesis of the short stature. The hypothesised reduced GH secretion has not been demonstrated in all cases. Above all an early appearance of the adulthood typical secretory GH pattern has been hypothesised (5). This finding suggested a gonadal involvement in the GH reduced peaks.

Veldhuis et al. proposed the absence of plasma oestrogen as cause of appearance of GH reduced peaks in the puberty (6).

On the other side, the absence of plasma oestrogen could explain the impaired Insulin-like Growth Factor I (IGF-I) secretion from liver that we observe in the subjects affected by TS, in the puberal age. The oestrogen replacement therapy can restore the normal IGF-I plasma values (7). The oestrogen's may induce the increase in the GH secretion or in the synthesis of the IGF-I from the liver.

Liver morphology in TS has not been extensively studied. In literature only few cases are reported: a case of portal hypertension (8), two infantile cases of cholestasis (3), a case of portal fibrosis (9) and a case of "neonatal liver" (4).

Svlven et al. observed that an elevation of the liver enzymes occurred in more than 80% of their patients affected by TS. In none of them there was an evidence of alcohol abuse (10).

It has been hypothesised that a deficit of sex hormones throughout the first month of extrauterine life, like occurs in TS, could be responsible of the abnormalities of hepatic architecture and functions (11).

Otherwise, this deficiency has been hypothesised to have an important role in the liver GH-induced IGF-I secretion. In fact, the replacement therapy (ethyinil-estradiol 100 µg/daily p.o.) can restore the normal IGF-I plasma values (7).

The failure in the IGF-I response to recombinant hGH therapy, as described in this report, could suggest that the liver involvement have a primary role in this aspect. The ovarian failure and the prolonged oestrogen absence may be responsible of this impaired hepatic response. Probably an early diagnosis and the oestrogen replacement therapy, when reduced plasma levels are found, could prevent the liver modifications and improve the biological and clinical response to the hGH recombinant therapy.

REFERENCES

1. Goldman, B., Polani, P.E., Daker, M.G., Angell, R.R. (1982) Clinical and cytogenetic aspects of X chromosome deletions. Clin Genetics 21:36-52

2. Turner, H.H. (1938) A syndrome of infantilism, congenital webbed neck and cubitus valgus. Endocrinology 23: 566-574

3. Gardner, L.I. (1974) Intrahepatic bile stasis in 45,X Turner's syndrome. New Engl J Med 290:406

4. Ulissi, A. and Ricci, G.L. (1989) Hepatic histology in a case of Turner's syndrome. Ital J Gastroenterol 21:340-341

5. Massarano, A.A., Brook, C.G.D., Hindmarsch, P.C., Pringle, P.J., Teale, J.D., Stanhope, R., Preece, M.A. (1989) Growth hormone secretion in Turner's syndrome and influence of oxandrolone and et ethinil-oestradiol. Arch Dis Childh 64: 587-592

6. Veldhuis, J.D., Johnson, M.L. (1986) Cluster analysis: a simple, versatile and robust algorythm for endocrine pulse detection. Am J Physiol 250:E486-493

7. Cutler, L., van Vliet, G., Conte, F.A., Kaplan, S.L., Grumbach M.M. (1985) Somatomedin-C levels in children and adolescent with gonadal dysgenesis: differences from age-matched normal females and effect of chronic replacement therapy. J Clin Endocrinol Metab 60: 1087-1092

8. Szekely, A.M. (1976) Liver anomalies with portal hypertension associated with Turner's syndrome. Arch Anat Cytol Pathol 24:311-316

9. Calais, L., Pelaez, J.L., Ibarrola, B., Calleja, J.L., Lopez Varela, J., Perianes, J. (1966) Sindrome de Turner con afectacion hepatica. Riv Clin Esp 101: 134-136

10. Svlven, L., Hagenfeldt, K., Brondum-Nielsen, K. and von Schoultz, B. (1991) Middle-aged women with Turner's syndrome. Medical status, hormonal treatment and social life. Acta Endocrinologica 125:359-395

11. Gustafsson, J.A., Mode, A., Norsted, G. and Skett, P. (1983) Sex-steroids-induced changes in hepatic enzymes. Annu Rev Physiol 45:51-60

LHRH agonists and uterine fibroids: before hysterectomy and after myomectomy

P. Galli, A. Carani, A. Colombo, R. Delli Carpini, R. Guidetti, R. Fiozzi and D. Tavernari

Department of Obstetrics and Gynecology, Azienda USL Modena, Mirandola, Italy

---

INTRODUCTION

Buserelin, Goserelin, Leuprorelin and Triptorelin have been used a) to reduce the uterine fibroids' volume before surgical treatment and to reduce the blood loss during surgical therapy (1), b) as pharmacological alternative to myomectomy (2), c) in case of severe menorrhagia in women at high surgical risk (3), d) in the anaemic patients candidated to hysterectomy (4), and even e) to facilitate abdominal hysterectomy for the removal of uterine fibroids (5).

We refer our experience regarding LHRH agonists used before hysterectomy in patients with severe anaemia and before myomectomy in patients affected by infertility due to uterine fibroids.

MATERIAL AND METHODS

We used 3.75 mg of triptoreline (Decapeptyl) every 28 days in one group of 10 anaemic patients (Hb < 9 g)

candidated to hysterectomy because of severe menorrhagya resistent to any other pharmacological treatment and in another group of 10 infertile women candidated to myomectomy in order to reduce fibroids volume and blood loss during myomectomy.

RESULTS

The group of patients candidated to hysterectomy required 1-3 administrations of triptoreline before Hb would reach 9 g and hysterectomy could be performed. Various degrees of menorrhagia vere present during the 15-20 days following triptorelin first administration. Yet no patients were blood trasfused but all them underwent e.v. and oral iron and acidum tranexanicum administration. During the operation (abdominal hysterectomy in all the patients) no special advantages or problems were observed if compared to routine abdominal hysterctomies performed in patients who had no pre-treatment with triptorelin. No patients needed blood trasfusions surgery related.

The group of patients candidated to myomectomy required 3-6 administrations of triptorelin before a 30% reduction of the initial fibroids diameter could be obtained and myomectomy performed. In this group of patients we collected 1 hysterectomy (the first triptorelin treated patient) because of pathologist's indication (6) and 19 myomectomies. Differently from hysterectomies, we found great difficulties in myomectomies if compared with myomectomies performed in patients who had no GNRH analogous pre-surgical treatment.

CONCLUSIONS AND COMMENT

We concluded that triptoreline pre-hysterectomy treatment is very usefull in the cases of severely anaemic patients because allows a satisfactory improuvement in haematologic conditions. Yet triptoreline offers no special advantages during hysterectomy.

On the other hand we concluded that in case of myomectomy the triptoreline pre-surgical treatment cannot coexist with our surgical tecnique so that we do not pre-treat anymore patients planned for myomectomy. Instead we are persuaded that triptorelin may rather follow than precede myomectomy in order to prevent future growth of those little myomas impossible to detect and or to remouve during the operation. This our present supposition would nevertheless require confirmation.

REFERENCES

1) Gesenheus Th., Hackenberg R., Deichert U., Sturm S., Schulz K.D.: Treatment of uterine fibroids with the GnRH analog goserelin. Gynecol. Endocrin., 4,Suppl.2,41,Abs 61, 1990

2) Genazzani A.R., Uccelli E., Petraglia F., Adamo R., Volpe A.: Terapia della fibromatosi uterina. Aggiornamento del medico, 14, 535-541, 1990

3) Motta T., Vercellini P., Vendola N., Colombo A., Von Wunster S., D'Alberton A.: GnRH agonist for severe menorrhagia in women at high surgical risk. Gynecol. Endocrin., 4, suppl.2, 15,1990.

4) Vercellini P., Crosignani P.G.: Goserelin (zoladex) and the anemic patient. Br. J. Obstet. Gynaecol., 101,suppl.10,33-37,1994.

5) Lumsden M.A., West C., Thomas E., Coutts J., Hillier H., Thomas N., Baird T.: Treatment with the gonadotrophin releasing hormone-agonist goserelin before hysterectomy for uteine fibroids. Brit. J., Obstet. Gynaecol., 101, 438-442,1994.

6) Shaw R.W.: Mechanisms of LHRH analogue action in uterine fibroids. Horm. Res., 32, suppl 1, 150-153, 1989.

Insulin-like growth factors and steroidogenesis in polycystic ovarian syndrome

A. Porcelli, C. Taccani and N. Surico

University of Turin, Faculty of Medicine of Novara, Department of Medical Sciences, Clinic of Obstetrics and Gynecology, Turin, Italy

INTRODUCTION

The identification of the insulin and insulin-like growth factor I (IGF-I) role in ovarian androgens biosynthesis was one of the most interesting development of the last years.
Hyperandrogenism itself could be an important moment in hyperinsulinism induction.
More recently, insulin-resistence presence was showed also always in PCOS patients having a variable expression degree.
Adashi and others showed that insulin and IGF-I increase thecal cells response to LH.
Barbieri showed that ovarian stromal cells of PCOS patients respond to LH stimolation in androgenic direction with the presence of insulin in coltural medium. The IGF-I action starts a sensibilization mechanism also at granulosa cells level with a consequent amplification response even related to the FSH biochemical action.
The action of insulin comes true trough a fall of phosphorylation and de-phosphorylation reactions: it recognizes as the first moment the activation of the appropriate insulin receptor tyrosine-kinase.
From this, an activation of proteine phosphatase derives, and this causes the biological activity of glycogen synthetase and the inhibition of glycogenolysis. This mechanism causes an increase of androgenic secretion as a response to the amplification mechanism of gonadotropins cell sensibility at ovarian level.
Consequent insulin resistence contributes to start a self-keeping dysbolism also indipendently by another androgenic stimulation (See Table 1).
The expression degree of this pathogenetic mechanism is various instead of this syndrome and it recognizes some different external variables (diet type, related dysbolisms presence, patient hereditary habitus) such as important factors in conditioning this pathology evolution.

MATERIALS AND METHODS

Our pathological group was formed by 21 women with a PCOS diagnosis. A control group formed by 10 women disease-free was also considered. An acceptance was asked and obtained from the whole patient group. The middle age was 27 +/- 5 for the control group and 28 +/- 5 for the pathologic group.
A PCOS diagnosis was made thru classical parameters (LH/FSH >2 and free testosterone increase). The imaging (echography) was considered as an additional data. We used a Toshiba 5 MHz transvaginal probe for ultrasonography. In both studied groups we evaluated Body Mass Indexes (BMIs). Glucose metabolism was valued through glucose, insulin, fructosamine and HbA1c serum levels: we also valued glucose and insulin serum levels after OGTT.
With regard to OGTT, we determined and valued the area under curve (AUC) and the insulin serum level response at 2 hrs. from OGTT. We also valued in all different phases the glucose-insulin serum values ratio.

In overweight patients we considered some different distributions of body fat (upper body or abdominal type).

Insulin Growth Factor (IGF-1) and its Binding Protein (IGFBP-1) was valued through an immunoradiometric technique on human serum with special kits provided by Diagnostic System Laboratories Inc.-Webster-Texas-USA.

We also valued gonadotropins, E2, progesterone, PRL, cortisol, free and total testosterone, SHBG, DHEAS, 17OH progesterone, thyroid hormons and GH plasma levels. Our study was made at the Faculty of Medicine of Novara, with the cooperation of the Ospedale Maggiore Analysis Laboratory, Novara. We always used a preselection protocol for our patients, which included severe criteria of exclusion or inclusion in our trial. IGF-I and IGFBP-I were related to themselves and to different considered markers to evaluate an eventual statistic significance.

RESULTS

In PCOS patients group, the considered parameters serum values were on average higher than control group. In Figure 1 we clearly show that there is a significant difference between the PCOS group and the control group with reference to FSH, LH, PRL, DHEA-S and Testosterone plasma concentrations. We can also show that the plasma average in the PCOS group with hyperprolactinemia is different as to the normal group. An analytic study of the linear correlations gave a positive result about a significative correlation between DHEA-S and PRL in PCOS group. In fact, the DHEA-S values (5,9+/-3,2 , SD) correspond to PRL middle values (24,2 +/-8,2 , SD). A graphic rapresentation of the whole parameters serum values (see Fig. 1) shows that an increased LH middle concentration correspond to an increased PRL middle concentration and that there is an inversion of the middle ratio related to the control group. At the same time, a significative DHEA-S increase is much more related to PCOS patients group with hyperprolactinemia.

Table 1 shows the middle plasma values of the considered hormonal parameteres with a Standard Deviation: also in this case, a direct comparison shows a parallel trend between LH, PRL, DHEA-S used as markers, in PCOS and control groups. Glucose metabolysm, glycemic percentual middle values, HbA1c, fructosamine and insulin were not significative, except for a restricted number of cases in which there was a strong hyperandrogenism related to an excessive weight increase and to a middle-high degree of hyrsutism. In these cases, there was an alteration of OGTT related to an increased insulin resistence, with some basal values and insulinemic profile (under stimulation) clearly pathologic. In obesity cases, a direct positive correlation was showed between insulin serum values (hyperinsulinemia) and SHBG serum values. The insuln response to OGTT was significative (p >/=0,01) if related to a serum SHBG trend inversion and to a fat increase. In PCOS patients group in which we valued IGF-Iα with IGFBP-1, we compared the obtained results to PCOS standard parameters: in particular, IGF-Iα and IGFBP-1 were related between themselves and to the most important considered parameters of the other groups. Table 2 shows the relation coefficients (R) between IGF-Iα and IGFBP-1 and between the considered endocrinological markers. At first, the relation between IGF-Iα and IGFBP-1 was significative (R=0,6047).

So, were significative also the other relations between IGF-Iα and DHEA-S (R=0,4570) and between IGF-Iα and free Testosteron (R=0,2740).

We also showed other significative relations between IGFBP-1 and LH (R=0,3186), between IGFBP-1 and FSH (R=0,5307), IGFBP-1 and E2 (R=0,56426), IGFBP-1 and PRL (R=0,4817), and, at least, between IGFBP-1 and DHEA-S (R=0,6527).

We also showed some negative relations between IGF-Iα and progesterone (R=0,2548, in luteal phase) and between IGF-Iα and SHBG (R= 0,0346) and also between IGFBP-1 and progesterone (R=0,034).

The insulin response to OGTT (as the area under the curve) increased in PCOS patients related to control group. The glycemic response to OGTT (AUC) was also higher in PCOS group than in control group even if the increase was very lower. At last, insulin concentration values were higher in PCOS group than in control group after 2 hrs from OGTT.

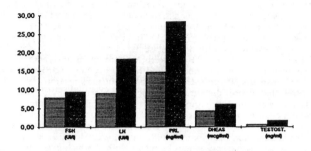

FIG.1
Average variations in PCOS and in control group patients

CONTROL GROUP		PCOD GROUP		
FSH	7,1±1,9	FSH	8,5±2,1	UI/L
LH	8,2±1,8	LH	16,8±3,2	UI/L
PRL	12,1±5,3	PRL	24,2±8,2	ng/ml
DHEAS	4,8±1,9	DHEAS	5,9±3,2	ng/ml
TEST.	0,6±0,3	TEST.	1,5±0,5	ng/ml

TAB.1
Plasma middle values of hormonal levels and their standard deviations

IGF1

IGFBP1	R=0,6047
DHEAS	R=0,4570
TEST.	R=0,2740
PROG.	R=-0,2548
SHBG	R=-0,0346

IGFBP1

LH	R=0,3186
FSH	R=0,5307
E2	R=0,5642
PRL	R=0,4817
DHEAS	R=0,6527
PROG.	R=-0,034

TAB.2
Correlation factors related to considered markers

199

CONCLUSIONS

From our results we showed an evident relation between adrenal and ovaric hyperandrogenism. DHEA-S determination is a significative marker of adrenal androgenic secretion as reported in litterature by many authors (Lobo). An excessive DHEA-S secretive response was obtained through a stimulation with ACTH, in some significative percentages of PCOS patients, after a suppression test with desametasone.

However, PRL action causes an androgenic hypersecretion through an interaction with some specific adrenal receptors, that it causes obesity and hyrsutism. The androgens peripheral aromatization with its consequent hyperestrogenism conditions a secretion increase of PRL and LH at pituitary level, that causes the basal dysendocrinia.

We also want specify that many authors supposed that there is a relative dopamine deficiency in these patients, which causes the hyperprolactinemia, that is consequent to a subthalamic disfunction. This mechanism is also known in the alteration of gonadotropines secretion. Is our opinion that this phenomenon principally conditions an excessive LH serum increase in the early follicular phase, with some consequent secretive "spikes" which make impossible the dominant follicle secretion through a follicular recruitment interference. At last, the insulin tolerance alteration can be related to hypertrichiasis and to fat increase: this mechanism can be explained through a probably insulin action on the ovarian function. Studied hyperinsulinism could cause the androgenic hypersecretion through a direct receptorial mechanism and also through a "cross-mediate" action on IGF-I receptors (Nagamani). The presence of some specific IGF-I receptors in stromal cells of healthy woman ovary was reported in litterature. In PCOS the number of these cells could strongly increase such as the number of IGF-I specific receptors: from this fact derives a consequent hypersecretion related to the presence of hypertrichiasis and to fat increase. Women with a little weight increase and a little hyrsutism would have a less concentration of specific binding sites for IGF-I and this could be the first cause to maintaine a normal insulin resistence. There is an evident direct relation between IGFBP-I and ovarian steroid secretion and so, it shows that the LH response increase is more evident in PCOS women with alterated glycidic metabolism. At the same time, adrenal hypersecretion shows a parallel trend and this evidences that the IGF-Iα action, made through its binding protein, is like a "metabolic switch" of the patologic mechanism.

REFERENCES

ADASHI EY, RESNIC CE, D'ERCOLE AJ, SVOBODA ME, VANWYK JJ
Insulin-like growth factors as intra-ovarian regulators of granulosa cell growth and function
Endocrine Rev. 6;400-420   1985

AYERS JWT
Differential response to adrenocorticotropin hormon stimulation in PCOD with high and low
DHEAS levels
Fertil. Steril. 37;645-9   1982

BALLARD J, BAXTER R, BINOUX M
On the nomenclature of IGF binding proteins
Acta Endocrinol. 121;751-2   1990

BALLARD J, BAXTER R, BINOUX M
Report on the nomenclature of IGF binding proteins
J Clin Endocrinol Metab 74;1215-6   1992

BARBIERI RL, MAKRIS A et Others
Insulin stimulates androgen accumulation in incubations of ovarian stroma obtained from
women with hyperandrogenism
J Clin Endocrinol Metab 62;904-9   1986

BARBIERI RL, SMITH S, RYAN KJ
The role of hyperinsulinemia in the pathogenesis of ovarian hyperandrogenism
Fertil. Steril. 50;197-212   1988

BLUMENFELD Z and LUNENFELD B
A potentiating effect of growth hormon on follicle stimulation with human pituitary
menopausal gonadotropine in a panhypopituytary patient
Fertil. Steril. 52;328-331 1989

CARLSTROM K, GERSHAGEN S, RANNEVIK G
Free testosterone and testosterone SHBG index in hirsute women: a comparison of diagnostic
accurancy
Gynecol Obstet Invest 24; 256-61 1987

CARMINA E, KOYAMA T, CHANG L, STANCZYK FZ, LOBO RA
Does ethnicity influence the prevalence of adrenal hyperandrogenism and insulin resistance
in PCOS ?
Am-J-Obstet-Gynecol 1992 DEC; 167(6): 1807-12

CATALDO NA, GIUDICE LC
Follicular fluid IGFBP profiles in PCOS
J Clin Endocrinol Metab 1992 MAR 74(3): 695-7

CHEUNG AP, CHANG JR
Polycystic ovary syndrome
Clin Obstet Gynecol 33, 3:655 1990

CROSBY PDA, RITTMASTER RS
Predictors of clinical response in hirsute women treated with spironolactone
Fertil. Steril. 55;1076-1081 1991

DAUGHADAY WH, ROTWEIN P
IGF 1 and 2. Peptide messanger ribonucleic acid and gene structures, serum and tissue
concentrations
Endocrine Rev 10; 68-91 1989

DUNAIF A, GREEN M
Insulin administration alters gonadal steroid metabolism
J Clin Invest 83; 23-29 1989

DUNAIF A, GRAF M et Others
Characterizations of groups of hyperandrogenic women with acanthosis nigricans and
impaired glucose tolerance
J Clin Endocrinol Metab 65: 499-507 1987

ELKIND-HIRSCH KE, VALDES CT, MC CONNEL TG, MALINAK LR
Androgen responses to acutely increased endogenous insulin levels in hyperandrogenic and
normal cycling women
Fertil. Steril. 55;486-490 1991

ERICKSON GF, MAGOFFIN DA, DYER CA, HOFEDITZ C
The ovarian androgen producing cells: a review of a structure function relationship
Endocrinol Rev 6;371-99 1985

FILICORI M
Increased insulin secretion in patients with multifollicular and polycystic ovaries and its
impact on ovulation induction.
Fertil. Steril. 62;279 1994

GARGOSKY SE, HASEGAWA T, TAPANAINEN and others
Urinary IGF's and IGFBP's in normal subjects, GH deficiency, and renal disease
J Clin Endocrinol Metab 1993 JUN; 76(6): 1631-7

HOFFMAN D, LOBO RA
The prevalence and significance of elevated DHEA-S levels in anovulatory women
Fertil. Steril. 42;76-81 1984

KATZ E, RICCIARELLI E, ADASHI EY
The potential relevance of GH to female reproductive physiology and pathophysiology
FERTIL-STERIL 1993 JAN; 59(1): 8-34

KAZER RR, UNTERMAN TG, GLICK RP
An abnormality of the GH/IGF-I axis in women with PCOS
J Clin Endocrinol Metab 71: 958-62 1990

KIDDY DS, SHARP PS, WHITE DM and others
Differences in clinical and endocrine features between obese and non obese subjects with
PCOS: an analysis of 263 consecutive cases
Clin Endocrinol 32; 213-20 1990

LOBO RA
The syndrome of hyperandrogenic cronic anovulation IN:"Infertility, contraception and
reproductive endocrinology"
Blackwell Pubblications-3rd Ed.: 447-87 1991

MASON HD, MARTIKAINEN H, BEARD RW, ANYAOKU V, FRANKS S
Direct gonadotropinic effect of GH on E2 production by human granulosa cells in vitro
J Endocrinol 126; R 1-4 1990

NAGAMANI M, STUART CA
Specific binding sites for IGF-I in the ovarian stroma of women with PCOD and stromal
hypertecosys
Am J Obstet Gynecol 163; 1992-97 1990

PCOS and surrenalic function

A. Tolino, S. Ronsini, M. Pellicano, A. Petrone and C. Nappi

Department of Gynecology and Obstetrics, University of Naples "Federico II", Naples, Italy

INTRODUCTION

Non-classical late-onset forms of congenital adrenal hyperplasia (CAH) are generally caused by 21-hydroxylase (21-OH), 3-ß-hydroxy-delta5-steroidodehydrogenase or, less frequently (1,2), 11-hydroxylase deficiency (11-OHD).

These three enzymatic defects have similar clinical features and are not easily distinguishable from other types of hirsutism or ovarian polycystosis. To correctly diagnose these pathologies, hormonal measurements are necessary.

CAH-21OHD is more frequent in caucasians (3,4), reaching an incidence of 30% in selected populations (5,6). On the other hand, CAH-11OHD is less frequent and only few combined forms of 21-OHD and 11-OHD have been described.

MATERIALS AND METHODS

One-hundred and twenty patients (mean age 22±5 years

203

range 16-28 years) affected by oligomenorrhea and/or hirsutism and/or acne were included in this study. Patients were recruited among those attending the gynecological endocrinology service of our clinic. Menstrual disorders were represented by amenorrhea (>= 6 months) or oligomenorrhea (intervals between menses 35-180 days). Sixty-seven patients presented acne and oligomenorrhea. Onset of hirsutism was referred by all patients at the age of 13-24 years and all presented normal pubertal development. Ferryman and Gallway score for all patients was bewteen 8 and 24 (7,8). No cases of virilization were observed and all patients had normal blood pressure.

Patients underwent clinical examination, pelvic ultrasonography and PRL, A, T, DHEA-S, E2, 17-OHP, F, S, DOC, 21DF, FSH, LH, SHBG plasma levels evaluation. The samples were collected at 8:00 A.M. in early follicular phase (3rd-6th day of the cycle). An ACTH stimulation test (0.250 mg of synthetic alfa1-24-ACTH e.v.) was also performed evaluating, after 60 minutes, 17-OHP, S, DOC T, A, DHEA-S, F and 21DF plasma levels.

Patients were defined affected by PCO when presenting an ultrasonographic pattern of polycystic ovaries, i.e. 10 or more follicles (15 if TV-USG), ranging 2 to 8 mm in diameter arranged around or dispersed through an increased amount of stroma, as decribed elsewhere (9-13). Diagnosis of CAH-21OHD was performed according to Dewailly et al. report (14). High S plasma levels and an S/F ratio higher than 2SD after ACTH stimulation test, and thus high levels of DOC, were indicative of "mild form" CAH (15).

Twenty women (mean age 24±6 years, range 26-32 years)

with normal menstrual cycle and without any sign of hirsutism volunteered as controls. No subject from the control group had a history of endocrine disorders in close relatives nor took drugs (oral contraceptives included).

Statistical analysis was performed using the Student's "t" test.

RESULTS

All patients showed an ultrasonographic pattern of PCO. Basal 17OHP plasma levels resulted lower than 5 ng/ml in all patients. Diagnosis of CAH-21OHD was performed in 18 cases (15%) and "mild form" CAH in six (5%). No differences were detected in basal and post-ACTH testing cortisol plasma levels among the three groups. T, A, and DHEA-S plasma levels found in subject affected by enzymatic defects were characteristic of an hyperandrogenic condition compared to controls, but similar among the different enzymatic deficiency.

17OHP plasma levels after ACTH stimulation were significantly higher in CAH-21OHD patients (121.1±42.7 nmol/l) compared to control group (4.6±2.8 nmol/l) and "mild-form" CAH 11-OHD patients (6.1±0.9 nmol/l) (p<0.0005). S plasma levels resulted elevated both in "mild-form" CAH-11OHD (16±3.4 nmol/l) and in CAH-21OHD patients (17.9±4.1 nmoli/l) compared to controls (5.1±4 nmol/l). DOC plasma levels were significantly higher in "mild form" CAH-11OHD patients compared to controls (3450±1640 and 1650±480 pmol/l respectively, p<0.0005). 21DF plasma levels resulted signficantly higher in CAH-21OHD patients compared to controls (21.2±7 and 1.2±0.7 nmol/l, respectively, p<0.0005).

DISCUSSION

Our data demonstrate an increase of S after ACTH stimulation in patients with CAH-21OHD, toghether with a concomitant presence of increased 11-OHD. This circumstance has been described by other authors (3,16,17); various hypothesis have been proposed, but the exact physiopathogenetic mechanism has not been defined.

We know that the genes that codify 21-OH and 11ß-OH are localized respectively on cromosomes 6 and 8 (18) therefore it is highly improbable that women with a mutation inducing CAH-21OHD may present an other mutation.

We also have to exclude the hypothesis of a peripheral conversion of 17OHP in excess in compound S, because there is no correlation between 17OHP and S serum levels.

Another hypothesis that we may rationally bring out is that these patients have a relative deficit of 11ß-hydroxilase caused by an excess of steroids not 11-hydroxilate different from S.

In particular, the excess of 17OHP may occupy 11ß-OH enzyme with production of 21 DF, that is infact increased also in our researh, competing with S in its trasformation in F. Another hypothesis entails that the excess of S depends on a real relative ipofunction of 11ß-OH amplified by the already described phenomena of overload.

This ipofunction might be "acquired" for the negative interference of androgens on 11ß-OH (19-21), but might be also dependent from an autoselection of a deficitary gene, as a compensation of the increased natriuresis present in 21-OH deficits.

For what concerns patients with MF CAH 11ß-OHD we want underline that the initial absence of hypertension in these patients might depend on their young age, because we know that age, stress and sodium intake are all factors risk of hypertension.

We can conclude that 21-OH and 11ß-OH deficits are relatively frequent in our study (15% and 5%, respectively) and that these patients need to be screened by ACTH stimolous test, not only for improving the treatment, but also for the possible development of hypertension.

REFERENCES

1) Gabrilove JL, Sharma DC, Dorfman RL: Adrenocortical 11ß-hydroxilasi deficiency and virilism first manifest in the adult women. New Engl J Med, 272, 1189-94, 1965.

2) Guthrie GP, Wilson EA, Quillen DL, Jawad MJ: Adrenal androgen excess and defective 11ß-hydroxylation in women with idiopathic hirsutism. Arch Int Med, 142, 729-35, 1982.

3) Blankstein J, Faiman C, Reyes FI, Schroeder ML, Winter JS: Adult-onset familial adrenal hyperplasia 21-hydroxilase deficiency. Am J Med, 68, 441-8, 1980.

4) Speiser PW, Dupont B, Rubistein P, Piazza A, Kastelan A, New MI: High frequency of non classical steroid 21-hydroxylase deficiency. Am J Hum Genet, 37, 650-57, 1985.

5) Chetkowski RJ, De Fazio J, Shamonki I, Judd HL, Chang RJ: The incidence of late-onset congenital adrenal hyperplasia due to 21-hydroxylase deficiency among hirsute women. J Endocrinol Metab, 58, 595-8, 1984.

6) Chrousos GP, Loriaux DL, Mann DL, Cutler GB Jr.: Late-onset 21-hydroxilase deficiency mimicking idiopathic hirsutism or polycystic ovarian disease: an allelic variant of congenital virilizing adrenal hyperplasia with a milder enzimatic defect. Ann Intern Med, 96, 143-8, 1982.

7) Ferriman D, Gallway J: Clinical assessment of body hair growth in women. J Endocrinol Metab, 21, 1440-7, 1961.

8) Morris DW: Hirsutism. Clin Obstet Gynecol, 12, 649-53, 1985.

9) Adams J, Franks S, Polson DW, Mason HD, Abdulwahid NA, Tucker M, Morris DW, Price J, Jacobs HS: Multifollicular ovaries: clinical and endocrine features and response to pulsatile gonadotrophin releasing hormone. Lancet, 2, 1375-8, 1985.

10) Adams J, Polson DW, Franks S: Prevalence of polycystic ovaries in women with anovulation and idiopathic hirsutism.

11) Fox R, Corrigan E, Thomas PA, Hull MGR: The diagnosis of polycystic ovaries in women with oligoamenorrhea:

predictive power of endocrine tests. Clin Endocrinol, 34, 127-31, 1991.

12) Parisi L, Tramonti M, Casciano J, Zurli A, Gazzarrini O: The role of ultrasound in the study of polycystic disease. J Clin Ultrasound, 10, 167-72, 1982.

13) Swanson N, Saverbrei EE, Coopeberg PL: Medical implications of ultrasonically detected polycystic ovaries. J Clin Ultrasound, 9, 219-22, 1991.

14) Dewailly D, Vantyghem-Haudiquet MC, Sainsar C, Buyat J, Cappoen JP, Ardaens C, Radacot A, Lefrebe J, Fossati P: Clinical and biological phenotypes in late-onset 21-hydroxilase deficiency. J Clin Endocrinol, 63, 418-23, 1986.

15) Geva TE, Hurwitz A, Vecsei P, Palti Z, Milwdiski A, Rosler A: Secundary biosynthetic defects in women with late-onset congenital adrenal hyperplasia. New Engl J Med, 323, 855-63, 1990.

16) Gandy HM, Keutmann EH, Izzo AJ: Characterization of urinary steroids in adrenal hyperplasia: isolation of metabolites of cortisol, compound S and deoxycorticosterone from a normotensive patient with adrenogenital syndrome. J Clin Invest, 39, 364-77, 1960.

17) Newmark S, Dluhy RQ, Williams GH, Pochi P, Rose LI: Partial 11- and 21-hydroxylase deficiency in hirsute women. Am J Obstet Gynecol, 127, 595-98, 1977.

18) New ML, White PC, Pang S, Dupont B, Speiser PW: The adrenal hyperplasia. In: Scriver CR, Beaudet AL, Sly WS, Valle D eds 6th. Mc Graw Hill, New York, 2, 1881-917, 1989.

19) Fraghacan F, Nowaczynski W, Bertranan E, Kalina M, Genest J: Evidence of in vivo inhibition of 11ß-hydroxilation of steroids by dehydroepiandrosterone in the dog. Endocrinology, 84, 98-103, 1969.

20) Mc Call AL, Stern J, Dale SL, Melby JC: Adrenal steroidogenesis: methyandrostenediol-induced hypertension. Endocrinology, 103, 1-5, 1978.

21) Sharma DC, Forchielli E, Dorfman RI: Inhibition of enzimatic steroid 11ß-hydroxilation by androgens. J Biol Chem, 238, 572-5, 1963.

The side-effects of oral hormonal contraceptives

N. Costin, I.V. Surcel, A. Rosca and S. Parastie

1st Department of Obstetrics and Gynecology, University of Medicine, Cluj-Napoca, Romania

The social-economicaly changes of the society, of the family as concept and the progress of the medicine have promoted new elements in the *Family Planning* (FP).

In Romania the FP have became present after 1989, when the interest of the couples for the contraception have evidently increased.

With all their advantages, the contraceptive methods have every one some inconveniences. To know really and deeply this disadvantages is very useful for the client and doctor in the same time, facilitating the choice of the most indicated contraceptive method. Even if, the disadvantages of the contraceptive methods are not so important, they remaind a reality, which must be considered, especially today when the contraception is free in our country.

The major intention of this article is to ilustrate the most frequent complications found in our practice of oral contraception usage.

Materials and Method:

We have a retrospective study on 3 years (1990-1992) and 551 women, using oral contraception.

The selection of the cases was made by the use of the same type of oral contraceptive more than 1 year, and the return for controls periodicaly.

The main parameters of our study are:

1. The group age
2. The origin area of the cases
3. Profession
4. Parity
5. Type of used contraceptives

211

6. The modification of the menstrual flow
7. The corporeal weight
8. The intermenstrual bleedings
9. The libido changes

Major findings and discution of the results:

1.The age group (table 1.) - we can see what the prevalent group is between 21-29 years, the most sexual and reproductive activity age.

Table 1 The age distribution of cases

Age group	Nr. cases	%
Under 20 years	41	7.30
21-29 years	254	45.76
30-39 years	201	36.21
Over 40 years	59	10.63

2. Following the origin area (table 2.), prevalent is the group of urban area patients - 496 cases (90.01%).

Table 2 Origin area

Area	Nr. cases	%
Urban area	496	90.01
Rural area	55	9.98

3. Following the profession (table 3.) the prevalent group is that of the worker women 225 cases (46.27%) succeed by housewifes 131 cases - 23.77%, office workers 47 cases, than the women with university studies, technicians.

Table 3 The profession of the patients

Profession	Nr. cases	%
Housewifes	131	23.77
Workers	255	46.27
Technicians	39	7.07

Office workers	47	8.52
University studies	44	7.98
University students	10	1.81
College students	9	1.63
Other professions	16	2.90

4. Following the parity, in our study are prevalents the multiparous women (table 4.), 409 cases - 74.22 % . This group uses the contraceptives to avoid unwanted pregnancy but also for birth spacing. The multiparous women use the oral contraception primarily for pregnancy prevention.

Table 4 The parity of the patients

Parity	Nr.cases	%
Nuliparous	142	25.77
Multiparous	409	74.22

5. As the types of oral contraceptives (table 5.) evidently the most common oral contraceptive in Romania is the Schering's *Microgynon* - used in our study by 78 % of the cases. This is followed by the Hungarian Richter's product *Ovidon* - 10.8 % then by *Marvelon* and *Femodene* - 1.8 %, *Minulet* - 1.9 %, *Diane 35* under 1 %.

Table 5 Type of oral contraceptives

Contraceptive	Nr.cases	%
Microgynon	430	78.30
Ovidon	60	10.80
Marvelon	20	3.62
Femodene	10	1.80
Cilest	5	0.90
Minulet	11	1.90
Rigevidon	1	0.10
Diane 35	5	0.90

6. The menstrual flow is not evidently influenced (table 6.); the Microgynon is reducing it (5 %).

Table 6 Changes of the menstrual flow

Contraceptive	Total cases	Increased flow	%	Decreased flow	%	No changes	%
Microgynon	430	4	0.93	20	4.65	406	94.41
Ovidon	60	5	8.33	1	1.66	54	90.00
Marvelon	20	0	0.00	1	5.00	19	95.00
Femodene	10	2	20.00	0	0.00	8	80.00
Cilest	5	2	40.00	0	0.00	3	60.00
Minulet	11	2	18.18	1	9.09	8	72.70
Rigevidon	1	0	0.00	0	0.00	1	100.00
Diane 35	5	0	0.00	0	0.00	1	100.00
Stediril	5	0	0.00	0	0.00	1	100.00
Trinordiol	4	0	0.00	0	0.00	4	100.00
From total cases	551	15	2.73	23	4.17	513	93.10

7.The corporeal weight (table 7.) is influenced, increasing in 14 cases using Microgynon (3.25 %), but insignificant with Ovidon.

Table 7 Weight changes

Contraceptive	Inc.	%	Dec.	%	No Change	%
Microgynon	14	3.25	2	0.46	414	96.27
Ovidon	1	1.66	1	1.66	58	96.66

8. The intermenstrual bleedings (table 8.) are most frequently at Microgynon - 7 case (1.62 %) and Cilest (40 %) and not significant with Ovidon (1.62 %).

The rest of contraceptives are not significantly used to obtain a general conclusion.

Table 8 Intermenstrual bleedings

Contraceptive	Total cases	Bleedings	%
Microgynon	430	7	1.62
Ovidon	60	1	1.66

Marvelon	20	0	0.00
Femodene	10	0	0.00
Cilest	5	2	40.00
Minulet	11	0	0.00
Rigevidon	1	0	0.00
Diane 35	5	0	0.00
Stediril		0	0.00
Trinordiol		0	0.00
From all cases		10	1.81

9. Regarding the libido changes, these are better as increasing 2.35 % as decreasing 0.90 %

Table 9 Libido changes

Contraceptive	Increased libidow	%	Decreased libido	%	No changes	%	Total	
Microgynon	12	2.79	4	0.93	414	96.27	430	
Ovidon	0	0.00	1	1.66	59	98.33	60	
Marvelon	0	0.00	0	0.00	20	100.00	20	
Femodene	0	0.00	0	0.00	10	100.00	10	
Cilest	0	0.00	0	0.00	5	90.90	5	
Minulet	1	9.09	0	0.00	10	100.00	11	
Rigevidon	0	0.00	0	0.00	1	100.00	1	
Diane 35	0	0.00	0	0.00	5	100.00	5	
Stediril	0	0.00	0	0.00	5	100.00	5	
Trinordiol	0	0.00	0	0.00	4	100.00	4	
From total cases	15	2.35	5	0.90	533	96.73	551	

10. Other parameters not presented on tables are:
- the nausea snesation is only in 1.81 %
- the headaches - 3.08 %
- the breast tenderness - 1.63 %
- the venous troubles, most frequents at the Ovidon users - 1.66 %

- the nervosity - 8.33 % at the Ovidon users and 3.72 % at Microgynon, 1 on Marvelon and 2 cases on Cilest.

Conclusions:

1. Even the side effects are present in 10.16 %, the discontinuity of the contraceptive usage is only 3.08 % in our study.
2. As the complications, these are most frequent in the usage of Microgynon, but not so significant, because of the prevalent use of this product in Romania. These are first the decreasing of the menstrual flow, the increasing of the corporeal weight, nausea, headaches but the increasing of the libido.
3. For Ovidon - the increasing of the menstrual flow, intermenstrual bleedings, venous troubles, depresion and the decreasing of the libido.
4. Even the side-effects ate most frequent at Ovidon's usage, the discontinuity is prevalent at Microgynon's usage.
5. The pregnancies, occured under contraceptive use are correspondents at the oral contraceptives failure rate (here under 1 %) and is because of the inaccurate use of the pills.

REFERENCES

1. Aitken,J. (1988). Future developments in contraception. *The Practitioner.*
2. Baudet, J.H. (1990). La contraception, un acte medical. *Revue de Formation Du Medecine Generaliste, vol.97.*
3. Beaumont, V., Beaumont, L.(1989). La risque vasculaire des contraceptifs oraux - realite et mecanisme. *Presse Med., pp.18, 24, 25, 1203-1206, 1249-1253.*
4. Darolle, R. (1982). La contraception orale aujourd'hui. *Encycopedie Medico-Chirurgicale, vol.53. no.4.*
5. Hatcher, R.A., Kowal, D., Gvest, F. (1989). Contraceptive technology. *International Edition, Atlanta, Georgia, USA, Printed Matter Inc.*
6. Lambotte, R, Remacle, P. (1990). La contraception hormonale. *Clinique Gynecologique et Obstetricale. Universite de Liege.*
7. Teodoru, G.C. (1985). Efectele secundare ale contraceptiei. *Editura Medicala, Bucuresti.*
8. Warton, C, Blackburn, R. (1988). Lower-Dose Pills. *Oral Contraceptives Population Reports, Series A, no.7, pp. 1-31.*
9. Warren, P.N. (1973). Metabolic effects of contraceptive steroids. *American J.Med.Sci., pp. 1, 256, 5-21.*
10. Zbranca, E. (1990). *Contraceptia. Editura Junimea, Iasi.*

Effect of medroxyprogesterone acetate on ornithine decarboxylase activity in human endometrial tissue and in MCF7 cells

G. Visca, R. Bellino, M. Tessarolo and A. Lanza

Department B of Gynecology and Obstetrics Institute, University of Turin, Turin, Italy

---

BACKGROUND

Ornithine decarboxylase, key enzyme of the polyamines biosintesis, has been recently proposed as a protooncogen, being the polyamines closely connected in the physiological and pathological mechanisms of cell growth

AIMS

To determine the effect of medroxiprogesterone acetate (MPA) treatment on ODC activity in tumor cells in vivo and in vitro.

METHODS

a) In vivo

Since 1980 all the endometrial adenocarcinoma treated at the Department B of Institute of Obstetrics and Gynecology, University of Torino had been given preoperatory 1 gr medroxiprogesterone acetate (MPA) per os for 30 days, 1 gr for the next two months and 500 mg for the following 12 months.

In 30 cases (mean age 61.2 12.30- minimum 31, maximum 72) the follow-up was held for 60 months. Grade of the tumor was calculated on the basis of :

- architectural (score 1 to 3),
- nuclear grading (score 1 to 3)
- No. of mitosis every 10 high resolution fields (score 1 to 3 for mitosis less then 5, between 5-10, more then 10).

We defined G1 with a score <4, G2 if >4 and <7, G3 >7.

We determinated ODC activity in samples of human endometrial tissue drawn from these patients before MPA treatment through hysteroscopic biopsy or D&C, and after the treatment on the surgical piece.

The tissue was immediately freezed and omogeneized with 0.15 M HCl in Ultra Turrax within 20 minutes.

● Part of the omogenenate was centrifugated at 12000 x g for 10 minutes and the supernatant was used for the misuration of *ODC activity* according to Janne and Williams-Adams method (1).

CO_2 formed by (1-C) D L-ornithine after 60 minutes in shaking incubator, was bloked with 0.5 ml of tricloroacetic acid at 40% and then fixed with 0.1 ml of NCS (Nuclear Chicago Solubilizer) contained in the reaction chamber and in the end quantified in a toluenic solution of PPO-POPOP with a scintillator counter.

● *Polyamines* had been determinated adding parts of the supernatant with 1.6 diaminoexane and dansilated at chamber temperature. The dansil-polyamines had been extracted with 1 volume of

benzene. After air evaporation of the organic phase, the polyamines solubized with 100 ul of acetonitrile had been analyzed using HPLC with the method described by Colombatto (2)
• For the hybridation in situ of the *ODC mRNA* the hystological sections of the samples had been deparaffinated and rehydratated and then treated with HCl 0.02 N for 10 minutes, washed with PBS for 5 minutes , then with PBS-Triton 0.01% for 2 minutes, then PBS again for 5 minutes.
After the tratment with K proteinase (250MCGgr/ ml with PBS) at chamber temperature for 10 minutes, the sections have been washed with cold PBS, incubated with formaldeide at 4% in PBS at chamber temperature for 5 minutes and disidratated with 1 minute alcool passages at 50, 70, 95, 100, and then dried in oper air for few hours.
The sections had been covered with pre-hybridation solution (Formamide 50%; SSC 20 x 4% ; Dextran solfate 5%; sperma salmon DNA 0.5 mg/ml; tRNA E.Coli 0.25 mg/ml ; Denhardt's solution 1 x), and then incubated for 1 hour in humid chamber.
This solution has been substituted with the hybridation one (Formamide 50 x ; SSC 20 x 4% ; Dextran solfato 5% ; sperma salmon DNA 0.5 mg/ml; tRNA E.Coli 0.25 mg/ml ; Denhardt's solution 1 x ; Probe 50 ng / ml) containing the oligonucleotide 5'-ACA-GCC-GCT-TCC-TAC-ATG-GAA-3' with the apten Digossigenin (DIG) (Boehringer Mannheim) through tailing with DIG-11-dUTP and the enzyme Terminal transferase with a tail containing at least 5-10 molecules of DIG-dUTP (by Perkin Elmer S.p.A.) and then incubated at 39° in humid chamber for one night.
Then the sections have been washed with 2x SSC containing 0.1 % SDS for 20 minutes then, with 0.2 x SSC containing 0.1% SDS for 20 minutes and in the end two times with 0.16 x SSC with 0.1 % SDS for 20 minutes, all at chamber temperature.
Sections had then been washed again with TRIS 0.1 M HCl + 0.15 M NaCl pH 7.5 and incubated for 30 minutes in TRIS 0.1 M HCl + 0.15 M NcCl pH 7.5 + Blocking reagent Boeringer Mannheim GmbH.
The previous reagent was then sustituted with the monoclonal antibody anti-dgossigenine (Clone 17 C) 1:250 and left 30' in incubation.
The sections were then newly washed 3 times for 3 minutes with TRIS-HCl 0.1 M + 0.15 M NaCl pH 7.5 and treated with anti-Mouse Vector 1:200 for a whole night.
The sections were again washed 3 times for 3 minutes with TRIS-HCl 0.1 M + 0.15 M NaCl pH 7.5 and incubated with Avidine-Biotine Alkaline fosfatase for 1 hour.
The sections had been washed with TRIS k/ pH 9.5 for 5 minutes and developed with 5-brome-4-clore-3-Inolyl Phosphate / Nitro Blue Tetrazole (BCIP/NBT) for 10 minutes until the reaction became clear.
Sections had been washed with distilled water and contercolurated with methyle green for 5 minutes , washed with water and loaded on glicerine.(3)

b) In vitro
We studied the effect of MPA on Ornithine decarboxylase activity in MCF7 cells grown in DMEM without fenol red and bovine fetal serum at 10%.
MCF7 is a human tumor cell line hormone responsive.
The cells been distribuited in the dishes at a density of 4000 cells per cm2 and cultivated for 3 days in DMEM and 5% bovine fetal serum treated with dextrane and active carbon (DCC serum).
After 3 days the medium was changed and Estradiol 10-10 M and medroxiprogesterone acetate 5uM have been added.
• To evaluate *ODC activity* the cells were sonicated in Tris-HCl 0,1 M (pH 7.5) containing EDTA (0.1 mM) and ditiotreitolo (2.5 mM).
The estract had been centrifugated for 20' at 20000 x g at 4 °C.
ODC activity has been determined on the supernatant.
• For the *polyamines* determination cells were harvested in percloric acid 0.2 N, and then centrifugated at 20000 x g for 10'.
Fractions of the supernatant had been added with 1,6 diaminoexane (internal standard) and dansilated at room temperature in a dark place for 16-18 hours before being analyzed by HPLC with the partially modified Stefanelli method.
The dansilderivated were separated on a Resolve C18 column (5um; 150 x 3.9 mm) through a mobile phase made with water, acetonitrile and methanolo in a 5:3:2 proportion (phase A) and acetonitrile and methanole in 3:2 proportion (phase B)
At time zero A was 72%, after 17 min A was 45%. At the 32nd minute A was 25% and remained such for the next 5'.
The rivelator used was a fluorimetre.

218

●   *Northern Blot* : RNA was obtained from cells by guanidine tiocianate and phenol/clorophorm estraction as previously described by other Authors.(4)

RNA was then separated on a 1% agarose gel containing formaldeyde 2.4 M and then transfered to a nylon membrane. The membrane had been prehybrydated with the prehybrydation buffer Rapid-hyb for 1 hour at 65° C.

The hybridation took place at the same conditions for 2 hours and 30' using as a probe the cDNA for the human ODC of 1900 bp labelled by random printing with the Pharmacia kit Ready to go 32P α dCTP and purified with a Bio Spin Cromatografy Column by BioRad.

The membrane was then washed at room temperature in 2 x SSC (Standard Saline Citrate)/SDS 0.1%, once at 65 ° C in SSC 2x / SDS 0.1% and once at 65° C in 0.1 x SSC / SDS 0.1% before exposition at 70 ° C on Hyperfilm-HP for 18-24 hours.

●   Proteins had been determinated using the method described by Lowry and others

●   For the *Western blotting* the cells were harvested in SDS sample buffer (TRIS-HCl 50 mM, pH 6.8, ditiotreitolo 100 mM, 2% SDS, 0.1% bromophenole blue, 10% glicerole) and loaded on a 8% poliacrilamide/bisacrilamide minigel for a SDS-PAGE.

The gel run at 200 V for 45 min. Then the transfer to nitrocellulose was performed at 50 V for 1 hour . The nitrocellulose was then washed with PBS (Phosphate Saline Buffer) an bovine seric albumine at 3%.

Then it followed incubation with rabbit antiserun anti-ODC diluited 1:1000 for 2 hours, washing to take away the unbounded antibody , incubation with the secondary antibody conjugated with the alkaline phosphatase, washing and reaction for the alkaline phosphatase to evidence the ODC band.

DISCUSSION

a) In vivo

The relationship between the expression of ODC mRNA before the treatment with MPA and the hystologic response of the tumor after the treatment (responders are all the cases with tumor reduced or disappeared) was not significative ($p = 0.41$).

However the majority of the non-responders cases was positive for the ODC mRNA.

The relationship remains not significant after MPA treatment, even if the total amount of the non responders cases is in the group with the expressed ODC mRNA, in spite of the adjuvant treatment.(tab 1)

Table 1 : relationship between the expression of ODC mRNA before and after treatment with MPA and the hystologic

response of the tumor to the terapy

	responders	not-responders
ODC mRNA + before MPA	11	7
ODC mRNA + after MPA	14	8
ODC mRNA - before MPA	4	1
ODC mRNA - after MPA	6	0

On the contrary ODC mRNA is related with the reduction of more than 50% of the mitosis after the treatment with MPA (Tab 2).

The cases which showed a decreased number of mitosis had also a low RNA expression. (Tab 3)

There is no relationship between the entity of the ODC mRNA and the survival before MPA (tab 4).

Table 2 : MPA effect on mitosis (decrease > 50%)

	responders	not-responders
ODC mRNA +	6	12
ODC mRNA -	5	0

Mantel- Haenszel : $\kappa2 = 6.67$; $P = 0,009$
Fisher : $P = 0,01$

Table 3 : Relationship between mitosis and mRNA

	responders	not-responders
ODC mRNA +	8	12
ODC mRNA -	7	1

Mantel- Haenszel : $\kappa2$ =5,00 ; P =0,02
Fisher : P = 0,02

Table 4 : Relationship between ODC mRNA expression before MPA and the survival

	NED	DOT
ODC mRNA +	12	6
ODC mRNA -	5	0

In the same way after MPA treatment its expression does not relate with survival.(tab 5)

Table 5 : Relationship between ODC mRNA expression after MPA and the survival

	NED	DOT
ODC mRNA +	15	5
ODC mRNA -	7	1

The relationship between survival and ODC mRNA is not significant either before (tab 4) or after the MPA treatment.(tab 5)
The diminuished activity of ODC caused by MPA (considernig positive a cut off of 20 nM CO_2 /g/h) correlated to survival (tab 6) and the diminuition of the mitosis(tab 7) is instead much significant.

Table 6 : Relationship between ODC activity and survival

	ODC activity < 20 nM CO_2 /g/h	ODC activity > 20 nM CO_2 /g/h
NED	21	3
DOT	0	6

Mantel- Haenszel : $\kappa2$ = 16,92 ; P =0,00003
Fisher : P = 0,0001

Table 7 : Relationship between ODC activity and mitosis decrease

	ODC activity < 20 nM CO_2 /g/h	ODC activity > 20 nM CO_2 /g/h
responders	16	1
non responders	5	8

The relationship between grading and ODC mRNA positivity before the treatment is not significant, but all the G3 cases show an immunostaining for the ODC mRNA(tab 8)

Table 8 : Relationship between ODC mRNA expression and grading

	G1-G2	G3
ODC mRNA +	13	5
ODC mRNA -	5	0

Fisher : P = 0,01

We evaluated ODC activity in the 30 patients before and after the hormonal treatment.
In the scarcely differentiated carcinomas the increase of the activity is 79 times the menopausal tissue one: in the G1 and G2 carcinomas it is 32 times the menopausal endometrium
In the well differentiated carcinomas the MPA treatment causes a 10 times decrease of ODC activity, taking the neoplastic tissue to values similar to the endometrial intermediate proliferative or advanced secretory phases.

The moderately differentiated carcinomas treated with MPA generally reacted with a decrease of ODC activity, although this reduction did not seem significant.

In the scarcely differentiated carcinomas we did not observe any reduction of ODC activity after MPA treatment.

In our 30 cases ODC activity diminished for the effect of MPA. On the whole this diminuition is not significant for the mixing of G1-G2-G3, but it becomes considerably significant ($p=0.000002$) for the matched dates, that is confronting case with case.(Table 9)

As far as the polyamines are concerned, even the putrescine concentration diminished for the MPA effect in the G1-G2 adenocarcinomas and it did not change for the G3 (tab 10)

Table 9 : Relationship between grading and ODC activity before and after MPA treatment

	No of cases	ODC nM CO_2 g/h/37°C
G1 before MPA	10	119 ± 18
after MPA	10	11.5 ± 4.9
G2 before MPA	10	143 ± 42
after MPA	8	67.5 ± 65
G3 before MPA	5	315 ± 25
after MPA	6	425 ± 418

Table 10 : Polyamines before and after MPA

	No. cases	putrescine nM/g	spermine nM/g	spermidine nM/g
G1 before MPA	15	314 ± 120	528 ± 48	286 ± 75
after MPA	15	123 ± 82	294 ± 65	270 ± 58
G2 before MPA	9	284 ± 63	615 ± 102	344 ± 12
after MPA	9	84 ± 63	496 ± 105	305 ± 67
G3 before MPA	6	372 ± 70	612 ± 85	386 ± 82
after MPA	6	302 ± 65	340 ± 48	496 ± 99

We did not find any significative relationship between grading and putrescine decreased concentration. Among the three grading the difference is not statistically significant.

In the G1 carcinomas after MPA treatment, the spermine concentration diminished to the half reaching the physiological values of an endometrium during weakly proliferative phase or weakly secretive phase.

Spermine concentration in G1-G2 tumors reduced after hormonal treatment and it showed values 5 times lower than before the treatment.

Spermidine concentration in G1 tumors was rather low, similar to that of normal endometrium in advanced secretive phase.

In G2 tumors it is similar to the perimenopausal endometrium, with signs of estrogenic stimulation and in the G3 it is little higher.

The MPA treatment doesn't reduce the concentration of spermidine.

b) In vitro

We studied MPA effect on MCF7 cells proliferation with progestinic receptors .

We cultivated the cells in a medium without fenol red because of its small estrogenic activity, and we treated the serum to eliminate the majority of the steroid hormones, and we let the cells to stand for at least 48 hours in a medium without steroids (DMEM without fenol red and 5% DCC serum) to deprive them of the steroids.

In order to observe MPA effects on cell growth and on ODC activity is necessary the simultaneus presence of Estradiol because the progestinic receptors are expressed just in presence of estrogens.

It was necessary to find the proper estradiol concentration to permit the expression of the progestinic receptors, and consequentely of MPA effect, and to avoid the execessive cell growth, because the estrogens stimulate MCF7 proliferation.

Such a concentration was of 10-10 M

Cells were cultured for 48 hours with different MPA concentrations.

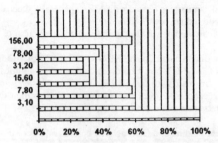

Fig. 1: Inhibiting effect of MPA on ODC activity in MCF7 cells

The maximum inhibition on ODC activity has been observed at a 31.2 μM.(Fig 1)
This concentration was used to follow ODC activity at different times of incubation with MPA.(Fig. 2)
The maximum inhibition is observable after 48 hours of incubation in presence of MPA.
After 48 hours the cells show only 30% of the ODC activity left compared to the controls and the cell growth is inhibited by 30%.
After this all the cells had been cultured for 48 hours in order to study the regulation of the ODC.
At 48 hours we analized the polyamines (fig 3).

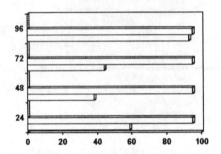

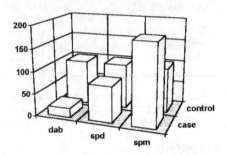

Fig . 2 : Course in time of ODC activity inhibition with
31.2 μM of MPA

Fig. 3 : MCF7 cells polyamines production after 48 hours of MPA treatment at 31.2 μM

Putrescine and spermidine decreased while spermine increased.
This could be explained considering that the lack of putrescine, which is a precursor of spermidine, leads to a decrease of the latter and that the amount of spermidine into the cells before MPA addition is converted to spermine by the addition of an aminopropilic group using as a donor decarboxylated-SAM.
We tried to find out how MPA rules ODC activity.
Experiments to determine ODC halflife in MCF7 control cells and in MPA treated cells were held
We incubated the cells with cicloesimide 200 μg / ml for 20, 40 and 60 minutes but no substantial change in the halflife has been observed.
Norther Blot experiments on total RNA had also showed that there is no change in the amount of mRNA codifying for ODC in both 48 and 96 hours conditions.(Photo 1)
ODC reduction due to MPA confirms the reduced metabolic tissue activity.
Even if MPA causes a decrease in ODC activity, this effect is not at a transcriptional level.
We also wanted to verify if the modification was due to a change in the translational rate in ODC mRNA, but no differences were observed.(Photo 2)
This means that the ODC mRNA is translated at the same speed, being present in the same quantity in the two different conditions.

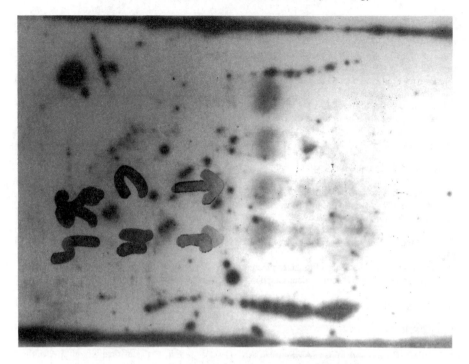

Photo 1 : ODC mRNA Northern Blot Analysis in MCF7 cells

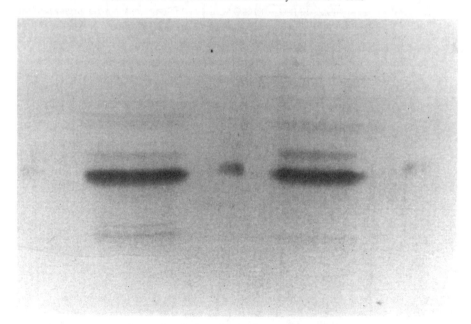

Photo 2 : ODC Immunoblotting Analysis in MCF7 cells

CONCLUSIONS

In vivo we demonstrated that:
- on 19 cases in which ODC activity was less than 20 nM of $CO_2/g/h$, 12 (63%) had still the expression of ODC mRNA
- in those cases in which ODC remains high after hormone therapy, ODC mRNA is always expressed in more than 40% of the cells.
- the presence of a high ODC after MPA treatment is coupled with a high number of mitosis or of relapses and of death, which means the cases with a more aggressive tumor
- the expression of ODC mRNA, both in the cells of the bioptical sample before the hormonal tratment and in the cells of the operative piece after the tratment , is accompanied by a persistence of mitosis.
It is also intresting to point out that all the cases with no signal for mRNA have a low ODC activity.
In vitro we demonstrated that :
- after 48 hours the MCF7 cells show only 30% of the ODC activity left compared to the controls and the cell growth is inhibited by 30%.
- mRNA and its protein are not modificated in the MCF7 cells treated with MPA even if it is possible to observe a reduction in ODC activity.

We conclude that MPA reduces ODC activity both in vivo (endometrial carcinoma) and in vitro (MCF7 cells).
It is still to know at which level this takes place.
The reduction of the ODC activity could happen through a post-translational mechanism.

Ackowledgment : the authors thank Pharmacia / Farmitalia Carlo Erba

REFERENCES

1. JEANNE J. and WILLIAMS-ASHMAN (1971): " On the purification of L-Ornithine decarboxylase from rat ptrostate and effects of thiol compounds on the enzyme". *Biol. Chem.*, 246, 1725

2. COLOMBATTO S. ,PEZZALI D.C., GRILLO M.A.(1987) : Selenium and polyamine metabolism : different effect of selenite on liver and bursa of Fabricious ornithine decarboxylase activity. Int. J. Biochem 19: 725-728

3. GAN F. , GESELL M.S., MOSHIER J.A., ALOUSI M., LUK G.D. (1992): "Detection of Ornithine decarboxylase mRNA in Human Hepatocellular Carcinoma by In Situ Hybritization". *Epith. Cell. Biol.*, 1, 13-17 .

4. PUISSANT C. , HOUDEBINE L.M. (1990): *Biotecniques* 8, 148-149 ;

Disturbances in the hypothalamic-pituitary-gonadal axis of depressed fertile women compared to normal controls

B. Hartmann, W. Baischer, G. Koinig, A. Albrecht, S. Kirchengast, J. Huber and G. Langer

Department of Gynecologic Endocrinology and Department of Psychiatry, University of Vienna, Vienna, Austria

THE PITUITARY-GONADAL-ADRENAL AXIS

Several anormalities of anterior pituitary and target endocrine gland hormone secretion patterns have been reported in patients with the endogenous subtype of major depression (1,2).
The most prominent and well studied of these anormalities involves hyperactivity of the hypothalamic-pituitary- adrenal cortical axis that has been reported to occur in up to 50 % of patients with endogenous depression (3,4). Since the symptoms of menopausal depression often coincide with alterations in plasma concentrations of sex-steroids, it frequently has been suggested that the influence of gonadal steroids on brain function is implicated in the pathophysiology of this special syndrome (5,6).
We therefore investigated depressed fertile women, as there are only a few studies testing the Hypophyseal-Gonadal Axis in this patient group. Our aims were to assess whether patients suffering from an endogenous depression would differ from healthy controls in any dimension of this endocrine axis and whether antidepressant drug treatment would have an influence on hormonal parameters, with an eventual effect on treatment outcome. Additionally we tried to asses a relationship between hormone-levels and the severity of depressive syndrome.

TWENTY DEPRESSIVE PATIENTS WERE COMPARED TO TEN NORMAL CONTROLS

Study procedures started on the first day after menstruation in the early follicular phase. The patients had to be drug free for at least 5 days not to use any hormones as well as to have a regular menstrual cycle. Baseline hormone levels and the GnRH-Test as well as psychometric evaluation using the Hamilton depression scale (7) were carried out: The patients had to answer different questions according to the result they were cathegorized, if they were suffering from an endogenous depression and if yes additionally about the severity of the disease: HAM-D scores had to be 14 points or more before treatment.

ANTI-DEPRESSANT MEDICATION: CLOMIPRAMINE

Twenty women aged from 21-43a, with endogenous depression completed the study procedures. Mean HAM-D score before treatment was 22,1 points. Following the baseline visit, including HAM-D test and GnRH test, all of them received an antidepressant medication consisting of 50-250mg (mean 125mg/d) Clomipramine per day throughout the study period.
Ten normal healthy volunteers were selected analogously and age matched with the patients and underwent the same testing procedure.

THE GnRH STIMULATION TEST

All hormonal investigatons were performed during the early follicular phase one day after menstruation. Blood samples for determination of estradiol, progesterone, testosterone, Prolactin (PRL), LH and FSH were obtained after an overnight fast by installing an intravenous catheter. Following the baseline collections at 8:30 a.m., the GnRH-test was performed stimulating hormonal response by injection of 50mcg synthetic GnRH, which was repeated 60 minutes later. After another 40 minutes, blood for measurements of stimulated LH and FSH was taken. The serum was separated by centrifugation and stored at -70 C until asseyed. Serum testosterone, estradiol and progesterone were determined by means of commercially available radioimmunological assays, LH by fluor immunoassay, FSH and PRL by enzymic immunoassay. Results of the GnRH-test Delta-LH and Delta-FSH, defined as response to the GnRH administration were computed as the difference between the highest level at 20, 40 or 60 minutes after the injection of 50 yg GnRH and the basal level

HAMILTON DEPRESSION SCORE: 12 PATIENTS RECOVERED

The assessment of treatment outcome - with definition of recovery as HAM-D scores < 9 following 5 weeks of treatment - 12 patients recovered and 8 non-recovered within the observation period . At the end of the 5 week's period the initial procedures were repeated. Statistical analyses were performed by use of non-parametric methods: to test group differences the Mann-Whitney U test was applied, a measure of association was obtained by the Spearman rank correlation. Both tests were carried out with two-sided alternatives at 5% significance level.
Statistical analyses showed significantly elevated basal serum levels of testosterone in the untreated patients relative to healty controls, while patients on clomipramine treatment still showed testosterone levels higher than normals but this difference no longer reached statistical significance.

LH, FSH, PRL AND DELTA FSH, LH LEVELS

No significant differences could be observed regarding estradiol, progesteron and PRL, LH and FSH between untreated patients and normal controls.

Table. Hormone concentrations (mean±SEM) of patients before and under clomipramine medication versus normal controls

---

	Patients untreated	Patients treated	Controls healthy
estradiol (pg/ml)	65,9±12,4	51,3±8,44	69,4±10,8
progesterone (ng/ml)	0,40±0,04	0,55±0,17	0,43±0,05
testosterone (ng/ml)	0,63±0,6*	0,56±0,08	0,42±0,04
LH (mU/ml)	4,74±0,57	4,69±0,84	4,42±0,99
FSH (mU/ml)	7,05±1,37	5,49±0,47	6,88±0,68
PRL (ng/ml)	8,19±1,66	10,2±1,54*	5,82±0,54
Delta-LH (mU/ml)	36,8±6,99	26,1±4,99	30,3±5,28
Delta-FSH (mU/ml)	7,73±1,04	5,25±0,77*	9,34±1,62

---

* denotes significant difference to controls (p<0,05)

Significant differences between clomipramine treated patients and controls were found with regard to PRL, due to the anti-depressant therapy knowing to augment PRL-levels and in regard to Delta-FSH, which proved to be lower in patients under clomipramine therapy. No difference was found in Delta LH and Delta FSH between untreated patients and normal controls.

SERUM ESTRADIOL CONCENTRATIONS

Regarding the neuroendocrine findings versus clinical characteristics in untreated depressive women a significant negative correlation between serum estradiol concentrations and the degree of severity of their HAM-score could be observed: Patients with more severe symptoms, expressed by higher HAM-D scores showed lower estrogen concentrations.

SIGNIFICANTLY HIGHER PLASMA TESTOSTERONE LEVELS WERE FOUND IN UNTREATED DEPRESSIVE WOMEN

In summary, our results showed essentially normal serum levels of pituitary gonadotropins but significantly higher testosterone levels in untreated depressive women: In the patient group, lower estradiol was associated with higher degrees of severity of depressive syndrome. Elevated PRL levels following clomipramine medication have been described earlier[8]. These results are consistent with some but not all previous data on patients with major depression: Altschule and Tillotson [9] used methyl-testosterone successfully in the treatment of depressed patients. They concluded that testosterone in large doses is followed by remission of symptoms in many patients with all types of depression. Sherwin [10] demonstrated that women on estradiol and testosterone substitution therapy "feel more composed, elated, and energetic" than those who where given estradiol alone. However, other studies have failed to demonstrate any additional benefit over estrogens alone, some even demonstrate androgenetic side effects such as severe hirsutism, decreased libido and depression [11,12]. Amsterdam et al [13] did not find any deviations of basal and GnRH stimulated LH, FSH and estradiol in fertile depressive women while Vogel et al [14] reported an increase in the testosterone-estradiol ratio in depressed females; Contrary to our results Vogel et al demonstrated an increase of both steroids, estradiol and testosterone, in depressive premenopausal women.

ESTROGEN/ANDROGEN RATIO - THE ANSWER ?

A plethora of questions may be raised concerning the levels of testosterone and possible psychiatric related effects. The data reviewed suggest that androgenetic steroids may both, relieve and cause depression. Some researchers have found that androgens are effective anti-depressants. Many other data, however, suggest that androgens may cause depression in some instances. Our data also confirm a relationship between testosterone concentrations on one hand and low estrogen concentrations on the other. Maybe the ratio of androgen to estrogen is the determinant.
Since there is little data currently available on androgenetic steroids and possible psychiatric related effects, further study is needed, particuluarly on biological mechanisms, which may help to explain the relationships between androgenic steroids and various behavioural effects.

REFERENCES

1. Carroll, B.J. (1978). Neuroendocrine function in affective disorders. In Lipton MA, DiMascio A, Killam KF, eds. *Psychopharmacology: A generation of progress.* New York, NY: Raven Press;487-497
2. Checkley S.A. (1980). Neuroendocrine tests of monoamine function in man: a review of basic theory and its application to the study of depressive illness. *Psychol. Med.;* 10, 35-53
3. Schulte H. , Oldfield E. , Loriaux D.L. (1984). Psychiatric implications of basic and clinical studies with corticotropin releasing factor. *Am. J. Psychiatry.;*141, 619-627
4. Pfohl B. , Sherman B. , Schlechte J. , Stone R. (1985). Pituitary/adrenal axis disturbances in psychiatric depression. *Arch. Gen.Psychiatry.*42, 897-903
5.Clare A.W. (1985). Hormones, behaviour and the menstrual cycle. *J. Psychosom. Res.;*3, 225-233
6. Eriksson E., Sundblad C., Lisjö P., Modigh K., Andersch B. (1992). Serum levels of androgens are higher in women with premenstrual irritability and dysphoria than in controls. *Psychoneuroendocrinology* ;17, 195-204
7. Hamilton M. (1960). A rating scale for depression. *J. Neurol. Neurosurg.Psychiat.;*23, 56-62

8. Anand V. S. (1985). Clomipramin-induced galactorrhoea and amenorrhoea. *Br. J. Psychiat.*;147, 87-88

9. Altschule M.D., Tillotson K.J. (1948). The use of testosteron in the treatment of depression. *N. Engl. J. Med.*;239, 1036-1038

10. Sherwin B.B. (1988). Affective changes with estrogen and androgen replacement therapy in surgically menopausal women. *J. Affect. Disord.*;14, 177-187

11. Urmann B., Pride S.M., Yuen B.H. (1991). Elevated serum testosterone, hirsutism and virilism associated with combined androgen-estrogen hormone replacement therapy. *Obstet. Gynecol.*;77, 595-598

12. Pope H.G., Katz D. (1987). Bodybuilder´s psychosis. *Lancet* ;i, 863

13. Amsterdam J.D., Winokur A., Caroff S., Snyder P. (1981). Gonadotropin release after administration of GnRH in depressed patients and healthy volunteers. *J. Affect. Disord.*;3, 367-380

14. Vogel W., Klaiber E.L., Broverman D.M. (1978). Role of the gonadal steroid hormones in psychiatric depression in men and women. *Prog. Neuro-Psychopharmcol.*;2, 487-503

SECTION 2

Fertility and Sterility

Clinical aspects of preimplantation diagnosis

P.N. Barri, A. Veiga, M. Boada, J. Santaló, F. Vidal and J. Egozcue

Reproductive Medicine Service, Department of Obstetrics and Gynecology, Institut Universitari Dexeus, Grup d'Investigació en Embrions Preimplantacionals Humans (GIEPH), Spain

Introduction

In order to be effective, a preimplantation diagnosis technique should be sufficiently specific and sensitive to obtain information from a single biopsied blastomere. Likewise the diagnosis should be quick so that the embryos do not need to be frozen and painstaking to safeguard the viability of the biopsied embryos.

Preimplantation diagnostic techniques now constitute a real alternative to prenatal diagnosis (HANDYSIDE et al., 1992). So far, the only possibility of avoiding the birth of off spring affected by genetic diseases or chromosomic abnormalities was by carrying out a prenantal diagnosis by means of chorion villus sampling or amniocentesis and a later induced abortion if the foetus was affected.

Indications

Indications for preimplantation diagnosis are the same as for prenatal diagnosis. Nevertheless, given the complexity of the technique we would recommend proposing this technique only to couples at high genetic risk. Some authors (MUNNE et al., 1993-b) propose preimplantation diangosis by means of an aneuploidy test in patients over 38 years.

Clinical changes in the IVF cycle for preimplantation diagnosis

When a preimplantation diagnosis program is carried out, it involves important changes in the IVF team. These changes can only be assimilated by IVF teams which are wide-ranging, a expert and with regular results.

a) Changes in team size

In order to cover all the stages of the process it is essential to include molecular biologists, clinical geneticists, obstetricians and pediatricians in the IVF team normaly comprising gynecologists and biologists.

b) Changes in team mentality

Due to the larger size of the team, it is essential to sacrifice character traits of each member to reach the appropiate harmony in daily work.

c) Changes in the IVF cycle

Follicular growth stimulation will have to be more intense in order to obtain more oocytes which will lead to more embryos available for biopsy. Likewise it will be useful to delay HCG administration in order to achieve a high percentage of mature oocytes.

Embryo replacement takes place one day later (day 3 after ovum pick-up) and at a time which depends on the molecular biology laboratory and on its speed in delivering results of the embryo biopsies.

In these cases, embryo transfer should be as atraumatic as possible given that these biopsied embryos are more sensitive to mechanical traumatisms. Some authors recommend the administration of antibiotics and corticoids after embryo transfer in these patients.

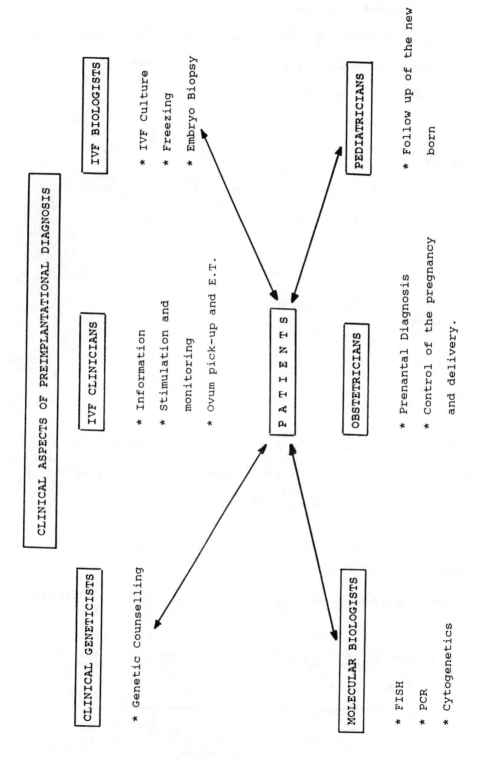

CLINICAL ASPECTS OF PREIMPLANTATIONAL DIAGNOSIS

CLINICAL GENETICISTS

* Genetic Counselling

IVF CLINICIANS

* Information

* Stimulation and monitoring

* Ovum pick-up and E.T.

IVF BIOLOGISTS

* IVF Culture

* Freezing

* Embryo Biopsy

PATIENTS

MOLECULAR BIOLOGISTS

* FISH

* PCR

* Cytogenetics

OBSTETRICIANS

* Prenantal Diagnosis

* Control of the pregnancy and delivery.

PEDIATRICIANS

* Follow up of the new born

d) Changes in the control of pregnancy

If a pregnancy is achieved, it is necessary to add to normal echographic and biochemical tests, a prenatal diagnostic test which by means of a chorion willus sampling or amniocentesis can confirm the diagnosis of the preimplantation evaluation.

Conclusion

Preimplantation diagnosis techniques already make up a clinical reality in some centers. However there are still some problem areas which must be eliminated

* Complexity and results of IVF

                        - Ovarian hyperstimulation

* Risk of   - Multiple pregnancy

                        - Abortion

* Failure of embryo biopsy

* Diagnostic error

Although the futur will help to solve these problems, we believe that, for the time being, these techniques should be reserved to reference centers which will receive enough cases to accumulate experience and to develop each technique.

Bibliography

1.- HANDYSIDE A.H., LESKO J.G., TARIN J.J., WINSTON R.M.L., HUGUES M.R. (1992)

Birth of a normal girl after IVF and preimplantation diagnostic testing for cystic fibrosis.

N. ENGL. J. MED. 327:594-598

2.- LIEBAERS I., SERMON K., LISSENS W., LIU J., DEVROEY P., TARLATZIS B., VAN STEIRTEGHEM A. (1992)

Preimplantation diangosis

HUM.REPROD. 107-110

3.- MUNNE S., LEE A., ROSENWAKS Z., GRIFO J., COHEN J. (1993)

Diagnosis of major chromosome aneuploidies in human preimplantational embryos.

HUM.REPROD. 8:2185-2191

4.- VEIGA A., SANTALO J., VIDAL F., CALDERON G., GIMENEZ C., BOADA M., EGOZCUE J., BARRI PN (1994)

Twin pregnancy after preimplantation diagnosis for sex selection: case report

HUM. REPROD. Vol.9 No.11 (In press)

Usefulness of cytogenetics in preimplantation diagnosis

A. Veiga

Servei de Medicina de la Reproduccio, Departament d'Obstetricia i Ginecologia, Institut Universitari Dexeus, Barcelona, Spain

INTRODUCTION
Preimplantation diagnosis can be actually performed with the use of the polymerase chain reaction (PCR) or fluorescent in situ hybridization (FISH). There is a considerable need for chromosome analysis of preimplantation embryos not only for couples who carry balanced translocations but also to detect chromosomal imbalance, major cause of of abnormal embryonic development. Cytogenetic analysis is still scarcely used due to the technichal difficulties that arise when trying to obtain good chromosome preparations from preimplantation biopsies. To obtain good chromosome preparations, embryo blastomeres must remain alive after the biopsy and the fixation method must produce good enough metaphase plates to be able to count the chromosomes. The ideal situation would be the obtention of good quality chromosome spreads to apply banding or painting techniques.

MATERIAL AND METHODS
Embryos coming from 1PN, ≥3PN zygotes, heavily fragmented embryos or cleaved embryos when no pronuclei were observed, coming from the Institut Dexeus IVF programm not suitable for transfer or freezing were used for embryo biopsy. The zona pellucida was drilled with acid Tyrode's solution. One or two blastomeres were gently removed from each embryo. After the biopsy, the embryos as well as the removed blastomeres were kept in antimitotic culture overnigth (vinblastine sulfate, 10^{-7}M) to obtain metaphase chromosomes. The zona pellucida was removed with the use of pronase and the rest of the blastomeres were disaggregated (short incubation in Ca^{2+} Mg^{2+} to compare technical efficiency between this material and biopsied blastomeres. Fixation was performed according to a modification of Tarkowski's method but using 10% human serum in distilled water as hypotonic treatment.

RESULTS
Biopsies were performed in 104 embryos, with an overall success rate of 79.8%. Eight embryos were kept in culture and 6 of them continued to cleave (75% surviving rate). Statistically

TABLE I
Efficiency of chromosome preparations from biopsied human
embryos.

type of embryo	nb of biopsies processed	fixed biopsies	chromosome prep.	interphase nuclei	loss
N	10	10 (100%)	1[a*] (10%)	6[b] 60%)	3[a] (30%)
2PN	17	15 (88.2%)	7[a+] (46.6%)	6[a] (40%)	2[b] (13.4%)
3PN	49	49 (100%)	10[a*] (20.4%)	29[b] (59.2%)	10[a] (20.4%)
NF?	7	7 (100%)	0	4 (57.1%)	3 (42.9%)

Within each column values with different superscripts (+,*) are
significantly different, P¼ 0.05
Within each row values with different superscripts (a,b) are
significantly different, P¼ 0.05

significant differences were observed when comparing the
proportion of chromosome preparations obtained depending on the
type of embryo biopsied (table 1).The differences in the
percentage of interphase nuclei and embryonic loss were not
statistically significant. A higher proportion of chromosome
preparations were obtained from 2PN embryos (46.6%) than from 1PN
(10%) and 3PN (20.4%) embryos. A higher proportion of interphase
nuclei were obtained from 1 PN and 3PN embryos (59.2%) with
respect to chromosome preparations and embryonic loss. In 2 PN
embryos the embryonic loss was lower (13.4%).

The results obtained with disaggregated embryos show no
statistically significant differences in the percentage of
chromosome preparations or embryonic loss when comparing the
different type of embryos but a lower proportion of interphase
nuclei (19.4%) was observed in 2PN embryos as compared with 3PN
(47%). A higher proportion of embryonic loss was also observed
in 2PN and 3PN embryos as compared with the percentage of
chromosome preparation obtained in each group.
Comparing the proportion of chromosome metaphases from biopsied
and disaggregated embryos, a lower percentage is obtained when
disaggregating the embryos. By contrast, a statistically higher
proportion of embryonic loss was observed when disaggregating 2PN
and 3PN embryos.
Overall,when chromosomes were obtained, 75% of the metaphase
plates were suitable to be analyzed by counting the
chromosomes.

The efficiency in obtaining good chromosome spreads has not yet
reached the figures to allow clinical use.Technical improvement
is needed; the use of normal cleaving embryos may also permit to

improve the results obtained. Unstransferable embryos may not the best material to use to improve the technique.

A combination of cytogenetics and FISH is proposed to reach the diagnosis even when chromosome spreads are not obtained or their quality is not good enough. An appropriate schedule that fits with clinical application is proposed:
- Embryo biopsy on the evening of day 2 (between 4 and 8 cell-stage).
- Overnight culture in medium + antimitotic.
- Chromosome preparations early in the morning.
- Results from cytogenetic analysis at 10 A.M.
- FISH at 11 A.M. (4 h hybridization).
- FISH analysis and results early evening.
- Transfer in the evening of day 3.

BIBLIOGRAPHY
- Tarin JJ, Handyside AH: Embryo biopsy strategies for preimplantation diagnosis. Fert Steril 59:943-952 (1993).
- Veiga A, Calderon G, Santalo J, Barri PN, Egozcue J:Chromosome studies in oocytes and zygotes from an IVF programme. Hum Reprod 2:425-430 (1987).
- Vidal F, Veiga A, Barri PN, Egozcue J, Santalo J: CYFISH: Cytogenetics plus FISH in preimplantation diagnosis. Am J Hum Gnenet 53 suppl A 1470 (1993).
- Veiga A, Santaló J, Vidal F, Calderón G, Giménez C, Boada M, Egozcue J, Barri P.N. Twin pregnancy after preimplantation diagnosis for sex determination: a case report. Hum Reprod 9, 2156-2159 (1994).

Factors affecting the selection of human embryos for transfer in an IVF–ET program

S.M. Walker

Assisted Reproduction Unit, University Hospital of Wales, Cardiff, UK

The last decade has seen a World-wide escalation of in vitro fertilisation and embryo transfer. Major advances have occurred in relation to ovarian stimulation and more recently micro injection of sperm , both subzonal (SUZI) and latterly directly into the ooplasm, intracytoplasmic sperm injection (ICSI).

Human embryo implantation however, remains an enigma. Much of the evidence was initially indirectly derived from the maternal environment. More recently assay of the supernatant from pre-embryo culture has demonstrated the in vitro production of immunosuppressants (Daya and Clark 1986).

The clinical pregnancy rate resulting from IVF-ET per treatment cycle has only increased by approximately 6% during the years 1985-1992 despite a gross increase in the number of procedures undertaken (Human Fertilisation and Embryology Authority 1994). One important factor in relation to the global success rates of IVF-ET is the increasing number of units involved in the provision of treatment, many of whom undertake relatively few procedures. Nonetheless, well established units still experience an excess embryo loss in the order of 20% of cycles, when compared with natural conception and an embryo loss of approximately 90% overall following transfer. Embryos are generally selected for transfer on the basis of morphological appearances and cleavage rate. Recent in vitro studies of human cumulus-corona cell proliferation (Gregory et al 1994) and 11ß hydroxysteroid dehydrogenase activity of the human granulosa-lutein cells (Michael et al 1993) have shown a relationship to the subsequent outcome of IVF-ET. Thus two aspects of follicle cell function have been identified which provide useful prognostic indicators for embryo implantation and consequently have implications for clinical management.

References

Daya, S. and Clarke, D.A. (1986)
Immunosuppressive factor produced by human embryos in vitro.
N. Eng. J. Med. 315, 1551-1552.

Human Fertilisation and Embryology Authority Third Annual Report (1994)
HMSO London.

Gregory, L., Booth, A.D., Wells, C. and Walker, S.M. (1994)
A study of the Cumulus-corona cell complex in in vitro fertilisation and embryo transfer; a prognostic indicator of the failure of implantation.

Michael, A.E., Gregory, L., Walker, S.M., Piercy, E.C., Antoniw, J.W., Shaw, R.W., Edward, C.R.W., Cooke, B.A. (1993)
Ovarian 11 hydroxysteroid dehydrogenase; ;a potential indicator of conception by in vitro fertilisation and embryo transfer.
Lancet 342, 711-712.

Implantation

K. El-Farra and J.G. Grudzinskas*

Queen Mary's University Hospital, Roehampton and *The Royal London Hospital, London, UK

INTRODUCTION:

Implantation means that the conceptus has completely left the " external milieu" i.e., the uterine lumen, and is definitely embedded in the uterine mucosa. This implies that an intense tissue remodelling by growth factors/cytokines and proteases induced by embryo-maternal interactions and endocrine events (1) exists to permit the penetration of the blastocyst. We shall discuss here the inter-relationship between the endometrium and early conceptus with special reference to cytokines.

THE PROCESS OF IMPLANTATION:

The metabolic and cellular events in the secretory phase of the human endometrium prepare it for implantation of the conceptus (2). The maternal recognition of fertilisation leads to the maintenance of luteal function by human chorionic gonadotrophin (hCG) (3). The nidation process can be divided in three stages: it begins with fixation-adhesion of the blastocyst, then penetration of the trophoectoderm cells between epithelial cells occurs. Lastly intrusion in the subepithelial zone is effected. Fixation-adhesion of the blastocyst to the surface epithelium is in some way a biologic paradox (4) There appears to be no other population of epithelial cells which seem to adhere by their apical poles. There is evidence of a reduction in the electronegative charge of the apex of surface cells during the nidation window. In addition, the presence of fucose, galactose, and acetylgalactosaminyl residues in the epithelial cells are likely to play a role. Little is known about the actual mechanisms of adhesion and just as enzymatic activation is probably needed for blastocyst hatching, the adhesion phenomenon is probably also dependent on an enzymatic molecular rearrangement at the surfaces of both cell types.

Lindenberg et al (5) described penetration as one of the earliest events after adhesion, in in-vitro experiments of endometrial epithelial cell and blastocyst cocultures, the first phenomenon being a displacement of epithelial cells by trophoblasts. Subsequently, the trophoblastic cells send long protrusions between epithelial cells leading to an obvious rupture of lateral tight junctions and the adjacent endometrial cells showing increased cellular activity. Thus, the contact between primary trophoplast and the subepithelial zone is established.

TROPHOBLAST-ENDOMETRIUM RELATIONSHIP:

It has long been noted that the cellular changes in the endometrium which accompany successful pregnancy are superficially similar to chronic inflammation, e.g., wound healing, a process that is beneficial to the survival of the species. Implantation involves extensive modifications of the embryo and the endometrium and is induced by contacts between the embryo and the uterus, and by extracellular signals which affect both blastcyst and the uterine epithelium.(6).

The uterine mucosa comprises four types of cells which are eventually involved in the contact with the early embryo-placental unit and almost exclusively with the primary trophoblast which completely surrounds the embryo. These cells are the epithelial cells of the surface epithelium, the epithelial gland cells, the stromal (decidual) cells, and the stromal lymphoid cells. The role of the surface epithelial cells seems to present a surface suitable for blastocyst adhesion, to separate from each other during the initial stage of implantation and to multiply in order to cover the area where the blastocyst is growing. Epithelial cells probably carry messages from the adhering blastocyst to the different compartments of the mucosa. Epithelial glandular cells have secretory products which serve as nutrients for the growing embryo (glycoproteins) or as carrier proteins for important molecules such as pregnancy-associated endometrial α_2 globulin (α_2 PEG) [also

246

known as placental protein14 (PP14)] for retinol a substance essential for cell growth and organ differentiation (7).

Following attachment to the endometrial surface, trophoblast penetrates the epithelium and its basement membrane (8). Contact is thus established with the underlying stroma, which also becomes differentiated under the influence of hormones (decidualisation). This process is not evident until some 5 days after contact between the human embryo and the stroma has occurred. Decidual tissue is secretory and a paracrine relationship is established between the mother and her embryo. Decidual cells produce prolactin (PRL) and insulin-like growth factor binding protein-1 (IGFBP-1) [also known as placental protein 12 (PP12)] (2& 10-12).

THE ROLE OF CYTOKINES/ GROWTH FACTORS IN IMPLANTATION:

Peptide growth factors were first identified 16 years ago (13). Initially divided into growth factors and cytokines, it is now clear that this distinction is arbitrary because of the pleiotrophic actions of many peptides. The role of cytokines in implantation may be divided into three sections. Firstly, they mediate the actions of steroids in preparing the receptivity of the endometrium. Secondly, maternal growth factors expressed in Fallopian tube epithelial cells and endothelial cells may have direct actions on the embryo. Finally, the decidual changes that accommodate the embryo are likely to be mediated by cytokines or growth factors (14).

There is considerable evidence that cytokines and factors that they induce are associated with oestrogen and progesterone regulated preparation of the uterus for blastocyst implantation (15). The synthesis of macrophage colony stimulating factor (CSF-1) and interleukin 1 (IL-1) is directly induced by hormones. Other inflammatory-type factors are more likely to be induced secondarily, probably through the action of IL-1. Successful implantation is likely to be dependent on production of several inflammatory-type factors such as histamine, prostaglandins, leukaemia inhibitory factor (LIF), and platelet activating factor (PAF), CSF-1 and IL-1. IL-6 and tumour necrosis factor-α (TNF-α) are not required. Since TNF is able to promote production of growth factors as well as to stimulate fibroblasts and endothelial cell stimulation, it is postulated that TNF might also play a role in the endometrial-trophoblast mutual control.

In order for implantation to occur, the blastocyst must attach to the endometrium. IL-1 is a major inducer of adhesion receptors. IL-1, which has been shown to be expressed at its highest concentration at implantation sites (15), could induce adherence receptors in uterine epithelial cells and, in doing so, facilitate blastocyst attachment. High levels of platelet-derived growth factor (PDGF) mRNA are seen in decidualization in the mouse.

Epidermal growth factor (EGF) has been found in the human endometrium and the decidua (16), and immunoreactive EGF has been identified in human placental sections and placental extracts (17). In the mouse, EGF protein and mRNA have been identified in uterine epithelial cells. The description of a strain of mice lacking the epidermal growth factor receptor (EGF-R) by T. Magnuson (18), where the embryos develop normally to blastocyst stage, but fail to implant, suggest that embryonic EGF-R is required for normal implantation. The EGF-R has a family of ligands, and data from Dey and S.R. Glasser (18) indicate that at least two members - amphiregulin and heparin-binding EGF- are present in the uterus in the implantation phase.

Transforming growth factor-α (TGF-α) mRNA expression was found exclusively in the decidua of the rat uterus from days 7 to 15 of gestation. TGF-α peptide was found to have a broad distribution in human decidual cells, villous and extravillous cytotrophoblast cells, and villous syncytiotrophoblast cells throughout pregnancy (19). It was also shown that exogenous TGF-α stimulated proliferation of first trimester human trophoblast cells *in vitro*. These results suggested that TGF-α may represent a key molecule at the fetomaternal interface with a growth promoting function for the placenta. The presence of TGF-β at the human fetomaternal interface and its critical role in the regulation of numerous trophoblast functions: proliferation, differentiation and invasion has been demonstrated (20). It was further demonstrated that TGF-β, derived from the decidua, and to a minor extent from the trophoblast, controlled trophoblast invasion by upregulating tissue inhibitor of metalloprotease (TIMP)-1 mRNA and protein. Trophoblast functions such as proliferation and invasion require stringent control in a spatial as well as a temporal manner. It is possible that opposing actions of certain peptides e.g., EGF/ TGF-α on the one hand and TGF-β on the other provide some of this control.

Insulin-like growth factors (IGFs) or somatomedins are polypeptide hormones which specifically bind to receptors on cell membranes and to soluble binding proteins. A number of binding proteins (IGFBPs) have been identified in various body compartments. The identification of IGFBP-1 [PP12] as a major secretory product of decidualized endometrium suggests that studies of the IGFs and their binding proteins are important to our understanding of implantation, (for review see 21&22). Hustin and colleagues (10) have described the expression of IGFBP-1 in relation to implantation. They concluded that implantation of the conceptus may be an important mechanism in the early expression of IGFBP-1 but not that of PP14. IGF-BP might compete with IGF-1 at the trophoblast receptor level and inhibit IGF-1 action. Of considerable interest is the real possibility that IGF-BP production could be delayed until largely after implantation. This decidual protein could then be involved in the regulation of trophoblastic extension within the gestational endometrium (4).

CONCLUSION

Although cytokines may be detected in other normal tissues, e.g., brain, the cytokine concentrations that are detected in the uterus are much higher than in non-reproductive tissues during pregnancy. Studies are needed to identify the key factors which orchestrate endometrial cytokine/growth factor expression and to seek ways of modulating their actions so as to improve implantation rates in women.

REFERENCES

1 Hearn, J. P.(1986). The embryo-maternal dialogue during early pregnancy in primates. *J.Reprod. Fertil.*, **76**, 809-819

2. Fay, T.N. & Grudzinskas J.G. (1991). Human endometrial peptides: a review of their potential role in implantation and placentation. *Hum Reprod*, **6**, 1311-1326

3. Lenton, E.A. (1988). Pituitary and ovarian hormones in implantation and early pregnancy. In Chapman M., Grudzinskas, J.G., Chard T. (eds) *Implantation: biological and clinical aspects*, pp. 17-32 Springer Verlag, London.

4. Hustin J. & Franchimont P.(1992). The endometrium and implantation. In Barnea E.R. (eds). *The first twelve weeks of gestation*. 26-42. Springer-Verlag, Heidelberg.

5. Lindenberg S., Hyttel P., Sjogren A., Greve T. (1989). A comparative study of attachment of human bovine and mouse blastocysts to uterine epithelial monolayer. *Hum Reprod* **4**, 446-456

6 Nieder, G.L., Macon, G.R. (1987). Uterine and oviductal secretion during early pregnancy in the mouse. *J. Reprod. fertil*, **81**, 287-294

7. Bell S.C. (1988). Secretory endometrial/decidual proteins and their function in early pregnancy. *J. Reprod. Fertil. [Suppl.]* **36**, 109-125

8. Denker, H.-W. (1990). Trophoblast-endometrial interactions at embryo implantation: a cell biological paradox. In Denker H.-W. and Aplin J.D. (eds.) Trophoblast invasion and endometrial receptivity. *Trophoblast Res.*,**4**, 3-29. Plenum Medical, New York, London.

9. Bell, S.C. (1988). Synthesis and secretion of proteins by the endometrium and decidua. In Chapman M., Grudzinskas J.G. and Chard T. (eds.) *Implantation. Biological and clinical aspects*. pp. 95-118. Springer- Verlag, London.

10. Hustin J., Philippe B., Teisner B. & Grudzinskas J.G. (1994). Immunohistochemical localisation of two endometrial proteins in the early days of human pregnancy. *Placenta* **15**, 701-708.

11. Chard T. & Grudzinskas J.G. (1992). Pregnancy protein secretion. *Seminars in Reprod. Endocrin.*, **10**, 61-71.

12. Seppala M., Anguvo M., Koistinen R., Ruttenen, L. & Julkunen M. (1991). Human endometrial protein secretion relative to implantation. *Bailliere's Clin. Obstet. Gynaecol.* **5**, 61-72.

13. Carpenter G. and Cohen S. (1979). Epidermal growth factor. *Annu. Rev. Biochem.*,**48**, 193-216.

14. Charnock-Jones D.S., Sharkey A.M., Rajput-Williams J., Burch D., Schofield, J.P., Fountain S.A., Boocock, C.A. and Smith S.K. (1993). Identification and localisation of alternately spliced mRNAs for vascular endothelial growth factor in human uterus

and steroid regulation in endometrial carcinoma cell lines. *Biol. Reprod.*, **48**, 1120-1128

15. Wood G.W. (1994). Role of uterine cytokines in pregnancy. *Trophoblast Reseach,***8**, 486-501.

16. Haining R.E.B., Schofield J.P., Jones D.S.C., Rajput-Williams J., and Smith S.K. (1991). Identification of mRNA for epidermal growth factor and transforming growth factor-α present in low copy number in human endometrium and decidua using reverse transcriptase-polymerase chain reaction. *J. Mol. Endocrinol.* **6**, 207-214

17. Bissonnette F., Cook C., Geoghegan T., Steffan M., Henry J., Yussman M.A., and Schultz G. (1992). Transforming growth factor-α and epidermal growth factor messenger ribonucleic acid and protein levels in human placentas from early, mid, and late gestation. *Am. J. Obstet. Gynecol.* **166**, 192-199

18. Aplin J.D. (1995). Meeting report: Molecular and cellular aspects of peri-implantation processes, Boston, Massachusetts 15-18 July 1994. *Placenta.* **16**, 109-111

19. Lysiak J.J., Han V.K.M. and Lala P.K. (1993). Localization of transforming growth factor (TGF)-α in the human placenta and decidua: Role in trophoblast growth. *Biol. Reprod.* **49**, 885-894.

20. Graham C.H., Lysiak J.J., McCrae K.R., and Lala P.K.(1992). Localization of transforming growth factor-β at the human fetal-maternal interface: Role in trophoblast growth and differentiation. *Biol. Reprod.***46**, 561-572.

21. Bell S.C. (1986). Secretory endometrial and decidual proteins: studies and clinical significance of a maternally derived group of pregnancy associated serum proteins. *Hum Reprod.* **1**, 129-143

22. Koistinen R., Kalkkinen N., Huhtala M-L, Seppala M., Bohn H., and Rutanen E-M (1986). Placental protein 12 is a decidual protein that binds somatomedin-binding protein from human amniotic fluid. *Endocrinology.* **118**, 1375-1378

In vitro gamete micromanipulation and intracellular ionic changes

L. Leybaert and H.T. Depypere

Laboratorium voor Normale en Pathologische Fysiologie and Vrouwenkliniek, Universiteit Gent, Gent, Belgium

Different *in vitro* micromanipulation techniques have recently been developed to assist and improve fertilization in the case of extreme male infertility. Distinction can be made between zona drilling (ZD), which consists of drilling a hole in the zona pellucida (ZP) with an acidified tyrode solution, partial zona dissection (PZD), which consists of mechanically disrupting the ZP with a sharp microneedle, subzonal sperm insertion (SUZI) and intracytoplasmic sperm injection (ICSI). These techniques are schematically summarized in Fig. 1.

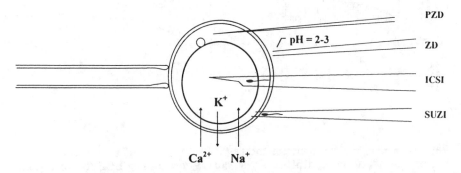

Fig. 1. Micromanipulation methods used in assisted fertilization.

A potential drawback of these methods is that they are rather invasive to the oocyte, with the possible consequence of a disturbance of the transmembrane ion gradients that exist for calcium, potassium and sodium. In many somatic cells a disturbance of the transmembrane ion gradients results in impairment of cell function, eventually followed by cell death. In the case of an oocyte, it is known that fertilization is followed by subtle changes in intracellular free calcium and pH, which play an important role in the normal progression of embryo development. Therefore, it is possible that a disturbance of intracellular ion concentrations results in disturbed embryo development.

In the present work, we have investigated intracellular ionic changes associated with ZD and ICSI.

ZD is a technique that uses an acidified medium (titrated to pH 2-3) to drill a hole in the ZP. This technique was initially developed with mouse oocytes, in which it was found to improve fertilization even at very reduced sperm concentrations and to result in normal subsequent development of the embryos (1). In human oocytes, ZD also improved fertilization but the technique seemed to have a detrimental effect on embryo survival. Payne et al. (2) have reported that one quarter of the embryos showed signs of cytoplasmic degeneration, whereas such degeneration barely occurs in the absence of micromanipulation. No clinical pregnancies have furthermore been obtained with ZD, suggesting that it is not well suited for human oocytes. The aim of the present experiments was to determine whether the extent of intracellular pH (pH$_i$) change associated with ZD was more pronounced in human oocytes.

In a first set of experiments we have measured pH$_i$ changes during ZD of mouse oocytes, using pH-sensitive microelectrodes (3). During ZD the pH$_i$ signal showed a rapid shift in acid direction, over approximately 0.1 to 0.2 pH units (Fig. 2A).

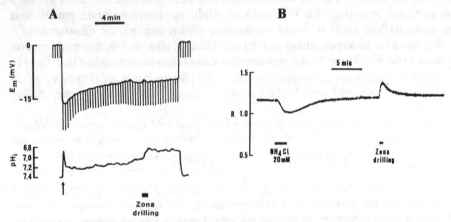

Fig. 2. A. Example of a pH$_i$ measurement in a mouse oocyte using a pH-sensitive microelectrode. Oocyte impalement (arrow) illustrates the negative membrane potential (E$_m$) and the slightly more acid pH$_i$. Zona drilling resulted in a rapid acid shift over approximately 0.2 pH units. Little recovery occurred because there was no superfusion and hence no washout of the acid drilling solution. Zona drilling had no influence on E$_m$.

B. Example of a pH$_i$ measurement in a human oocyte using BCECF. No absolute pH values are given; an upward deflection corresponds to a pH change in acid direction. The short exposure to ammonium chloride (NH$_4$Cl) was used for calibration purposes. Zona drilling resulted in a rapid acid shift over approximately 0.3 pH units. The signal showed subsequent recovery because the oocyte was superfused in these experiments.

Reproduced with permission, from reference 3.

The mean pH change over 20 cells amounted to 0.16 ± 0.02 pH units (mean $\pm$ S.E.M.).

In a second set of experiments we measured pH_i changes associated with ZD of human oocytes. Human oocytes were obtained from the IVF unit of the university hospital and consisted of cells that failed to fertilize. Experiments were performed between 48 and 52 h following oocyte pick-up. In these experiments pH_i was measured using the fluorescent pH-sensitive indicator BCECF. This technique was used because it is less invasive to the cell, which was necessary with regard to the limited number of oocytes available. ZD resulted in a rapid shift in acid direction over approx. 0.3 pH units (Fig. 2B). The mean pH_i change over 14 cells was 0.36 ± 0.10 pH units, significantly higher (P<0.05) than in mouse oocytes.

In summary, the experiments show that ZD is associated with a modest intracellular acidification which is more pronounced in human oocytes than in mouse oocytes. Although methodological differences (oocyte retrieval procedure, pH_i measurement) preclude a possible comparison of the two experimental groups, there are some arguments to expect indeed a larger pH_i change during ZD of human oocytes. First, the perivitelline space in human oocytes is much smaller compared to mouse oocytes, so that the drilling pipette is much closer to the oolemma. Second, ZD takes a much longer time in human oocytes compared to mouse oocytes, so that exposure to the acid drilling solution is much longer.

The question then arises whether a pH_i change in the order of 0.3-0.4 pH units is sufficient to account for a detrimental effect on embryonic development. This is certainly too small to result in dramatic effects like protein denaturation. It must however be kept in mind that the pH_i changes observed in this study give an idea of the average pH_i change over the cytoplasm; it is possible that the pH_i change is much more pronounced close to the plasmamembrane. Payne et al. (2) have indeed reported morphologic changes of the oolemma facing the drilling pipette.

A possible link between a modest acidification and oocyte degeneration may reside in the important role of pH_i as a metabolic regulator. Studies in mouse but also in human oocytes have shown that exposure to a solution with pH 2-3 can induce parthenogenetic activation (4). Parthenogenetic activation has however not been reported following ZD (5). In lower vertebrates like frog, fertilization is followed by an intracellular alkalinisation (6). No data are available on post-fertilization pH_i changes in human oocytes. Possibly the pH_i change induced by ZD somehow disturbs the physiology of further embryonic development.

In conclusion, these experiments show that ZD is associated with a modest intracellular acidification that is more pronounced in human oocytes. This possibly plays a role in the high incidence of cytoplasmic degeneration that is observed following ZD of human oocytes.

In a second part of the study we have measured the changes of the intracellular free calcium concentration ($[Ca^{2+}]_i$) associated with ICSI. ICSI is the most invasive micromanipulation technique and yet, a little contradictory, it results in the highest fertilization rates (7). Fertilization with this technique deviates very much from physiologic fertilization since interaction of the spermatozoon with the ZP and oolemma is circumvented. This suggest that oocyte activation, which is necessary for subsequent embryo development, is caused by factors different from sperm-membrane interactions. Experimental work in different species has shown that an increase of $[Ca^{2+}]_i$ plays a central and essential role in oocyte activation (8-10). During the procedure of ICSI, a large increase of $[Ca^{2+}]_i$ can be expected because of the destruction of the oolemma or intracellular membranes with leakage of calcium from the extracellular space or from intracellular stores into the cytoplasm where $[Ca^{2+}]_i$ is extremely low. In addition phenomena like calcium-induced calcium release may further exacerbate this increase of $[Ca^{2+}]_i$. This is what is observed when for example a neuron is impaled, even with a submicron pipette. It can thus be hypothesized that impalement of an oocyte with the rather thick (7 μm) ICSI pipette results in an increase of $[Ca^{2+}]_i$ with subsequent oocyte activation. The aim of this study was to determine the extent of $[Ca^{2+}]_i$ change associated with the procedure of ICSI.

We used mouse oocytes in this study; $[Ca^{2+}]_i$ was measured using the calcium-sensitive fluorescent indicator fura-2. Normal fertilization by incubating the oocytes with mouse spermatozoa resulted in approximately 80 % of the cells (on a total of 96 cells) reaching two cell stage. A normal oscillatory calcium response was observed in approximately 40 % of the cells (Fig. 3A).

A first series of experiments was performed to investigate the effect of impalement of the oocyte with an ICSI pipette and injection of approximately 1 pl of medium, without a spermatozoon (the medium contained 2 mM calcium).

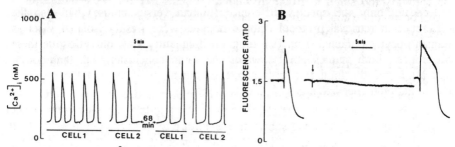

Fig. 3. Example of $[Ca^{2+}]_i$ measurements in mouse oocytes using fura-2.
A. Oscillatory changes of $[Ca^{2+}]_i$ in 2 mouse oocytes following incubation with mouse spermatozoa. **B.** No absolute values are given in this recording; upward changes correspond to a $[Ca^{2+}]_i$ increase. Impalement of the oocyte was associated with a small artefactual depression of $[Ca^{2+}]_i$ due to cell displacement and compression. After penetration, a short period of suction was applied to check access to the cytoplasm and this was followed by medium injection. Two different responses were observed. The left- and and rightmost trace show cells that responded with a large increase of $[Ca^{2+}]_i$, to approximately 1 μM, followed by partial recovery. All these cells subsequently lysed. Lysis corresponds to the sharp drop of the signal caused by leakage of the indicator out of the cell. The middle trace shows a cell that did not show any change of $[Ca^{2+}]_i$, not in the acute period (except for the artefactual change) as shown here and not in a late period 4 h after impalement (not shown). Recordings during successful injection, i.e. injection not followed by cell lysis, of a mouse or human spermatozoon showed a time course as in the middle trace, i.e. no change of $[Ca^{2+}]_i$ occurred.

Two different responses were observed upon penetration with the pipette (Fig. 3B). Approximately 44 % of the cells (on a total of 45 cells) showed a large increase of $[Ca^{2+}]_i$, followed by a period of recovery; all these cells subsequently lysed. Approximately 56 % of the cells did not show any change of $[Ca^{2+}]_i$, not in the acute period and not in a late period 4 h after impalement.

A second series of experiments was performed to investigate the effect of ICSI, i.e. impalement and injection of a spermatozoon, on $[Ca^{2+}]_i$. Some experiments were performed with injection of a mouse spermatozoon. The problem with mouse spermatozoa is that these are far more difficult to inject than human spermatozoa, due to a slightly different morphology. Hence it was more difficult to perform the ICSI procedure successfully, i.e. without subsequent cell lysis. In 7 successful attempts of ICSI with a mouse spermatozoon, no acute change of $[Ca^{2+}]_i$ could be observed. We also performed ICSI with a human spermatozoon, which is more simple to perform and hence is more appropriate as a model for ICSI as it is used in the human. In 24 successful attempts of ICSI with a human spermatozoon, no changes of $[Ca^{2+}]_i$ could be observed, not in the acute period and not in a late period 4 h after ICSI.

In summary, the experiments show that successful application of the ICSI procedure does not result in acute changes of $[Ca^{2+}]_i$ in mouse oocytes. These findings stand in contrast to the findings of Tesarik et al. (11) who reported that the ICSI procedure, with or without injection of a spermatozoon, is associated with an acute increase of $[Ca^{2+}]_i$ in human oocytes. However, this increase of $[Ca^{2+}]_i$ was not sufficient to activate the oocyte. There are, again, methodological differences that make a comparison between both studies difficult. There is indeed not only the species difference (human versus mouse) but also the difference in retrieval protocol (mouse oocytes were freshly isolated whereas human oocytes obtained from IVF units are frequently 48 h old). Despite these differences, both studies point towards the same conclusion, i.e. that oocyte activation and the high fertilization rate of human ICSI are not the result of manipulation induced changes of $[Ca^{2+}]_i$.

References.

1. Depypere, H.T., McLaughlin, K.J., Seamark, R.F., Warnes, G.M. and Matthews, C.D. (1988). Comparison of zona cutting and zona drilling as techniques for assisted fertilization in the mouse. *J. Reprod. Fert.* **84**, 205-11.
2. Payne D., McLaughlin, K.J., Depypere, H.T., Kirby C.A., Warnes, G.M. and Matthews, C.D. (1988). Experience with zona drilling and zona cutting to improve fertilization rates of human oocytes in vivo. *Hum. Reprod. Fert.* **6**, 423-31.
3. Depypere, H.T. and Leybaert, L. (1994). Intracellular pH changes during zona drilling. *Fertil. Steril.*, **61**, 319-23.
4. Johnson, M.H., Pickering, S.J., Braude, P.R., Vincent, C., Cant, A. and Currie, J. (1990). Acid Tyrodes can stimulate parthenogenetic activation of human and mouse oocytes. *Fertil. Steril.*, **53**, 266-70.

5. Edirisinghe, W.R., Wales, R.G., Chapman, H.M. and Yovich, J.L. (1991). Assisted fertilization of mouse oocytes and preliminary results of human oocytes using zona drilling. *J. In Vitro Fertil. Embryo Transfer* **8**, 48-55.
6. Busa, W.B. and Nucitelli, R. (1984). Metabolic regulation via intracellular pH. *Am. J. Physiol.* **246**, R409-38.
7. Payne, D. (1994). Embryo viability associated with microassisted fertilization. *Baillières Clin. Obstet. Gynaecol.* **8**, 157-175.
8. Tesarik, J. (1994). Calcium and oocyte maturation. How the spermatozoon awakens the oocyte: lessons from intracytoplasmic sperm injection. *Hum. Reprod.* **9**, 977-8.
9. Swann, K., Homa, S. and Caroll, J. (1994). An inside job: the rsults of injecting whole sperm into eggs supports one view of signal transduction at fertilization. *Hum. Reprod.* **9**, 978-80.
10. Taylor, C.T. (1994). Calcium signals and human oocyte activation: implications for assisted concenption. *Hum. Reprod.* **9**, 980-4.
11. Tesarik, J., Sousa, M. And Testart, J. (1994). Human oocyte activation after intracytoplasmic sperm injection. *Hum. Reprod.* **9**, 511-8.

Effect of follicular fluid on sperm motility, acrosomal reactivity and chemotactic response

A. Revelli, P. Tacconis, M. Modotti, C. Ansaldi, M. Balerna* and M. Massobrio

Istituto di Ginecologia e Ostetricia, Cattedra D, Università di Torino, Ospedale Mauriziano "Umberto I" di Torino, Italy and *Laboratorio di Andrologia, Endocrinologia Ginecologica, Ospedale "La Carità" di Locarno, Switzerland

INTRODUCTION

During its migration in the female genital tract, the male gamete encounters several fluids with which it interacts. In the upper part of the salpinx, some of these fluids mix constituting a biochemical "milieu" which is known as the "fertilization milieu at the fertilization site". This biochemical environment is composed of approximately equivalent parts of peritoneal fluid (PF) and follicular fluid (FF), which are mixed with little amounts of tubal fluid.

Differently from tubal fluid, PF and FF can be easily obtained during assisted reproduction procedures, and thus have been extensively studied. Unfortunately, the results of such researches have often been conflicting. PF, for instance, has been reported either to slightly enhance or depress sperm motility as function of the experimental conditions (1, 2), and a sperm imobilizing factor has been isolated from the PF of infertile women (3). FF, in turn, has been claimed either to inhibit sperm motility (4) or to exert stimulating effects on both sperm motility and acrosomal reactivity (5, 6). The sperm-stimulating properties of FF have been attributed mainly to its content of progesterone (P), which is approximately 125 folds greater than in PF (7). In fact, it was shown that steroid-stripped FF loses its sperm-stimulating effects (8), but soon after the addition of P these are promptly recovered (9). Moreover, progesterone binding sites have been identified inside the membrane of the anterior part of the sperm head, which covers the acrosomal cap (10, 11). Some authors also claim that FF is able to attract chemically human spermatozoa (12); this effect could be accomplished by means of a family of N-formylated peptides (13).

Hereby are presented the results of our work about the effects of FF (and PF) on some sperm characteristics, such as motility, acrosomal reactivity, and chemotactic response. In

259

some of the following "in vitro" studies, we tried to better approximate the "in vivo" conditions testing both "pure" PF and FF, and some volumetric combinations of PF and FF from the same woman (14, 15). Moreover, we attemped to verify if P could be the substance which is responsible for the effects on sperm motility, and thus we tested on sperm PF supplemented with exogenous progesterone (7). Finally, we tested "in vitro" the ability of FF to attract chemically human spermatozoa. Overall, we demonstrated that, at least in our experimental conditions, FF stimulates sperm motility and acrosomal reactivity, but has limited chemotactic effect. Moreover, P can be only partially responsible for the FF-mediated increase of sperm motility.

FOLLICULAR FLUID AND SPERM MOTILITY

Methods

Twenty infertile women partecipating the GIFT program were enrolled in the study and underwent superovulation with hMG plus hCG. At the time of pick-up laparoscopy, PF and FF were aspirated in sterile conditions, centrifuged (1500 X g, 10 min, RT), filtered (0.22 mcm) and freezed at -20°C until tested. Subsequently, in paired experiments, PF and FF were incubated separately or in given volumetric mixtures (PF/FF 75/25, 50/50, 25/75) with swim-up sperm suspensions from normospermic patients. Sperm progressive velocity and the percentage of motile gametes were measured by multiple exposure photography at time = 0, 2.5 and 5 hours.

Results

FF always stimulated progressive motility and substained the number of motile gametes, as function of time, better than PF or the PF/FF combinations (Fig. 1; $p<0.05$). This motility-enhancing effect was particularly evident after 5 hours of incubation. Anyway, it was observed already at t=0. Both PF and PF/FF mixtures did better than the control medium (B2-Menezo) only at t=5 hours.

Conclusions

FF transmits motility-enhancing signals to spermatozoa, whereas PF can transmit either positive, negative or neutral signals (noise signals). The volumetric combination of FF and PF that occurs in the tubal environment at ovulation can therefore result in synergic or antagonistic effects on sperm motility.

IS PROGESTERONE RESPONSIBLE FOR THE FF-MEDIATED INCREASE IN SPERM MOTILITY?

Methods

PF coming from five sterile women superovulated with gonadotropins in a GIFT program was supplemented with exogenous progesterone (P) in order to obtain P concentrations comparable to those observed in FF. Eleven normal sperm samples were then incubated with

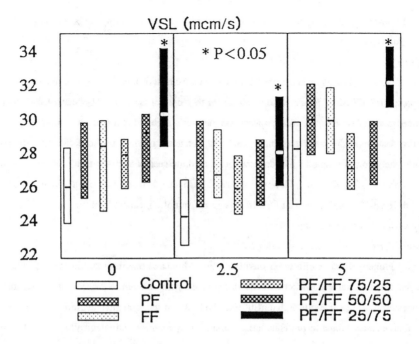

Fig. 1. Sperm velocity straight linear (median and 95% c.i.) after incubation with PF, FF and their mixture, as function of time.

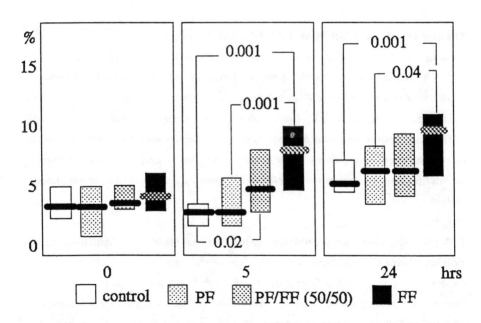

Fig. 2. Percentage of acrosomal reaction (median and 95% c.i.) after incubation with PF, FF and their mixture, as function of time.

these PF with/without exogenous P, and sperm motility was assessed by CASA at time = 0, 2.5, 5 and 24 hours.

Results

Overall, there was no constant trend for enhancement or inhibition of sperm motility in P-supplemented PF when compared to native PF or to a control medium (B2-Menezo). P generally induced a negative effect on those sperm samples with high velocities in the native PF, and a positive effect on those sperm samples demonstrating low motility in the native PF. In other words, the incorporation of P into the incubation medium seemed to result in a "tuning" of sperm velocity around 30-50 mcm/s. However, a given sperm sample reacted differently when incubated with different PFs and, reciprocally, different semen samples incubated with the same PF showed very variable motility patterns.

Conclusions

P exerts variable effects on sperm motility. This can arise from the fact that each sperm sample contains several subpopulations of gametes with different sensitivity to progesterone (progesterone receptor content), but also from the fact that in a complex medium, such as PF or FF, P is variably bound to proteins that modulate the amount of its biologically active fraction. Therefore, P can be a motility-enhancing factor, but probably its activity depends both from biochemical conditions encountered in PF or FF (e. g. the albumin content, the concentration of other motility-influencing factors), and from individual characteristics of the semen.

EFFECT OF FF ON ACROSOMAL REACTIVITY

Methods

Twenty-three women enrolled in the GIFT program were superovulated with GnRH-A, pFSH and hCG. At laparoscopy, PF and FF were taken in sterile conditions, centrifuged, filtered and stored as previously described. Given volumetric combinations of PF and FF (100/0, 50/50, 0/100) were incubated with swim-up sperm suspensions from normal semen specimens, and the precentage of acrosomally reacted spermatozoa was assessed at time = 0, 5 and 24 hours. A modified triple-stain (16) method was used to determine the occurrence of acrosomal reaction (AR).

Results

Compared with an albumine-free control medium (Earle's solution), moderate but significant increases of AR were observed as function of the relative content of FF in the incubation medium, as well as function of time. In contrast, when PF alone was present in the incubate, no stimulating (or inhibiting) effects on AR were registered. The FF-mediated stimulation of acrosomal reactivity although evident as a trend at earlier times, was statistically significant after at least 5 hours of incubation (Fig. 2; $p < 0.05$).

Conclusions

FF, alone or diluted by PF, seems to induce some rapid and time-dependent processes which finally lead to AR. It is likely that before ovulation PF acts maintaining spermatozoa in an unreacted status, thus preventing the occurrence of a premature AR, useless for fertilization. Afterwords, at ovulation, the entrance of FF in the ampulla is able to stimulate the occurrence of AR in the presence of the oocyte.

IS FOLLICULAR FLUID ABLE TO ATTRACT CHEMICALLY SPERMATOZOA?

Methods

Semen specimen coming from 40 normospermic and 14 dyspermic patients were treated with a standard swim-up procedure in HTF medium. Afterwards, dedicated chemotactic chambers (Costar, Como, Italy) were prepared as follows: 500 mcl sperm suspension with known sperm concentration were put in the bottom well, and 60 mcl of HTF or FF in the upper well. The chambers were then left at 37°C in 5% CO_2 atmosphere and spermatozoa were allowed to migrate to the upper well through a 8 mcm multipore membrane. Sperm concentration in the upper well was determined after 30 minutes by a Hamilton Thorn analyser.

Results

An average of 48% of spermatozoa were recovered in the upper well when a normal semen was used, while with pathological semen specimens the recovery rate was only 18%. No statistical differences were observed comparing FF and the control medium, even if a trend towards a better performance of FF could be noticed with normal specimens. Results did not substantially change after diluting FF or prolonging the incubation to 2 hours. An extreme variability in the recovery rate was noticed from one semen to the other, as well as from one FF to the other.

Conclusions

In our experimental setting a significant chemotactic effect of FF on sperm was not confirmed. Unfortunately, no known sperm chemoattractants are commercially available, and thus we could not use them as positive controls. Therefore, an insufficient sensitiveness of the method can not be ruled out. Further experiments are needed to better clarify this issue.

REFERENCES

1. Soldati, G., Piffaretti-Yanez, A., Campana, A., Marchini, M., Luerti, M., Balerna, M. (1989). Effect of peritoneal fluid on sperm motility and velocity distribution using objective measurements. *Fertil. Steril.*, **52**, 113

2. Guidi, F., Revelli, A., Soldati, G., Stamm, J., Massobrio, M., Piffaretti-Yanez, A., Balerna, M. (1993). Influence of peritoneal fluid from spontaneous and stimulated cycles on sperm motility *in vitro*. *Andrologia*, **25**, 71

3. Soldati, G., Piffaretti-Yanez, A., Medici, G., Eppenberger, U., Balerna, M. (1993). Purification of a factor from human peritoneal fluid that is able to immobilize spermatozoa. *Human Reprod.*, **8**, 428

4. Mukherjee, A.B., and Lippes, J. (1972). Effect of human follicular and tubal fluids on human, mouse and rat spermatozoa in vitro. *Can. J. Genet. Cytol.*, **14**, 167

5. Falcone, L., Soldati, G., Piffaretti-Yanez, A., Marchini, M., Eppemberger, U., Balerna, M. (1991) Follicular fluid enhances sperm motility and velocity in vitro. *Fertil. Steril.*, **55**, 619

6. Tesarik, J. (1985) Comparison of acrosome reaction-inducing activities of human cumulus oophorus, follicular fluid and ionophore A23187 in human sperm populations of proven fertilizing ability in vitro. *J. Reprod. Fertil.*, **74**, 383

7. Modotti, M., Togni, G., Medici, G., Revelli, A., Stamm, J., Piffaretti-Yanez, A., Massobrio, M., Balerna, M. (1994). Effect of peritoneal fluid supplemented with exogenous progesterone on sperm motility *in vitro*. *Human Reprod.*, **9**, 303

8. Mbizvo, M.T., Burkman, L.J., Alexander, N.J. (1990). Human follicular fluid stimulates hyperactivated motility in human sperm. *Fertil. Steril.*, **54**, 708

9. Morales, P., Llanos, M., Gutierrez, G., Kohen, P., Vigil, P., Vautman, D. (1992). The acrosomal reaction-inducing activity of individual human follicular fluid samples is highly variable and is related to the steroid content. *Human Reprod.*, **7**, 646

10. Tesarik, J., Mendoza, C., Moos, J., Carreras, A. (1992). Selective expression of a progesterone receptor on the human sperm surface. *Fertil. Steril.*, **58**, 784

11. Revelli, A., Modotti, M., Piffaretti-Yanez, A., Massobrio, M., Balerna, M. (1994). Steroid receptors in human spermatozoa. *Human Reprod.*, **9**, 760

12. Ralt, D., Manor, M., Cohen-Dayag, A., Tur-Kaspa, I., Ben-Shlomo, I., Makler, A., Yuli, I., Dor, J., Blumberg, S., Mashiach, S., Eisembach, M. (1994). Chemiotaxis and chemiochinesis of human spermatozoa to follicular factors. *Biol. Reprod.*, **50**, 774

13. Gnessi, L., Fabbri, A., Silvestroni, L., Moretti, C., Fraioli, F., Pert, C.B., Isidori, A. (1986). Evidence for the presence of specific receptors for N-formyl chemiotactic peptides on human spermatozoa. *J. Clin. Endocrinol. Metab.*, **63**, 841

14. Revelli, A., Soldati, G., Stamm, J., Massobrio, M., Topfer Petersen, E., Balerna, M. (1992). Effect of volumetric mixtures of peritoneal and follicular fluid from the same woman on sperm motility and acrosomal reactivity *in vitro*. *Fertil. Steril.*, **57**, 654

15. Revelli, A., La Sala, G.B., Gallicchio, D., Modotti, M., Piffaretti-Yanez, A., Massobrio, M., Balerna, M. (1995). Effect of peritoneal fluid, follicular fluid, and their volumetric mixture on acrosomal reactivity *in vitro*. *Fertil. Steril.*, **63**, 200

16. De Jonge, C.J., Mack, S.R., Zaneveld, L.J.D. (1989) Synchronous assay for human sperm capacitation and the acrosome reaction. *J. Androl.*, **3**, 232

Folliculogenesis with recombinant FSH stimulation

F. Ubaldi, J. Smitz, A. Van Steirteghem and P. Devroey

University Hospital, Dutch-Speaking Brussels Free University (Vrije Universiteit Brussel), Belgium

Follicle stimulating hormone (FSH) during the follicular phase controls major ovarian morphological and cellular events. It induces the activation of the adenylate cyclase system,.[1] it prompts the induction of luteinizing hormone (LH) and prolactin receptors on granulosa cells and the activation of the steroidogenic enzymes needed for progesterone biosynthesis.[2] While there is no debate about the fundamental role played by LH mid-cycle surge, there is controversy about the amount of LH necessary to support steroid production prior to ovulation. FSH and growth factors rather than LH appear to be crucial to follicular growth and development. It has been calculated that resting levels of LH in serum should be sufficient for an adequate stimulation of theca cells[3] and exogenous LH is therefore not necessary during controlled ovarian hyperstimulation (COH) in gonadal women presenting basal elevated or normal serum LH concentrations. This assumption has been confirmed by several studies in which gonadotropin-releasing hormone agonists (GnRH-a) have been used in combination with human purified FSH preparations containing less than 1% of LH. Successful development of multiple follicles and normal implantation rates have been reported in such cases.[4]

On the other hand, several studies during the last few years have indicated the possible negative effect of a high follicular phase LH concentration on oocyte quality, fertilization and early gestation.[5-6]

Recombinant FSH: structural and biological characteristics

The rationale behind the use of preparations containing as little LH as possible is the avoidance of exogenous administration of a hormone that can elevate endogen LH level [7] which might have a negative effect on oocyte quality.[5-6] Small amounts of LH (<1%) are present in human FSH preparations. Recently, a biochemically pure molecule with biological properties very similar to those of human urinary or pituitary FSH has been obtained.[8] This molecule, called recombinant FSH, is obtained by transfecting a genomic clone containing the entire coding sequence for both FSH subunits into Chinese Hamster Ovarian (CHO) cells.[8] The rec-FSH mass, its polypeptide backbone and the glycosylation essential for bioactivity is very similar in both glycoproteins.[9] This molecule is of extreme biochemical purity (it contains 60 times less protein per injection).[9] This high degree of purity allows the rec-FSH preparation to be given subcutaneously. The intrinsic LH bioactivity of rec-FSH is negligible.(less than one-tenth that of pure urinary hormone).[10] The specific bioactivity of rec-FSH is >10.000 IU FSH/mg of protein. With regard to the biological properties, no differences have been observed between pituitary or urinary FSH.[10]

Clinical application

From a phase-I study to assess safety and pharmacokinetic/ pharmacodynamic properties of rec-FSH performed recently in gonadotropin-deficient volunteers, [11] it appears that rec-FSH is safe, non-immunogenic and well tolerated and that its half-life is comparable to that of natural FSH. However, minimal amounts of LH to induce an appropriate steroidogenesis are requested. Rec-FSH fails to induce an adequate rise in estradiol in hypogonadotropic hypogonadal women.[12] On the other hand, rec-FSH induces adequate follicular development and endocrine profile in normally menstruating and in World Health Organization (WHO) group II anovulatory women. Moreover, successful pregnancy and birth have been reported in such cases. [13-14]

With the aim of assessing the efficacy of rec-FSH in stimulating multiple follicular development in induced ovulation and in in-vitro fertilization and embryo transfer (IVF/ET), two comparative randomized multicentric studies have been performed in normal menstruating women.[15-16] In both studies similar results have been obtained when rec-FSH and urinary FSH were compared. According to these data, it seems that the minimal amount of LH (<1%) present in natural FSH preparations are not really determinant for the induction of follicular development.

Gonadotropin-releasing hormone agonists are frequently combined with menotropins for COH in IVF/ET and related assisted-reproduction techniques. Continuous administration of GnRH-a induces a reversible state of hypogonadotropic hypogonadism whose intensity is related to the agonists' structure-receptor interaction, elimination half-life, dosage and route of administration.[17] With the aim of assessing weather low endogenous basal LH levels obtained after pituitary desensitization are able to induce adequate steroidogenesis and related reproductive processes when GnRH-a is used in

Table 1. Median (range) endocrine values on the day of hCG

	Treatment group				
	I	**II**	**III**	**IV**	**V**
FSH	21	13	15	17	17
(IU/l)	(14-26)	(4-17)	(7.6-24)	(9.1-27)	(10-30)
LH	5.1	2.3	1.3	1.2	1.6
(IU/l)	(1.2-20)	(0.5-7.1)	(0.5-7.1)	(0.8-3.5)	(0.5-2.7)
E2	1101	1899	1749	1749	1531
(pg/ml)	(684-2467)	(984-2640)	(683-1749)	(633-1768)	(1058-3350)
P	0.5	0.3	0.6	0.5	1.1
(ng/ml)	(0.2-1.6)	(0.2-1.3)	(0.1-1.5)	(0.2-1.3)	(0.3-4.5)
Inhibin	9.7	10.3	9.1	13.2	12.2
(IU/l)	(7.6-20.5)	(3.7-14.2)	(1.7-23.1)	(6.5-20.3)	(6.8-24.1)

From Devroey P. et al.,[18]

combination with rec-FSH for COH, a pilot study in which various GnRH-a/rec-FSH regimens were compared was carried out.[18]

A total of 50 couples were involved in this study. Five different stimulation protocols were compared: rec-FSH alone (group I), rec-FSH in combination with buserelin intranasaal spray, 4 x 150 mg per day, in a short (group II) or in a long protocol (group III) and rec-FSH in association with tryptorelin depot 3,75 mg i.m. (group IV) or daily subcutaneous injections of 200 mg (group V). Age, weight and

Table 2. Mean (±SD) number of oocytes recovered, embryos transferred and pregnancies

	Treatment group				
	I	II	III	IV	V
Oocytes/retrieval	9.4±7.6	9.0±3.2	10.7±4.8	10.4±4.7	11.1±3.6
Embryos/transfer	2.3±0.8	2.8±0.4	2.7±0.6	2.6±0.7	2.5±0.7
Transfers	7	7	11	8	10
Clinical pregnancies	0	3	2	4	1
Ongoing pregnancies	0	3	2	2	1

From Devroey P. et al.[18]

height of the patients were comparable, as were median baseline levels of E2, P and inhibin. In all women, treatment with rec-FSH induced multiple follicular growth. Increases in estradiol and inhibin were also obtained but their levels on the day of hCG revealed no significant differences in the five groups of patients (table 1). In group I, a reduced mean number of preovulatory follicles >17mm was observed. This might be due to the fact that in this group premature LH surge occurred in 3 out of 9 patients, so that they received hCG prematurely. The mean number of oocytes retrieved was comparable and the clinical and the ongoing pregnancy rates were 23.2% and 18.6% per transfer (table 2). Data from this study demonstrate that GnRH-a/rec-FSH therapy is effective and safe but further clinical studies to compare this with urinary FSH will be required in order to assess possible significant differences in short-term and long-term protocols.

CONCLUSIONS

From clinical data it appears that in gonadal women rec-FSH is as effective as natural human FSH in inducing follicular development and successful pregnancies either with ovulation induction or with assisted procreation. Endogenous circulating LH levels, therefore, are able to induce adequate steroidogenesis. This is also true when pituitary desensitization has been induced by continuous use of GnRH-a. No significant differences have been noted between different GnRH-a/rec-FSH regimens and no adverse effects have been observed. The possibility of injecting rec-FSH subcutaneously with no pain at all represents a significant clinical advantage as self administration is much easier and is well tolerated by patients.

REFERENCES

1. Steinkampf, M.P., Mendelson, C.R., and Simpson, E.R. (1987). Regulation by follicle stimulating hormone of the synthesis of aromatase cytochrome P-450 in human granulosa cells. Mol Endocrinol, 1, 465-471
2. Erickson, G.F., Wang, C. and Hsueh, A.J.W. (1979). FSH induction of functional LH receptors in granulosa cells cultured in a chemically defined medium. Nature, 270, 336-339
3. Doerr, P. (1979). Relationship between saturation of LH receptors and steroidogenic response in isolated rat granulosa cells. Horm. Metab. Res., 11, 181-182
4. Neveu, S., Hedon, B., Bringer, J., Chinchole, J., Arnal, F. and Viala, J. (1987). Ovarian stimulation by a combination of a gonadotropin-releasing hormone agonist and gonadotropins for in vitro fertilization. Fertil. Steril., 47, 639-643
5. Stanger, J.D. and Yovich, J.L. (1985). Reduced in vitro fertilization of human oocytes from patients with raised basal luteinizing hormone levels during the follicular phase. Br. J. Obstet. Gynaecol., 92, 385-392
6. Homburg, R., Armar, N.A., Eshel, A., Adams, J. and Jacobs, H.S. (1988). Influence of serum luteinizing hormone concentrations on ovulation conception and early pregnancy loss in polycystic ovarian syndrome. Br. Med. J., 297, 1024-1026
7. Mizunuma, H., Takagi, T., Honjyo, S., Ibuki, Y. and Igarashi, M. (1990). Clinical pharmacodynamics of urinary follicle-stimulating hormone and its application for pharmacokinetic simulation program. Fertil. Steril., 63, 440-445
8. Keene, J.L., Matzuk, M.M., Otani, T., Fauser. B.C., Galway, A.B. and Hsueh, A.J. (1989). Expression of biologically active human follitropin in chinese hamster ovary cells. J. Biol. Chem., 246, 4769-4775
9. De Boer, W. and Mannaerts, B. (1990). Recombinant follicle-stimulating hormone II. Biochemical and biological characteristics. In Crommelin, D.J. and Skellekens, H. (eds.) From clone to clinic, developments in biotherapy, pp.253-259. (Dordrecht, The Netherlands: Kluwer Academic Publishers)
10. Mannaerts, B., De Leeuw, R., Geelen, J., Van Ravestein, A., Van Wezenbeek, P., Shuurs, A. and Kloosterboer, H. (1991). Comparative in vitro studies on the biological characterisics of recombinant human follicle-stimulating hormone. Endocrinology, 129, 2623-2630

11. Mannaerts, B., Shoham, Z., Schoot, D., Fauser, B., Bouchard, P., Harlin, J., Jacobs, H. and Rombout F. (1993) Single-dose pharmacokinetics and pharmacodynamics of recombinant human follicle-stimulating hormone (Org 32489) in gonadotropin-deficient volunteers. Fertil. Steril., 59,108-114
12. Schoot, D., Mannaerts, B., Lamberts, S., Bouchard, P., Fauser, B. (1992). Human recombinant follicle-stimulating hormone induces growth of preovulatory follicles without concomitant increase in androgen and estrogen biosynthesis in a woman with isolated gonadotropin deficiency. J. Clin. Endocrinol. Metab., 74, 1471-1473
13. Devroey, P., Van Steirteghem, A., Mannaerts, B. and Coelingh Bennink, H. (1992) Successful in vitro fertilization and embryo transfer after treatment with recombinant human FSH. Lancet, 339, 1170-1171
14. Homnes, P., Giroud, D., Howles, C., and Loumaye, E. (1994). Recombinant human follicle-stimulating hormone treatment leads to normal follicular growth, estradiol secretion, and pregnancy in a World Health Organization group II anovulatory woman. Fertil. Steril., in press
15. Homburg, R. (1994) Efficacy of recombinant human follicle stimulating hormone Gonal-F for inducing ovulation in WHO II anovulatory patient. Preliminary results of a comparative multicentre study. In VIIIth World Congress on In Vitro Fertilization and Alternate Assisted Reproduction - Kyoto, Japan, Sept 1993 (New York: Serono Symposia, Raven Press), in press
16. Loumaye, E., Alvarez, S, Barlow, D. et al. (1994). Efficacy of recombinant human follicle-stimulating hormone (Gonal-F) for stimulating multiple follicular development in assisted reproductive technologies. In VIIIth World Congress on In Vitro Fertilization and Alternate Assisted Reproduction - Kyoto, Japan, Sept 1993, (New York: Serono Symposia, Raven Press), in press
17. Brogden, R.N., Buckley, M.M.T. and Ward, A. (1990). Buserelin. A review of its pharmacodynamic and pharmacokinetic properties, and clinical profile. Drugs, 39, 399-437
18. Devroey, P., Mannaerts, B., Smitz, J., Coelingh-Bennink, M., Van Steirteghem, A. (1994) Clinical outcome of a pilot efficacy study on recombinant human FSH (Org. 32489) in combination with various GnRH agonist regimens. Hum. Reprod. (in press)

Use of gonadotropins for assisted reproductive techniques

G. De Placido, C. Carravetta, C. Alviggi, A. Mollo, C. La Rusca and C. Cadente Colucci

I Department of Obstetrics and Gynecology, School of Medicine "Federico II", University of Naples, Naples, Italy

Gonadotropins have been widely used in the treatment of hypotalamic-pituitary isufficiency (group I OMS) and dysfunction (group II OMS). In the last decade the hormonal control of multiple follicular growth for assisted reproductive techiniques represented a new important therapeutic use of LH and FSH.

The outcome of an IVF program depends on ovarian stimulation protocol that is directed toward increasing number and quality of oocytes retrived, of embryios replaced, and enhancing successful implantation and early embryionic development in utero.

The use of FSH and LH for controlled ovarian hyperstimulation (COH) has been originally based upon the two-cells hypothesis (1). According to this theory the cooperation of both gonadotropins is required for follicular growth and ovulation. HMG (human Menopausal Gonadotropin), containing equal amounts of FSH and LH (75 IU/ampule), has been the first drug employed in Gn induced cycles.

The introduction of pure FSH has led to the rivalutation of the role of the LH in the ovulatory process. There is no debate about the importance of the mid-cycle preovulatory LH surge, which leads to the resumption of meiosis by inhibiting the production of OMI (Oocyte Maturation Inhibitor), and to the follicular rupture and ovulation.

Although several reports describing the use of LH in the follicular phase of the menstrual cycle have appeared in the literature, the contribute of this gonadotropin to events which occur prior to ovulation is controversial (2). In 1984 Kenisberg showed that pure FSH can induce multiple follicular development in primates after gonadotropin suppression by GnRH antagonist (3). Furthemore it has been demonstrated that pure FSH without LH can initiate and mantain E2 production and allow oocyte maturation in normal ovulatory women (4).

In 1988 Couzinet et Al. reported stimulation using pure FSH in hypotalamic-hypogonadal women. They concluded that FSH alone may allow follicular maturation and E2 production when negligible amounts of LH (secreted endogenously or administered exogenously) are present (5). Clinical and basic science observations support this conclusion: in 1991, based on the hypothesis that less then 1% of LH receptors need to be occupied to elicite a maximal steroidogenic response, Chappel and Howels observed that resting levels of LH (after GnRHa) provide maximal support for thecal cells (2). On the other hand, it must be cconsidered that complete absence of LH occurs in only 1.2 % of infertile patients affected by hypotalamic-hypogonadism.

Several studies show that the use of FSH without added LH during the follicular development can improve the IVF outcome. In 1985, Bernardus et Al. first reported an increase in oocyte recovery, as well as an improvement in transfer and pregnancy rates, parallel with the increase in the ratio of exogenous FSH to LH (6). In 1986, Polan et Al. (7) observed that ovulation induction with FSH compared with hMG results in a significant increase in on-going pregnancies.

Other clinical and experimental evidences suggest that high basal concentration of LH during the preovulatory period are not only unnecessary for follicular development but may result deleterious to post-ovulatory events. An association between high levels of serum LH and early pregnancy loss as well as reduced pregnancy rates has been described in normal ovulatory women (8), in patients with polycystyc ovarian disease (PCOD) (9) and in infertile women treated with clomiphene citrate (10). Jacobs et Al. (11) first hypothesized that elevated levels of LH during the follicular phase prior to the LH surge may prematurely inhibit OMI, which would result in a premature resumption of meiosis and in the ovulation of post-mature oocytes. Other reports (12) suggest that increased E2 serum levels during the follicular development may lead to impaired endometrial function and implantation.

The presence of LH during ovulation induction seems to alter thecal androgen metabolism, resulting in a significant shift in follicular fluid androgen levels (7). Similiar observations have been reported in our later studies (13) conducted in order to assess the clinical outcome in two groups of patients hyperstimulated with FSH or hMG. In spite of similiar pregnancy and implantation rates, we observed an increase in the abortion rate in women stimulated with hMG (tab.1).

Tab. 1

FSH vs hMG IN IVF
OUTCOME

	Group A (Pure FSH)	Group B (hMG)
• P.R. / cycle	26.7%	25.7%
• Multiple pregnancy	2	3
• Implantation rate	9.0%	9.0%
• Ongoing preg. / cycle	23.3%	17.1%
• Abortion rate	1/8 (12.5%)	3/9 (33.3%)
• Biochemical preg.	o	2

IVF Unit-Dept. OB/GYN
School of Medicine
"Federico II" Naples - Italy

Fig. 1

FSH vs hMG IN IVF
E_2 IN FOLLICULAR FLUID

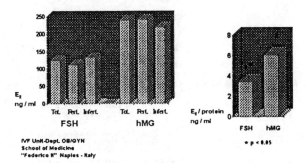

IVF Unit-Dept. OB/GYN
School of Medicine
"Federico II" Naples - Italy

* p < 0.05

Fig. 2

FSH vs hMG IN IVF
TESTOSTERONE IN
FOLLICULAR FLUID

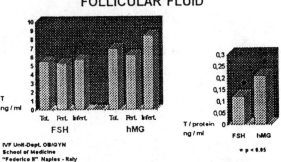

IVF Unit-Dept. OB/GYN
School of Medicine
"Federico II" Naples - Italy

* p < 0.05

A possible explanation can derive from what we observed in follicular fluids in which we studied steroid and protein content, comparing results between fertilized and unfertilized oocytes. Estradiol and testosterone were found to be significantly lower in FSH group when we expressed the concentration as nanograms per miligram of protein (fig. 1,2).

Premature luteinization is another deleterious effect of high basal LH in follicular phase on successful pregnancy. Several reports suggest that lower pregnancy rates may be a consequence of abnormal endometrial environment and receptivity, while it has been shown that premature luteinization in COH has no adverse effect on oocyte and, hence, embryo quality (14).

These evidences supports the contention that an amplification of ovarian physiology based on high level of FSH and low level of LH in follicular phase may improve the IVF outcome.

In the next future the availability of recombinant FSH and LH will make possible the performance of highly personalized protocols, which could result in a significant raise in the success rates.

REFERENCES

1) FALCK B. (1987). Site of production of oestrogen in rat ovary as studied by microtransplants. Acta Physiol Scand. 47, 163: 1-101.

2) CHAPPEL S.C., HOWELS C. (1992). Reevaluation of the roles of luteinizing hormone and follicle-stimulating hormone in the ovulatory rocess. Hum Reprod. 6(9): 1206-1212.

3) KENIGSBERG D. et Al. (1984). Medical hypophysectomy.I. Dose response using a gonadotropin realisig hormone antagonist. Fertil Steril. 42: 112-114.

4) JONES S.J. et Al. (1985). The effect of follicle-stimulating hormone without additional luteinizing hormone on follicular stimulation and oocyte development in normal ovulatory women. Fertil Steril. 43: 696-702.

5) COUZINET B. et Al. (1988). Stimulation of ovarian follicular maturation with pure follicle-stimulating hormone in women with gonadotropin deficiency. J Clin Endocrinol metab. 66: 552-556.

6) BERNARDUS R.B. et Al. (1985). The significance of the ratio in follicle-stimulating hormone and luteinizing hormone in induction of multiple follicular growth. Fertil Steril. 43: 373-378.

7) POLAN L.P. (1986). Ovulation induction with human menopausal gonadotropin compared to human urinary follicle-stimulating hormone result in a significant shift in follicular fluid androgen levels without discernible differences in granulosa-luteal cell function. J Clin Endocrinol Metab. 63: 1284-1291.

8) REGAN L. et Al (1989). Hypersecretion of LH and spontaneous miscarriage: a field study. J Endocrinol. 123: Abstr. 28.

9) *HOMBURG R. et Al. (1988). Influence of serum luteinizing hormone concentrations on ovulation, conception, and early pregnancy loss in polycystyc ovarian syndrome. Br Med J. 297: 1024-1027.*

10) *SHORHAM (SCHWARTZ) et Al. (1990). Hormonal profiles following clomiphene citrate therapy in conception and nonconception cycles. Clin Endocrinol. 33:271-278.*

11) *JACOBS H.S. et Al. (1987). Profertility uses of LHRH agonist analogues. In Vickery B.H. and Nestor I.J. (eds), LHRH and its Analogues: Contraception andTherapeutic Application, MTP Press, Lancaster: 303-319.*

12) *FORMAN R. et AL. (1988). Evidence for an adverse effect of elevated serum estradiol concentrations on embryo implantation. Fertil Steril. 49: 118-122.*

13) *DE PLACIDO G, ZULLO F. et Al. (1993). Confronto tra FSH puro ed hMG nella induzione della superovulazione per FIVET. In: FSH purificato nella terapia della sterilità; Estratto da "Nuovi orientamenti in fisiopatologia ostetrica e ginecologica. CIC Edizioni Internazionali. 57-62.*

14) *HOFMANN G.E. et Al. (1993) Premature luteinization in controlled ovarian hyperstimulation has no adverse effects on oocyte and embryo quality. Fertil Steril. 60: 675-679.*

Use of pFSH for controlled ovarian hyperstimulation in an IVF-ET program

M. Salvatori, M.R. Sgherzi, P.G. Artini*, G. Regnani, P. Traversi** and C. Battaglia

Università degli Studi di Modena, Istituto di Fisopatologia della Riproduzione Umana, Modena, *Università degli Studi di Pisa, Clinica Ostetrica e Ginecologica, Pisa and **Ospedale Dalmati, Sant'Angelo Lodigiano, Italy

INTRODUCTION

In IVF-ET programs, several stimulation protocols can be used to induce multiple follicular development and increase the pregnancy rates (1).

Human menopausal gonadotropin (hMG) have been widely used to induce controlled ovarian hyperstimulation (COH) and estrogen synthesis by granulosa cells (2).

Recent reports suggest that purified follicle stimulating hormone (pFSH) is able to support adequate folliculogenesis without using exogenous luteinizing hormone (LH) (3,4).

The aim of the present study was to compare, in IVF-ET patients, the results of two different COH protocols by using pFSH alone or in association with hMG.

MATERIAL AND METHODS

Forty women with irreparable tubal disease (N=20) or hormonal disfuctions (N=20) (LH/FSH ratio >2) were randomly assigned to either one of two treatment protocols: 22 patients were treated with pFSH (Group A), and 18 with pFSH plus hMG (Group B).

Hypogonadotropic hypogonadism was previously induced by subcutaneous administration of LHRH-analogue (Suprefact, Hoechst, Germany: 0.3 mg x 2/daily).

In the group A, from the first day of cycle until human Chorionic Gonadotropin (hCG) administration, 150 IU/daily (two ampoules) of pFSH (Metrodin, Serono, Italy: 75 IU/ampoule) were intramuscolar (im) administrated. In group B, the treatment started with pFSH (150 IU/daily), from the first to the third day of the cycle, and continued with im administration of pFSH plus hMG (Pergonal, Serono, Italy). The amount of Metrodin and Pergonal ampoules, in both protocols, was individually adjusted on the basis of plasma estradiol levels and ultrasonographic evaluation of follicular growth. Ovulation was induced by im injection of 10,000 IU of hCG (Profasi, Serono, Italy) when evidence of mature follicles was obtained (i.e. estradiol > 200 pg/ml/ follicle of ≥ 17 mm in maximum diameter). During the study were assayed the plasma levels of LH, FSH, estradiol (E2) and progesterone (P). Oocytes were collected, about 35/h after hCG administration, by a transvaginal echographic route.

For the study we analysed: days of stimulation, amount of gonadotropin used, number of recruited follicles, number of collected oocytes, degree of oocytes maturation, and pregnancy rate.

Based on oocyte-cumulo-corona complex morphology and appearance, oocytes were classified as: mature, intermediate, immature and atretic (3).

Seminal fluid treatment, insemination and embryo-transfer were performed with standard tecniques. After embryo-transfer the patients received progesterone supplementation (Gestone, Pabyrn, Italy: 100 mg on alternate days). Pregnancy was diagnosed by ultrasonographic evidence of the gestational sac. Biochemical pregnancies were not considered.

RESULTS

Comparing the results of the two different treatments, we found that stimulation period was longer (11.3±1.0 days vs 9.8±0.4 days) and the number gonadotropin ampoules was greater (27±1.8 vs 23±0.9) in group A than in group B. Similarly, the number of follicles with a ≥ 15mm diameter was significantly higher in the group A than in the group B (9.2±1.3 vs 6.1±0.7; p<0.05). The number of mature follicles was not significantly higher in patients submitted to pFSH than patients treated with pFSH + hMG (10.6±1.1 vs 7.2 ± 0.8; p< 0.01).

The fertilized oocytes were significantly increased in group A when compared to group B (7.7 ± 0.7 vs 5.9 ± 0.9; p< 0.05).

Significantly higher amount of immature oocytes was observed in group A in comparison to group B (4.1±1.2 vs 2.1±0.9; p< 0.05). No significant differences in plasma hormonal levels was found. The cancellation rate (2.1% vs 1.8%) and pregnancy rate (18.2% vs 16.6%) was similar in both group. No ovarian hyperstimulation occurred during the study.

DISCUSSION

In the present study there were no significant differences between the two COH protocols in relation to the stimulation days, the number of used ampoules and the number of mature oocytes. We agree with other authors(5) that neither LHRH-agonists or LHRH antagonists are able to completely suppress pituitary endogenous production of gonadotropins. We suggest that the theca cells necessitate very low LH amounts to produced androgens, which are subsequently aromatized, by the granulosa cells, into estrogens (6).

The numbers of immature oocytes produced were significantly higher in group B when compared to group A. This suggests that pharmacological doses of LH may induce an abnormal intrafollicular secretion of androgens which may impair oocyte growth.

Follicular development was more uniform and, probably, steroidogenesis more effective in the pFSH treated group. This suggests that: a) the LH pulsatile secretion is not necessary for follicular growth; and b) the low FSH levels achieved during pFSH stimulation allow an adequate ovarian production of androgens/estrogens levels.

In conclusion, the present study showed that even better results in follicular number and oocytes maturity are acheivable by pFSH stimulation, no improvements pregnancy rate were obtained.

REFERENCES

1. Grillo,M., Buck, S., Freys, I., and Mettler, L. (1989). Results of the use of a pure urinary FSH stimulation regimen in patients unsuccessfully treated with hMG in an in vitro fertilization program. Gynecol Obstet Invest 28, 169-173

2. Venturoli, S., Orsini, L.F., and Paradisi, R. (1986). Human urinary follicle-stimulating hormone and human menopausal gonadotropin in induction of multiple follicular growth and ovulation. Fertil Steril 45, 30-34

3. Jones, G.S., Acosta, A.A., and Garcia, J.E. (1985). The effect of follicle-stimulating hormone on follicular stimulation and oocyte development in normal ovulatory women. Fertil Steril 43, 696-700

4. Russel, J.B., Polan, M.L., and De Cherney, A.H. (1986). The use of pure follicle-stimulating hormone for ovulation induction in normal ovulatory women in an in vitro fertilization program. Fertil Steril 45, 829-834

5. Loumaye, E. (1990). The control of endogenous secretion of LH by gonadotropin-releasing hormone agonist during ovarian hyperstimulation for in vitro fertilization and embryo transfer. Hum Reprod 357-376

6. Shoam, Z., Balen, A., Patel, A., and Jacobs, H. (1991). Results of ovulation induction using human menopausal gonadotropin or purified follicle-stimulating hormone in hypogonadotropic hypogonadism patient. Fertil Steril 56, 1048-1053.

The luteal support in stimulated cycles

C. Montoneri, F. Nardo and G. Zarbo

University of Catania, 2nd Institute of Gynecology and Obstetrics, Ascoli – Tomaselli Hospital, Catania, Italy

---

Pharmacological induction of ovulation may cause the formation of an insufficient corpus luteum. Therefore, it is a common habit to support the luteal phase by administering progesterone or chorionic gonadotropin.

A preparation with progestinic effects, recently put on the market, may be administered intravaginally. So, the aim of the present study was to evaluate the efficacy of the different types of treatment.

269 women (from sterile couples) were included in the study and underwent controlled ovarian hyperstimulation (COH). They were divided into four groups, according to the type of luteal support employed.

group A (57 subjects):
COH (control group)
fertilization by artificial insemination using husband's semen (AIH)

group B (57 subjects):
COH + intravaginal administration of progesterone (100 mg/d) for 14 days, starting on day 2 after insemination
fertilization by AIH

group C (53 subjects):
COH + intramuscularly administration of progesterone (100 mg/d IM) for 14 days, starting on day 2 after insemination
"in vitro" fertilization and embryo transfer

group D (102 subjects):
COH + hCG (2.000 IU/mL IM) at day 18, 21, 23, 26 of the cycle
fertilization by AIH

The characteristics of the four groups were similar, although the number of subjects of group D was higher and group C was the only group that underwent IVF+ET (tab.1).

The data were subjected to paired Student's t-test for statistical analysis.

Tab. 1 - Characteristics of the four groups

	group A	group B	group C	group D
N. of cases	57	57	53	102
Mean age (women)	31,0 ± 6,0	29,9 ± 6,0	31,5 ± 5,2	29,6 ± 6,2
Mean age (men)	35,8 ± 4,7	34,2 ± 4,7	34,8 ± 5,0	32,9 ± 6,1
Duration of sterility	6,2 ± 3,4	5,8 ± 2,8	8,7 ± 4,5	7,0 ± 3,6
N. of cycles of COH	128	128	85	200
N. of cancelled cycles	15 (11,71%)	13 (10,15%)	22 (26,50%)	25 (12,37%)
Twin pregnancies	3 (5,26%)	5 (8,77%)	3 (5,66%)	7 (6,86%)

Causes of sterility are reported in fig. 1. Obviously a high incidence of anovulatory sterility is observed in group D and of tubal sterility in group C. Furthermore, 23 to 72% of cases shoved a male factor etiology. In all cases of group A and B it was not possible to detect any female factor of sterility and women were apparently healthy.

The protocol used for COH is shown in fig. 2. The results are presented in fig. 3. Although statistical analysis did not show any significant difference compared with the control group (probably due to the low number of subjects), it is interesting to observe that group B, which was treated with intravaginal progesterone, showed the highest percentage of pregnancies and a low incidence of undesirable effects (fig. 4). In addition women generally preferred this type of treatment to intramuscular administration.

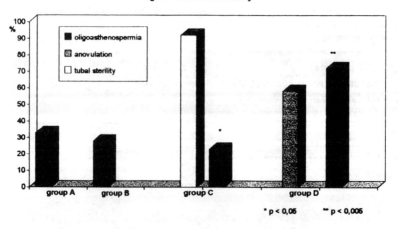

fig. 1 - Causes of Sterility

* p < 0,05   ** p < 0,005

fig. 2 - Protocol of Controlled Ovarian Hyperstimulation

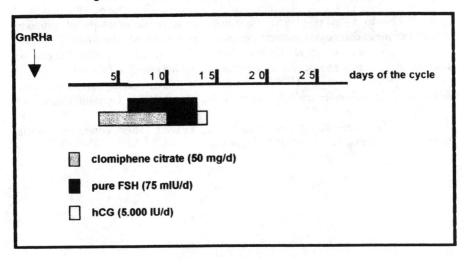

fig. 3 - Incidence of Pregnancies and Abortions

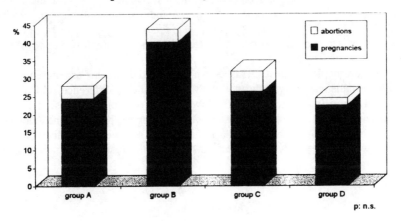

fig. 4 - Undesirable Effects

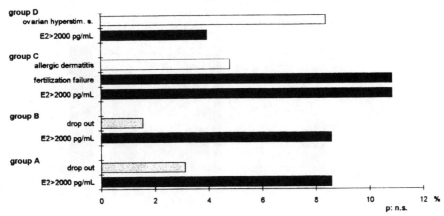

REFERENCES

1. Nardo F. et al. (1988). Inseminazione artificiale omologa ed induzione dell'ovulazione in coppie con partners oligospermici. *Fisiopatol. Riproduz.*, **6**, 49-51

2. Lo Presti L. et al. (1989). Protocolli di induzione dell'ovulazione per tecniche di fecondazione assistita. *Mediterranean J. Gynaecol.*, **1**, 269-273

3. Nardo F. et al. (1994). Résultats de l'insémination intrautérine après induction de la croissance multiple des follicoles. Revue Franç. Gynécol. Obstét., **89**, 382-386.

4. Montoneri C. et al. Results of IVF/ET after controlled ovarian hyperstimulation and oocyte donation (in press).

Endometriosis: impact on fertility

A. Caruso, G. Paradisi and A.M. Fulghesu

Department of Obstetrics and Gynecology, Catholic University of Rome, Rome, Italy

Abstract

Endometriosis is a gynecologic disease that affects women in their reproductive years, associated with marked subfertility. The accepted theory postulated is that endometriosis follows retrograde menstruation, but much laboratory and clinical evidence suggests that endometriosis is more complex than this. Abnormalities in both cell-mediated and humoral immunity have been found in endometriosis. Pelvic adhesions, distorted anatomy, and ovarian or tubal damage compromise fertility in moderate and severe stages of the disease. Alterations of the ovulatory process, ovum capture and sperm function, can possibly be related to increased macrophage activity and high peritoneal content of prostaglandins, cytokines and other secretory products. It can also be responsible for infertility in all degrees of endometriosis.

A long period without childbirth and the rate of disease in women studied for infertility similar to that found in parous women, are two epidemiologic factors which make the etiopatogenesis of endometriosis still discussed. Moreover, endometriosis must be treated when the extent of the disease may interfere with future fertility.

Introduction

Since the sixties, endometriosis has been considered a risk factor for fertility. Many studies have been made to consider the real impact of that pathology on infertility. The lack of a sure correlation between the role of the disease and pregnancy rate, the impossibility of knowing the exact prevalence of endometriosis and the lack of certainty about etiopathogenesis made difficult a correct valutation of the whole problem. Obviously, also the therapeutic approach to endometriosis reflects a scarcity of information on the condition, so that there are various choices of therapeutic methods. Following the latest studies, we will illustrate the "state of art" research on the impact of endometriosis in fertility.

Classification and pregnancy rate

During the last 20 years, several classifications have been proposed to provide prognostic significance in the evaluation of endometriosis severity. Acosta[1] in 1973, Kistner[2] in 1977 and the American Fertility Society[3] (AFS) in 1979 classified the rate of endometriosis based on the extention and location of lesions. The AFS classification, reviewed further[4] in 1985, is accepted by major authors. It is based on the localization and extention of lesions and identified 4 stages of the disease: minimal, mild, moderate and severe. It has been demonstered that some patients affected by severe endometriosis are fertile and, conversely, some patients with mild disease are infertile[5-7]. In fact, this kind of classification doesn't consider the functional aspect of lesions. Recent studies seem to modify classic theories about various aspects of endometriosis. "Atypical" implants of endometriosis have been shown to be more active in hormonal production than black implants; the latter are the forms usually evaluated at laparoscopy but they do not show any active production of prostaglandins[8,9]. The importance of the "atypical" forms and microscopic lesions may invalidate diagnostic criteria and even the revised American Fertility Society classification[4,10]. So it is clear that in all the studies that use the AFS classification there isn't a real correlation between the degree of disease and pregnancy rate.

Prevalence

Many factors in literature influence the calculation of the incidence of endometriosis. The principal ones are: type of surgical procedure; indication for surgery; type of hospital involved; "atypical" endometriosis.

Type of surgical procedure: the surgical approach including the abdominal and vaginal way and, recently, the laparoscopic way. It is clear that the vaginal method doesn't permit a complete pelvic vision; moreover, the choice of a specific type of surgical procedure leads to a patient selection that doesn't permit a homogenity of data 11,12.

Indication for surgery: more reliable estimates of the prevalence of endometriosis in the general population[13] can be based on laparoscopic observation of groups not at particular risk for the disease[14]. Parous, asymptomatic women requesting voluntary sterilization constitute the only large-scale group, to undergo laparoscopic pelvic visualization. Furthermore, data derived from the presumably normal cohort, are not necessarily directly generalizable to the entire premenopausal female population.

Type of hospital involved: cases studied in first level centres will show a minus frequency of endometriosis respect to the other cases studied in third level centres where we find a "selected" pathology.

"Atypical" endometriosis: it has been proven that its biochemical potential is greatly superior to those of the black implants[8]. However, only in recent years, have the so called atipical lesions, acquired a clinical importance. It continues to be difficult to make a classification for "atypical" endometriosis.

Etiology

Over the past 10 years, there has been a renewal in interest for retrograde menstruation. It is proven that endometrial cells have the capacity to adhere and proliferate. Whether these cells became implanted and accepted by peritoneal immune mechanism is not yet confirmed. A few evidence[15,16] supports the concept that the amount of retrograde menstruation is an important mediating factor in the pathogenesis of endometriosis and associated to infertility. The lack of an accurate method to quantify the degree of retrograde menstruation is the disturbing factor in studying the association between retrograde menstruation, endometriosis and infertility.

The other possible etiology is the mesothelial mataplasia.

Pathogenesis of sterility

When endometriosis involves the ovaries and causes adhesions that don't permit the tubaric motility and the tubal-oocyte pick-up, there will probably be sterility problems; whereas, information on the role of peritoneal factors in infertility are uncertain. Prostaglandins could be a factor of infertility in their endometriosis sites. They cold alterate tubaric motility, and cause a defect of ovum pick-up, LUF sindrome and endocrine luteal disturbance. However, it isn't yet demonstrated that endometriosis women have high levels of prostanoids in their peritoneal fluid, in respect to other steril women. The observations made on experimental endometriosis in animals show that infertility decreases after indometacin treatment[17]; so probably prostaglandins are involved in endometriosis infertility.

Also the immunity system could be another factor of endometriosis infertility. Humoral and cellular immune mechanisms are involved in the clearing of the peritoneal cavity from regurgitated menstrual debris. Some papers have demonstrated that in the case of endometriosis patients the assault on the system may be too extensive or too aggressive, and the defence mechanisms may be flawed; for

these reasons, viable endometrial fragments may implant.
Even hyperactivation of the immune system will not allow for
complete removal of the deposits in some patients, and these
will be the ones to develop clinical endometriosis. This
hyperactivated immune response may be reflected in an
increased number and an increased activational state of the
peritoneal macrophages[18,19] (with the ensuing production of:
cytokines, growth factors, prostaglandins, complement
components, hydrolytic enzymes and fibronectin), in
increased activation of T cells[20] (and reduced Natural
Killer activity), in increased antibody production to
autologous cells by B cells, and in a hostile, in fertility
terms, peritoneal environment. A few authors have recently
stated that endometriosis could be considered an autoimmune
disease[21,22]. This is based on the evidence that women with
endometriosis showed the same immunological profile as women
with unexplained infertility.

Obviously, all these hypothesis need further
confirmations. Even now, their role in respect to
infertility associated to endometriosis will be very
interesting for future studies.

Discussion

From literature it is evident that, on one side,
endometriosis-infertility relation is indubitable, and on
the other side it is not easy to establish the cause-effect
relationship and estimate its impact on fertility. Recently
it has been shown that the risk of endometriosis grows in
proportion to the time of last birth[23]; thus, endometriosis
may be a consequence of a long period without pregnancy.
Furthermore, the rate of disease in women studied for
infertility, has been found similar to that found in women
with one or more pregnancy[24].

Despite the lack of basic knowledge about the condition,
varies therapeutic methods have been proposed. They vary
from expectant management to medical ovarian suppression in
minimal or mild disease, and from endoscopic treatment to
conservative surgery in moderate and severe stages.

In our opinion that endometriosis must be treated when the extent of the disease may interfere with future fertility; on the contrary, when the extention is mild or minimal it would be better to proceed with expectant management.

In conclusion, other studies are necessary to clear up numerous questions that endometriosis poses and to which it is not yet possible to give a definitive answer.

References

1) Acosta, A.A., Buttram, V.C., Franklin, R.R. and Besch, P.K. (1973). A proposed classification of pelvic endometriosis. Obstet. Gynecol., 42, 19-22

2) Kistner, R.W., Siegler, A.M. and Behrman, S.J. (1977). Suggested classification for endometriosis: relationship to infertility. Fertil. Steril., 28, 1008-14

3) The American Fertility Society (1979). Classification of endometriosis. Fertil. Steril., 32, 633-38

4) The American Fertility Society (1985). Revised American Fertility Society classification of endometriosis. Fertil. Steril., 43, 351-2

5) Jones, H.W. and Jones, G.S. (1982). Endometriosis. In Jones, H.W. and Jones, G.S. (eds.) Gynecology, 3rd edn., pp. 353-8. (Baltimore: Williams & Wilkins)

6) Wheeler, J.M., Johnston, B.M. and Malinak, L.R. (1983). The relationship of endometriosis to spontaneous abortion. Fertil. Steril., 39, 656

7) Guzick, D.S., Bross, D.S. and Rock, J.A. (1982). Assessing the efficacy of the American Fertility Society's classification of endometriosis: application of a dose-response methodology. Fertil. Steril., 38, 171

8) Vernon, M.W., Beard, J.S., Graves, K. and Wilson, E.A. (1986). Classification of endometriotic implants by morphologic appearance and capacity to synthesize prostaglandin F. Fertil. Steril., 46, 801

9) Nisolle, M., Berliere, M., Paindaveine, B., Casanas-Roux, F., Bourdon, A. and Donnez, J. (1990). Histological study of peritoneal endometriosis in infertile women. Fertil. Steril., 53, 984

10) Schenken, R.S. (1994). Endometriosis classification for infertility. <u>Acta Obstet. Gynecol. Scand.</u>, <u>159</u>, 41-44

11) Goldman, M.B. and Cramer, D.W. (1990). The epidemiology of endometriosis. <u>Prog. Clin. Biol. Res.</u>, <u>323</u>, 15-31

12) Houston, D.E., Noller, K.L., Melton, L.J.III, Selwyn, B.J. and Hardy, R.J. (1987). Incidence of pelvic endometriosis in Rochester, Minnesota, 1970-1979. <u>Am. J. Epidemiol.</u>, <u>125</u>, 959-69

13) Kirshon, B., Poindexter, A.N. and Fast, J. (1989). Endometriosis in multiparous women. <u>J. Reprod. Med.</u>, <u>34</u>, 215-7

14) Moen, M.H. and Muus, K.M. (1991). Endometriosis in pregnant and non pregnant women at tubal sterilization. <u>Hum. Reprod.</u>, <u>6</u>, 699-702

15) Bartosik, D., Jacobs, S.L. and Kelly, L.J. (1986). Endometrial tissue in peritoneal fluid. <u>Fertil. Steril.</u>, <u>46</u>, 796-800

16) Kruitwagen, R.F.P.M., Poels, L.G., Willemsen, W.N.P., De Ronde, I.J.Y., Jap, P.H.K. and Rolland, R. (1991). Endometrial epithelial cells in peritoneal fluid during the early follicular phase. <u>Fertil. Steril.</u>, <u>55</u>, 297-303

17) Golan, A., Dargenio, R. and Winston, R.M.L. (1986). The effect of treatment on experimentally produced endometrial implants. <u>Fertil. Steril.</u>, <u>46</u>, 954-8

18) Olive, D.L., Weimberg, J.B. and Haney, A.F. (1985). Peritoneal macrophages and infertility: the association between cell number and pelvic pathology. <u>Fertil. Steril.</u>, <u>44</u>, 772-7

19) Dunselman, G.A.J., Hendrix, M.G.R., Bouckaert, P.X.J.M. and Evers, J.L.H. (1988). Functional aspects of peritoneal macrophages in endometriosis of women. <u>J. Reprod. Fertil.</u>, <u>82</u>, 707-10

20) Oosterlynck, D.J., Cornillie, F.J., Waer, M., Vandeputte, M. and Koninckx, P.R. (1991). Women with endometriosis show a defect in natural killer activity resulting in a decreased cytotoxicity to autologous endometrium. <u>Fertil. Steril.</u>, <u>56</u>, 45-51

21) Gleicher, N. (1994). The role of humoral imunity in endometriosis. <u>Acta Obstet. Gynecol. Scand.</u>, <u>159</u>, 15-17

22) Dmowski, W.P., Gebel, H.M. and Braun, D.P. (1994). The role of cell-mediated immunity in pathogenesis of endometriosis. <u>Acta Obstet. Gynecol. Scand.</u>, <u>159</u>, 7-14

23) Moen, M.H. (1991). Is a long period without childbirth a risk factor for developing endometriosis? <u>Human Reprod.</u>, <u>6</u>, 1404-7

24) Rawson, J.M.R. (1991). Prevalence of endometriosis in asymptomatic women. <u>J. Reprod. Med.</u>, <u>36</u>, 513-5

Superovulation and pregnancy rate in minimal and mild endometriosis

R. Agostini, S. Galossi, G. Pesce, A. Quinzi and G. Traficante

I Clinic of Obstetrics and Gynecology, University of Rome "La Sapienza", Rome, Italy

INTRODUCTION

Infertility is probably almost 20 times more common in endometriosis but the relationship between them is unclear. Several pathogenetic hypotheses have been advanced and it's possible that more than one of it may contribute to produce unexplained infertility and increased pregnancy loss.

Numerous endocrine alterations, alterated oocyte transport, abnormalities of fertilization and implantation, luteal phase defects have been found in many but not in all women affected by endometriosis.

Some authors found LUF syndrome associated with endometriosis but the frequency seems no higher than that found in other patologies (1-2) while some others observe repetitive abnormal follicular growth and low estradiol production (3). Lower LH receptor concentrations in ovarian follicles, abnormal LH patterns, second LH surge have been observed by cheesman (4) ' 82; decreased progesterone production or increased progesterone levels on day 6th to 9th of the cycle have been reported too (5).

Studies on women undergoing in vitro fertilization demostrated lower implantation rate in endometriotic women than in those affected by tubal desease, suggestive of the presence of a factor that inhibits implantation (6). The study of the structure and ultrastructure of the preovulatory endometrium of endometriotic women showed the existance of many alterations not revealed in the controls . Such alterations founded in 50% of the studied cycles of endometriotic normo-ovulating women were:

heterogeneity of the surface epithelium (during follicular phase), decreased ciliated cells; non ciliated cells ratio, incomplete ciliogenesis and reduction in cellular heigth probably due to an alterated expression of the estradiol receptors on the cells causing a decreased sensitivity of the endometrium to the normal estrogenic stimulation.

These morphological alterations could depend also on an immunological phenomena involving endometrium and triggered by the presence of ectopic implants (7) . To investigate about these thesis we performed the following study.

MATERIALS AND METHODS

We admitted to the study 90 women 23-38 years old, with laparoscopic diagnosis of mild and minimal endometriosis (American Fertility Society Classification) attending our center. Before laparoscopy all women underwent a comprensive infertility investigation including : basal body temperature measurements, serial measurements of plasma progesterone and prolactine , endometrial biopsy on day 24th-26th of the cycle .hysterosalpingografy, post coital test, semen analysis of the partners. To obtain superovulation we treated:

Group A : 20 women for 3 cycles with Clomiphene Citrate 100 mg/day from day 2nd to 6th of the cycle.

Group B: 70 women for 3 cycles with FSH purified 75UI/day + HCG 10000UI.

Follicular growth was monitored by serial sonografy using an endovaginal probe 5Mhz; HCG 10000UI was given when the diameter of the lead follicle was 20-22mm. Progesterone concentrations were measured on the day of HCG administration and 4-6-8 days later.

Pregnancy was defined as the presence of the serum concentration of beta HCG>5mUI/ml associated with a delay in menses.

Vaginal ultrasonography was performed in all patients with elevated levels of betaHCG after 6 weeks of amenorrhea to document the intrauterine presence of the gestational sac no ovarian.

RESULTS

In group A we obtained 45 ovulatory cycles (75%) while in group B the ovulatory cycles were 201 (95,7). A total of 5 pregnancies occurred (5,5) of all treated women and 7,14 % of patients treated with FSH. All pregnancies occurred with normospermic partner (69 normospermic and 21 mild oligospermic partners) and in the group B, in four pregnancies live enfants have been delivered, one ended in abortion at week 10.

CONCLUSION

We treated the patiens only for 3 cycles and this could be a short period of study, but our data and those of other authors suggest that only early cycles have the better chances of success (8).

We observed that pharmacological treatment do not improve pregnancy rate in endometriotic women; infact only 5 pregnancies occurred the percentage (7,14) obteined is lower than any other reported with Clomiphene Citrate (14-43% Cittadini Gysler) (9-10) and with FSHp (16-72% Tyler-March) (11-12).

Supposing that infertility in endometriosis is due to ovulatory dysfunctions it was to be expected that during superovulation induction the incidence of these abnormalities woud decrease and consequently pregnancy rate improve. We did not obtain improvement of the pregnancy rate so the failure has to be attributed to other factors. Always more concrete become the hypothesis of an immunological cause or concause that may involve either cellular or humoral immune function both peripherally and locally in the peritoneum and in the endometrium.

The presence of ectopic implants could cause an autoimmune reaction against endometrium to give evidence to this thesis there are the findings of immunoglobulin igG-igA antiendometrium and C3-C4 complement deposits in endometrial mucosa of these patients, the increase and faster attivation of peritoneal macrophages and finally the observation that often one or more immunological defects may precede the occurence of endometriosis in the same patien (13).

BIBLIOGRAPHY

1) BROSENS IA, KOINC KX PR; CORVELYN PA: " A study of plasma progesterone, estradiol 17 beta, prolactin and LH levels, and of the luteal phase appearance of the ovaries in patients with endometriosismand infertility " Br. J. Obst. Gyn. 85: 246, 1978.

2) BMOWSKI WP, RAO RR, SCOMMEGNA A: " The luteinized unruptared follicle syndrome and endometriosis " Fert. and Steril. 33:30, 1980.

3) LEWINTMAL D, FURMAN A, BLANKSTEIN J, CORENBLUM B, SHALEV J, LUNENFELD B: "Subtle abnormalities in follicular development and hormonal profile in women with unexplained infertility " Fert. and Steril. 46: 833, 1986.

4) CHEESEMAN KL, CHEESEMAN SD, CHATTERTON RT, COMEN MR : " Alterations in progesterone metabolism and luteal function in fertile women with endometriosis " Fert. Steril. 40: 590,1983.

5) AYERS JWT,BIRNEBAUM DL MENON KML: " Luteal phase dysfunction in endometriosis : elevated progesterone levels in peripheral and ovarian veins during the follicular phase " Fert. and Steril. 47: 925, 1987.

6) YVOCH JL, MATSON PL, RICHARDSON PA ; HILLIARD C: " Hormonal profile and embryo quality in women with severe endometriosis treated by in vitro fertilization and embryo transfer " Fert. and Steril. 50: 308, 1988.

7) FEDELE L, MARCHINI M, BIANCHI S, DAORTAM, ARCAINIL, FONTANA PE: " Structural and ultrastructural defects in preovulatory endometrium of normo-ovulating inferile women with minimal and mild endometriosis " Fert. and Steril. 53: 989. 1990.

8) DODSON WC, WHITESIDES DB, HUGHES CL JR, EASLY HA III, HANEY AF: " Superovulation with intrauterine insemination in the treatment of infertility: a possible alternative to gamete intrafallopian transfer and in vitro fertilization " Fert.and Steril. 48: 441-5, 1987.

9) CITTADINI E, AMODEO G, PALERMO R, GUASTELLA G, BENIGNO m : " Clomiphene Citrate with and without hmg in the induction of ovulation and superovulation in gynecological endocrinology " GENAZZANI A.R. ed VOLPE A., FACCHINETTI F. p. 429.

10) GYSLER M, MARCH CM , MUSHELL DR JR, BAILEY ES: " A decad e experience with an individualizated Clomiphene treatment regimen includingf its effect on post coital test " Fert. and Steril. 37: 161, 1982.

11) TYLER E: " Treatment of anovulation with menotropis " Jama 205: 86, 1968.

12) MAROM CM: " Improved pregnancy rate with monitoring of gonadotropin therapy by three modalities " Am J Obst. and Gyn. 156 : 1473, 1987.

13) GLEICHER N: " Endometriosis : a new approach is needed " Hum. Reprod 7: 821, 1992.

The surgical treatment of recurrent endometriosis

L. Fedele, S. Bianchi, M. Candiani, M. Busacca and M. Vignali

Università degli Studi di Milan, Centro per lo Studio e la Cura dell'Endometriosi, Milano, Italy

Endometriosis is generally defined as a progressive disease that may be locally invasive and tends to recur after treatment. Based on this concept, definitive surgery was considered for years as the only logical treatment option. However, various studies, particularly that of Meigs published in 1953, demonstrated a low recurrence rate after conservative surgery (1). This finding suggested that recurrence might not be inevitable and raised the question of which conservative procedures were most appropriate.

The natural history of endometriosis, however, is still unclear and poorly documented. That it is progressive is widely accepted, but data supporting this view are not unequivocal. The currently most accredited pathogenetic theory, that of retrograde menstruation, would explain progression of the disease and the occurrence of ex novo lesions after conservative treatment. In fact, even after all foci apparent at treatment are eliminated, the patient would remain at risk of developing new implants because of the persistence of retrograde menstruation. The appearance of ex novo endometriotic lesions after adequate treatment, however, is also compatible with the theory of coelomic metaplasia. The mechanisms, including metaplasia of cells originating from the coelomic epithelium, may be repetitive.

The results of a prospective study (2) and those of two cross-sectional investigations (3, 4) seem to suggest that the formation of ex novo implants is a relatively limited phenomenon whereas single foci appear able to evolve, at least in some women. An important aspect of endometriosis is the existence of macroscopically invisible, but histologically demonstrable, lesions in apparently intact peritoneal areas (5). Such microscopic foci have been detected also in women apparently free of endometriosis. They could progress and give rise to clinically appreciable lesions, interpreted as new areas of ectopic endometrium.

Based on these considerations, it is clear that many endometriosis recurrences could represent evolution of lesions invisible at time of treatment. Disease persistence may also be due to lack of recognition of visible but subtle lesions (frequently documented in recent years), lack of identification of subperitoneal lesions, or incomplete surgical treatment.

The exact recurrence rate of endometriosis after conservative surgery is not known. Rates from 2% to over 50% have been reported in literature. The uncertainty surrounding the true recurrence rate after conservative surgery is due primarily to the lack of specific prospective long-term studies. Only a few trials have included a systematic repeat laparoscopy to document any recurrences; unfortunately, in most cases the second laparoscopy was generally performed too soon to obtain long term data. Other studies have provided results based on the reappearance of symptoms as a measure of disease recurrence. In most cases, follow-up was variable and incomplete, and visual documentation of endometriosis recurrence by laparoscopy or laparotomy was obtained only in selected patients. The recurrence rates after conservative surgery at laparotomy and laparoscopy are quite similar, varying from 2% to 51% and from 2% to 33%, respectively. However, a reliable comparison of the two surgical approach cannot be made, because the women treated at laparoscopy generally had less severe endometriosis. In the largest study published so far, Punnonen observed a reoperation rate of 15% in a six- to ten-year follow-up of 903 surgically treated patients (6). Wheeler and Malinak (7) found a recurrence rate of 10% in their 423 patients. The cumulative recurrence rate at 5 years was 20%. Redwine recently calculated the interval and cumulative recurrence rates in 359 women with stages I-IV endometriosis treated by excision through the laparoscope and followed for a mean of 2 years (8). He demonstrated recurrence or persistence od the disease in 53 (43%) of 81 reoperated women, for a a five-year cumulative recurrence rate of 10% among the original group of 359 women.

THE MANAGEMENT OF RECURRENT ENDOMETRIOSIS

The available therapeutic options for recurrent endometriosis are substantially the same as those used to treat the disease initially. No pathogenetic or histologic difference has been demonstrated between initial and recurrent endometriotic lesions. However, in the case of recurrent endometriosis, the gynecologist will obviously choose therapeutic measures that carry the least risk of further recurrence. Thus, definitive surgery may be considered even for women under 40 and those with such extensive disease that complete resection is not feasible. Also, unilateral adnexectomy may be deemed appropriate if the condition of the ovary appears incosistent with normal function; this operation may be performed with greater confidence if the controlateral adnexa appear normal. In women with severe pain symptoms, pelvic denervation should be combined with conservative surgery in very selected cases. There are no data indicating whether laparatomy is better than laparoscopy for treating conservatively recurrent endometriosis. The choice of therapy for recurrent endometriosis should take into account: (a) the patient's symptoms; (b) the extent of disease; (c) the desire to maintain menstrual and/or reproductive function. Furthermore, the presence of important associated diseases may influence treatment decisions. A particular subset of patients are those with infertility associated with stage III/IV recurrent endometriosis. In these patients we prefer to perform conservative surgery (at laparotomy or laparoscopy according to the operator's experience and skill) with the aim to obtain complete removal of the disease and restoration of pelvic anatomy (9). If elimination of the disease is not possible, it is useful when performing diagnostic laparoscopy to carry out surgical maneuvers (mobilization of the ovaries, lysis of adhesions, emptying of endometriomas) that may favor the succes of a subsequent assisted reproduction technique.

REFERENCES

1.   Meigs, J.V. (1953). Endometriosis - etiologic role of marriage and parity; conservative treatment. *Obstet. Gynecol.*, **2**, 46-53

2.   Thomas, E.J., Cooke, I.D. (1987). Impact of gestrinone on the course of asymptomatic endometriosis. *Br. Med. J.*, **294**, 272-4

3.   Redwine, D.B. (1987). The distribution of endometriosis in the pelvis by age groups and fertility. *Fertil. Steril.*, **47**, 173-5

4.   Konninckx, P.R., Meuleman, C., Demeyere, S., Lesaffre, E., Cornillie, F.J. (1991). Suggestive evidence that pelvic endometriosis is a progressive disease, whereas deeply infiltrating endometriosis is associated with pelvic pain. *Fertil. Steril.*, **55**, 759-65

5.   Murphy, A.A., Green, W.R., Bobbie, D., de la Cruz, Z.C., Rock, J.A. (1986). Unsespected endometriosis documented by scanning electron microscopy in visually normal peritoneum. *Fertil. Steril.*, **46**, 522-4

6.   Punnonen, R., Klemi, P., Nikkanen, V. (1980). Recurrent endometriosis. *Gynecol. Obstet. Invest.*, **11**, 307-12

7.   Wheeler, J.M., Malinak, L.R. (1983). Recurrent endometriosis: incidence, management and prognosis. *Am. J. Obstet. Gynecol.*, **146**, 247-53

8.   Redwine, D.B. (1991). Conservative laparoscopic excision of endometriosis by sharp dissection: life table analysis of reoperation and persistent or recurrent disease. *Fertil. Steril.*, **56**, 628-34

9.   Candiani, G.B., Fedele, L.,Vercellini, P., Bianchi, S., Di Nola, G. (1991). Repetitive conservative surgery for recurrence of endometriosis. *Obstet. Gynecol.*, **77**, 421-4

Atypical laparoscopic appearances of peritoneal endometriosis

S. Dessole, G. Ambrosini, M. Dei, A. Scapinelli and N. Vargiu

Institute of Obstetrics and Gynecology, University of Sassari, Sassari, Italy

In laparoscopy, the peritoneal endometriotic typical lesion appears as a flat or raised area, of darkened colour either black or bluish, with a puckered aspect and of variable dimensions, from that of a pin head to several centimeters in diameter. When these pigmented lesions are found, the diagnose is easy.

Peritoneal endometriosis can also appear, however, with nonpigmented lesions, that have atypical characteristics. These lesions can appear as a flat whitish area, a raised red area, polypoid excrescences, subovarian adhesions, brown discoloured areas, circular peritoneal defects, petechial peritoneum, or hypervascolarized areas.(1)

The aim of this study is to evaluate several aspects of these atypical peritoneal lesions seen during laparoscopy in patients with pelvic endometriosis which was confirmed histologically.

MATERIALS AND METHODS

We examined 25 women, between the ages of 21 and 37 years (mean=26), undergoing laparoscopy for infertility or pelvic pain in whom, the histologic exam, performed on the biopsies, demonstrated pelvic endometriosis.

These biopsies were performed on both the typical lesions, macroscopically endometriotic, and on the nonpigmented peritoneal lesions and in particular, on the raised red lesions, polypoid excrescences, subovarian adhesions, circular peritoneal defects, and peritoneal opaque areas.

All biopsy specimens were immediatly fixed in formaldehyde and sent to a pathologist for histological exam.

In this study, the microscopic criteria used to define an endometriotic lesion were the presence of endometrial epithelium, or glandular or stroma tissue.

We evaluated the incidence of atypical lesions and their histological characteristics related to different macroscopic appearances, as well as their localization.

RESULTS

Typical lesions were found in 19 cases (76%) and atypical lesions were found in 23 cases (92%) of the 25 patients suffering from pelvic endometriosis. Both lesion types were found in 17 cases (68%). (Table 1)

Table 1. Appearances of endometriosis during laparoscopy.

	N.	%
ENDOMETRIOSIS	25	(100)
"Typical" lesion	19	(76)
"Subtle" lesion	23	(92)
"Typical and subtle" lesions	17	(68)

Biopsies were performed on 48 nonpigmented peritoneal lesions (Table 2). The presence of endometrial epithelium, glandular and stroma tissue, was found in 25 lesion samples (52%), tissue containing one of the two endometrial components, glandular or stroma, was found in 8 samples (17%). In the remaining 15 samples, non endometriotic alterations were found, or more precisely; 7 cases (15%) of inflammatory reaction, 5 cases (10%) of mesothelial cell proliferation and 3 cases (6%) of small mesenteric cysts.

The presence of endometriotic tissue was found to be different in relation to the macroscopic aspect of the peritoneal lesions during laparoscopy (Table 3).

Table 2. Laparoscopic biopsies of non-pigmented peritoneal lesions

Biopsies	N.	%
Glands and stroma	25	(52)
Glands or stroma	8	(17)
Inflammatory reactions	7	(15)
Mesothelial cell proliferation	5	(10)
Mesenteric cyst	3	(6)
Total	48	(100)

Table 3. Laparoscopic appearances of peritoneal lesions and endometriosis

Lesion		Endometriosis	
	N.	N	%
White opacified peritoneum	10	9	(90)
Red flame-like lesion	14	13	(93)
Glandular lesion	8	6	(75)
Subovarian adhesion	4	2	(50)
Yellow-brown patches	3	2	(66)
Circular peritoneum defect	3	0	-
Vescicular excrescences	6	1	(16)
Total	48	33	(68,7)

Endometriotic tissue was found in 93% of the red, flame-like lesions, 90% of the raised whitish lesions, in 75% of the lesions with a glandular aspect, 50% of the subovarian adhesions, 16% of the polypoid excrescences and not found in the cases of the circular peritoneal defects.

Table 4.Biopsy specimen localization of subtle endometriotic lesions.

Localization	N	%
fossa ovarica	3	(9)
pouch of Douglas	7	(21)
uterosacral, Douglas	10	(30)
broad ligament	9	(28)
uterovesical fold	4	(12)
Total	33	(100)

The atypical peritoneal endometriotic lesions were localized prevalently at the level of the uterosacral ligaments, in the Douglas pouch and in the posterior of the broad ligament, less frequently in the uterovesical fold and fossa ovarica (Table 4).

DISCUSSION

Numerous studies in the past decade (2-5) have described the polymorphic aspects of atypical peritoneal endometriotic lesions. These lesions seem more active in the invasion of the extracellular matrix with respect to the typically pigmented lesions.(6-9). These last would represent the final consequence of the proliferation cycle in the hemorrhagic formation, with hematic pigmentation and scarring phenomena (7,10). This can be confirmed by the frequent appearance of "atypical lesions together with typical lesions as the continued evolution of nonpigmented lesions. Moreover, the atypical lesions appear more frequently in younger women, while those pigmented in older women (11).

In our cases, atypical lesions were found in 96%, while pigmented lesions were found in 76%, and both were found in 68% of the cases.

In the last few years, the frequence of atypical endometriosis found during laparoscopy has increased notably (4), especially in women with infertility or with pelvic pain, reaching 60% (12).

Jansen and Russell in 1986 (2) were the first to describe, using biopsy techniques, a series of lesions that did not have the typical aspects, with bluish or black pigmentation, but that had, histologically, characteristics of endometriosis .

The prevalence of endometriosis in peritoneal lesions was near 70% in our study, in fact typical endometrial epithelium, glands and stroma, were present in 52% of the biopsies; glandular epithelium or stroma in 17%. On first viewing, numerous other lesions can be confused with atypical foci of endometriosis, therefore visual suspicions should always be followed by biopsy with histologic exams.

The prevalence of endometrial epithelium changes in relation to the morphological aspect of the lesion. In our case reports, red, flame-like lesions and peritoneal whitish lesions demonstrated an elevated percentage (>90) of endometrial epithelium.

The localization of the atypical endometrial lesions was prevalent in the Douglas pouch peritoneum and in the posterior of the broad ligament, less frequently at the peritoneum level of the fossa ovarica or at the uterovesical fold. This occurs because the ovaries become involved in the endometriotic process later in the reproductive age and in older women (13).

Nonpigmented peritoneal lesions should be classified as mild endometriosis. It is not yet clear if this early form of endometriosis should be considered an expression of the disease or a normal condition that can occur intermittently in most women of fertile age (14).

REFERENCES

1. Brosens J, Donnez J and Benagiano (1993). Improving the classification of endometriosis. Hum. Reprod., 8,1992-1995.

2. Jansen RPS & Russell P (1986). Non pigmented endometriosis : clinical, laparoscopic and pathologic definition. Am. J. Obstet. Ginec. 155,1154-1159.

3. Stripling MC, Martin DC, Chatman DL, Zwaag RV & Poston WM (1988). Subtle Appearence of endometriosis. Fertil. Steril. 49,427-431.

4. Martin DC, Hubert GD, van Der Zwaag R & El-Zeky FA (1989). Laparoscopic appearence of peritoneal endometriosis. Fertil. Steril. 51,63-67.

5. Moen MH & Muus KM (1991). Endometriosis in pregnant and non-pregnant women at tubal sterilisation. Hum. Reprod. 6,699-702.

6. Vernon MW, Beard JS, Graves K, Wilson EA (1986). Classification of endometriosis implants by morphologic appearences and capacity to sinthesize prostaglandin F. Fertil. Steril. 46,801-806.

7. Nisolle M, Paindaveine B, Bourdon A et al. (1990). Histologic study of peritoneal endometriosis in infertile women. Fertil. Steril. 53,984-988.

8. Donnez J, Nisolle M & Casanas-Roux F.(1992). Three-dimensional architectures of peritoneal endometriosis. Fertil. Steril. 57,980-983.

9. Spuijbroeck MDEH, Dunselman GAJ, Menheere PPCA and Evers JLH (1992). Early endometriosis invades the extracellular matrix. Fertil. Steril. 58,929-933.

10. Brosens IA, Puttemans P, Deprest and Rombauts Luk (1994). The endometriosis cycle and its derailments. Hum. Reprod. 9,770-771.

11. Redwine DB (1987). Age-related evolution in color appearence of endometriosis. .Fertil. Steril. 48,1062-1963.

12. Koninckx PR, Meuleman C, Demeyere S , Lesaffre E and Cornille F (1991). Suggestive evidence that pelvic endometriosis is a progressive

disease, whereas deeply infiltrating endometriosis is associated with pelvic pain. Fertil. Steril. **55**,759-765.

13. Redwine DB (1987).The distribution of endometriosis in the pelvis by age groups and fertility. Fertil. Steril. **47**,173-175.

14. Koninckx PR (1994). Is mild endometriosis a disease? Is mild endometriosis a condition occurring intermittently in all women? Hum Reprod **9**,2202-2211.

Hysteroscopy in infertile women

V. Benedetto, V. Palmara, M. Micalizzi, G. Zona, J. Leonardi and R. Leonardi

Department of Gynecology, University of Messina, Italy

INTRODUCTION

A great number of data can be obtanied with hysteroscopic investigation and these regard the difference anatomic districts (1, 2, 3), thus permitting an observation in vivo of the cervical canal, of the disposition of the palmate folds, of the eventual polyps, sinechiae and cervical isthmus incontinence; it also permits the diagnosis of hypoplasia and uterine malformations, it evidence intracavitary pathology and the morpho-functional modification of the endometrium during the different phases of the mestrual cycles; furthermore it allows the observation of the uterus-tube junction area and the conformation of the area next to the tubes.

Hysteroscopic investigation have evidenced the frequent presence of adhesion on patients suffering of amenorrhea, of secondary oligo-amenorrhea, recurrent abortion or unclear infertility, especially in those cases where it was difficult by other means to reveal them, that is when they were not very dense and of little extension.

NATERIAL AND METHODS

These are the results we collected from January 1988 to July 1994 at the hysteroscopy department of the Istitute of Gynecology, University of Messina.

During that period 572 patients, who were affected by infertility or sterility, aged between 20 and 38 years, underwent hysteroscopic investigation. We preferred doing investigation during the proliferative phases, that is between the 8th and 13th day of the cycle, because the uterine orifice and isthmus are hypotonic and the endometrium is thin and tends to bleed less easily; also the visualization of the uterine cavity and of tubaric ostium is better.

A Hammon hysteroscopy (diameter 4mm, length 25cm) (9) was used to do investigation; a CO_2 hysteroinsufflator was used to distend the uterine cavity, preselecting an average endouterine pressure of 40mmHg (never above 80mmHg) at a flow rate of 30/50 ml/m', a cold ligthgenerator of 150 watts (10) provided the ligth.

The patients sent to the department had benn previously treated with 10 mg of diazepam and 0,5 mg of atropine i.m., 30 minutes before investigation.

RESULTS

The studypopulation consisted of 572 infertile women, ranged in age from 20 and 38 years, that underwent a full investigation which included a hystory and phisical examination, detection of ovulation by ultrasound and serum progesterone essays, post-coital test and analyses, hysterosalpingography. A normal uterine cavity and cervical canal were found in 192 (33,6%) of the 572 patients, while some abnormality was found in the remaining 380 (66.4%). (Tab. I)

Of the 380 patients with abnormal findings,148 (25,9%) had cervical canal abnormalities, 232 (40,5%) uterine cavity abnormalities. (Tab. II)

Of the total number (572 patients), 58 (10,13%) had cervical synechiae, 14 (2,44%) cervical incompetence, 64 (11,18%) cervical polyp, 12 (2,09%) endocervical mucosa alterations (Tab. III), 82 (14,33%) had uterine hypoplasia, 36 (6,29%) uterine synechiae, 30 (5,24%) submucosus fibroids, 42 (7,34%) uterine malformations, 32 (5,59%) endometrial polyps and 10 (1,74%) emdometrial hyperplasia. (Tab. IV)

During investigation it was possible to lyse not very thick synechiae with the extreme point of the hysteroscope or to remove small polyp-like formations found in the cervical canal with curettes (21 out 62) (Tab. III).

The same thing was done for thin vascular pons of the uterine cavity (9 out of 36), for small polyps (7 out of 32) and for small myomas (5 out of 30). (Tab. IV)

In order to subject the other patients to myomectomy or polypectomy with resector, an elective hospitalization was programmed. The uterine malformations were found: 2 (0,34%) bicornuate-bicervix uteri with vaginal septum, 2 (0,34%) bicornuate-bicervix uteri; 3 (0,52%) bicornuate uteri, 10 (1,74%) complete uterine septum and 25 (4,37%) uterine sub-septum of various degrees. (Tab. V)

The hysteroscopy diagnosis was preceedede by hysterosalpingography; the most serious abnormal pathologies were confirmed by celioscopy.

It was possible to resect the septum, in part or totally, for all the patients with a complete septum or sub-septum (10 out of 25 cases respectively).

We believe that hysteroscopy constitutes a valuable method in the investigation of infertility, as it is a relatively simple and safe procedure that gives accurate findings of uterine cavity and cervical canal abnormalities.

Tab. I: <u>PATIENTS EXAMINED</u>

total infertile women	572 (age >20 <38)	
withouth pathology	n° 192	33,60%
with some pathology	n° 380	66,40%

Tab. II: <u>WOMEN WITH SOME PATHOLOGY</u>

total women	380	
cervical canal abnormalities	148	25,90%
uterine cavity abnormalities	232	40,50%

Tab. III: <u>CERVICAL CANAL ABNORMALITIES</u>

cervical canal synechiae	58	10,13%
cervical incompetence	14	2,44%
cervical canal polyps	64	11,18%
cervical mucosa alterations	12	2,09%

Tab. IV: <u>UTERINE CAVITY ABNORMALITIES</u>

uterine ipoplasia	82	14,33%
uterine synechia	36	6,29%
submucosus fibroids	30	5,24%
uterine malformations	42	7,34%
endometrial polyps	32	5,59%
endometrial hyperplasia	10	1,74%

Tab. V: <u>UTERINE MALFORMATIONS</u>

bicornuate-bicervix with vaginal septum	2	0,34%
bicornuate - bicervix uteri	2	0,34%
bicornuate uteri	3	0,52%
complete uterine septum	10	1,74%
uterine subseptum	25	4,37%

<u>REFERENCES</u>

1 Flamigni C. et Al. (1985). Uterine pathology and infertility. Acta Europ. Fertil. 16, 1
2 Perino A., Mencaglia L., Hamou J.E. et Al. (19). Hysteroscopy for metroplasty of uterine septu:
3 Scarselli G., Tantini C., et Al. (1983). Microhysteroscopy and infertility. In " Hysteroscopy ". van der Pas H. et Al. (Edts) MTP Press Publisher, Boston, p.151.
4 Taylor J.P., Haman J.E. (1983). Hysteroscopy. J. Reprod. Med. 28,166.
5 Valle R.F. (1980). Hysteroscopy in the evaluation of female infertility. Am. J. Ostet. Gyn. 137,425.
6 Siegler A.M. (1977). Hysterography and hysteroscopy in infertile patients. J. Reprod. Med. 18, 143
7 Sugimoto O. (19). Diagnostic hysterography and hysteroscopy in infertile patients. J. Reprod. Med.
8 Taylor P.J., Cumming D.C. (1979). Hysteroscopy in 100 patients. Fertil Steril 31, 301.
9 Hamou J. (1984). Hysteroscopie et microcolpohysteroscopie. Atlas et Traité. Palermo COFESE Publisher.
10 Siegler A.M., Kemmann E.K., Gentile G.P. (1976). Hysteroscopy procedures in 257 patients. Fertil. Steril. 27, 1267
11 De Jong P., Doel F., Falconer A. (1990). Outpatients diagnostic hysteroscopic. Br. J. Obst. Gyn. 97, 299

Reproductive outcome after hysteroscopic metroplasty

N. Colacurci, A. Mollo*, C. Carravetta*, R. Sagliocco*, T. Santoro and G. De Placido*

*II Università degli Studi di Napoli, II Cattedra di Ginecologia e Ostetricia and *Università "Federico II" di Napoli, I Cattedra di Ginecologia e Ostetricia, Naples, Italy*

INTRODUCTION

The septate uterus is associated with the highest incidence of reproductive failure such as abortion and premature delivery (1). Several studies showed very poor reproductive performances where the malformation is not treated (2). Successfull pregnancy outcome is significantly improved by metroplasty ranging from 5 to 90% (3).

At present the hysteroscopic metroplasty should be considered as a first choice treatment of the septate uterus if compared to the abdominal approach, because of its well-known advantages, such as the short hospitalization required, reduced morbidity, avoided laparotomy and hysterotomy, low risk of pelvic adhesions, more chances of vaginal delivery.

In this five years retrospective study we analysed the reproductive outcome of 69 patients with septate uterus who underwent hysteroscopic metroplasty.

SUBJECTS AND METHODS

From March 1990 to October 1994, a total of 69 patients, with different degrees of septate uterus, underwent hysteroscopic metroplasty. We performed the hysteroscopic metroplasty on 2 total septate uterus with two apparent cervix, 11 total septate uterus, 54 subtotal septate uterus and 2 communicating septate uterus, according to 1984 Toaff's Classification (4). In the 13.2% of these cases the sepatate uterus was associated to organic intracavitary pathology, such as polyps, myomas or adhesions, and the surgical procedure was therapeutical for both indications.

A number of 48 patients out of the total had an obstetrical hystory of recurrent miscarriage or fetal wastage, while 21 women had a hystory of primary infertlity. In the infertile patients the operation was performed during diagnostic laparoscopy or in preparation of IVF techniques.

In all the cases the operative procedures was performed by means of a 26 F resectoscope (Karl Storz GmbH, Tuttlingen, Germany) with specific loops electrode. The cutting current was set at 50-70 W. The uterine cavity was distended using an urological solution of sorbitol-mannitol at an inflow pression of 60-90 mm of Hg. The operative time length was measured from the insertion of the resectoscope to its final extraction.

The effectiveness was evaluated by hysterosalpingogrphic or hysteroscopic checks two months after the operations.

RESULTS

The surgical time ranged from 10 to 42 minutes, including the cases of interventions with polyps or myoma slicing.

Post-operative hysterosalpingogram or hysteroscopic examination showed a normal cavity with a little fundal notch, wich was less than 1 cm wide in 85.5% of the cases, while in 10 cases it was more than 1 cm wide.

In two cases a second surgery was needed: in both cases the first procedure was made whitin 60 days after a miscarriage of more than 12 weeks, when the two emicavity were not yet simmetrical. We did not observe complications, either during the operation or in post-operative time.

We observed 46 pregnancies, with two sets of twins, and a miscarriage rate of 13%.

Table 1.   Reproductive Outcome Post-Surgery

	Recurrent fetal wastage	Infertility	Total
Total cases	48	21	69
Pregnancies	40	6	46
single	38	6	
twins	2	-	
Miscarriages	6	-	6 (13%)
Delivery < 36 W with live birth	4	1	5 (10.8%)
PROM	2	-	2
Term delivery	28	3	31 (67.4%)
cesarean section	13	2	15 (48.3%)
vaginal delivery	15	1	16 (51.7%)
Pregn. ongoing	2	2	4 (8.6%)

We performed 13 cerclages; our personal indication to cerclage are as follows:

- a present obstetrical situation of cervical incompetence
- an incompetence demonstrated by HSG performed out of pregnancy
- a personal hystory of more than 3 miscarriages or preterm delivery before the 30th week with fetal wastage.

Table 2. Preterm delivery rate in patient with or without cerclages

Pregnancies	46
Cerclages	13 (28.2%)
Preterm delivery with cerclage	1/13 (7.6%)
Preterm delivery without cer.	4/33 (12.1%)

The modality of term pregnancy deliveries, wich often were not attended by our group, were cesarian sections in 48% of the cases and vaginal delivery in the 52%. The preterm delivery rate ranges from 21.1% in women without cerclage, to 7.6% in women with cerclage.

DISCUSSION

Several different methods and instruments for the hysteroscopic transection of uterine septum have been applied , including scissors (semirigid or rigid), resectoscope or Laser (Nd:YAG or KTP or Argon). Various Authors have analized the pregnancy outcome after hysteroscopic metroplasty when that had been performed with different methods. Fedele et al. (5) compared the results obtained with the three different thecniques: they performed 80 procedures with microscissors, 10 with Argon Laser and 12 with resectoscope. Their conclusion was: "the reproductive outcome was not affected by the method of septal incision or by surgical intracavitary morphology". Cararach et al (6) compared the results obtained when the operation was performed by scissors, 17 cases, with those performed by resectoscope, 53 cases, and they found no difference in the evolution of the pregnancy in the two groups, but they noticed that the pregnancy rate after the removal of the septum with scissors was grater than after the division of the septum by means of the resectoscope. They suggested, according to Hamou (7) and Duffi (8), that electrosurgery might cause thermic damage of the vasculature of the myometrium, which could negatively affect the development of the endometrium covering the excised septal areas.

The choice of the technique seems to depend on different reasons: operating time, cost of instrumentations, familiarity of the surgeon with the technique, rate of complications. The operating time depends on the semplicity of the technique and on the possibility of having an optimal vision during the whole time of the procedure: the resectoscope is certainly the faster surgical procedure, with the best vision and, therefore, with a low rate of complication.

313

Moreover, the instruments costs is very low, when compared with laser. For these reasons our personal experience, begun in 1990, is based only on the use of resectoscope.

In our opinion, and according to different Autrhors (4-5), the more than 1 cm wide residual notch observed in 10 cases (14.5%), does not influence either the frequence of miscarriage or the reproductive outcome. Furthermore we must remember the posssibility of having an uterine rupture during pregnancy after metroplasty, even if the surgical procedure has not provoked immediate complication (9). It is for this reasons that we prefere leaving a little fundal notch, possibly less than 1 cm wide.

With regard to the modality of delivery, the indication for cesarian section for the other gynecologists who assisted the delivery, was not the metroplasty itself, but the "precious pregnancy" after a pathological obstetrical hystory.

The last aspect to be taken into consideration is the indication to cervical cerclage. There are two opposite position on the subject: on one side Abramovic claims that it is needed in all cases of mullerian malformation, on the other side some claim it is necessary only in real, documented cases of cervical incompetence. Fedele in 1993 performed the 23.6% of cerclage and found that the cerclage significantly modified the preterm delivery:from 21% in women without cerclage to 7% in women with cerclage. Our results show that in women with cerclage the rate of preterm delivery was lower than that referring to women without. This difference was not statistically significant.

REFERENCES

1) Fayez JA (1986). Comparison between abdominal and hysteroscopic metroplsty. Obstet Gynecol, 78:213-20

2) Musich JR, Behrman SJ (1978). Obstetric outcome before and after metroplasty in women with uterine anomalies. Obstet Gynecol, 52:63-8

3) Choe JK, Baggish MS (1992). Hysteroscopic treatment of septate uterus with Neodimium-YAG laser. Fertil Steril, 57:81-4

4) Toaff ME, Toaff AS, Toaff R (1984). Communicating uteri, review and classification with introduction of two previously unreported types. Fertil Steril 41:661

5) Fedele L, Arcaini L, Parazzini F, Vercellini P, Di Nola G (1993). Reproductive prognosis after metroplasty in 102 women: lifle-table analysis. Fertil Steril, 59:768-72

6) Cararch M, Penella J, Ubeda A, Labatisda R (1994). Hysteroscopic incision of sepatate uterus: scissors versus resectoscope. Human Reproduction, 9:87-9

7) Hamou J. Courants haute frèquence en hystéroscopie et microcolpohystéroscopie opératoire. Contracept Fertil Sexual, 16:737-41

8) Duffi S, Reid PC, Sharp F (1991). In vitro study of uterine electrosurgery. Obstet Gynecol, 78:213-20

9) Lobaugh ML, Bammel BM, Duke D, Webster BW (1994). Uterine rupture during pregnancy in a patient with a hystory of hysteroscopic metroplasty. Obstet Gynecol, 83:838-40

Laparoscopic treatment of adnexal torsion

S. Dessole, P.L. Cherchi, M. Farina, G. Ambrosini and M. Dei

Institute of Obstetrics and Gynecology, University of Sassari, Sassari, Italy

Adnexal torsion is a rare gynecological emergency, that if not diagnosed and treated quickly, can cause necrosis of the affected organs, peritonitis and possibly threaten the life of the patient (1).

The incidence of this clinical entity is low. Hibbard (2) reported that during a 10 year period, 3772 patients required an emergency operative procedure and adnexal torsion was found in 2.7% of these patients. In another study by Bruhat (3), 0.38% of the 10,000 laparoscopies performed revealed an adnexal torsion. Twelve to eighteen per cent of adnexal torsions occur during pregnancy (1,4-6).

The torsion can be complete or incomplete, can involve either or both the ovary and Fallopian tube. If incomplete, the venous and lymphatic circulation are the first to be disturbed, with the resulting enlargement of the organ. But, if quickly corrected, before venous and arterial thrombosis, the affected organs can be recovered.

If the torsion is complete and persistent, the degradation can progress rapidly until arterial occlusion with ischemia of the organ, which becomes cyanotic, with necrosis and possible infection and peritonitis (1).

Precise diagnosis and rapid treatment are essential if the adnexa and its endocrine and reproductive functions are to be preserved.

Sudden pain in the lower quadrant of the abdomen or the presence of an adnexal mass, which is painful to the touch, are nonexclusive characteristics of such a condition; consequently, a correct diagnosis is made in only 38-66% of the cases (2).

315

The use of ecographic and laparoscopic examinations, today widely available, permits a surgeon to make an early diagnosis, if the surgeon has a well-grounded suspicion. (7-9).

Adnexal torsion is a gyneacological emergency, that in the past was treated with laparotomy, often preceded by a laparoscopic diagnosis. The treatment consisted of the extirpation of the necrotic adnexa, to avoid the risk of thromboembolism or more rarely, in its untwisting and anchorage by suture (2).

The developments in laparoscopy, in the last ten years, have reduced the diagnostic time and have modified the treatment of this pathology, that, usually, occurs during the reproductive age.

We report three cases in which laparoscopic procedures were used.

CASE 1

The patient P.M., 25 years of age, was sent to us by her general physician for pain in the right iliac region, present for several days and accentuated in the last two hours. Physical examination revealed tenderness on palpation in the right lower quadrant and a tumor in the right adnexal position.

Ultrasonic examination showed the presence of a dishomogeneous mass of approximately 5 cm of diameter.

An adnexal torsion was suspected. Laparoscopy confirmed the presence of the right adnexa twisted of 540 degrees, cyanotic and edematous.

After the adnexa was untwisted, quick effects of the tubal perfusion were demonstrated. The normal colouring of the tube was restored, while the ovary showed no appreciable change.

The colour and consistancy of the ovary are not always indicative of irreversable ischemic damage. Consequently, to evaluate the residual eutrophic ovarian tissue, laparotomy was performed, which confirmed the irreversible damage of the ovarian parenchyma.

CASE 2

The patient P.N., 37 years of age, multiparous, had a colic-like pain on the left side for a period of 48 hours with an exacerbation of 1 hour.

Pelvic examination disclosed initial rigidity,spasm and pain on lower quadrant palpation with no evidence of a mass in the genital tract .

A sonographic examination did not demostrate alterations to the genital tract. As there was a modest amount of liquid in the cul de sac of Douglas, a hemorrhage of an ruptured ovarian cyst was hypothesized.

Laparoscopy demonstrated the presence of an ovarian fibroma of 5 cm in diameter, peduncled and twisted on its axis, attached to the abdominal wall, pulling the tube and the ovary, twisting them 180 degrees. After the fibroma was separated from the abdominal wall, the adnexa untwisted itself and after cutting off the peduncle , the fibroma was extirpated through a small abdominal breach.

CASE 3

The third case is a young nullipara, 20 years of age, with intense pain in the right iliac region, extending to the homolateral side, present for several hours and accompanied by nausea and vomiting. The pelvic examination demonstrated tenderness to superficial palpation and a right adnexal mass.

The ultrasonic examination showed a dishomogeneous mass greater than 5 cm in diameter in the cul de sac of the Douglas.

A right adnexal torsion with an ovarian cyst was suspected.

The following laparoscopy confirmed the presence of an enlarged, cyanotic and twisted right adnexa, with ovarian cyst. An untwisting was performed. It is important to evaluate the recovery of the hematic perfusion after such a procedure.

The risk of thromboembolism mentioned above, related to the untwisting, resulted as being more theoretical than real.

The cystectomy performed on an ischemic ovary, edematous and fragile, is sometimes difficult and can lead to an additional lesion of the undamaged parenchyma.

Therefore, several authors (1) recommend performing a simple aspiration of the cystic content and revaluation of the ovary after 6-8 weeks. If the cyst persists, a laparoscopic procedure should be performed.

CONCLUSIONS

Adnexal torsion is a rare but not uncommon occurance, usually occurs during the reproductive age. This condition must be diagnosed and treated quickly to preserve the intergity of the reproductive system. Laparoscopy is particularly helpful because it allows diagnosis and adequate surgical treatment.

REFERENCES

1. Nichols D.H.,Julian PJ (1985).Torsion of the adnexa. Clin. Obst. Gynec.28,375-380

2. Hibbard l(1995). Adnexal torsion.Am J Obstet Gynecol. 152,456-461.

3. Bruhat MA,Mage G., Pouly JL,Manhès H,Canis M,Wattiez A (1989):- Coelioscopie operatoire. MEDSI/McGraw-Hill,

4. Walker PA (1962). A case of torsion of the fallopian tube in pregnancy. J. Obstet. Gynecol. Br. Commonw. 69,112-114

5. Korenz Z & Bichacho S(1967). Torsion of pregnant tube. J Obstet Gynecol Br Commonw. 74,603-604

6. Chambers J T, Thiagarajah, S and Kitchin J D (1979):Torsion of the normal fallopian tube in pregnancy. Obstet Gynecol 54:487-489

7. Helvie M., Silver T. (1989). Ovarian torsion:sonographic evaluation. JCU 17,327-32

8. Bider D, Mashiach S, Mordechai D, Kokia E, Lipitz S and Ben-Rafael Z. (1991): Clinical, surgical and pathologic findings of adnexal torsion in pregnant and non pregnant women. Surgery, Gynecology Obstetrics, , 173,363-366

9. Warner M,Fleischer A, Edell S, Theine G, Bundy A Kurtz a et al (1985): Uterine Adnexal torsion: sonographic findings. Radiology 154:773-75

10. Zweizig S, Perron J,Grubb D, Mishell D (1993):Conservative management of adnexal torsion. Am J Obstet Gynecol 168:1791-5

11. Oelsner G, Bider D, Goldenberg M, Admon D, Mashiachs (1993). Long-term follow-up of the twisted ischemic adnexa managed by detorsion. Fertil Steril 60,976-9.

Idiopathic sterility and intratubaric insemination

R. Agostini, D.R. Ambrosio, C. Ban, M.T. Filosofi and A. Quinzi

I Clinic of Obstetrics and Gynecology, University of Rome "La Sapienza", Rome, Italy

INTRODUCTION

In the last few years a large number of studies have been carried out on sterility due to "tubal factor" and new insemination techniques have suggested, if there are indications, important alternative methods to solve sterility. Our assumption was that disorders of the intramural trait of the salpinx can influence fecundation. The intramural trait of the salpinx has a muscular structure similar to a sphincter which does not represent an autonomous-independent morphologic and functional unity, but is very important for the coordination and transport of the fertilized ovum and the sperm. This structure is frequently characterized by a tortuous lumen with a 2 mm mean diameter and it is very sensitive to the action of different hormonal flows: oestrogens, prostaglandins, progesterone, adrenergic substances which influence its functional and contractile activity. In the past it was already noted that by resecting the uterus-tubal junction the number of spermatozoids augmented at ampullar level and cases of polyspermia were recorded. This was probably due to a selective mechanism acting on spermatozoids.

Starting from the above mentioned considerations we were able to carry out a technique which could allow us to deposit the prepared sperm beyond the tubal ostium in the salpinx. This technique is already used by means of hysteroscopy for intratubal deposition of gametes instead of GIFT. However, apart from the mechanical drawing of the oocyte and its transfer before or after fertilization (which implies a non operable ampullar tubal occlusion), we have always to consider that intratubal deposition of the seed is also indicated in cases of inexplained sterility, cervical mucus hostility or oligospermia. On the other hand the majority of authors agree that the higher the prepared spermatozoids are deposited, the greater is the number of pregnancies achieved. Intratubal insemination is useful in several conditions such as the surpassing of the tubal ostium if a functional pathology exists, the insemination of the only pervious tube, the insemination of homolateral tube in respect to the dominant ovarium. Similar results have been achieved both in Clomiphene or HMG + HCG stimulated cycles and in cases of cervical mucus hostility. If disorder of the tubal angle exists the guided cannulation of the salpinx by hysteroscopy is required, but this technique may be difficult also for experienced people and, in addition, it is troublesome for the patient and is not without risks. In normal cases selected by hysteroscopy, tubal cannulation can be performed also through echography-guided tactile sensation. Some authors have already expressed their favourable opinion on this aggressive technique which gives appreciable results. This technique requires an excellent personal experience and it is important that a preliminary hysterosalpingography reveals a non excessively tortuous lumen at isthmic level. It is necessary to be provided with: a sensitive echography apparatus, a good Teflon catheter guide about 28 cm long and with a 1.8 mm diameter, an obturator of malleable metal, a second flexible Teflon catheter about 33 cm long with a 1 mm diameter and tightening in the last 3 centimetres until it reaches a diameter of 0.66 mm. With the patient in the Trendelnburg position, through echography-scanning, after uterine horns are localized, the catheter is passed along the posterior wall of the uterus trying to put the apex near to the intramural trait of the salpinx. Through the tactile sensation the catheter is put forward and subsequently the internal catheter containing the gametes is pushed for about 3-4 cm up to the ampullar region. The homolateral pain that the patient feels when the internal catheter enters is a good indicator. In many cases the catheterization of the salpinx is not successful. In cases of inexplicable sterility the intratubal deposition of the seed by echography-guided tactile sensation has given 35% of pregnancies (Donna E. et al.). However this technique is not always successful and without risks such as salpingitis and empyema of Douglas, as pointed out by the authors. Moreover it is not indicated for the deposition of the fertilized oocyte. Khan A.J.(1992) has proposed the perfusion of capacitated spermatozoids in the salpinx in concomitance with the pharmacological super ovulation.

MATERIALS AND METHODS

We have studied 48 couples suffering from sterility. Of these 37 couples suffered from inexplicable sterility and 11 had a sterility due to insufficient cervical factor.

We came to these conclusions after undergoing couples to routine analyses which are carried out when sterility is diagnosed. The sampling and the following research were performed at the "Conjugal Sterility Centre" of the 1st Institute of Obstetrics and Gynaecology (University of Rome "La Sapienza") during 1993 and 1994. First of all we induced super ovulation with Clomiphene citrate and purified FSH. We administered

10.000 of LH at the given timing. The insemination was carried out after 34-36 hours from the injection of HCG. After pre-medication with 10 mg of Diazepam, 1 hour before the operation, the woman was put in the Trendelenburg position. The cervix uteri was accurately disinfected and washed with HAM F10. A double-thick Kremer probe with a very slight terminal end was put in the uterine cavity and the cervix uteri was closed with a pair of Ellis pincers the jaws of which were covered with rubber. Magendie pincers can also be used. We applied to the catheter a syringe with 4 cc of suspended spermatozoids treated with the swim-up method in use for FIVET. We injected the suspension at 1 cc per minute. The woman had to rest in bed for 1 hour. In order to avoid the oocyte drainage due to perfusion it was necessary that the administration of 10000 UI of HCG was well monitored so as to allow the insemination shortly before the bursting of the follicle.

RESULTS

The 48 sterile couples were treated with 116 cycles of intratubal spermatic perfusion. They were all suffering from inexplained sterility or from insufficient cervical factor. The partners' seminal fluids had normal qualitative and quantitative values.

We have eliminated 19 cycles because oestradiol blood levels were higher than 4000 pg/ml and echography showed more than 4 follicles. With these treatments 15 intrauterine pregnancies were obtained; 8 women aborted between the V and the VIII week of pregnancy; 13 women went on with their pregnancy and 6 women had given birth to healthy foetus. No ectopic pregnancies were recorded and there was one twin pregnancy.

Eight women became pregnant after the first cycle of treatment. About the half patients became pregnant after two cycles of treatment. In no case were complications or sepsis reported.

CONCLUSIONS

In conclusion, we think that in cases of transfer of oocytes or tubal angle pathology it is preferable to perform intratubal insemination under hysteroscopic control. On the other hand, in cases of inexplained sterility or insufficient cervical factor it is preferable to perform simpler and less aggressive techniques: intratubal insemination with echography-guided tactile sensation and tubal perfusion with capacitated sperm. These techniques (performed as we described) give favourable results.

It is very important that insemination is performed before the bursting of the follicle, otherwise the oocyte is drained out. However this technique gives better results than intrauterine insemination and intraperitoneal insemination. In our opinion, only after having performed at least three cycles of intratubal perfusion which are cheap and almost safe, we advise the sterile couple to follow other types of assisted fecundation.

REFERENCES

1- AGOSTINI R, CRISAFULLI M L, MAFFEI RM "Accorgimenti tecnici di microchirurgia nel reimpianto tubarico". Il Giornale di Chirurgia Vol VI N6, 606, 1985

2- ALLEN, N.C., HERBERT, C.M.,III, MAXSON, W.S., ROGERS, B.J., DIAMOND, M.P., WENTZ, A.C. (1985) Intrauterine insemination: a critical review. Fertil Steril., 44, 569-580.

3- BAUER O, VAN DER VEN H, DIEDRICH K, AL-HASANI S, KREBS D, GEMBRUCH U: Preliminary results on transvaginal tubal embryo stage transfer (TV-TEST) without ultrasound guidance. Hum Reprod 5:553, 1990.

4- BERGER GS: Intratubal insemination. Fertil Steril 48:328, 1987.

5- BYRD, W., ACKERMAN, G.E., CARR, B.R., EDMAN, C.D., GUZICK, D,S., McCONNELL, J.D. (1987) Treatment of refractory infertility by transcervical intrauterine insemination of washed spermatozoa. Fertil Steril., 48: 921-927.

6- COHEN, J. and de MOUZON, J. (1990) Outcome of IVF-pregnancies in Europe. Second Joint ESCO-ESHRE meeting, Milan. Hum Reprod. Suppl I. Abstr. 111.

7- COULAM, C.B.., MOORE, S.B., O' FALLON, W. (1988) Investigating unexplained infertility. Am. J. Obstet. Gynecol. 158, 1374-1381.

8- CROSIGNANI, PG, WALTERS, D.E. and SOLIANI, A. (1990) The ESHRE multi-centre trial on the treatment of unexplained infertility. Second Joint ESCO-ESHRE meeting, Milan. Hum Reprod. Supl I. Abstr. 51.

9- DONNA E. PRATT. ERIC BIEBER. RANDALL BARNES. " Transvaginal intratubal insemination by tactile sensation : a preliminary report. " Fertil. Steril. Vol. VI n° 5, 984, 1991.

10- HORVATH, P.M., BOHRER, M., SHELDEN, R.M., KEMMANN, E. (1989) The relationship of sperm parameters in superovulated women undergoing intrauterine insemination: Fertil Steril 52, 288-294.

11- JANSEN RPS, ANDERSON JC: Catheterization of the fallopian tube from the vagina. Lancet 2:309, 1987.

12- KHAN A. J. DURING V. SOUNDE A. MOLNE K. " Fallopian tube sperm perfusion used in a donor insemination programme. " "Human Reproduction. " Vol. 7, n° 6, 806, 1992.

13- LUCENA E, RUIZ JA, MENDOZA JC, ORTIZ JA, LUCENA C, GOMEZ M, ARANGO A: Vaginal intratubal insemination (VITI) and vaginal GIFT, endosonographic technique: early experience. Hum Reprod 4:658, 1989.

14- MEDICAL RESEARCH INTERNATIONAL and the SOCIETY for ASSISTED REPRODUCTIVE TECHONOLOGY: In vitro fertilization -embryo transfer in the United States: 1988 results from the IVF-ET Registry. Fertil Steril 53:13, 1990.

15- OVERSTREET, J.W., HANSON, F.W., BRAZIL, C., OBASAJU, M.F., WILEY L.M., CHANG, R:J. (1988) Antisperm antibodies in women receiving intrauterine insemination. Endocrine Fertility Forum 1, 2.

16- PATTON, P.E., BURRY, K.A., NOVY, M.J., WOLF, D.P. (1990). A comparative evaluation of intracervical and intrauterine routes in donor therapeutic insemination. Hum Reprod, 5: 263-265.

17- PUNJABI, U., GERRIS J., van BIJLEN, J., DELBEKE, L., GIELIS, M., BUYTAERT, Ph., (1990) Comparison between different pre-treatment tecnhiques for sperm recovery prior to intrauterine insemination, GIETor IVF. Hum. Reprod, 5, 75-83.

18- RISQUEZ F, BAYER P, ROLET F, MAGNANI M, GUICHARD A, CEDARD L, ZORN JR: Retrogade tubal transfer of human embryos. Hum Reprod 5:185, 1990.

19- SERHAL, P.F., KATZ, M., LITTLE, W., WORONOWSKI, H. (1988) Unexplained infertility-The value of Pergonal superovulation compined with intrauterine insemination. Fertil Steril., 49, 602-606.

20- SHELDEN, R., KEMMANN, E., BOHRER, M., PAQUALE, S (1988) Multiple gestation is associated with the use of high sperm numbers in the intrauterine insemination specimen in women undergoing gonadotropin stimulation. Fertil Steril., 49, 607-610.

21- SHER, G., KNUTZEN, V. K., STATTON, C.J., MONTAKHAB, M.M., ALLENSON, S.G. (1984) In vitro sperm capacitation and transcervical intrauterine insemination for treatment of refractory infertility. Phase 1, Fertil Steril., 4, 260-264.

22- SUNDE, A., KAHN, J.A. (1988) Intrauterine insemination with pretreated sperm. A collaborative report: Hum Reprod 3, Supl:2, 69-73.

Psychological and clinical aspects of assisted reproduction with donor semen

G. D'Ambrogio, P.G. Artini, A.A. de Micheroux, M. Tarabusi*, V. Cela, C. Parri, C. Battaglia* and A.R. Gennazzani

*Department of Obstetrics and Gynecology, University of Pisa, Pisa and *Department of Obstetrics and Gynecology, University of Modena, Modena, Italy*

Introduction

Long-standing infertility has a negative effect on psychological functioning, which results in emotional distress and sexual and marital problems (1-5). The main psychological problem facing infertile couples appears to be anxiety. Cook et al. (6) reported that in couples embarking upon infertility treatment, both men and women showed high levels of anxiety compared with the general population. Although anxiety was high, depression was not found to be a problem. Women show higher anxiety, depression, loss of self-esteem, feeling of guilt, neuroticism, social and sexual and marital problems than men. The meaning and emotional consequences of infertility may differ in some respects for women and men. For women an important reason for distress associated with infertility may be the lack of fulfilment of the central role of motherhood. Furthermore, research has demonstrated that many infertile men feel guilty because of their inability to give proof of their manhood and act as real fathers (7). One consequence of lack of fertility may be an associated loss of confidence in sexuality. Infertile individuals report that others commonly assume a sexual cause for infertilty, in particular, that men are sexually inadequate. The diagnosis of infertility blocks and immediately paralyzes a man's emotional life, it represents a strong attempt to the image of himself to the ideal of his ego. He falls a prey to the distress of being abandoned and refused by his partner. He falls barren and fallacious. He feels angry, depressed, inferior and lacks desire. How a men elaborates this wound of infertility, mourns the lack of his own biological son and faces the wishes, phantoms, plans of his partner, from the quality of reaction to inner, conjugal dialogue will emerge the most appropriate alternatives. Generally speaking, men mostly suggest the alternative of donor insemination to their female partners. They feel guilty because unable to let their partner reach pregnancy and delivery and regard these events as extremely important to a woman's achievement.

The aim of the present study was to evaluate the psychological aspects of infertile couples who underwent repeated failed cycles of donor insemination - intracervical (ICI) or intrauterine insemination (IUI) with donor semen, in order to address the couples, to psychological counselling and psychotherapy for the treatment of psychological disturbances related to infertility, and to gametes intrafallopian transfer (GIFT) as assisted reproduction technique procedure for the treatment of infertility.

Patients and methods

Patients.   The study was conducted with 32 couples, whose age ranged from 25 to 42 years old. The primary indications for heterologue insemination were azoospermia in 14 cases and severe oligoasthenozoospermia in 18 cases. Before the psychometric measures and the GIFT procedure took place, all the couples failed to conceive after 12 cycles of ICI or IUI with donor semen.

Assisted reproduction procedure. All female patients were verified to have patent tubes by hysterosalpingogram and diagnosed free from endocrine disorders. Ovarian stimulation was induced with gonadotropin-releasing hormone agonist, triptorelin i.m. (Decapeptyl 3,75 mg, Ipsen, Italy), long protocol, on the first day of the cycle, followed by the administration of follicle stimulating hormone 150 IU (Metrodin, Serono, Italy) from the 3rd day of the cycle until the day of human chorionic gonadotropin (hCG) administration. Follicular maturation was assessed by periodic vaginal ultrasound and serum estradiol concentration. When a number of two to five follicles reached a minimum preovulatory diameter of 16 millimeters and 17β-estradiol concetration exceeded 500 pg/ml, hCG 10,000 IU (Profasi, Serono, Italy) was injected. Oocyte retrieval was carried out 36 hours after hCG injection by means of transvaginal aspiration. Crossed match donor semen was prepared by swim-up and Percoll technique prior to the procedure. The GIFT procedure was carried out by laparoscopy. A catheter with a 1 ml syringe was used for laparoscopic transfer. The catheter was loaded with two to five oocytes and 300,000 to 500,000 motile spermatozoa in a total volume of $\leq$ 25 μl. Gamete were transferred to a position at least 3-4 cm into the fimbriated end of the tube. All the assisted technique procedure using donor semen were performed in a private clinic for infertility in observance of the Italian Law, as heterologue insemination procedure is not allowed in public health structure.

Psychometric measures.   The couple underwent, individually:

1) an individual structured interview concerning psychological items;

2) State Trait Anxiety Inventory in Y-1 and Y-2 form [8]. It is a self report questionnaire, comprising two different sets of twenty questions describing feelings of tension worry or apprehension. One set of questions deals with how the respondents feel at the time (state) and the other with how they generally feel (trait). Therefore, "state anxiety" is defined as the general tendency of an individual to be upset in stressful situations, or as the mean level of long-term anxiety; it is considered as a personality trait.

326

3) Westbrook Coping Scale [9]. It is a self-report scale for the evaluation of personal coping strategies to stress condition.

4) Questionnaire about the motivation leading to the choice of the partner [10].

The individual interview and the psychometric tests were administered after the failure of the 12 cycles of ICI and before the initiation of the GIFT procedure.

Results

After the first cycle of GIFT using donor semen, 22 couples had a starting pregnancy, with a pregnancy rate of 69%, and the remaining 10 couples failed to conceive.

As far as the psychological and psychosexual measures of the study are concerned, all the couples reported a worsening in sexual intercourse with variable loss of libido in all cases, anorgasmy (3 cases) and dispareunia (1 case) in women.

State anxiety was higher than trait anxiety in 13 couples (41%) and it was significantly correlated to the time from the diagnosis. State anxiety score higher than the average score of the Italian population was directly correlated to relative trait anxiety levels higher than the average. Individuals who had trait anxiety score higher than the average also showed higher state anxiety score. Both trait anxiety and state anxiety resulted significantly higher in women than in men. Individuals with higher score of trait and state anxiety more frequently showed a depressive adaptive coping style. Men showed more frequently than women an active coping style and, finally, men showing score of trait anxiety higher than the average, usually adopted coping depressive style in response to stressful situation.

Discussion

The stress response is not only caused by the aversive nature of the stressor, but especially by the ability of the organism to deal with the stressor. If an individual can cope successfully with the environmental challenge, little or no stress is experienced. Coping strategies rather than the nature of the stressor will determine whether or not stress is experienced by an individual [11]. Long-term infertility leads to depression in subjects with less effective coping mechanism. The major difficulty facing couples during infertility treatment is anxiety; couples whose treatment was unsuccessful instead risk depression. Therefore, anxiety is thought to be developing in response to a future threatening event such as stressful treatment or fear that treatment will fail, while depression result from loss, the loss of a potential child, in the case of infertile couples whose treatment was unsuccessful. The state anxiety stress response can be considered as the expression of the acute ineffectiveness of the used coping strategies. In the acute stress situation women with high depressive coping score also show high state anxiety levels. Therefore, a chronic ineffectiveness of coping with the infertility problem in general will result in an acute ineffectiveness of coping with the specific stress of the repeating procedures of assisted reproduction.

Coping mechanisms are believed to be essential in psychological functioning and are likely to affect psychological adjustment. The use of avoidance coping strategies has been associated with greater emotional distress in infertile couples than those using approach coping strategies such as seeking information about their treatment or making a plan of action (6, 12). It seems, therefore, that approach coping strategies are positively related to adaptation to infertility and in couples who have failed to conceive as a result of assisted reproduction. Coping mechanisms are used to reduce the harmful effects of stress which can be psychological or biological. The coping mechanisms themselves can also activate some dimensions of the stress response.

Subjects showing high levels of trait anxiety and state anxiety specifically related to a given stressful situation, generally react with a depressive coping style and low self-esteem, and particularly women use cognitive and emotional coping strategies involving social support seeking and approval in order to attenuate the psychological effects of the stressor, and not to remove the cause.

The hope of achievement is replaced by the bereavement of the loss of the imaginary son who was not born, leading to deep silence between the couple [13]. This stage is followed by a fase in which, having forgotten the wound, the couple undergoes other attempts with less emotional involvement and more sense of reality. The acceptance followed by a series of failure is a common attitude although the definite bereavement may give way to deep-saved sorrow in the soul and the life of the couple.

In recent years, there has been a move towards counselling for couples receiving infertility treatment, which raises the question of the form the counselling should take. There is no systematic research concerning the most effective form of counselling for infertile couples. In addition, little is known about the efficacy of different styles of counselling for these couples. As mentioned above, the most common problem for couples undergoing treatment is anxiety, which suggest that anxiety management training could be beneficial, in addition to more general counselling, such as the re-thinking of negative thought patterns [14]. Furthermore, helping couples to use approach coping strategies as opposed to avoidance strategies is likely to be helpful. Couples themselves should be stimulated to find some ways to confront and cope with their infertility. These include becoming mentally prepared by anticipating bad news at each stage of treatment, seeking information about treatment, seeking support from others and planning a course of action in order to increase their feelings of control [15].

GIFT is an assisted reproduction technique, characterized by higher risk, cost and invasiveness but, on the other hand it has much more higher efficacy than artificial insemination techniques, ICI or IUI [16]. Therefore, we suggest that GIFT could be used after 12 cycles of failed intracervical or intrauterine insemination in infertile couples with a stable psychological profile; in infertile couples with high anxiety levels (trait anxiety) and a high depressive coping style GIFT should be performed after a lower number (six or eight) or failed cycles of donor insemination.

References

1. Kraft A. D., Palumbo J., Mitchell D., Dean C., Meyers S., Wright-Schmidt A. The psychological dimension of infertility. *Am. J. Ortopsychiatry* 1980; 50: 618.

2. Drake T. S., Grunert M. A cycle pattern of sexual dysfunction in infertility investigations. *Fertil. Steril.* 1979; 32: 542.

3. Utian W. U., Goldfarb J. M., Rosenthal M. B. Psychological aspects of infertility. In: Dennerstein L. and Burrows G. D. (Eds.), Handbook of Psychosomatic Obstetrics and Gynecology. Elsevier Biomedical Press, Amsterdam, 1983, p. 199.

4. Menning B. E. The emotional needs of infertile couples. *Fertil. Steril.* 1980; 34: 313.

5. Seibel M. M., Taymor M. L. Emotional aspects of infertility. *Fertil. Steril.* 1982; 37: 137.

6. Cook R., Parson J., Mason J., Golombok S. Emotional, marital and sexual problems in couples embarking upon AID and IVF treatment for infertility. *J. Reprod. Infant. Psycol.* 1989; 7: 87.

7. David A., Avidan D. Artificial insemination by donor: clinical and psychological aspects. *Fertil. Steril.* 1976; 27: 528.

8. Spielberg C. D. State-Trait Anxiety Inventory: A comprehensive bibliography. Palo Alto, California, U.S.A., Consulting Psychologist Press, 1983.

9. Demyttenaere K. Psychoneuroendocrinological aspects of reproduction in women. Peeter Press, Louvain, 1990.

10. Pallanca G. F., Baldaro Verde J., Carrer F. Il sintomo sessuale e la sua evoluzione in rapporto alla scelta del partner ed alla risposta alla frustrazione in una situazione di ricerca-intervento. *Sessuologia* 1982; 6: 419.

11. Vogel W. H. Coping, stress, stressors and health consequences. *Neuropsychobiology* 1985; 13: 129.

12. Stanton A.L., Tenne H., Affleck G., Mendola R. Coping and adjustment to infertility. *J. Soc. Clin. Psychol.* 1992; 11:1.

13. Baram D., Tourtelot E., Muechler E., Huang K. E. Psychosocial adjustment following unsuccessful in vitro fertilization. *J. Psychosom. Obstet. Gynecol.* 1988; 9: 181.

14. Callan V. J. and Hennessey J. F. Strategies for coping with infertility. *Br. J. Med. Psychol.* 1989; 62: 343.

15. Golombok S. Psychological functioning in infertility patients. *Hum. Reprod.* 1992; 7: 208.

16. Kovacs G. T., King C. The use of gamete intra-fallopian transfer with donor spermatozoa after failed donor insemination. *Hum. Reprod.* 1994; 9: 859.

Psychological counselling in the infertile couple

P. Pezzella and L. Cersosimo

A GI CO Associazione Ginecologi Consultoriali, Rome, Italy

INTRODUCTION

It is showed that during the long period of infertility
management, emotional and psychological factors play an
important role and influence the course and results of
treatment.
The psychological counseling is an important moment in
diagnosis and treatment of the infertile couple.
Medical research on sterility has demonstrated a
relation between organic and psychological aspects and
unproductiveness. Recent studies in psychological field
have attributed some situations of infertility to psychological problems. But also when is an organic
disease, the consequences of the infertility on the
psychological life are many.
Besides the psychological disorder is qualitatively
different according to infertile cause. For this reason
the clinical acticity suggest medical and psychological
intervention to infertile couple.
In this paper, the following aspects will be discussed:
the infertility investigation, male psychological
infertility, female psychological infertility, the psychologist role in equipe.

THE INFERTILITY INVESTIGATION

The clinical tests of an infertile couple includes very
medical procedures (sperm analysis, postcoital test,
laparascopy, hysterosalpingografy, basal body temperature), but at the same time, it must be kept in mind

the psychological and emotional aspect of man and woman.
When the technical approaches reports that there are
not organic to conception, it need find the cause of
problem in psychological aspects.
In cases of unexplained infertility there are psychological conflicts: therefore it is extremely important to
evalue the factors following:
1) global personality structure
2) psyco-dinamic of the affective life and of the relationship of couple.
3) motivation and ambition to maternity or paternity
4) socio-cultural attributed to maternity or pathernity
5) presence of conflicts or of pathologies of the psyche

MALE PSYCHOLOGICAL INFERTILITY

The psychological causes of infertility in male partner
are the following:

1) sexual impotence connectd to psychological pathology
of the erection or to psychological disorders of the
ejaculation
2) conflicts with the partner as the "white marriage"
3) psychopathologies

These emotional aspects discussed have consequences on
the fertility playing an important part.

FEMALE PSYCHOLOGICAL INFERTILITY

The psychological causes of infertility in the female
partner are the following:

1) negative experienced about sexual intercourse
2) inibition of the sexual drive
3) unconscious fear of to dead during the childbirth
4) dissatisfaction against to partner
5) sexual life and attitude to the passiveness
6) sexual life and absence of tenderness

These psychological problems alter the physiological
processes that the will lead to a pregnancy.

ROLE OF PSYCHOLOGIST IN INFERTILE COUPLE

It should be kept in mind that, in our culture, fertility, masculinity, and potency are often related; and
it is wellknow the traditional relation between
sexuality and reproduction.

The infertile woman to have feelings of failure and uselessness.

The coscience of being infertile arouses refusal, anger, depression in the partners. The unproductiveness is seen as an invalid condition. The infertile couple seems oppresed by a sense of guilt and feels ashamed for its own infertility.

Psychological intervention is necessary to sustain the couple during the treatment needed to achieve a pregnancy.

The psychological counseling is characterized as an "helping relation" which promotes in the couple the management of its own problems.

CONCLUSIONS

Concerning infertility we have made some interesting observations.

The investigation, the diagnostic tests, and the long treatment of infertility cause great stress in the couple. Therefore it is important to help the couple's partners for to make a good relantionship, that they could discuss problems and fantasies about their condition. Besides the couple will be encouraged to accept the sexuality without procreation.

Often the sexual life of the couple decline instead it is very important that the sexual activity and sexual pleasure remains.

For these reasons the medical and psychosexual approach is the best for the management of infertile couple.

REFERENCES

-Berrazon N. et al.: "Stress, sexual satisfaction and marital adjustment in infertile couples.
J Sex Marital Ther 1992 winter; 18 (4): 273-84
- Fenelli A., Lorenzini R.: Clinica delle disfunzioni sessuali. Roma, NIS, 1991
- Gilmore D.: La genesi del maschile. Modelli culturali della virilita'. Firenze, La nuova Italia, 1993
- Havelock E.: Psicologia della maternita'. Roma Newton-Compton, 1971
- Jones H.W. et al.: "The infertile couple"
N Engl J Med 1993 Dec; ", 239 (23): 1710-5
- Moynihan C.: "A history of couselling"
J R Soc Med 1993 Jul; 86 (7): 421-3
-Rosenthal M.B.: "Infertility;psychotherapeutic issues"
New Dir Ment Healt Serv 1992; (55): 61-71

Recurrent spontaneous abortion: epidemiology and prospective management

V. Trojano, R. Alfonso and N. Veloce

Università degli Studi di Bari, Clinica Ostetrica Ginecologica Iª, Policlinico, Bari, Italy

SUMMARY

The authors have reported the results of a study on 2100 patients who experienced recurrent spontaneous abortion.
This study occurred at the Gynaecological and Obstetrician Clinic of Bari University between January 1991 to December 1994. From accurate examination of the various etiological causes (metabolic disorders, infectious, endocrine disorders, immunologic, cytogenetic, disformation, environment and psychogenic) results demostrated abortions that's occurred "sine causa" are still present in a reasonably high rate of causes (24%) and that only detailed studies with the understanding of therapeutic protocol is one able to reduce that type of pathology.

INTRODUCTION

Recurrent spontaneous abortion is defined when a spontaneous abortion occurs after at least two consecutive pregnancies outcome in spontaneous abortion without next sons birth alive. Actually to calculate the relative incidence of this pathology is very difficult. In fact the rates of recurrent spontaneous abortion reported in medical literature varies considerably. During the period of this study by Obstetrician Clinics of "USL BA/9" in Bari recorded an increase of 7.1%. This rate was processed by the national statistics office (ISTAT). It is

Table 1   Rate of abortive risk in patients with a history of
spontaneous abortion

| Authors | AFTER | | |
	I abortion	II abortion	III abortion
MALPAS	22%	38%	73%
EASTMAN	13%	37%	84%
WARTBURTON e FRASEN	24%	26%	32%

important to emphasize that the risk of spontaneous abortion
increases when there has been a history of abortion in the
patient (Table 1). In order of importance the risk factors are:
- age (< 19 years > 35 years);
- exposure of specific species of pathogenic noxae in the
  working environment;
- period of gestation (up until the 12th week).
In the last fifteen years, 2100 women with this pathology by the
Puglia region were selected for this multicentric study. The
frequency of recurrent spontaneous abortion in respect to
various other diagnostic etiological noxae would be reported in
a description of single etiological factors.

METABOLIC CAUSES (18.33%)

The patohology of glycogen metabolism is seen like a metabolic
disorder of glycogen as the direct action of insulin on the
placental receptors (1) which regulate the transport of amino
acids and glucose at this level.

ENDOCRINAL CAUSES (3,5%)

-- Alteration of prolactin hormonal dosages;
- Insufficient levels of luteinic hormones at the commencement
  and end of the ovarian cycle;
- The pathology of corticoadrenal functionality agrreing that
  ipo like iper;
- Endocrinal   alterations   of   autoimmunologic   etiology
  (thyroiditis of Hashimoto). (2)

INFECTIOUS CAUSES (6,2%)

- Mycoplasma Hominis and Ureaplasma Urealithicum have the capacity to colonise the endometrium and to determine chomosomic aberrations;
- This microorganism have been isolated cervical secretions of patients studied with an abortion related fever in foetal tissue, in ejaculation and in prostatic secretions;
- Chlamydia Trachomatis appear to play an important role which leads to sterilization and infertility causing a specific endometritis. (3)

IMMUNOLOGIC CAUSES (6,1%)

There are several theories which explain the etiology of these causes:
- a diminishing of the maternal immobilising antibodies; (4,10)
- a production of the antiembryon and antiplacenta autoantibodies; (5)
- a maternal desensitization by this types of antibodies which could be achieved with intradermal injection of X-irradiated (50 gy) paternal mononuclear cells; (4)
- the presence of immunoglobulins M and G inhibiting the coagulation nominated LAC (Lupus anti-coagulant).
Patients with levels of LAC present a tendency to develop characteristic thombotic fits associated with RSA due to small occlusions occurring in the utero-placental and/or in the foetal-placental flow. (6,7,8)

CYTOGENETIC CAUSES (10,3%)

The balanced translocations appear to be mainly involved in this type of etiology, but also minor chomosomic anomalies and genetic mutations appear to have a casual role in this etiology. (5,9)

"MULLERIAN" CAUSES (21,4%)

Due to these congenital anomalies or those acquired by the ovular chamber, or like cervico isthmical anomalies dysfunctions of traumatic, constitutional and dysfunctional types. (5,9)

ENVIRONMENTAL CAUSES (7,6%)

Intoxication of lead and mercury chronic, of organic solvents (benzene, toluol, etc) and anaesthetic gases (9,11).

Table 2   Etiologycal factors determined and related rate in the
          patients examined with a history of R.S.A. Patients
          cured and related rate for each etiologycal factor

Etiologycal factors	CASES			
	Selected	(%)	Cured	(%)
METABOLIC	385	(18.33)	245	(63.6)
ENDOCRINAL	74	(3.50)	48	(64.9)
INFECTIOUS	130	(6.20)	47	(36.2)
IMMUNOLOGIC	128	(6.10)	–	
CYTOGENETIC	216	(10.20)	–	
MULLERIAN	450	(21.40)	293	(63.2)
ENVIRONMENTAL	160	(7.60)	–	
PSYCHOGENIC	65	(3.1)	18	(26.6)
"SINE CAUSA"	492	(23.57)	267	(54.3)
	2100	(100)	918	(43.7)

PSYCHOGENIC CAUSES (3,1%)

The research by Roscharch test, three types of women were
isolated:
- immature women who are dependent and who tend to repress their
  emotions;
- active women, dynamic and independent who reject their female
  role and display a pronounced competitiveness with males;
- women with important Oedipus complex not yet resolved from
  their infancy. All of these women mentioned during
  psycho-therapeutic sessions that their spontaneous abortion
  gave their a "sense of freedom" (12).

CONCLUSION

The multifactorial pathogenesis of the RSA often makes it
difficult to determine the causes and therefore it becomes
difficult to find a specific therapy.
The present study allowed the researchers to individualise in a
lot of patients the etiological causes of their pathology with
the possibility to establish a specific therapeutic treatment.
The achieved results (Tab. 2) were encouraging even though about
24% of abortions remained "sine causa".
From all of this information it is necessary to coordinate
scientific research with clinical practice, programming
multicentric studies which can promote a diagnostic and
therapeutic univocal approach and always more valid in the
resolution of this pathology.

REFERENCES

1. Coluccia. E., Altavilla. A., Restaino. A., Causio. F., Battarino.O. (1984). Aborto ripetivo e dismetabolismo glicidico. La nuova stampa medica italiana. 4, n.2, 77

2. Lattanzi. V., Ciampolillo. A., Vincenti. C., Salluzzi. G., Giorgino. R. (1984). Studio della funzione tiroidea nell'aborto ripetitivo. LXIII Congr. Naz. Soc. Ital. Ginecol. e Ostet. Arch. Atti, 687. Milano

3. Witkin and Leolger. (1992). Antibodies to Chlamydia Trachomatis in sera of women with recurrent spontaneous abortions. Am. J. Obstet.Ginecol.,167, n.1, 135-138

4. Koji Aoki et al. (1993) Clinical evaluation of immunotherapy in early pregnancy with X-irradiated paternal mononuclear cells for primary recurrent aborter. Am. J. Obstet. Gynecol., 3, 649-652

5. Plouffe et al. (1992). Etiologic factors of recurrent abortion and subsequent reproductive performance of couples: have we made any progress in the past 10 years?. Am.J.Obstet.Gynecol., 167, n.2, 313-319

6. Carreras, L.O., Defreyn, G., Machin, S.J. et al. (1981). Arterial trombosis, intrauterine death and "Lupus anticoagulant":detection of immunoglobulin interfering with prostacyclin formation. Lancet, 244

7. De Mitrio. V., Loiacono. R., Lomuscio. S., Cagnazzo. G. (1987). Ricerca del "Lupus Anticoagulant" nell'aborto abituale e/o morte fetale intrauterina: un utile test di screening per la sua evidenziazione: Comun. Semin. Inver. Aggiorn. in Gineco. e Ostet. Arch. Atti, 245. Madonna di Campiglio

8. Laurentaci, G. (1990). Aspetti immunologici della riproduzione. Bari

9. Candiani, G.B. (1990). Aborto spontaneo ricorrente (A.S.R.): patogenesi multifattoriale. Atti Simp. Inter. "Protocolli diagnostici e teraspeutici in Ost. e Ginec. Bari

10. Coulam. (1992). Immunologic tests in the evaluation of reproductive disorder: a critical review. Am. J. Obstet. Ginecol., 167, n.6, 1844-1850

11. Candiani. G.B. et al. (1980). Ann. Ost. Gin. Med. Pern. Vol. CI, n. 5. Aborto Abituale

12. Tanburro. G.A., De Donatis. T., Pasqual Marsettin. E., Tota. A. (1984). Psicodinamica dell'aborto ripetitivo. LXIII Congr. Naz. Soc. Ital. Ginecol. e Ostet. Arch. Atti, 245. Milano.

Antiphospholipid syndrome and spontaneous recurrent abortion

V. Benedetto, J. Leonardi, R. D'Anna, G. Zona, F.V. Ardita, A. Mancuso and R. Leonardi

Department of Gynecology, University of Messina, Italy

INTRODUCTION

In "Spontaneous Recurrent Abortion" (SRA), pregnancy loss can be the only symptom of autoimmune disease, but not rarely it is associated with systemic eritematosus lupus and sclerodermia.

In some of these patients pregnancy loss can be associated with the presence of antiphospholipid antibodies as lupus anticoagulant (LAC) and anticardiolipin antibodies (ACA), that are responsible of thrombofilia and probably placental tronbosis and necrosis. (1, 2, 3, 6)

MATERIALS AND METHODS

In our outpatients clinic for immunologic infertility 150 women with SRA have been referred from January 1992 to November 1994, and 107 (71,33%) of them have completed the diagnostic protocol; 85 (56,66%) of 107 patients have primary SRA, 22 (14,66%) have secondary SRA. (2, 4, 5) (Tab. I)

12 (14,10%) of 85 patients with primary SRA have had two recurrent pregnancy losses, 52 (61,17%) three recurrent pregnancy losses and 21 (24,70%) four or more pregnancy losses. (Tab. II)

15 of 22 patients with secondary SRA have had two abortions after a normal delivery at term and 7 have had 3 recurrent abortions after a normal delivery at term. (Tab. III)

All the 107 patients received from the day after the first BhCG positive test onward 1-1,6 mg/kg/die of aspirine (85 - 100 mg/die) and 15-25 mg/die of prednisolone. (7, 8, 9, 10) (Tab. IV)

The patients continued the treatment until the end of pregnancy.

RESULTS

The study of the two groups, primary and secondary SRA, have given favoureble results.

In the group of women with primary SRA we had 36 (42,35%) pregnancies in all, 7 (19,44%) in women with two recurrent pregnancy losses, 23 (63,88%) in women with three pregnancy losses and 6 (16,66%) in women with four or more pregnancy losses. (11) (Tab. V)

On 36 pregnant patients with primary SRA, 16 brought the delivery at term with alive infants, 7 had a pre-term delivery with one fetal death due to a considerably premature birth 4

Tab. I: **TOTAL PATIENTS**

selected patients	107	71,33%
primary SRA	85	56,66%
secondary SRA	22	14,66%

Tab. II: **PRIMARY SRA**

2 pregnancy losses	12	14,11%
3 pregnancy losses	52	61,17%
4 pregnancy losses	21	24,70%

Tab. III: **SECONDARY SRA**

2 pregnancy losses	15	68,20%
3 pregnancy losses	7	31,80%

Tab. IV: **THERAPY**

aspirine	65 - 100 mg / die
prednisolone	15 - 25 mg / die
gamma - globulin	400 mg / kg/ die

Tab. V: **36 TOTAL PREGNANCIES - PRIMARY SRA 42,35 %**

2	pregnancy	losses 7	19,44%
3	pregnancy	losses 23	63,88%
4	pregnancy	losses 6	16,66%

Tab. VI: **RESULTS OF 36 PREGNANCIES WITH PRIMARY SRA**

at - term	16	44,44%
pre - term	7	19,44%
miscarriages	4	11,11%
on going	9	25,00%

Tab. VII: **RESULTS OF 22 PREGNANCIES WITH SECONDARY SRA**

at - term	4	18,18%
pre - term	3	13,63%
miscarriages	3	13,63%
on goimg	2	9,03%

Tab. VIII: **5 PATIENTS TRESIATED WITH GAMMA - GLOBULIN**

at - term	3	60%
on going	2	40%

had spontaneous miscarriages during the first 18 weeks of gestation and 9 pregnancies are still going on, 5 of these already at their third trimester of gestation. (Tab. VI)

12 of 22patients with secondary SRA had treated pregnancies: 4delivered at term, 3 had preterm delivery with 2 alive infants, 3 had spontaneous miscarriages during the first 18 weeks of gestation and 2 pregnancies are still going on, one of these two is already at the third trimester of gestation. (Tab. VII)

We considered a therapeutic failure the seven miscarriages occurred in pregnancies; we have treated successive pregnancies in these women with i.v. G-globulin. (12, 13)

The treatment protocol includes two i.v. infusion of 400 mg/kg/die G-globulin as soon as possible after the first positive b.hCG test and successive one intravenous infusion every 21-28 days until the 34° th week of pregnancy. (Tab. III)

The results obtained giving the patients IgG e.v., were of 5 pregnancies, 3 of these had delivery at term, 2 are still going on, and no pre-term delivery or miscarriage. (Tab. VIII)

The data of our study on patients who had recurrent abortions with immunological pathogenesis seemed interestimg to us even in the absence of a control group.

All infants born during our study were free of congenital defects and treatment did not produce adverse effects on mothers or infants.

REFERENCES

1 Tho S.P.T., McDonough P.G. (1987). Recurrent pregnancy loss. In "Ginecology. Principles and practies", Z.rosenwarks, F.Benjamin, M.L.Stone (Eds) McMillan, New York, pag. 262
2 Scott R.J., Rote N.S., Bronch W. (1987). Immunologic aspects of recurrent abortion and fetal death. Obstet. Gynecol, 70: 645 - 656.
3 Mowbray J.F., Underwood J.L.E. (1985). Immunology of abortion. Cli. exp. Immunol. 60: 1-7.
4 McIntyre J.A., McConnachie P.R., Taylor C.G. (1984). Clinical immunologic and genetic definitions of primary and secondary recurrent spontaneous abortions. Fertil. Steril. 42: 849 - 855
5 Coulam C.B., McIntyre J.A., Faulk W.P. (1986). Reproductive performance in women with repeated pregnancy lossed and multiple partners. Am Reprod Immunol Microbiol. 12: 10.
6 Branch W., Scott J.R., Kocheour N.H. (1985). Obstetrics complications associated with lupus anticoagulant. N. Engl. J. Med. 313: 1322 - 26.
7 Scott J.R., Rote N.S., Branch D.W. (1988). Immunological aspects of recurrent abortions and fetal death. Obstet. Gynecol. 70: 645.
8 Branch W., Silver R.Blackwell J. (1992). Outcome of treated pregnancies in women with antiphospholipid syndrome: an update of the Utah experience. Obstet. Gynecol. 80: 614
9 Cowchock S., Reece A., Balaban D. (1992). Repeted fetal losses associated with antiphospholipid antibodies: a collaborative randomized trial prednisone with low - dose heparin treatment. Am. J. Obstet. Gynecol. 166: 1318.
10 Kwak J.Y.H., Gilman - Sachs A., Beaman K.D. (1992). Reproductive out-come in women with recurrent abortion of alloimmune and autoimmune causes: preconception versus postconception treatment. Am. J. Obstet. Gynecol. 166: 1787.
11 Scott J.R., Rote N.S., Branch D.W. (1988). Immunological aspects of recurrent abortion and fetal death. Obstet. Gynecol. 70: 645.
12 Sacher R.A.,King J.C. (1988). Intravunes Gamma-Globulin in pregnancy. Obstet. Gynecol. Survey. 44: 25-34.
13 Cittadini C.,Montemagno U., Pardi G., Perino A., et al. (1991). Procol for the diagnostic and therapeutic management of recurrent alloimmune abortion. ACTAEuropea fertilitatis. 22: 267-274.

Intrauterine auto-erotic movements: preparation to coping mechanisms – a case report

C. Battaglia, P.G. Artini*, M. Salvatori, M.R. Sgherzi, P. Traversi** and A. Volpe

Università degli Studi di Modena, Istituto di Fisiopatologia della Riproduzione Umana, Modena, *Università degli Studi di Pisa, Clinica Ostetrica e Ginecologica, Pisa and **Ospedale Dalmati, Sant'Angelo Lodigiano (MI), Italy

INTRODUCTION

Ultrasonographic determination of fetal gender is quite accurate from 20 gestational weeks on. Attempts to document fetal sex serve numerous important purposes. Careful analysis of the fetal perineum may detect: ambigous genitalia (1); cases with discrepant ultrasonographic and chromosomal data regarding fetal gender (testicular feminization) (2); documentation of different sex in twin pregnancies (dizygoticity). Furthermore, among fetuses at risk for X-linked pathologies, identification of a female fetus excludes the possible incidence of the disorder. For these reasons and for the parents' desire to know the fetal sex, the sonologist should assess the fetal gender during the prenatal ultrasonographic evaluations (3).

In the present report we illustrate a case of fetal "masturbation" (4) serendipitously observed during a routine fetal ultrasound scan at 29 gestational weeks.

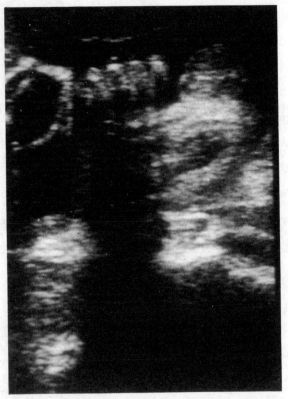

Figure 1: Axial oblique section through low fetal pelvis. The fetus is grasping his erected penis.

Case report.

A 26 years-old, gravida 1, para 0, after the first and second trimester scan which revealed a pregnancy consistent with amenorrhea and with no visible fetal malformations, presented for the third routine fetal ultrasound scan at 29 gestational weeks. The fetal examination was performed in a quite room with the patient in a semirecumbent position with a 15° tilt to the left side, by using 3.5 MHz linear transducer (Ansaldo AU 540. Genova, Italy). At an axial oblique section through low pelvis we evidenced a fetus grasping his erected penis (Fig.1) miming masturbation movements.

These movements were repetitive and lasted 8 minutes later. Afterwards the penis remained in erection for other 3 min. Gross fetal movements were observed. During the examination period an axial scan lightly caudad to the one commonly used for the determination of the biparietal diameter revealed both orbits. The observation of fetal lens showed intermittent synchronous eye movements (IEM activity). The fetal biometry corresponded to the gestational age. One week later, at a follow-up sonogram, after maternal informed consent, the penile activity was observed for two hours. While scanning the penis became erect and remained in that posistion for 7 min. No "masturbation" was observed. Rapid and synchronous eyes movements (REM activity) (5) associated to few gross fetal body movements were observed during the erection. The penis "detumescens" was associated to micturition and bladder reduction in lumen size. At 40 completed weeks a normal 3470 grs male infant was born by spontaneous vaginal delivery. The Apgar score was 10 at 1 and 5 min interval. Postnatal penile activity was not evaluated.

Discussion

In the present report we showed a case of fetal "masturbation" serendipitously observed. These intrauterine "auto-erotics" movements were done during a fetal waking state as confirmed by IEM. Furthermore, at a follow-up ultrasonography scan, an intrauterine penile erection not associated to masturbation activity was evidenced during a phase of active sleep.

Fetal movements emerge early during the first trimester of pregnancy and from their beginning onwards are specific, well recognizable by ultrasounds, and closely resemble those observed after birth (6,7). In fetal development, several basic types of reflexes can be elicited: avoiding and/or protective, feeding, grasping, genital and simulated respiratory. During the first 12 weeks of gestation, only the simplest components of these basic reflexes can be obtained and these appear in a very stereotyped manner. With advancing development, they become more varied and complex. The functional development of the reflexes is closely correlated with the morphological development and differentiation of the nervous system. Exteroceptive and proprioceptive sensory receptors are probably the first to become functional. Accordingly, reflex responses to stimulation around the mouth occur first. These are later followed by responses to genito-anal and, ultimately, to palmar-plantar stimulation. Motor fibers and effectors are the final components of the reflex arc to become functional. However, muscle contraction may be elicited by direct tactile stimulation even before the reflex arc is completed (8). Motor behaviour is the first language and expresses the answer to pain, fright and pleasure.

We speculated that in the studied case, the fetus after a penile erection, probably while a phase of active sleep, waked up, occasionally elicited a palmar reflex, and grasped his penis. Afterwards "masturbation" started.

It is impossible to evaluate the fetal consciousness of the act. Several behavioural forms imply cortical function during fetal life. Various cognitive, coordinative and associative capabilities in response to visual and/or auditory stimuli are an expression of fetal cortical function. In 1920 Freud wrote that "...Eros operates from the beginning of life and appears as a life instict in opposition to the death instinct". Few years later Ferenczi assumed that exists pleasure in intrauterine life to which all individuals want to return throughout their life. Furthermore, other authors successively hypothesized a prenatal libidinal phase of development which implies psychic activity. Otherwise, the research of pleasure, during the fetal life, would be a primordial preparation to ultilize the "transitional object". In other words it would be considered an attempt of the fetus to estinguish some emotionally unpleasant experiences. Furthermore, this fetal consoling capability would be considered the precursor of the subsequent "Ego strength", or the precursor of the ability to tolerate the anxiety during the adult life.

For a refined clinical interpretation further and extensive researches are necessary to verify the correlation between pleasure/distress signals and fetal motor language.

REFERENCES

1. Cooper C, Mahony BS, Bowie JD. Prenatal ultrasound diagnosis of ambigous genitalia. J Ultrasound Med 4:433, 1985.

2. Stephens JD. Prenatal diagnosis of testicular feminisation. Lancet 2:1038, 1984.

3. Bronshtein M, Rottem S, Yoffe N, et al. Early determination of fetal sex using transvaginal sonography: technique and pitfalls. JCU 18:302, 1990.

4. Meizner I. Sonographic observation of in utero fetal "masturbation". J Ultrasound Med 6:111, 1987.

5. Arduini D, Rizzo G, Giorlandino C, et al. The development of fetal behavioural states: a longitudinal study. Prenat Diagn 6:117, 1986.

6. Visser GHA, Prechtl HFR. Movements and behavioural states in the human fetus. In : Fetal and neonatal development. Jones CT,ed. Perinatology Press (Ithaca,NY). p581, 1988.

7. Roodenburg PJ, Wladimiroff JW, van Es A, Prechtl HFR. Classification and quantitative aspects of fetal movements during the second half of normal pregnancy. Early Hum Dev 25:19, 1991.

8. de Vries JIP, Visser GHA, Prechtl HFR. The emergence of fetal behaviour I. Qualitative aspects. Early Hum Dev 7:301, 1982.

Chronic anovulation: therapeutical strategies and clinical results

A.M. Mattei, P. Monti, B. Bocconcello, M. Serrani, V. Liprandi and P. Capetta

V Department of Obstetrics and Gynecology, University of Milan, Milan, Italy

Chronic anovulation seems to be the main cause for infertility in 25-30 % of women in fertile age. Hyperprolactinemia is frequently (15-20%) found to be the primary reason for anovulatory infertility but the chronic use of short or long-acting dopaminergic compounds has been demonstrated to be effective not only in normalizing serum prolactine levels, but also in restoring regular, ovulatory menses in the great majority of the patients (70-85%) [1, 2, 3].

The use of GnRH agonists (GnRH-a) as adjuncts to ovulation is now common. In patients with hypothalamic-hypogonadism the use of GnRH pulsatile infusion represents the choice treatment, with ovulatory rate more than 85% and pregnancy rate average 65% [4]. Particular considerations have to be discussed when polycistic ovarian syndrome is concerned [5].

In this particular clinical condition even therapy with antiestrogens or very small amounts of HMG may induce multiple and unorganized follicular growth, rising up to the various degrees of ovarian hyperstimulation syndrome [6].

In these last years some authors started using a pre-treatment with GnRH analogs before starting the treatment with HMG or pulsatile GnRH.

These analogues are used in a variety of protocols as a means of enhancing the number and/or quality of follicles that can be stimulated, decreasing of premature luteinization rates, decreasing cancellation rates, eventually improving pregnancy rates [7].

Treatment with a gonadotropin-releasing hormone-agonist (GnRH) has been shown to create a hypogonadotropic hypogonadism condition with normalization of androstenedione and testosterone levels in Policistic Ovarian Syndrome (PCOs) [8].

Aim of our study is to refer our experience in the management of chronic anovulation comparing the results obtained in the treatment with HMG or pulsatile GnRH with or without pretreatment with Analogs.

MATERIALS AND METHODS

The study population consisted of 37 subjects with PCOs, 21 to 45 years aged (mean: 31.22), affected by I or II infertility who met all the following criteria:

- history of oligomenorrhea or amenorrhea since menarche;
- hirsutism (defined as Ferriman-Galwey score > 10);
- ovarian volume normal or greater with multiple subcortical follicles < 7mm (more than 10 follicles each);
- normal PRL, TSH, 17 hidroxyprogesterone and DHEA-S concentrations;
- documented tubal patency on hysterosalpingogram or direct visualization by laparoscopy;
- normal semen analysis from the sexual partner.

No subject was on any other therapy at the time of the study.

The Body Mass Index ranged from 16.7 to 33 Kg/m^2 (mean: 23).

Twenty-one patients were assigned to receive a pre-treatment period (2-4 months) with a single monthly injection of 3.75 mg of triptoreline, followed either by HMG / purified FSH or pulsatile GnRH infusion.

The 2nd group of patients -16 subjects- began the above mentioned ovulation induction without the pretreatment with GnRH agonists.

The stimulation either with gonadotropins and with pulsatile GnRH started in the 1st group on 45th day of the last triptoreline injection, while in the 2nd group on the 4th day after the onset of a spontaneous bleeding or -in patients with amenorrhea or oligomenorrhea- of the bleeding induced by 100 mg medroxyprogesterone intramuscolarly.

Gonadotropins were hMG (Pergonal; Serono, Rome, Italy) or purified human urinary FSH (Metrodin; Serono). They were given intramuscolarly and the dosage was adjusted individually according to the response as judged by the growth of the follicles as measured by ultrasonography.

The starting dose was 75 IU for the first days -because of the known risk of hyperstimulation in PCOs- the maximum daily dose was 150 IU, the dosage was then mantained until the leading follicle measured > 18 mm in diameter. Then the patient was given an intramuscolar injection of hCG (Profasi; Serono, 5000 IU)

Patients stimulated with pulsatile GnRH (Lutrelef Ferring Valeas - Milano) with micro-infusion pump (Zyclomat Ferring) at a dosage of 5-20 mcg i.v.

and a frequency of 60-90 minutes underwent a vaginal ecography every 48-72 hours starting on day 5th while urinary stick to detect LH surge were performed by the patient herself at home and referred to the clinical staff.

The study population has been allocated according to the below schedule:

A] HMG or purified FSH (*11 subjects*).

B] Pulsatile GnRH infusion (*5 subjects*).

C] HMG or purified FSH starting on 45th day of a 2-4 months pre-treatment period with single monthly injections of 3,75 mg of triptoreline (*7 subjects*).

D] Pulsatile GnRH infusion after GnRH agonist chronic pre-treatment as above illustrated (*16 subjects*).

Hormones analyses:
Serum PRL, LH, FSH and Progesterone concentrations were determined by RIA and IRMA methods.
In the first method commercial kits by Serono have been used and the interassay and intra-assay coefficients of variation (CV%) of PRL, LH, FSH and Progesterone were respectively: PRL = 3,1-2,7; LH = 4,3-4,9; FSH = 9,5-3,4; Prog=10-5. The sensitivity of the RIA dosages were respectively: PRL=1 ng/ml; LH=1,5 mIU/ml; FSH=1,5 mIU/ml; Prog=0,1 ng/ml.
In the IRMA method Maia-clone kits by Ares-Serono have been used, and the interassay and intra-assay coefficients of variation were respectively: PRL = 5.5-1,4; LH = 4,3-1,9; FSH = 2-1,2; Prog = 5,7-6,9. The sensitivity of the IRMA dosages were respectively: PRL = 0,30 ng/ml; LH = 0,30 mIU/ml; FSH = 0,27 mIU/ml; Prog = 0,08 ng/ml.

RESULTS

The results obtained in terms of ovulations' and pregnancies' rates are shown in the below table.
Six out of 11 patients (54 %) who were administered with HMG or purified FSH ovulated and 1 (9 %) conceived, while 4 out of 5 subjects (80 %) treated with pulsatile GnRH ovulated but no pregnancy was obtained. One subject administered with GnRH infusion and two patients treated with gonadotropins stopped the therapy because of cystic involutions.
In the "pre-treatment arm" 6 out of 7 women (85 %) treated with gonadotropins ovulated and 2 of them (29 %) conceived, as well as 9 out of 16 patients (56 %) administered with pulsatile GnRH ovulated and 5

pregnancies (31 %) were obtained. Two patients infused with pulsatile GnRH had to stop the treatment because of cystic involutions.

	Pre-treated gonadotropins	Pre-treated pulsatile GnRH	Gonadotropins	Pulsatile GnRH
Ovulations (%)	6 (85)	9 (56)	6 (54)	4 (80)
Pregnancies (%)	2 (29)	5 (31)	1 (9)	/

DISCUSSION

Our study allows a significant conclusion. Both the treatments (pulsatile GnRH or gonadotropins) are capable of inducing an appropriate follicular growth with certain ovulation, as demostrated by ovulation rates [8].
But the pre-treatment with Analogs followed by both therapies shows better results in terms of pregnancy rate. This is explained by the hypogonadotropic state achieved in PCO patients after the triptorelin administration. Our findings do not allow to estabilish which is the treatment of choice in PCO subjects CC resistant in terms of advantages: the ultrasonographic assessment is comparable, as well as the risk of hyperstimulation or cystic involution. Anyway our results can be considered only preliminary data, also satisfactory compared to more invasive treatment of PCO syndrome (criocoagulation, follicular aspiration).

REFERENCES

1] Crosignani PG, Ferrari C:
Dopaminergic treatment for hyperprolactinaemia.
Balliere's Clinical Obstetrics and Gynaecology 4: 441 - 455, 1990

2] Dalicin AC, Marshall JC:
Medical therapy of hyperprolactinemia. Endocrinology and metabolism.
Clinics of North America 18: 259 - 276, 1989

3] Tan SL:
Hyperprolactinemia and the management of related tumors.
Current Opinion in Obstet. and Gynaecol. 2: 378 - 385, 1990

4] Mattei A, Galparoli C, Spellecchia D, Crosignani PG:
Induction of ovulation with pulsatile LHRH.
Acta Europea Fertilitatis 18: 267 - 269, 1987

5] Yen SSC, Vela P, Rankin J:
Inappropriate secretion of follicle-stimulating hormone in polycystic ovarian disease. J Clin Endocrinol 30: 435 - 442, 1970

6] Jansen RPS, Handelsman DJ, Boylan LM, Conway A, Shearman RP, Fraser IS: *Pulsatile intravenous gonadotropin-releasing hormone for ovulation-induction in infertile women. Safety and effectiveness with outpatient therapy.* Fertil. Steril. 48: 33, 1987

7] Scott RT, Navot D:
Enhancement of ovarian responsiveness with microdoses of gonadotropin-releasing hormone agonist during ovulation induction for in vitro fertilization. Fertil. Steril. 61: 880 - 885

8] Tanbo T, Dale PO, Kjekshus E, Haug E, Abyholm T:
Stimulation with human menopausal gonadotropin versus follicle-stimulating hormone after pituitary suppression in polycystic ovarian syndrome. Fertil. Steril. 53: 798 - 803, 1990

9] Dale PE, Tanbo T, Lunde O, Abyholm T:
Ovulation induction with low-dose follicle-stimolating hormone in women with the polycystic ovary syndrome. Acta Obstet. Gynecol. Scand. 72: 43 - 46, 1993

10] Filicori M, Flamigni C, Meriggiola MC, Cognigni G, Valdiserri A, Ferrari P, Campaniello E.
Ovulation induction with pulsatile gonadotropin-releasing hormone: technical modalities and clinical perspectives. Fertil. Steril. 56: 1 - 13, 1991

11] Filicori M, Campaniello E, Michelacci L, Pareschi A, Ferrari P, Bolelli G, Flamigni C:
Gonadotropin Releasing Hormone (GnRH) Analog suppression renders Polycystic Ovarian Disease patients more susceptible to ovulation induction with pulsatile GnRH. J. Clin. Endocrin. Metabol. 66: 327 - 333, 1988

12] Corenthal L, Von Hagen S, Larkins D, Ibrahim J, Santoro N:
Benefits of continuous physiological pulsatile gonadotropin-releasing hormone therapy in women with polycystic ovarian syndrome. Fertil. Steril. 61: 1027 - 1023, 1994

13] Larsen T, Falck Larsen J, Schioler V, Bostofte E, Felding C:
Comparison of urinary human follicle-stimulating hormone and human menopausal gonadotropin for ovarian stimulation in polycystic ovarian syndrome. Fertil. Steril. 53: 426 - 431, 1990

14] Sagle MA, Hamilton-Farley D, Kiddy DS, Franks S:
A comparative, randomized study of low-dose human menopausal gonadotropin and follicle-stimulating hormone in women with polycystic ovarian syndrome. Fertil. Steril. 55: 56 - 60, 1991

Comparison between u-hFSH conventional protocol and a personalized approach in controlled ovarian hyperstimulation

F. Zullo, C. Di Carlo*, M. Pellicano*, R. De Stefano*, P. Mastrantonio and C. Nappi*

Department of Gynecologic and Paediatric Sciences, Medical School of Cantanzaro, University of Reggio Calabria Ospedale "A. Pugliese", Cantanzaro and *Department of Gynecology and Obstetrics, University "Federico II" of Napoli, Naples, Italy

Introduction

A gonadotrophin controlled ovarian hyperstimulation (COH) with or without intrauterine insemination (IUI) has been shown effective in the treatment of infertility caused by anovulation, mild endometriosis or unexplained (1-3).

Stimulation of two to four follicles plays a key role in increasing the pregnancy rate (single or twin) without raising significantly the rate of triplets and ovarian hyperstimulation syndrome (OHS) (1-4).

In this regard it is extremely useful to consider single parameters to define the best gonadotrophin starting dose to obtain the maturation of two to four follicles.

On the basis of a previous study of our group (5) we suggest to personalize the approach to COH using the body mass index (BMI) and the body fat distribution expressed as waist/hip ratio (WHR).

We have then organized a randomized cross-over

comparison between u-hFSH COH conventional protocol and a personalized approach.

Materials and methods

We studied a population of 42 infertile women, with an anovulatory, endometriosis or unexplained infertility lasting more than two years, excluding tubal and male factor.

We performed at these patients a total of 175 cycles.

The personalized protocol (group A) has the following starting doses:

-for women with BMI < 19, 37,5 IU/day of u-hFSH;

-for patients with BMI between 19 and 25 (both normoovulatory and PCOS) 75 IU/day;

-for women with BMI > 25 (both normal and PCOS) and with a feminine body fat distribution (WHR < 0.8) 150 IU/day doubling the dose in absence of ovarian response after 7 days;

-for PCOS patients with BMI > 25 and WHR > 0.8 a low dose protocol starting with 75 IU/day and increasing the dose of 37.5 IU/day in absence of ovarian response every 7 days.

The conventional protocol (group B) has a starting dose of 75 IU/day of u-hFSH doubling the dose after 7 days in absence of ovarian response.

A step-up approach was anyway present in both group up to the administration of hCG when 1 to 4 follicles (cancellation when more than 4) were more than 18 mm mean diameter. Thirtysix hours after hCG administration a timed intercourse was prescribed or they underwent an intrauterine or intraperitoneal insemination after swin-up semen preparation (6).

Patients were randomized to group A and B and when not getting pregnant during the first cycle they were crossed to the apposite protocol.

Statistic evaluation was performed by chi-square test and Student t-test when appropriate.

Results and discussion

Clinical parameters related to the camparison of group A and B are reported in Tab.1. Ovulation rate was not different between the two groups. Number of monofollicular ovulations was higher but not significantly in group A and so the cancellation rate was higher using the personalized approach but again not significantly.

Not different between the two groups were peak E2 serum levels and number of u-hFSH ampoules used.

Lenght of stimulation (number of days) was significantly higher (p<0.01) in cycles with conventional protocol.

Pregnancy rate/cycle was significantly higher in the group of cycles (A) treated by a personalized protocol and abortion rate not different between group A and B.

The better pregnancy rate in group A can be interpreted either as dependent or the higher rate of multifollicular ovulation in this group, or as a faster reach of FSH treshold value envolving a more physiologic oocyte maturation.

Actually the lower stimulation lenght in group A could be explained on the basis of a better responder group but this selection bias should have been avoided by the crossover experimental design.

Confirmed from these preliminary data is that a slightly more aggressive protocol (1-4) on the basis of a more

TABLE 1

	Conventional (A)	Personalized (B)	p
N° cycles	87	88	
N° ovulatory cycles	71 (81.6%)	78 (88.6%)	
N° monofollicular cycles	43 (60.5%)	32 (39.5%)	ns
N° cycles 2-4 follicles	28 (39.5%)	46 (60.5%)	ns
N° cancellated cycles	16 (18.3%)	10 (10.5%)	ns
E2 (pg/ml)	394±201	472±315	ns
Lenght stimulation (days)	16.4±4.8	12.2±4.1	p<0.01
Ampoules of u-hFSH	18.1±6.3	16.1±5.9	ns
N° pregnancies	67	18	
singles	6	12	
doubles	1	6	
triplets	-	-	
% pregnancy/cycle	8.0	20.4	p<0.05
% = /ovulatory cycle	9.8	23.1	ns
N° evolutive pregnancies	5	14	
% abortion	28.6	22.2	ns
N° mild/severe OHS (%)	1(1.1%)	2(2.3%)	ns

adapt starting dose (thanks to easily evaluable parameters such as BMI and WHR) permit to obtain a better number of single and bigemin pregnancies, without any important increase of incidence of plurime pregnancies and of ovarian hyperstimulation syndrome.

References

1) Mascarenhas L, Khastgir G, Davies WAR, Lee S: Superovulation and timed intercourse: can it provide a reasonable alternative for those unable to afford assisted conception? Hum Reprod, 9, 67-70, 1994.

2) Aboulghar AM, Mansour RT, Scrour GI, Amin Y, Abbas AM, Salah IM: Ovarian superstimulation and intrauterine insemination for the treatment of unexplained infertility. Fertil Steril, 60, 303-6, 1993.

3) Corson GH, Kemman E: The role of superovulation with menotropins in ovulatory infertility. Fertil Steril, 55, 468-77, 1991.

4) Gratton RJ, Nisker JA, Daniel S, Toth S, Gunter J, Kaplan BR, Tummon IS, Yuzpe AA: An aggressive phylosophy in controlled ovarian stimolation cycles increases pregnancy rates. Hum Reprod, 8, 528-31, 1993.

5) Zullo F, Di Carlo C, Pellicano M, Catizone C, Mastrantonio P, Nappi C: Superovulation with urinary human FSH: correlations with body mass index and body fat distribution. In Press on Gynecol Endocrinol.

6) Sher G, Knutzen VK, Stratton CJ, Montakhab MM, Allenson SG: In vitro sperm capacitation and transcervical intrauterine insemination for the treatment of refractory infertility: phase I. Fertil Steril, 41, 260-64, 1984.

Pelvic endometriosis with histological aspects of perineural involvement: case report

A. Azzena, G. Cerri, R. Salmaso*, F. Vasoin, C. Vasile and A. Ferrara

Università degli Studi di Padova, Istituto di Ginecologia ed Ostetricia "G.B. Revoltella" and *Istituto di Anatomia Patologica, Padova, Italy

SUMMARY

A case of endometriosis involving the right utero-sacral and the large ligaments; in which non neoplastic endometrial glands were present in the perineural space is reported.

In the past, epithelial invasion of the peri-neural space was considered evidence of the presence of malignancy.

Rodin and coll. however concluded that the perineural space is not a lymphatic space and its involvement may also represent the extension of non neoplastic benign cells into a lower resistance tissue.

Peri-neural invasion has been reported in benign conditions of the breast, including chronic cystic disease and sclerosis adenosis.

It is important to stress that the perineural invasion in endometriosis must not be interpreted as evidence of malignancy.

Key words: Pelvic endometriosis; Perineural involvement.

INTRODUCTION

Endometriosis consists of the presence of functional endometrium outside its normal site in the liming of the uterine cavity; adenomyosis is the presence of the endometrial cells at myometrial level (1) ("endometriosis interna").

In order to explain the ectopic presence of the endometrial tissue, a lot of theories of

363

histogenesis of endometriosis have been suggested: a) retrograd menstruation and direct implantation which assumes that ectopic endometrial tissue is transplanted from the uterus to a pathologic location within the peritoneal cavity by way of the uterine tubes; b) methaplasia of the ectopic epithelium (Meyer, Novak, Meigs, Ranney) which postulates that dormant immature multipotential cells of the embryonic coelomic liming, common in the central area of the pelvis may persist in adult life and under cyclic oestrogenic stimulation these cells undergo methaplasia and may form endometrial tissue (this theory may explain the occasional implants of endometrium within the peritoneum, in the pleura, in the extremities and even in other areas of the body); c) blood or lymph propagation of the endometrial cells; d) post surgical spread of endometrial tissue; e) combination of transplant and in site theories.

Tab. 1 illustrates the most frequent clinical findings of endometriosis (symptoms and signs).

The most common manifestation of endometriosis is pain and the chief complication is infertility. It is useful to remember the so-called "4 D" of endometriosis: dysmenorrhea, dispareunia, disuria and dyschezia.

Many women with a personal history of infertility and sterility; during the routine gynecologic controls may discover the disease.

The most used routine examination for diagnosing endometriosis are shown in Tab. 2.

The progress and widespread of new endoscopic techniques as laparoscopy provided better visualization and it became important to diagnose not only the classic hyperpigmental lesions but also all the endoscopic aspects of unpigmented endometriosic lesions (Tab.3) (4-6).

Accurate classification or staging, by laparoscopy or laparotomy is of paramount importance in the investigation and management of endometriosis.

The American Fertility Society proposed a staging of the disease in order to realize a pratical and accurate approach and to determin the real effectiveness of the various treatments suggested by different Auhtors (Tab.4) (7).

The therapy of endometriosis may be pharmacological (Progestogens, Danazol, GnRH Analogues); in this case is taken into consideration the hormonal sensitivity of the endometrial tissue, the local factors which influence the symptomatology and therefore, at least partly, this type of medical treatment acts on the pain nervous terminations.

The medical approach is suggested in all the symptomatic patients whithout endometriomas or adnexal adhesions (8-14).

Patients with endometriomas with a large spread of the disease must be surgically treated (possibilly by laparoscopic tecniques); surgery can be associated with a previous medical therapy which reduces the size and activity of the ectopic tissues, facilitates asportation and decreases the possibility of post-surgical implants spread;

Tab. 1: High frequency signs and symptoms in pelvic endometriosis

SYMPTOMS   SIGNS

- Infertility   - Reduced uterine mobilization
- Pelvic pain   - Douglas pouch nodes
- Dysmenorrhea   - Uterosacral ligaments nodes
- Dyspareunia   - Increased adnexal size
- Menstrual disorders   - Reduced adnexal mobilization
- Bladder symptomatology   - Eventual   visible   foci (clinical   exam,
                                    colposcopy)
- Bowel disturbs

Tab. 2: Diagnostic methods in pelvic endometriosis

- Ultrasound   - MNR
- Laparoscopy   - TAC
- Lapoarotomy   - Immunoscintigraphy - CA-125 assay

Tab. 3: Endoscopic aspects of non pigmented endometriosic lesions

- Red flame-like lesion   - White opacification
- Glandular excrescence   - Subovarian adhesions
- Petechial peritoneum   - Yellow-brown peritoneal patches
- Hypervascularization areas   - Circular peritoneal defect

from: Nisolle M., Donnez J., Casanas-Roux F. (1994): Medical therapy of endometriosis: histomorphologic effects and rationale for surgery. Endometriosis and pelvic pain: time of review. Ed. by Crosignani P.G., Vercellini P. The Parthenon Publishing Group.

pharmacological approach may also be used after the surgery, in order to eliminate the residual disease (15,16).

CASE REPORT

S.M. 33 years old; mother with cardiac pathology, menarche at 13 years of age, regular menstrual cycles complains of secondary dysmenorrhea during the last 7 years, PARA 2012.

During a routine gynecologic control, at the pelvic examination a fibrous pelvic right parametrial mass has been revealed; the uterus had normal size and mobility and the adnexal zones were normal.

The patients underwent surgery: during the pelvic inspection a fibrous, 5 cm diameter mass was pointed out; its location was at the right parametrial level and compression of the omolateral ureter (which became sthenotic in the point where it came in contact with the pelvic mass and dilated upper the sthenosis) was noted.

The pelvic mass strongly infiltrates the bladder and reaches the basis of the parametrium.

Previous preparation of the pararectal and paravescical space, isolation of the ureter in its pelvic portion, opening of the uretere's tunnel and isolation of the pelvic mass from the bladder and the cervix have been performed, in order to realize the asportation of the mass.

Despite of the ureter's isolation from the pelvic mass, it was taken into consideration its sthenotic portion and the lack of a good peristaltic activity so that an ureteral incannulation was decided subsequently.

The postoperative period presented no complications.

Four fibrous tissutal fragments, of increased consistence, the biggest of 3.5x1.5 cm were studied histologically. The histological findings consisted of adenosis "islands" formed by endometrial active glands and endometrial stroma. The presence of endometrial glands in the perineural spaces of numerous nerves is specific (Fig. 1-2).

DISCUSSION

In the past, the observation of an epithelial invasion of the perineural spaces was considered a paramount evidence of malignancy.

Subsequently, different Authors, demostrated the presence of various aspects of perineural invasion in the fibrocystic dysplasia and in the breast sclerosing adenosis.

The aim of this study was to describe the perineural presence of endometrial non neoplastic glands in a case of pelvic endometriosis.

Robin and coll. demonstrated, using immunohistochemical and electronic microscopical techniques, that the perineural space lack of endothelium is not a lymphatic space and therefore, its involvement may represent an extension through a minor resistence tissue. So that the invasion of the perineural zone must not be considered a sure malignancy criteria, invalidating in this way the classic theories.

The reported case of pelvic endometriosis allows us to stress the importance of this pathology which must not be underevaluated because of its rapid evolutive possibilities, with subsequent adhesions and compression of the anatomic proximal structures which

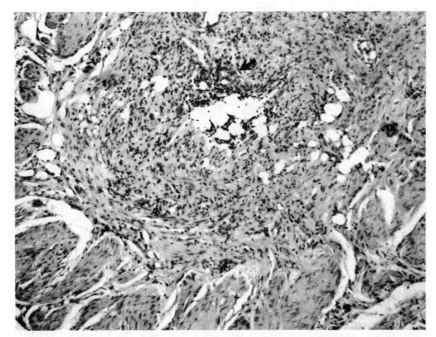

FIG.1 Fibrous fatty tissue with central ramification which appears focally infiltrated by endometriosis foci.

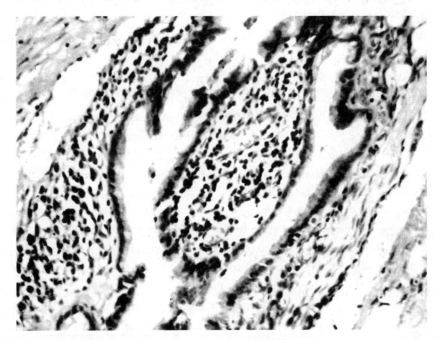

FIG.2 Perineural endometriosis foci; particular (E-E 60X).

improve the difficulty of the surgical approach, transforming a relative simple into a more complicated operation.

Therefore, all cases with dysmenorrhea, chronic persistant pelvic pain must undergo an accurate diagnosis in order to exclude endometrosis.

When the patients are in fertile age, it is even more important to realize an early, correct diagnosis, as they may desire a future pregnancy, which could be obtained in patients with endometriosis (the association between endometriosis and infertility is already well known).

The instrumental diagnosis of endometriosis includes ultrasounds (abdominal or vaginal), a simple non invasive diagnostic method; diagnostic laparoscopy, even if invasive, may become therapeutical and avoids laparotomy.

Laparoscopic diagnosis allows also the staging of the disease, in order to evaluate the reproductive capacities of the patients and to choose the most adequate assisted fertilization technique to be performed.

REFERENCES

1) Pescetto G., De Cecco L., Pecorari D., Ragni N. (1989): Manuale di Ginecologia ed Ostetricia, Volume I, II Edizione. Società Editrice Universo - Roma.

2) Ranney B. (1980): Endometriosis: pathogenesis, symptoms and findings. Clin. Obstet. Gynecol., 23, 865-80.

3) Mahmood T.A., Templeton A. (1991): Prevalence and genesis of endometriosis. Human. Reprod., 6, 544-9.

4) Martin D.C., Hubert G.D., Van der Zwaag R., El-Zeky F. (1989): Laparoscopic appearance of peritoneal endometriosis. Fertil.Steril., 51, 63.

5) Jansen R.P.S.,Russel P. (1986): Non-pigmented endometriosis: clinical laparoscopic and pathologic definition. Am. J. Obstet. Gynecol., 15, 1154.

6) Vercellini P., Bocciolone L., Vendola N., Colombo A., Rognoni M.T., Fedele L. (1991): Peritoneal endometriosis: morphologic appearance in women with chronic pelvic pain. J. Reprod. Med., 36, 533-7.

7) The American Fertility Society (1985). Revised American Fertility Society classification of endometriosis: 1985. Fertil. Steril., 43, 351-5.

8) Moghissi K.S., Boyce C. (1976): Management of endometriosis with oral medroxyprogesterone acetate. Obstet. Gynecol., 47, 265-7.

9) Luciano A.A., Turksoy N., Carleo J. (1988): Evaluation of oral medroxyprogesterone acetate in the treatment of endometriosis. Obstet. Gynecol., 72, 323-7.

10) Greenblatt R.B., Tzingounis V. (1979): Danazol treatment of endometriosis:long term follow-up. Fertil. Steril., 32, 518-20.

11) Barbieri R.L., Evans S., Kistner R.W. (1982): Danazol in the treatment of endometriosis:analysis of 100 cases with a 4-year follow-up. Fertil. Steril., 37, 737-46.

12) Lemay A:, Maheux R., Faure N., Jean C., Frazekas A.T. (1984): Reversible hypogonadism induced by a luteinizing hormone releasing hormone (LH-RH) agonist (Buserelin) as a new approach for endometriosis. Fertil. Steril., 41, 863-71.

13) Zorn J.R., Mathieson J., Risquez F., Comaru-Schally A.M., Schally A.V. (1990): Treatment of endometriosis with a delayed release preparation of the agonist D-Trp6-luteinizing hormone: long-tem folow-up in a series of 50 patients. Fertil. Steril., 53, 401-6.

14) Venturini P.L., Fasce V., Costantini S., Anserini P., Cucuccio S., De Cecco L. (1990): Treatment of endometriosis with goserelin depot, a long-acting gonadotropin-releasing hormone agonist analog: endocrine and clinical results. Fertil. Steril., 54, 1021-7.

15) Canis M., Mage G., Manhes H., Pouly J.L., Wattiez A., Bruhat M.A. (1989): Laparoscopic treatment of endometriosis. Acta Obste. Gynecol. Scand., 150 (Suppl.), 15-20.

16) Nezhat C., Crowgey S., Nezhat F. (1990): Videolaparoscopy for the treatment of endometriosis associated with infertility. Fertil. Steril.: 51, 237-40.

Strange histological findings of the uterine endometriomyosis: biological meaning

S. Cianci, A. Mangiacasale and L. Milluzzo

School of Specialization in Gynecology and Obstetrics II, University of Catania, Italy

---

An our hystomorphological research, still in progress, about endometriomyosis during pre- and postmenopausal climacterium, that we have developed on 317 uteri, that were removed for different reasons in the period 1992-93, in women aged from 40 to 79, has allowed to notice a percentage respectively of 76,63% and 52,63%. These percentages, that are very high, include minimum and extensive lesions.

We make use of term "endometriomyosis" when endometrial infiltration of myometrium affects both stroma and glandulas, event that happens much more frequently, and we keep the term "adenomyosis" for the cases that are characterized by the presence of glandulas without stroma.

In the contest of our investigations, we have noticed some exceptional hystomorphological kind of endometriomyosis:

1) total endometriomyosis, with complete uterine paries involvement;

2) ectopic lymphatic lacunas with abundant endometrial tissue;

3) endometriomyotic formations with realization of pseudo-uterine cavity and with glandulas that flow into cavity;

4) into a fetal uterus (30 weeks) there is a congenital endometriomyosis, nearer to perimetrium than endometrium.

In the our research it should come out that endometriomyosis is a physiological condition since it interests more than 70% of examined uteri.

There isn't any effective explanation to understand because, in some case, mucosa shows a clear enough outline as regards remaining myometrium, while, in other cases, it is wavy, with areas where endometrium penetrates more or less deeply, so much that it produces a real endometriomyosis.

Congenital fetal endometriomyosis, that probably is due to an irregular invagination of primitive coeloma into mesoderm, could be a good explanation for those forms that mime uterine cavities or that haven't a continuity with superficial mucosa.

SUMMARY

The authors find out of 317 removed uteri, during pre- and postmenopausal climacterium, an endometriomyosis' percentage respectively equal to 76,63% and 52,63%.

They describe some particular hystomorphological form and formulate some etiogenic consideration.

Menopause

Menopause and pregnancy: the woman's point of view*

M. Boulet

International Health Foundation, Brussels, Belgium

What makes a postmenopausal woman want to become a mother for the first time, or to repeat the experience of motherhood?

The state of being postmenopausal as such does not mean a great deal in this context. It usually evokes a picture of a woman aged around fifty, but it may also, unfortunately, include a woman who is aged only around 35. Is it then so strange that such a woman should yearn to have a child? At 35 years of age, a woman is of course not old, and women nowadays tend to have their children at around that age, sometimes even their first child.

I have also asked myself, as a woman witnessing our fast changing world, whether wanting a child at an advanced age is not in fact a case of snatching the opportunity that rapidly advancing technology in human reproduction research now offers, to take advantage of this unique and final chance to have a child. However, the contradiction here is that women who have already experienced motherhood appear to want a baby just as passionately and deeply as those who never have.

*This paper was initially presented in Paris at the 15th Anniversary Meeting of the AFEM (Association Française pour l'Etude de la Ménopause) in December 1994.

It is to be published in Reproduction Humaine et Hormones (in Press) and also in these proceedings of the 4th World Congress of Gynecological Endocrinology and 2nd Congress of the European Society for Gynecologic and Obstetric Investigation, Madonna di Campaglio (Italy) February 1995.

The actual situation is undoubtedly more complex, a mixture of a longing to be a mother once again and a blurred wish to hold on to the youth, power and femininity that a woman values so highly.

But this becomes part of another debate that I will leave to the psychologists, the philosophers and the geneticists.

I believe essentially that a woman has to be selfish. She may in fact have a hundred good reasons for wanting a child at a later age, for example the loss of a child, remarriage, questions of inheritance, or merely to know finally what it means to be a mother. But this selfishness - and I believe this with the same intensity - this selfishness has its limits, which are imposed by the rights of the very object of her selfishness: the child itself.

I do not want to be judgemental. But I do also think that parents owe everything to their children, perhaps more these days than at any time in the past, because now, thanks to modern contraception, a child should be a wanted child, and no longer an "accident".

What can parents aged around fifty or sixty offer? Love, yes, most probably to a suffocating degree, as well as material security and a certain serenity in regard to life, since most of it will be behind them.

One could always argue that many children are succesfully raised by their grandparents, and that everything goes well in such circumstances. At first sight, this may seem true. But has this ever actually been investigated? Has a survey ever been conducted? I personally know as many unfortunate as fortunate children in such situations.

Those older mothers and fathers - did they really think about what might become of their children if they, as parents, were to die early? The children would then join the ranks of the young orphans. What if they died when the children were 15-17 years old? A child of 15-17 still needs his or her parents just as much as a youngster of 7-10 years. The nature of the need may change, but not the need itself. A longing to be cuddled and for a reassuring presence changes into a need fo parental help, advice, backing and moral support.

Table 1:
Characteristics of the sample

1.	AGE	
	29-40 years	10% (21)
	41-50 years	32% (68)
	51-60 years	48% (102)
	61-70 years	10% (21)
2.	MENOPAUSAL STATUS	
	Premenopausal	14% (30)
	Perimenopausal	23% (49)
	Postmenopausal	62% (131)
3.	EDUCATION	
	Secondary level	50%
	University level	33%
4.	MARITAL AND FAMILY STATUS	
	Already had children	85%
	Living with husband/ partner	54%

Some will argue that the current trend in life - expectancy curves is upwards. And this is true, although fatal outcomes due to maternity are not uncommon and these increase with advancing age, as can be seen from the day-to-day medical statistics.

At the International Health Foundation we wanted to obtain more detailed knowledge of women's opinions on this topic around the world. A survey was accordingly undertaken among 213 women from 15 different countries.

The sample profile is shown in table 1.

Table 2 summarizes the geographical distribution of the sample.

The women were asked only one question: "What do you think of postmenopausal women who are determined to have a baby? Do you favour this attitude?". They were invited to comment briefly on their answer if they so wished.

Looking more closely at the "noes" (73%), it can be seen that 28% of the interviewees thought that from 50 years of age onwards it was difficult to adjust physically to the

Table 2:
Geographical distribution of the sample

WORLD REGIONS	

Europe
  Belgium
  Finland
  Great Britain
  Italy
  Spain
  Sweden
	55%

South-East Asia
  Hong Kong
  Indonesia
  Philippines
  Singapore
	21%

South America
  Argentina
  Brazil
  Peru
	11%

Australia	9%
USA	5%

demanding efforts needed to raise a young child - at that age women lacked the necessary energy; the age difference between mother and child was unacceptable; practical problems arose; financial, personality, conflictual and menopausal difficulties were experienced. Sixteen percent (16%) of the women thought it was contrary to nature; nature should not be forced; the women concerned were irresponsible; it was not in good taste; it was better to adopt a child.

Fifteen percent (15%) considered the women to be selfish; the children would be exposed to too many emotional problems; the children needed active parents in good health; it was tantamount to bringing orphans into the world; it was not fair on the children. As to health considerations, 4% thought it was potentially dangerous for the child (Down's syndrome; physical and genetic malformations). Four percent (4%) of the women thought that, economically speaking, it was a waste of money, that such fecundation problems were the preserve of younger women and that the money could better be used for cancer screening. If we now consider the positive answers, or at least the less negative ones, we find that 11% of the women (23) replied "yes", 10% (21) said "yes, but" and 6% (14) said "no, but" (Table 5).

Table 3:
Summary of the answers given

	Number	%
No	155	73
No, but	14	6
Yes	23	11
Yes, but	21	10
	213	100

Table 4:
Negative comments

For following reasons	%
Physical condition	28
Ethics	16
Child's welfare	15
Psychological impact	7
Child's health	4
Financial impact	4

Table 5:
Other comments

	Abs	%
Yes	23	11
Yes, but	21	10
No, but	14	6

The (more or less) positive comments thus referred to considerations regarding actual age at the menopause (2%), the women's health and usually sound financial situation (4%), and their maturity, which was seen as a positive contributor towards successful motherhood (8%). Some of the women interviewed referred to a life dream coming true, to the child as a new bond between an old couple (12%), and to the mixture of feelings involved, combining a sense of additional responsibility with one of immense joy (newly discovered in the case of a first child, and rediscovered otherwise). The respect that such a decision merits was also a subject of comment.

Table 6:
Answers given by the women interviewed according to age, menopausal status, marital status and parity (%)

Age	Yes	Yes, but	No, but
29-40	23	5	-
41-50	36	30	43
51-60	27	65	43
61-70	14	-	14
Menopausal status			
Premenopausal	13	3	3
Perimenopausal	14	8	8
Postmenopausal	8	12	7
Marital status			
Living with husband/ partner	10	10	7
Living alone	15	9	3
Parity			
Had children	10	10	8
No children	16	6	-

The profile of the women who answered "yes", "yes, but" or "no, but", might be summarized as follows (slide 6). In general, those who said "yes" were more often premenopausal and perimenopausal (13% and 14% respectively) than postmenopausal (8%). Indeed, postmenopausal women expressed less clear opinions by replying "yes, but" (12%).

Women living alone replied "yes" in 15% of cases, while "yes, but" was the answer of 10% of the women living with a husband or partner. As to parity, 16% of the childless women and 10% of those who had had children were more in favour of maternity after the menopause.

Age as an influencing factor was distributed as follows: 41 % of the women who replied "yes" were aged between 51 and 70 years, while 95% of the women who said "yes, but" and 86% of those who said "no, but" were between 41 and 60 years of age.
Educational level had no influence at all.

Conclusion

All the figures we obtained indicate very clearly that the majority of the women who participated in this survey were definitely opposed to pregnancy after the menopause.

But these are only opinions. There will always be those whose minds are made up, who have the financial means to fulfil their dreams and ambitions and who will go ahead and do what they want.

Laws and ethics are normally there to protect citizens against themselves. But these laws will never be a barrier to those who are really determined and the dividing line is easy to cross.

Personally, I do not believe such postmenopausal women will ever be very numerous. Neither do I believe in attempting to persuade such women against having a child. This would not be realistic. Women themselves must demonstrate their own sense of responsibility and draw on their own maturity and wisdom to reason their way through clearly to the right decision.

Accidents do not always happen to other people!

Medical journals and magazines are full of articles about motherhood and fatherhood in later life giving rise to problems such as malformations, trisomia, etc. To want a child at any price, whatever the risk, is in my opinion frankly shocking. But of course, such a fanatical desire to have a child is beyond any reasonable understanding!

To be absolutely honest, I would feel I was caught up in a nightmare if, at the age of 60, I was again faced with sleepless nights, teething miseries, the worry of childhood maladies and of course the generation gap (or gulf in this case) ... not to mention motorbike fever in the late teens (by which time I would be a mere 80 years of age!!).

<u>References</u>

Antinori S., Versaci C., Hossein Gholami G. et al. A child is a joy at any age. Human Reproduction, 1993, 8, 10, 1542-1544

Bossemayer R. Até quando reproduçao assistida? Ponto de Vista, (Communication personnelle), 1994.

Bowman M.C., Saunders D.M. Community attitudes to maternal age and pregnancy after assisted reproductive technology: too old at 50. Human Reproduction, 1994, 9, 1, 167-171.

Edwards R.G. Pregnancies are acceptable in post-menopausal women. Human Reproduction, 1993, 8, 10, 1542-1544.

Flamigni C. Egg donation to women over 40 years of age. Human Reproduction, 1993, 8, 9, 1343-1345.

How to give science a bad name. Comment. New Scientist, 1994, 1907, 3.

Italiaanse vrouw krijgt drieling. Algemeen Dagblad, 28/10/1994.

Mori T., Pregnancies in post-menopausal women. Post-menopausal pregnancy is permissible for women below 60 years of age. Human Reproduction, 1994, 9, 2, 187.

Oakley A. Time is power. The Lancet, Nov. 1988

Paulson R.J., Sauer M.V. Pregnancies in post-menopausal women. Oocyte donation to women of advanced reproductive age: 'How old is too old?' Human Reproduction, 1994, 9, 4, 571-572.

Sauer M.V. Extending reproductive potential in the older woman. In: Lobo R.A. (ed.) Treatment of the postmenopausal woman.: Basic and clinical aspects. Raven Press Ltd., New York, 1994, p. 35-46.

Sauer M.V., Paulson R.J. Quadruplet pregnancy in a 51-year-old menopausal woman following oocyte donation. Human Reproduction, 1993, 8, 12, 2243-2244.

Sauer M.V., Paulson R.J., Lobo R.A. Pregnancy after age 50: application of oocyte donation to women after natural menopause. The Lancet, 1993, 341, 8841, 321-323.

Solomon C. Warning: little kids are health hazard to the older parent. Middle-aged moms and dads complain of aching backs, colds, injuries and fatigue. Wall Street Journal, 8/11/1994.

Warnock M. A woman's right... Children of choice: Freedom and the New Reproductive Technologies by John A. Robertson. New Scientist, 1994, 1942, 36.

Acknowledgements

I would like to thank my many friends who helped me with the fieldwork, namely Roberto Bocanera (Argentina), Ronald Bossemeyer (Brazil), Carlo Campagnoli (Italy), Antonio Cano (Spain), Ronald Carter (Peru), Jean Coope (UK), Elizabeth Farrell (Australia), Ian Fraser (Australia), Andrea Genazzani (Italy), Julita R. Jalbuena (Philippines), Michael S. Marsh (UK), Anna-Maria Martits (Brazil), Terry McCarthy (Singapore), Santiago Palacios (Spain), Ingemar Persson (Sweden), Reijo Punnonen (Finland), Ratna S. Samil (Indonesia), David Sturdee (UK), Grace Tang (Hong Kong), Wulf Utian (USA), Henri Van Kets (Belgium), Eduardo F. Villario (Spain), Malcolm Whitehead (UK) and Lucio Zichella (Italy), as well as Ms Liliane Moeremans who assisted me with the statistical work and compilation of the files.

Late effects of menopausal ovarian failure: physiopathological and clinical aspects

M. Massobrio, M. Ardizzoja, M. Gallo and G. De Luigi

Clinica Ostetrica e Ginecologica, Università degli Studi di Torino, Turin, Italy

Cross-sectional studies of hormonal levels around the time of menopause show that 20-40% of women in the first 6-12 months after cessation of menses have estrogen concentrations consistent with the presence of functioning follicles. By 12-24 months estrogen concentrations fall into the postmenopausal range in most women, though some women still secrete significant amounts of estradiol.

Postmenopausal ovaries with evidence of stromal hyperplasia produce higher amounts of aromatizable androstenedione and estrogens than not hyperplasic stroma. Furthermore immunoreactive aromatase has been found in some stromal compartment of postmenopausal ovaries in which no follicle could be observed.

Both residual ovarian steroid production and aromatization potential by peripheric tissues can explain individual differences in the evidence and heaviness of climateric syndrome, particulary for what concerns long term symptoms as well as coronary heart disease and osteoporosis.

CORONARY HEART DISEASE

The concept that the menopause, or biological changes induced by it, is relevant to cardiovascular disease in women is probably based on simple inspection of the age curve for the incidence of and mortality from ischaemic heart disease in the two sexes. Data from the Framingham Heart Study (1) identify that any initial manifestation of coronary heart disease (CHD) occurs about a decade later among women than among men, with myocardial infarction occuring as much as 20 years later. In this study an increase in coronary heart disease incidence was demonstrable after both surgical and natural menopause and it was not restricted to younger women with premature menopause, whereas the Nurses' Health Study suggests that bilateral ovariectomy but not natural menopause increases the risk of CHD (2). This increase appears to be prevented by estrogen replacement therapy. Meta-analysis of 18 published studies confirm that estrogen replacement treatment protects against ischaemic heart disease (3).

Ovarian hormones have atherosclerotic-inhibiting and hemodynamic effects through actions on arterial and cardiac mechanisms which control blood flow. Hormone effects on arterial resistance, blood flow velocity and stability, vasodilator reserve capacity, and cardiac output have been reported.

Estrogen and progesterone receptors are present in the heart and in the wall of blood vessels and hormone receptor-mediated actions explain some of the hemodynamic effects of ovarian steroids reported in animal and human studies.

However a not ER-mediated mechanism must exist because:
- the inhibition of RNA synthesis doesn't modify estradiol-induced increase in uterine blood flow (UBF);
- estradiol hemodynamic effects appear to be too rapid for genomic mechanism.

Many investigations suggest that the acute effects of ovarian steroids are due to actions on vascular endothelium by modulating the release of vasodilators and vasoconstrictors, on ionic channels in cell membranes of vascular smooth muscle (VSM) cells and cardiac myocytes, and on neurotransmitter release at presynaptic junctions.

Williams et al. reported an increase in the coronary vascular response to Ach stimulation in ovariectomized cynomologous monkeys after estradiol-17B (E2) treatment. Intracoronary infusion of Ach caused constriction in the estrogen-deficient monkeys while constriction was not seen in monkeys receiving E2 (4).

Estrogen-induced uterine vasodilation has been shown to be antagonized by L-nitroarginine methyl ester (L-NAME), an inhibitor of EDRF (Endothelial-Derived Releasing Factor) synthesis. This finding further substantiates an endothelial-dependent mechanism.

Polderman et al. have recently reported that estrogen administration to patients undergoing male-to-female transsexual surgery led to a decrease in plasma levels of endothelin-1, a potent vasoconstrictor, while patients undergoing female-to-male transformation who received testosterone showed an increase in endothelin-1 levels (5).

E2 induces endothelial-independent relaxation in human coronary arteries "in vitro". In fact human epicardial coronary rings from patients undergoing heart transplantation, suspended in organ baths and exposed to E2 at physiological concentrations, show significant concentration-dependent relaxation. This effect was unaffected by the removal of the endothelium and no differences were seen after nitric oxide synthesis inhibition with L-NAME or indomethacin.

In addiction estrogens may exert several other antiatherosclerotic effects, as:
- reduction of cell adhesion molecules (CAMs) production by endothelium-leukocyte interaction;
- modulation of lipoprotein metabolism;
- increase in PGI2 production;
- reduction in smooth muscle and intima cell proliferation.

OSTEOPOROSIS

A reduction in estrogen levels after menopause is thought to be responsible for the accelerated bone loss and increased risk of osteoporotic fractures occuring in postmenopausal women. The bone loss due to estrogen deficiency is attributable to an increase in bone resorption, together with a smaller increase in bone formation.

Estrogens are generally considered to maintain bone mass through an antiresorptive mechanism, which has recently been shown to be partially explicable as a direct effect on bone. Estrogens induce cells of the osteoblastic (OB) lineage to inhibit osteoclastic (OC) bone resorption.

Proliferation and differentiation of OB and OC is a complex process, regulated by systemic and local growth factors. In women the availability of estrogens is an essential factor in the maintenhance of bone mass. A direct stimulatory effect of estrogen on OBs has been demonstrated. An intermediate factor between estrogens and bone cell metabolism is also plausible. Indirect effects of estrogen on bone can be identified in:

- an increase in 1-alfa-hydroxylase activity in the kidneys and in intestinal receptors for 1,25-dihydroxy-cholecalciferol, with a consequent increment in the intestinal resorption of calcium;
- an increase in calcitonin secretion by thyroid parafollicular cells: the bone eroding activity of OCs, which possess calcitonin receptors, is then inhibited (6);
- an increase in GH production and in osteoblastic synthesis of IGF-I: GH stimulates OB proliferation whereas IGF-I may induce the production of collagen by these cells (7);
- a reduction in osteoblastic synthesis of PGE2: among the different effects on bone metabolism exerted by this prostaglandin, its role in the coupling between OBs and OCs seems to be one of the most relevant (8,9);
- a reduction in synthesis of cytokines by circulating monocytes, OBs and stromal cells: cytokines and Colony Stimulating Factor (CSF) secreted by OBs and monocytes promote OC activity and preOC differentiation to OC (10).

It seems possible that the anabolic role of estrogen, in addition to its known antiresorptive effect, may be of relevance to the mechanism by which bone is lost in estrogen-deficient states and to therapeutic approaches to the postmenopausal bone loss in women.

REFERENCES

1 - Gordon T, Kannel WB et al. Ann Intern Med 1978;89:157.
2 - Colditz GA et al. N Engl J Med 1987;316:1105.
3 - La Vecchia C. Human Reproduction 1992;7 no.2:162.
4 - Williams JK et al. Circulation 1990;81:1680.
5 - Polderman KH et al. Ann Intern Med 1993;118:429.
6 - Reginster TY et al. J Clin Invest 1989;83:1073.
7 - Dawson-Hughes B et al. J Clin Endocrin Metab 1986;63:424.
8 - Raisz LG et al. Bone Miner Res 1984;2:286.
9 - Sakamoto S et al. Bone Miner Res 1986;4:49.
10- Horowitz MC. Science 1993;260:626.

Urodynamic diagnosis and ultrasound findings

L.D. Cardozo, V. Khullar, S. Hill and A. Yip

Urogynaecology Unit, Department of Obstetrics and Gynaecology, King's College Hospital, London, UK

OBJECTIVE:

Ultrasound enables the lower urinary tract to be visualised as well as the surrounding tissues. Transvaginal ultrasound has been used to measure bladder wall thickness and this appears from a pilot study[1] to be a non-invasive screening technique for detecting detrusor instability. A large blinded study has not been carried out. 3-D ultrasound allows assessment of the urethral sphincter in morphology as well as measurement of tissue volumes this may increase our understanding of the pathophysiology of urinary incontinence.

DESIGN AND METHODS:

Women with urinary symptoms were recruited prior to undergoing videocystourethrography (VCU). One hundred and eighty women had a transvaginal ultrasound (5MHz ATL) assessment of bladder wall thickness after voiding with postmicturition residual less than 50 mls and 70 women had a perineal 3D ultrasound scan with a 5 MHz probe (Kretz). The volume of the urethral sphincter and average bladder wall thickness was measured. If women had a mean bladder wall thickness greater than 5mm and detrusor instability was not diagnosed they underwent ambulatory urodynamics. The urethra, urethral sphincter and bladder neck were visualised in the sagittal plane. The urethral lumen and immediately adjacent tissues appear hypoechoic(black) this may extend from the urethral meatus to the bladder. This is surrounded along the mid length of the urethra by a homogenous round structure which thicker anteriorly than laterally or posteriorly. From pilot studies in cadavers, trucut biopsies of this area under ultrasound guidance have shown the tissue to be striated muscle. The structure is likely to be the rhabdosphincter.

RESULTS:

All the women (42) with urethral sphincter incompetence had a continuous hypoechoic area from the bladder neck to the urethral meatus. Also some of the women with severe genuine stress incontinence had breaks in the continuous circle of the "rhabdosphincter" and it was replaced by hyperechoic areas. This may indicate damage to the urethral sphincter. The "rhabdosphincter" was significantly smaller in women with urethral sphincter incompetence (Table 1).

	Urethral Sphincter Incompetence (n=42)	Competent Urethral Mechanism (n=28)	Mann Whitney U Test
Hypoechoic Volume/cm³	0.8 (0.4-1.3)	0.5 (0.3-0.8)	P = 0.03
Total Sphincter Volume/cm³	3.9 (2.3-4.7)	4.6 (3.4-6.1)	P = 0.02
True Sphincter Volume/cm³	2.8 (2.0-3.8)	4.1 (2.9-5.4)	P = 0.03

Table 1: Three dimensional ultrasound measurements of the urethral sphincter in women with urinary symptoms.

The hypoechoic volume was significantly larger in this group of women and this may relate to the pressure exerted by surrounding structures.

The diagnoses on videocystourethrography were:

Diagnosis	Detrusor Instabilit	Genuin e Stress Incont .	Mixed Incontin .	Sensory Urgency	Voiding Difficul t.	Normal UDS
Numbers	43	52	43	5	3	34

The positive predictive value of a mean bladder wall thickness greater than 5mm to diagnose detrusor instability is 94%(VCU and ambulatory tests combined). VCU in these women had a positive predictive value of 65%. In the group of women with a mean bladder wall thickness less than 3.5mm the positive predictive value for diagnosing genuine stress incontinence by VCU was 76% and by measurement of mean bladder wall thickness was 82%.

CONCLUSION:

Ultrasound may be useful in determining the pathophysiology of urethral sphincter incompetence as well as being a diagnostic tool. Measurement of bladder wall thickness with transvaginal ultrasound is a sensitive screening method for diagnosing detrusor instability in certain women and may be also be useful in excluding detrusor instability in a smaller group of symptomatic women.

1.A novel technique for measuring bladder wall thickness in women using transvaginal ultrasound

Khullar, V., Salvatore, S., Cardozo,L.D., Abbott,D., Kelleher,C.J. and Bourne,T.H. (1994) Ultra Obstet Gynaecol 4, 1-4.

Mammary changes during the menopausal transition

R. Pérez Sanz, L. Villavieja, P. de la Cueva, I. Morollón and F.R. Pérez-López

Departments of Obstetrics and Gynecology, and Radiology, Hospital Clínico and University of Zaragoza Faculty of Medicine, Zaragoza, Spain

INTRODUCTION

The mammary changes occurring during menopausal transition are related to both the aging process and to hormone changes. The breast responds to endogenous fluctuations of the sex steroids and some peptide hormones (1-3). Exogenous hormones may also have effects on the duct lobular unit (4-8). Early diagnosis and treatment of breast cancer and hormone replacement therapy are major tasks for gynaecologists for the next decades. In the present study we report the mammographic changes detected in women during the menopausal transition.

MATERIAL AND METHODS

We have studied the mammary characteristics in 35 women randomly selected from the gynaecologic outpatient clinic who had had two mammograms. The patients complained of mild to moderate mastalgia either in the premenstrual phase or for more prolonged periods. The first radiologic evaluation was carried out 25.3 ± 26.8 (mean ± SD) months (range 0-120 months) prior to either natural menopause (n = 30) or surgical castration (n = 5). The second mammographic exploration was carried out 66.6 ± 45.7 months (range 12-182 months) after the menopause.

The women had 2.5 ± 1.4 pregnancies and 2.1 ± 1.0 deliveries. One woman had secondary sterility and another one policystic ovaries. Previous mammary pathology included 3 cases of mammary abscess, telorrhea in 4 women and 10 women had previous mammary biopsies. Before the first mammogram 9 women had received some hormone treatment including combined contraceptive pills (n = 1), progestin during the luteal phase (n = 1), bromociptine (n = 1) and tamoxifen (1 patient for up to 17 months).

The mammographic exploration was performed with a senograph 600 T from General Electric with an automatic exposimetry and using Kodak's MIN-R film. Craneocaudal and medilateral views were obtained for the present study. The films were systematically evaluated by a experienced mammographer in one session without knowledge of the individual clinical characteristics, according to the following criteria:

1. Ratio parenchymal mass/total mammary volume: more than 50 %, 25-50 %, 5-25 %, and less than 5 %.
2. Wedge subcutaneous adipose tissue (expressed in mm) in the upper quadrant at 5 cm from the nipple in both the craneocaudal and the mediolateral views.
3. Subareolar ducts: not visible, partially visible, ducts are visible, all ducts very easily visible.
4. Nipple: normal, slightly retracted, retracted, very retracted.
5. General parenchymal pattern: low density, medium density or high density.
6. Blood vessels: not visible, slightly visible, visible, very visible. Calcified vessels: yes or not.
7. Calcifications: number, type and localization.
8. Skin characteristics: thickened skin: yes or not. Skin folds: yes or not.
9. Anterior fascia identification: not visible, slightly visible, visible, very visible.
10. Concomitant benign lesions.

RESULTS AND COMMENTS

The complete mammographic evaluation is presented in tables 1 to 3. The radiologic semiology of benign and malignant breast diseases have been widely detailed. However, limited information is available on the normal mammary changes occurring in healthy women. The studies of Wolfe (9-11) are based on mammograms from women submitted to biopsies or mastectomies. The marked variation in mammographic appearance of the breast structures in women who do not develop breast cancer makes it difficult to define "normal".

Table 1. Mammary characteristics in premenopausal (first) and postmenopausal (second) phases, and changes between both mammograms. * P<0.01 as compared to the first mammogram.

Mammogram	first	second	changes
1. Parenchymal mass/total breast volume:			
- > 50%	23	9	
- 25-50%	9	13	
- 5-25%	3	11	
- < 5%	0	2	
- No changes			13
- Changes in 1 degree			20
- Changes in 2 degrees			2
2. Adipose tissue in upper quadrant (mm):			
- Right craneocaudal view	13.6 ± 5.8	19.1 ± 8.6 *	
- Right lateral view	16.0 ± 6.8	20.4 ± 7.3 *	
- Left craneocaudal view	14.8 ± 7.4	18.2 ± 7.1 *	
- Left lateral view	16.7 ± 7.7	20.7 ± 8.6 *	
3. Subareolar ducts:			
- Not visible	13	5	
- Partially visible	21	15	
- Ducts are visible	1	13	
- All ducts very easily visible	0	2	
- No changes			13
- Changes in 1 degree			20
- Changes in 2 degrees			2
4. Nipple:			
- Normal	21	11	
- Slightly retracted	10	15	
- Retracted	4	8	
- Very retracted	0	1	
- No changes			20
- Changes in 1 degree			14
- Changes in 2 degrees			1

Table 2. Mammary characteristics in premenopausal (first) and postmenopausal (second) phases, and changes between both mammograms.

Mammogram	first	second	changes
5. *General parenchimal pattern:*			
- Low density	6	15	
- Medium density	8	11	
- High density	21	9	
- No changes			19
- Change in 1 degree			11
- Changes in 2 degrees			5
6. *Blood vessels:*			
- Not visible	5	3	
- Slightly visible	6	1	
- Visible	22	15	
- Very visible	2	16	
- No changes			11
- Change in 1 degree			19
- Changes in 2 degrees			3
- Changes to worse			2
- Calcified vessels	0	2	
7. *Calcifications:*			
- 0	9	5	
- < 5	11	11	
- 5-10	9	8	
- 10-20	3	7	
- > 20	3	6	
- No changes			22
- Change in 1 degree			13
- Anular calcifications	8	12	
- Amorph puntiform	23	25	
- Lineal calcifications	2	2	
- Microcystic calcifications	1	0	

Table 3. Mammographic findings in premenopausal (first) and postmenopausal (second) phases, and changes between both mammograms.

Mammogram	first	second	changes
8. Skin characteristics:			
- Thickened skin	2	7	
- Skin folds	2	2	
9. Anterior fascia identification:			
- Not visible	1	0	
- Slightly visible	11	6	
- Visible	21	10	
- Very visible	2	19	
- No changes			10
- Change in 1 degree			24
- Changes in 2 degrees			1
10. Concomitant benign lesions:			
- No pathology	6	4	
- Fibrocystic disease	25	25	
- Cysts	12	10	
- Retroareolar fibrosis	2	2	
- Ductocele	1	0	
- Fibroadenoma	1	3	
- Paget	0	1	
- Suspicious microcalcifications	0	1	
Global mammary evaluation:			
- Better mammary image			10
- Similar aspect			17
- Changes to worse			6
- New pathology			2

COMMENTS

The radiologic semiology of benign and malignant breast diseases have been widely detailed. However, limited information is available on the normal mammary changes occurring in healthy women. The studies of Wolfe (9-11) are based on mammograms from women submitted to biopsies or mastectomies. The marked variation in mammographic appearance of the breast structures in women who do not develop breast cancer makes it difficult to define "normal".

In our present preliminary study the mammograms were from women attending the outpatient clinic of Gynecology without specific symptoms although the gynecologist indicated breast radiology due to some doubts about inespecific clinical complaints. A high incidence of radiologic images compatible with fibrous mastopathies is detected in the women studied. The radiologic diagnosis of fibrocystic mastopathy exclusively affects the mammographic aspect of the glandular tissue by analogy with the the images obtained in women with the authentic clinical illness. Therefore, the term "fibrocystic mastopathy" of the radiologic semiology does not suppose a clinical reality nor does it correspond to a anatomopathological substratum. Furthermore, the women studied presented clinical symptomolgy making a mammographical study necessary, and, therefore, are possibly not strictly representative of "normal" women.

It seems that during the menopausal transition there is a reduction of parenchymal mass in benefit of fatty tissue which determines that other structures such as blood vesseles, anterior fascia or retroareolar ducts become more visible. In some cases the nipple's tendency to retract was observed, along with the appearance of dispersed calcifications of benign appearance in the parenquyma and arteriolare. In the post-menopause period the lower mammary density facilitates the detection of parenchymatous lesions. However, these date do not constitute an absolute criteria which could define how, when and to what extent a given woman will experience change on reaching the menopause. In order to carry out an in depth study of the physiological mammary evolution during the climacteric period, the evolutionary tendencies should be quantified in terms of time using objective criteria, with a larger population of women, and carrying out periodic studies.

REFERENCES

1. Andersson, I., Andrén, L. and Pettersson, H. (1978). Influence of age at first pregnancy on breast parenchymal patterns: A preliminary report. *Radiology*, **126**, 675-6

2. Grove, J.S., Goodman, M.J., Gilbert, F.I. and Mi, M.P. (1985). Factors associated with mammographic pattern. *Br. J. Radiol.*, **58**, 21-5

3. Leinster, S.J., Walsh, P.V., Whitehouse, G.H. and Al-Sumidae, A.M. (1988). Factors associated with mammographic parenchymal patterns. *Clin. Radiol.*, **39**, 252-6

4. Bland, K.I., Buchanan, J.B., Weisberg, B.F., Hagan, T. and Gray, L.A. (1980). The effects of exogenous estrogen replacement therapy of the breast: Breast cancer risk and mammographic parenchymal patterns. *Cancer*, **45**, 3027-33

5. Bergkvist, L., Tabar, L., Adami, H.O., Persson, I. and Bergström, T. (1989). Mammographic parenchymal patterns in women receiving noncontraceptive estrogen treatment. *Am. J. Epidemiol.*, **130**, 503-10

6. Berkowitz, J.E., Gatewood, O.M.B., Goldblum, L.E. and Gayler, B.W. (1990). Hormonal replacement therapy: Mammographic manifestations. *Radiology*, **174**, 199-201

7. Stomper, P.C., Van Voorhis, B.J., Ravnikar, V.A. and Meyer, J.E. (1990). Mammographic changes associated with postmenopausal hormone replacement therapy. A longitudinal study. *Radiology*, **174**, 487-90

8. Boyd, N.F., O'Sullivan, B., Fshell, E. *et al.* (1984). Mammographic patterns and breast cancer risk: Methodologic standards and contradictory results. *J. Natl. Cancer Inst.*, **72**, 1253-9

9. Wolfe, J.N. (1976). Breast parenchymal patterns and their changes with age. *Radiology*, **121**, 545-52

10. Wolfe, J.N. (1976). Breast patterns as an index of risk for developing breast cancer. *Am. J. Roentgenol.*, **126**, 1130-9

11. Wellings, S.R. and Wolfe, J.N. (1978). Correlative studies of the histological and radiographic appearance of the breast parenchyma. *Radiology*, **129**, 299-306

Parenteral versus oral replacement therapy with estrogens: an overview

A.E. Schindler

Department of Gynecology and Gynecological Oncology, University of Essen, Essen, Germany

INTRODUCTION

The route of estrogen application appears to have different effects when used for hormone replacement therapy in climacteric women. The metabolic consequences are dependent upon the route of application and the type of the estrogen used. The effect on climacteric symptoms is similar for different estrogens, however, dependent upon the dose applied.

The following estrogens and routes of applications will be discussed:

Oral estrogens: Conjugated (equine) estrogens 0,625-1,25 mg/day
        Estrone sulfate 1,5 mg/day
        Estradiol valerate 1-2 mg/day
        Micronized estradiol 2 mg/day

Transdermal estrogen: Estradiol
        a.) patch 0,05 - 0,10 mg/day
        b.) gel 1,5 - 3,0 mg/day

Oral administration of the above mentioned estrogens results in the absorbed steroid being delivered as a bolus to the liver, whereas the nonoral estrogen delivery systems (patch, gel) provide a nearly constant level (1). Nonoral hormone replacement therapy delivers estradiol in a manner similar to the ovary into the systemic circulation and achieves plasma values similar to those observed in women in the reproductive age during the normal menstrual cycle. However, oral estrogen result in daily peak and nadir values (2,3). In addition, meals do influence the circulating estrogen levels by changing

401

gut absorbtion and enterhepatic recirculation (4). Oral estradiol application results predominantly in a rise of estrone versus estradiol, while oral estrone or estrone sulfate as well as the large portion of estrone sulfate contained in the conjugated equine estrogens reaches the circulation to a large extend as estradiol (5,6,7). The differences of oral and transdermal estradiol hormone replacement are shown in Fig. 1.

Due to the differences in the first pass effect of oral estrogens on the liver versus transdermal estradiol there are marked differences in liver protein production such as SHBG, CBG, TBG, Vitamin D binding protein, renin, and factors of coagulation and fibrinolysis with will be eluded to later.

CLINICAL SYMPTOMS

There is general agreement that for instance transdermal estradiol (0,1 mg/day) appears to be equally effective as conjugated estrogens (0,625 or 1,25 mg/day) for controlling postmenopausal symptoms (8,9).

BLEEDING PATTERN

Transdermal estrogens or oral use of 0.3 - 1.25 mg/day of conjugated equine estrogens (dose according to symptoms) resulted in a similar frequency of withdrawal and breakthrough bleedings without and with gestagens (10)

BONE

The exellent effect of oral estrogens on bone has been shown manyfold (11). Recently, it was demonstrated that transdermal estradiol increases bone mass independently of age and time interval after menopause (12). Similar bone mass changes of 0.625 mg/day of conjugated equine estrogens and transdermal estradiol 50 μg/day induce with a 2.8% increase for 1 year similar effects while controls demonstrated a 1.9% decrease during the same time period (13). This is also true, when transdermal estradiol or oral estrogens are combined with gestagens (14,15). A control of the different bone areas is mandatory, since the change in the bone mineral content between the different bones varies greatly (10).

Recently, Lufkin and Ory (16) stated that transdermal E2 is more effective then oral conjugated equine estrogens in maintaining bone mineral density in women with osteoporosis who smoke. Because of the 1:1 ratio of E2/E1 transdermal E2-in addition- may eliviate headaches in patients previously receiving oral estrogens.

Patients with hypercholesterinemia, however, and no other lipid abnormality might be best treated by oral estradiol (16).

Fig. 1: Comparison of oral versus transdermal estradiol

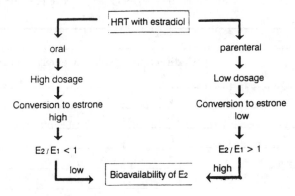

LIPOPROTEINS AND TRIGLYCERIDES

Transdermal estradiol with systemic potency similar to that of oral estradiol had no significant effect on HDL levels or metabolic rates. Thus, the first pass effect of oral estradiol or estrogens in the liver and/or the intestine appears to increase HDL, particularly HDL 3, by increasing HDL production and not by reducing HDL catabolism (17). The HDL/LDL ratio did not change with 50 µg/day of transdermal estradiol and rose significantly with 0,625 mg/day conjugated equine estrogens (18). Among the oral application of estradiol versus estrone sulfate different effects were seen.

Oral estradiol causes a significant increase of total cholesterol, HDL cholesterol, HDL2 cholesterol and triglycerides without effecting HDL. By contrast, estrone sulfate causes a significant decrease of total plasma cholestreol and LDL cholesterol and an increase of HDL cholesterol, HDL2 cholesterol but no change in total triglycerides concentrations (19). Overall, transdermal estradiol might be more beneficial in patients with hypertriglyceridimia and hepatobillary disorders (16).

CARDIOVASCULAR EFFECTS AND HEMOSTASTIS

Estrogen replacement therapy leads to about 50 % reduction in both morbidity and mortality from cardiovascular disease (CVD). At least death from stroke demonstrates a similar positive effect. This seems to apply to oral and transdermal estrogen treatment as well (19). Other factors than lipids may play a role. Recently, it was demonstrated that conjugated estrogens and transdermal estradiol increased factor VII concentration, factor VII antigen and the prothrombin fragment 1 + 2. Conjugated estrogens increased, however, factor VII antigen signifantly higher than transdermal estradiol, while plasminogen activator inhibitor (PAI), the thrombin-antithrombin complex (TAT) and antithrombin III were decreased by oral estrogens (21). A summary of results is shown in table 1.

Table 1: Risk factors of atherosclerosis and CVD and the effect of oral and transdermal estrogens (20)

Risk factor	Risk direction	Oral estrogens	Transdermal estradiol
HDL-2	↓	↑↑	↑
LDL-C	↑	↓	↓
TG	↑	↑	↓
Renin substrate	↑	↑	-
BP	↑	-	↓
Fasting insulinemia	↑	-	-
Vasodilators Prostacyclin	↓		↑
Vascular resistance Carotid artery	↑	?	↓

INSULIN AND GLUCOSE HOMEOSTASIS

Transdermal estradiol appears to cause less negative effects on glucose- and insulin metabolism than oral estrogens (22). Transdermal estradiol even did lead to a decrease of the insulin concentration and an increase in hepatic insulin clearance. Using the oral glucose tolerance test an inreased plasma insulin response was found with transdermal estradiol (23). The HBA 1C remains unchanged under estrogen replacement therapy (24).

INSULIN-LIKE GROWTH FACTOR (IGF-1) AND GROWTH HORMONE (GH)

Oral estrogens cause a reduction in circulating insulin-like growth factor 1 (IGF-1) and an increase in growth hormone. Transdermal estrogen replacement therapy leads to an increase of IGF-1 and no change in GH and GH-bindings proteins (25). IGF-1 probably is further decreased in its action by an increase in IGFBP's with oral estrogens but not with transdermal estradiol. The mitogenic potential of IGF-1 needs to be considered. Therefore, oral estrogens could be to some extent protective to the breast while the effect of the transdermal estradiol needs further studies (26). The long term effect of different binding of estradiol comparing the oral versus the transdermal route for instance on breast tissue but also on endometrium remains to investigated (27).

REFERENCES

1. Campell,S. and Whitehead, M.I. (1982). Potency and hepato cellular effects o estrogens after oral, percutanius and subcutanius administration. In van Keep, P.A., Utian W.H. and Vermeulen A. (eds) The controvercel climacteric, TP. 103-5, (MTB Pres Lancaster)

2. Powers, M.S., Schenkel, L., Darley, P.E., Good, W.R., Balestra ,J.C, and Place, V.A. (1985) Pharmacokinetics and pharmacodynamics of transdermal dosage forms of 17ß-estradiol: comparison with convential oral estrogens used for hormone replacement. *Am. J. Obstet. Gynecol.* 152, 1099-106

3. Scott, R.T. and Anderson, C. (1991). Pharmacokinetics of percutaneous estradiol: A corssover study using a gel and a transdermal system im comparison with oral micronized estradiol. *Obstet. Gynecol.* 77, 758-64

4. Englund, D., Heimer, G. and Johansson, E.D.B. (1984). Influence of food on oestriol blood levels. *Maturitas 6*, 71-5

5. Yen, S.S.C., Martin, P.L., Burnier, A.M., Czekala, N.M., Greaney, M.O. and Callantine, R. (1975). Circulating estradiol, estrone and gonadotropin levels following the administrion of orally active 17ß-estradiol in postmenopausal women. *J.Clin. Endocrinol.Metab.* 40, 518-21

6. Anderson, A.B.M., Sklovsky, E., Sayers, L. Steele, P.A., and Turnbull, A.C. (1978). Comparison of serum oestrogen concentrations in post-menopausal women taking oestrone suphate and oestradiol. *Brit. Med. J.* 3, 140-2

7. Schindler, A.E., Bolt, H.M., Zwirner, M., Hochlehnert, G. and Göser, R. (1982). Comparative pharmacokinetics of oestradiol, oestrone, oestrone sulfate and "conjugated oestrogen" after oral administration. *Arzneim.-Forsch./Drug Res.* 32, 787-91

8. Place, V.A., Powers, M. Darley, P.E., Schenkel, L. and Good, W.R. (1985) A double-blind comparative study of estraderm and premarin in the amelioration of postmenopausal symptoms. *Am. J. Obstet. Gynecol.* 152, 1092-9

9. Lauritzen, C. (1988). Vergleichende Prüfung einer transdermalen Östrogenverabfolgung mittels Pflasteranwendung gegen ein orales Östrogenpräparat. *Münch. Med. Wochenschr.* 130 (Suppl) 66-8

10. Runnebaum, B., Salbach, B. and von Holst, T. (1994). Orale oder transdermale Östrogensubstitutionstherapie im Klimakterium? *Geburtsh. u. Frauenheilk.* 54, 119-30

11. Cheang, A. Sitruk-Ware, R. and Utian, W.H. (1993). A risk-benefit appraisal of transdermal estradiol therapy. *Drug safety* 9, 365-79

12. Lufkin E.G., Heinz, W.W. William, W.M. Hodgson, S.F., Cotowicz, M.A., Laue, A.W. Judd, H.L., Caplan, R.H. and Riggs, B.L. (1992) Treatment of postmenopausal osteoporosis with transdermal estrogens. *Ann. Int. Med.* 117, 1-9

13. Castelo-Branco, C., Pons, F. and Gonzalez-Merlo, J. (1993). Bone mineral density in surgically postmenopausal women receiving hormonal replacement therapy as assessed by dual photon absorptiometry. *Maturitas* 16, 133-7

14. Adami, S., Suppi, R. Bertoldo, F., Rossini, M. Residori, M., Marscu, V. and Lo Cascio, V. (1989). Transdermal estradiol in the treatment of postmenopausal boneloss. *Bone Mineral* 7, 79-86

15. Stevenson, J.C., Custe, M.P., Ganger, K.F., Hillard, T.C., Lees, B. and Whitehead, M.I. (1990). Effects of transdermal versus oral hormone replacement therapy on bone density in spile and proximal famur in postmenopausal women. *Lancet* 335, 265-9

16. Lufkin, E.G. and Ory, S.J. (1994). Relative value of transdermal and oral estrogen therapy in various clinical situations. *Mayo Clin. Proc.* 69, 131-5

17. Walsh, B.W., Li, H. and Sacks, F.M. (1994) Effects of postmenopausal hormone replacement with oral and transdermal estrogen on high density lipoprotein metabolism. *J. Lipid Res.* 35, 2083-93
18. Adami, S., Rossini, M., Zamberlan, N., Bertoldo, F., Dorizzi, R. and Lo Cascio, V. (1993) Long-term effects of transdermal and oral estrogens on serum lipids and lipoproteins in postmenopausal women. *Maturitas* 17, 191-6
19. Colvin, P.L., Auerbach, B.J., Koritnik, D.R., Hazzard, W.R. and Applebaum-Bowden, D. (1990= Differential effects of oral eestrone versus 17ß-estradiol on lipoproteins in postmenopausal women. J. Clin. Endocrinol. Metab. 70, 1568-73
20. Cheang, A., Sitruk-Ware, R. and Samsioe, G. (1994). Transdermal oestradiol and cardiovascular risk factors. *Brit. J. Obestet. Gynecol.* 101, 571-81
21. Kroon, U.-B., Silfverstolpe, G. and Tengborn,L. (1994) The effects of transdermal estradiol and oral conjugated estrogens on haemostasis variables. *Thrombosis and Haemostasis* 71, 420-3
22. Stevenson, J.C., Crook, D. Godsland, I.F., Lees, B. and Whitehead, M.I. (1993) Oral versus transdermal hormone replacement therapy. *Int. J. Fertil.* 38 (Suppl), 30-5
23. Cagnacci, A., Soldani, R., Carriero, P.L., Paoletti, A.M., Fioretti, P. and Melis, G.B. (1992) Effects of low doses of transdermal 17 beta-eestradiol on carbohydrate metabolism in postmenopausal women. *J. Clin. Endocrinol. Metab.* 74, 1396-400
24. Mosnier-Pudar, H., Faguer, B. Guyenne, T.T. and Tchobroutsky, G. (1991) Effects of deprivation and replacement by percutaneous 17 beta estradiol and oral progesterone on blood pressure and metabolic parameters in menopause patients with non-insulin-dependent diabetes. *Arch. Mal. Coeur Vaiss.* 84, 1111-5
25. Weissberger, A.J., Ho, K.K.Y. and Lazarus, L. (1991) Contrasting effects of oral and transdermal routes of estrogen replacement therapy on 24-hour growth hormone (GH) secretion, insulin-like growth factor I, and GH-binding protein in postmenopausal women. *J. Clin. Endocrinol. Metab.* 72, 374-81
26. Campagnoli, C., Lesca, L., Cantamessa, C. and Peris, C. (1993) Long-term hormone replacement treatment in menopause: new choices, old apprehensions, recent findings. *Maturitas* 18, 21-46
27. Ricci, G., Marchesan, E., Malisano, M. Alberico, S., Pregazzi, R. Radillo, L, Dussi, R. and Mangiarotti, M.A. (1993) Circulating hormone levels in postmenopausal women receiving transdermal estrogen replacement therapy: comparison with oral administration (Abstr. of paper) Intern. Symp. on Women's Health in Menopause, Behav., Cancer, Cardiosvasc. Dis., Hormone Replacement Ther. Milan (Italiy), Sept. 69-29, 1993. Final Program and Abstr. Book. Milano, Univ. degli. Studi. s.a. 54

Comparison of oral and transdermal hormone replacement therapy: a multicenter study with a new transdermal system

J. Herold, B. Sajtos*, U.H. Winkler** and A.E. Schindler**

Gynecological Practice, Munich, *Rhône-Poulenc Rorer, Cologne and **Department of Gynecology and Gynecological Oncology, University of Essen, Germany

INTRODUCTION

Life expectancy for women in developed countries increased in average to 82 years. This leads to the fact, that women are living over a third of their lives after the menopause. Therefore the use of Hormone Replacement Therapy (HRT) to diminish the risk of major health disorders related to the lack of estrogens will be an increasing concern to gynecologists. The benefits of HRT in the prevention of postmenopausal osteoporosis (1-5) and cardiovascular diseases (6-10) are undeniable.

The majority of prescriptions for HRT are still for oral peparations, but this route of administration can be associated with adverse effects on carbohydrate and protein metabolism, presumably because of first-pass hepatic metabolism. On the other hand the cutaneous application of estrogen as a patch has several benefits including achieving steady state serum estrogen levels over the three to four day wearing period and achieving premenopausal serum estrogen levels and estrogen pattern.

At present, there is mainly one estradiol containing transdermal therapeutic system prescribed for postmenopausal HRT. In opposite to the conventional reservoir-based technology of this patch, where the estradiol is solubilized in an alcohol containing gel enclosed in a drug reservoir, a new Matrixpatch was recently developed. This new technology allows a much thinner, discrete and flexible transdermal system.

The aim of this investigation was to examine the efficacy, safety and acceptability of this new Matrixpatch in the treatment of menopausal complaints in comparison to the well established oral treatment with conjugated equine estrogens.

MATERIAL AND METHODS

In an open, randomized, parallelgroup, multicenter study 166 postmenopausal women in the age of 45-65 years were included by practicing gynecologists. Randomization was performed by telephone contact. Women were included with FSH levels >40 IU/L and at least 3 hot flushes per day measured during a 7-14 days screening period. Patients were excluded from the study if they had taken any hormonal replacement therapy within seven days before sreening; with known or suspected estrogen dependent malignancy; with undiagnosed vaginal bleedings or severe diseases of the renal, hepatic or cardiac system. Further exclusion criteria were known allergic reactions against transdermal systems und abuse of alcohol, drugs or nicotine. Written informed consent was obtained from all patients prior to the screening period.

The treatment period for both groups extended over 3 cycles of 28 days. Patients in the transdermal group recieved 6 patches (50 μg estradiol/day) twice weekly per cycle using a 3 week on/1 week off treatment regimen. A progestagen (medrogeston, 5mg/day) was to be taken during the last 11 days of the estrogen therapy. In the control group oral equine conjugated estrogen (0,625 mg/day) was applied with an additional progestagen (medrogeston, 5mg/day) in the same treatment regimen.

During the course of the study patients contacted the gynecologist 5 times. The main efficacy parameter, the number of hot flushes per day, was recorded in a patient diary. The intensity of other postmenopausal symptoms was registered by the Kuppermann Index. Estradiol and FSH levels were measured before the start of treatment and at the end of the third cycle. The tolerance of both treatments as well as the acceptance of the patch was monitored. By using the Clinical Gobal Impression Index (CGI) the gynecologist could judge the success of the therapy in terms of efficacy and safety.

RESULTS

The demographic data as well as the consumption of alcohol and nicotine was comparable in both treatment groups. Physiological menopause was observed in 90 % of the enrolled patients, 10 % were menopausal due to ovarectomy. 20 % of the patients in the control group discontinued the treatment prematurely, whereas all patients of the transdermal group finished the study according to protocol.

The mean number of hot flushes per day was reduced during therapy from 6.2 to 0.8 in the transdermal group and from 6.1 to 1.1 in the control group. The main effect of the therapy was noticed in both groups during the first cycle of therapy (1.7 hot flushes per day in the transdermal group, 2.2 in the control group). At the beginning of treatment the intensity of the postmenopausal symptoms measured by the Kuppermann Index was classified as moderate to severe in 81.7 % (transdermal group) and in 80.6 % (control group) of the patients. After the end of therapy 95.0 % of the patients in the transdermal group were free of symptoms whereas 5 % mentioned slight complaints. In the control group 90.7 % were free of symptoms whereas 9.3 % still suffered from slight to moderate symptoms. The influnce of both treatments on the intensity of the different postmenopausal symptoms described by the Kuppermann Index was similar with a slight advantage for the patch especially for the symptoms hot flushes, sweatening and lack of concentration. All differences were statistically not significant.

The blood levels of Estradiol and FSH before and after therapy are given in the following figure:

Fig. I: (Boxplot, n=68):

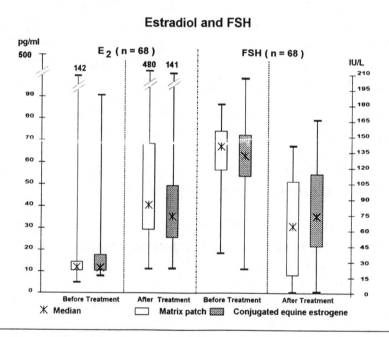

The overall trend of the study towards comparable results in both treatment groups was also observed for the CGI. Regarding the intensity of the postmenopausal symptoms a significant improvement could also be noticed in both groups by using this index.

The use of the patch was judged as very simple to simple by 88.3 %of the patients. 85.0 % asked for a continuation of the therapy with this patch. Only 15 % refused further transdermal therapy.

Both drugs were well tolerated. The rate of side effects was 17.2 % in the transdermal group and 20,7 % in the control group. Only 3.2 % of the patients in the transdermal group mentioned slight cutaneous side effects (redness, allergic reaction). Serious adverse events were reported in 1.6 % of the transdermal group and 3.2 % of the control group. Only in one case of the control group the relation to the medication was rated as possible (thrombosis).

CONCLUSION

Both drugs induced a clincally relevant reduction of the postmenopausal symptoms. Major differences concerning the efficacy did not exist. The clinical effect fit very well with the serum blood levels of Estradiol and FSH, which have been achieved with both application forms. The systemic tolerance of the new Matrixpatch was comparable to the oral control group. The rate of the cutaneous side effects was very low in comparison to the published data with other transdermal systems. Due to these results it can be stated that this new Matrixpatch is a convincing therapeutic alternative to the existing therapeutic tools, which is especially underlined by the high acceptance of this patch by the patients.

REFERENCES

1. T. A. Hutchinson, S. M. Polansky and A. R. Feinstein. Postmenopausal oestrogens protect against fractures of hip and distal radius. A case-control study. *Lancet*, 1979; 2: 705

2. R. Lindsay, D. M. Hart, J. M. Aitken et al. Long-term prevention of postmenopausal osteoporosis by oestrogen. Evidence for an increased bone mass after delayed onset of oestrogen treatment. *Lancet*, 1976; 1: 1038

3. N. Munk-Jensen, S. Pors Nielsen, E. B. Obel et al. Reversal of postmenopausal vertebral bone loss by oestrogen and progestogen: a double blind placebo controlled study. *Br Med J [Clin Res Ed]*, 1998; 296: 1150

4. R. L. Prince, M. Smith, I. M. Dick et al. Prevention of postmenopausal osteoporosis. A comparative study of exercise, calcium supplementation, and hormone-replacement therapy. *N Engl. J Med*, 1991; 325: 1189

5. M. E. Quigley, P. L. Martin, A. M. Burnier et al. Estrogen therapy arrest bone loss in elderly women. *Am J Obstet Gynecol*, 1987; 156: 1516

6. T. L. Bush, E. Barrett-Connor, L. D. Cowan et al. Cardiovascular mortality and noncontraceptive use of estrogen in women : results from the Lipid Research Clinics Program follow-up study. *Circulation*, 1987; 75: 1102

7. H. W. Gruchow, A. J. Anderson, J. J. Barboriak et al. Postmenopausal use of estrogen and occlusion of coronary arteries. *Am Heart J*, 1988; 115: 954

8. R. H. Knopp. Cardiovascular effects of endogenous and exogenous sex hormones over a woman's lifetime. *Am J Obstet Gynecol*, 1988; 158: 1630

9. R. A. Lobo. Cardiovascular implications of estrogen replacement therapy. *Obstet Gynecol*, 1990; 75 (Suppl): 18S

10. M. J. Stampfer, W. C. Willet, G. A. Colditz et al. A prospective study of postmenopausal estrogen therapy and coronary artery disease. *N Eng J Med*, 1985; 313: 1044

77

Estrogen–androgen hormone replacement therapy

M.M. Gelfand

Department of Obstetrics and Gynecology, McGill University and Jewish General Hospital, Montreal, Quebec, Canada

For many women, the middle years of 40-60 are a time that is relatively free from previous obligations surrounding child-bearing and rearing, offering new opportunities for educational and personal fulfilment -- at work, at home or in the community.[1] The physiological changes that result from a decrease in ovarian hormone levels, however, can have a significant impact on a woman's physical and mental health.

The postmenopausal period has been described as a time when a woman lives in a "catabolic milieu" or a state of breakdown of many of her physical systems.[2] Much emphasis has been placed on the use of estrogen replacement therapy (ERT) to alleviate the physical results of estrogen depletion, including urogenital atrophy, vasomotor symptoms, bone loss and adverse cardiovascular consequences.[3] Far too little attention has been given to changes that occur as a result of decreases in androgen production -- including impairment of a woman's emotional and sexual functioning. Despite the fact that recent research has demonstrated the positive impact of estrogen-androgen hormone replacement therapy (EA-HRT) on sexual interest and satisfaction, sense of well-being and osteoporosis, this therapy option is still not widely used or even discussed with patients.[4,5]

Lack of physician/patient discussion about the risks and benefits of hormone replacement therapy (HRT) and all available therapeutic options contributes to poor patient compliance, one of the major problems impeding successful therapy outcome. It is estimated that 50% of women taking ERT stop therapy within twelve months, and 20-30% never even have their prescriptions filled. This summary reviews the current research and clinical application of EA-HRT.

The frequency of ovulation slows after age 40, after which women experience various physical manifestations of declining estrogen production. This time in a woman's life, known

413

as the climacteric, ends with the cessation of menses, or menopause at age 48-55.[1]

For many years physicians focused solely on the consequences of estrogen depletion following menopause. We now know that progesterone levels fall as well, and that androgens - - also secreted by the ovary -- are decreased at this time.[3,6] Following menopause, a woman's total estrogen production decreases by 66%, and androgen production decreases by as much as 50%.[5] Surgically menopausal women experience an even greater decrease in androgen production.[3]

These hormonal changes bring 50-60% of women into their physician's office for relief of symptoms, including disturbances in menstrual pattern, vasomotor instability (hot flashes), vaginal atrophic conditions such as dyspareunia and pruritus, and psychological problems of anxiety, depression, decreased libido and insomnia.[1]

Many of these symptoms can result in a woman's decreased sense of well-being and can have a major impact on quality of life. While there is controversy over which of the psychological symptoms are estrogen-related, recent research has shown that the level of androgens is directly related to a woman's sense of well-being, energy, mood, and quality of life.[5]

In several double-blind, placebo-controlled crossover studies conducted in our clinic, we have shown that women who had a total hysterectomy and salpingo-oophorectomy showed improvement in energy, well-being, sexuality and depression after a parenteral dose of androgen along with estrogen.[7,8] Women who lose their ovaries suffer a precipitous fall in both estrogen and androgen levels, thus forming an ideal test group for the evaluation of estrogen and/or androgen administration on physical and psychological symptoms in women.

One study clearly demonstrated that estrogen alone was not more effective than placebo on energy level improvement or enhanced feelings of well-being. In contrast, increased testosterone levels had a positive effect on these factors as well as increasing appetite. The superior performance of the androgen-containing preparations may stem from the anabolic and energizing properties of this sex steroid, as well as the possibility that androgens may interact directly with the hypothalamus, pituitary and limbic system.[7,8]

In addition, Sherwin has reported that women taking combination estrogen/androgen were more composed, upbeat, and energetic than women who were taking estrogen alone or placebo.[9]

A primary role for an androgen component in HRT is in the augmentation of sexual motivation. Studies by Sherwin and Gelfand have demonstrated that sexual arousal is enhanced by the administration of exogenous androgens in postmenopausal women. In addition, the studies have shown that sexual fantasies increase and the level of sexual desire is heightened.

Another potential role of estrogen-androgen therapy is in delaying the onset of senile vaginal changes in postmenopausal women. Studies have revealed a link between sexual activity, increased levels of circulating androgens and a decrease in vaginal atrophy.[10]

A further advantage in adding androgens to HRT is its promise of decreased osteoporotic development beyond what estrogens can offer. Estrogens alone have been found to reduce the rate of bone loss following menopause. Estrogen slows the rate of bone remodelling and hence decreases the rate of bone loss. However, estrogen does not cause a noticeable increase in bone mass. Although an initial small increase may occur in the first two years of treatment, bone mass remains stable after this point.

The added effect of androgens is its stimulation of osteoblastic activity and also an anti-osteoclastic effect stemming from the peripheral conversion of androgens into estrone. Evidence continues to grow that intramuscular-administered androgens can increase bone mass and perhaps decrease fracture rates. Research has also related a decreased incidence of vertebral crush fractures to an increase in circulating levels of androgen.[11] Studies also indicated that injectable androgen increased Bone Mineral Content and Lean Body Mass while decreasing Fat Mass.[12]

Testosterone has been used in the supplementary treatment of breast cancer. It has been used in the management of endometriosis. It is possible that testosterone like Tamoxifen is an agonist on the endometrium and antagonist on breast tissue. We are reviewing the large numbers of patients in our clinical who have been on EA-HRT for 30 years. In a recent publication Lovell has stated that "in a menopause clinic practice of approximately 4,000 patients treated almost exclusively with subdermal (estradiol and testosterone pellets) or injection of estradiol and testosterone cypionate, a marked statistical difference (lower incidence) was found as compared to the general and other population groups...The author feels the principal variable is the inclusion of testosterone. Estradiol serum levels are maintained at 190-650 pg/dl."[13]

Clinical Guidelines for the Use of EA-HRT

Thinkograms III and IV[2] clearly demonstrate the positive and negative aspects of using EA-HRT or EA-HRT with added progestin.

CONCLUSION

It is clear that physicians need to address the full spectrum of menopause-related effects, not just the physical symptoms. It is also essential to devote enough time with patients to discuss all of the available options for hormone replacement therapy. The important role of EA-HRT in alleviating many of the symptoms of surgical and natural menopause can no longer be overlooked.

THINKOGRAM III

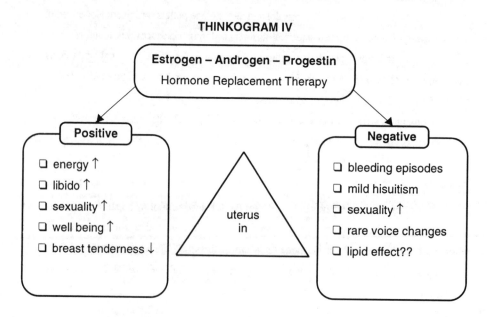

M.M. Gelfand. Estrogen-androgen hormone replacement therapy, Chapter 10. In *Hormone Replacement Therapy*, Donald P. Swartz (ed). Williams & Wilkins, Baltimore, Maryland, September 1992.

THINKOGRAM IV

M.M. Gelfand. Estrogen-androgen hormone replacement therapy, Chapter 10. In *Hormone Replacement Therapy*, Donald P. Swartz (ed). Williams & Wilkins, Baltimore, Maryland, September 1992.

REFERENCES

1. Speroff L. Menopause and hormone replacement therapy. Clin Geriatr Med Veb 1993;9(1):33-35.

2.ʹ Gelfand MM. Estrogen-androgen hormone replacement therapy. Hormone Replacement Therapy, DP Swartz (ed), Williams & Wilkins, Baltimore, MD, 1991.

3. Bachmann GA. Estrogen-androgen therapy for sexual and emotional well-being. The Female Patient 1993;18:15-16.

4. Hallstrom T. Sexuality in the climacteric. Clin Obstet Gynecol 1977:4.

5. Young RL. Androgens in postmenopausal therapy. Menopause Management, 5/1993:21-24.

6. Gelfand MM. When estrogen-androgen should be used in treating postmenopausal women. OBG Management supplement: S-6, S-7, S-8.

7. Sherwin BB, Gelfand MM. Differential symptom response to parenteral estrogen and/or androgen administration in the surgical menopause. Am J Ob Gyn January 15, 1985;151:159.

8. Sherwin BB, Gelfand MM, et al. Androgen enhances sexual motivation in females: a prospective, cross-over study of sex steroid administration in the surgical menopause. Psychosomatic Med, July 1985:47(2):339-351.

9. Sherwin BB. Affective changes with estrogen and androgen replacement therapy in surgically menopausal women. J Affect Disord 1988;14:177.

10. Leiblum S, Bachmann G, et al. Vaginal atrophy in the postmenopausal woman. JAMA, April 22/29, 1983;249:2198.

11. Longcope C, Baker RS, et al. Androgen and estrogen dynamics in women with vertebral crush fractures. Maturitas 1984;6:309.

12. Hassager C, Reis BJ, et al. Nandrolone decanoate treatment of postmenopausal osteoporosis for two years and effects of withdrawal. Maturitas 1989;11:4 305-317.

13. Lovell CW. Breast cancer incidence with parenteral estradiol and testosterone replacement therapy. Menopause - Abst North Am Menopause Soc 1994;1(3):150.

Effect of conjugated estrogens on skin thickness: a randomized, double-blind, placebo-controlled study

R. Maheux

Research Centre, Saint-François d'Assise Hospital and Department of Obstetrics and Gynecology, Quebec City, Quebec, Canada

Background: The number of women aged 60 years and older will approach 350 million by the year 2000 (1). During the past few decades, several studies have documented the deleterious impact of menopause on bone mass (2-3). Estrogen replacement therapy stops bone loss associated with menopause and can thus prevent the development of symptomatic osteoporosis and fracture (4,5). Despite a better understanding of the benefits of estrogen replacement therapy, on average only 15% of postmenopausal women in the U.S.A. receive estrogens (6). This disappointing figure can be partially explained by the fact that the medical profession has concentrated on climacteric diseases such as osteoporosis which, although quite important, are insidious and not readily apparent. Indeed, the less obvious benefits of estrogen replacement therapy has been stressed, whereas the visible ones on the skin have never been addressed in a randomized, placebo-controlled clinical trial.

Objective: The purpose of this study was to assess the effects of the oral administration of conjugated estrogens therapy on skin thickness in a randomized, double-blind, placebo-controlled study.

Study Design: Sixty postmenopausal women were randomly allocated to conjugated estrogens or placebo treatment for twelve months. Inclusion criteria were: Weight of ± 20% of the normal weight for age as predicted by the Metropolitan Life Insurance form; age from 50 to 75 years old; non-smoker; menopause confirmed by one of the following: 1) serum follicule-stimulating hormone (FSH) > 40 IU/L, 2) amenorrhea > 6 months with hot flushes, 3) a previous history of bilateral oophorectomy; no evidence of endometrial premalignant or malignant lesion confirmed by one of the following: i) previous hysterectomy, ii) normal endometrial biopsy, iii) negative medroxyprogesterone acetate challenge test (absence of vaginal bleeding after daily drug administration of 10 mg for 10 days) and endometrial thickness at ultrasound < 3 mm.
Exclusion criteria were: Skin disorders such as extensive burns, scars or psoriasis; a past or present history of Cushing syndrome; corticosteroid treatment; acromegaly; sclerodermia; lupus

erythematosus; rheumatoid arthritis; diabetes mellitus; thyroid disease; acute or severe chronic liver diseases; thromboembolic or ischemic cardiac disease; classic migraine; diastolic blood pressure > 95 mm HG; breast or endometrial cancer; pharmacologic treatment of hyperlipidemia.

Neither the participants nor the investigators were aware of the group allocation. Skin thickness was measured by ultrasound using an Acuson 128 (Acuson Corporation,Ca,U.S.A.), with a linear 7.5 megaHertz probe adjusted for thyroid resolution (lateral resolution, 0 mm, power =-3 decibels, 55 decibels= 2/2/0, gain = -17 to 23 decibels, depth of field= 4 cm). All tests were carried out by the same technician, video-recorded and interpreted by the same radiologist. Evaluations were performed at 3 sites: the right thyroid lobe between the common carotid and the right jugular vein, 2 cm below the umbilicus, and the right thigh 3 cm below the great trochanter. Skin thickness was measured by ultrasound at baseline, and after 6 and 12 months of treatment.

Bone mineral content of the lumbar spine (L2-L4) and femoral neck was measured by dual photon absorptiometry (Sophos, Sopha, Paris, France).

Hormones (FSH and LH) were measured in duplicate by double antibody radioimmunoassay (RIA), using kits obtained from Diagnosis Products Corporation (Los Angeles, CA, USA distributed by Inter Medico, Markham, Ontario, Canada). The lowest curve calibrators were 0.8 IU/l (2nd IRP 78/549) for FSH and 1.8 IU/l (WHO 1st IRP 68/40) for LH. Serum estradiol was measured by competitive immunoassay based on antibody-coated tubes (commercial kits: Coat-A-Count, Diagnosis Product Corporation, Los Angeles, CA, USA distributed by Inter Medico, Markham, Ontario, Canada). Hormonal assessments were not made available to the investigators prior to the completion of the study.

Cholesterol and triglyceride concentrations were measured with a Hitachi 705 analyzer using Boehringer Mannheim calibrators (Precical 62010, lot XLS-64) and reagents (Boehringer Mannheim Canada). High-density lipoprotein cholesterol (HDL-C) was evaluated using the heparin-MnCl2 precipitation method (7,8). Serum alkaline phosphatase was measured on a 704 BM/Hitachi system using Boehringer Mannheim calibrators and reagents. Both serum and 24-hour urine calcium determinations were performed using CIBA-CORNING calcium reagents (manufactured by Ciba Corning Diagnostics Corp. Oberlin, Ohio 44074 USA).

Twenty-four hour urinary hydroxyproline and creatinine were measured using Prockop and Udenfriend (9) and Jaffe methods respectively. Quality of life and adverse events were recorded at each visit and at the end of treatment.

Results: No inter or between-group differences were observed in their age, weigh and height.

A statistically significant (p<0.01) increase in skin thickness compared to baseline (T0), as measured by ultrasound was observed after 12 months of conjugated estrogen treatment at the level of the great trochanter, whereas no change in skin thickness occurred in the control group. Baseline skin thickness was 2.41 mm ± 0.07 and 2.45 mm ± 0.06 for the placebo and conjugated estrogens groups respectively (N.S); 2.44 mm ± 0.07 and 2.55 mm ± 0.07 after 6 months and 2.50 mm ± 0.06 and 2.73 mm ± 0.07 after 12 months of treatment. There was no significant differences in skin thickness at the thyroid and subumbilical levels, although a similar trend was observed.

In the placebo group, there were no significant changes in

circulating hormones, lipids, and in serum and urine biochemistry, whereas there was a significant (p<0.05) decrease in bone mineral content both at L_2-L_4 and femoral neck.

In the conjugated estrogens group, where serum E2 levels rose significantly above baseline (p<0.0001), there was no significant bone loss with a significant decrease in alkaline phosphatase (p<0.01). However urinary calcium and hydroxyproline/creatinine ratios did not change significantly. There was a significant increase in the HDL-C fraction (p<0.01). Quality of life was reported to be improved (p<0.05) in women treated with estrogen compared to the placebo group.

Eleven (11) women reported at least one episode of vaginal bleeding during the study and seven (7) others reported monthly withdrawal bleeding. All were in the conjugated estrogens group.

Six (6) women in the placebo group and one in the estrogens group reported worsening of their hot flushes. However, these differences are not statistically significant and none of the subjects required clonidine medication.

Conclusion: This is the first randomized, double-blind, placebo-controlled study addressing the effects of estrogen replacement therapy on skin thickness. A 11.5% increase (p<0.01) in skin thickness were observed after 12 months' administration of 0.625 mg of conjugated estrogens, without any significant change in the placebo treated.

These results may help postmenopausal women to better appraise the benefits of estrogen replacement therapy and provide further evidence of the potential of conjugated estrogens in preventing skin aging.

REFERENCES

1. Dickfalusy E. Introduction: Menopause, Developing Countries, and the 21st Century. In: Mishell DR, ed. Menopause: Physiology and pharmacology. Los Angeles: Year Book Medical Publishers 1987:1-19.

2. Lindsay R, Hart DM, MacLean A, et al. Bone response to termination of oestrogen treatment. Lancet 1978;i:1325-1327.

3. Brincat M, Kabalan S, Studd JWW, Moniz CF, de Trafford J, Montgomery J. A study of the decrease of skin collagen content, skin thickness, and bone mass in the postmenopausal women. Obstet Gynecol 1987;70:840-5.

4. Linsay R, Hart DM, Clark DM. The minimum effective dose of estrogen for prevention of postmenopausal bone loss. Obstet Gynecol 1984;63:759-763.

5. Lindsay R, Hart DM, Aitken JM, et al. Long-term prevention of postmenopausal osteoporosis by oestrogen. Lancet 1976;i:1038-1041.

6. Fox R. More than hot flushes, editorial. Lancet 1991;338:917-8.

7. Warnick GR, Cheung MC, Albers JJ. Comparison of current methods for high-density lipoprotein cholesterol quantification. Clin Chem 1979;25:596-604.

8. Ruiz-Albuisac JM, Velasquez E, Montes A. Differential precipitation of isolated human plasma lipoproteins with heparin and manganese chloride. Clin Chem 1988;34:240-43.

9. Prockop DJ, Udenfriend S. A specific method for the analysis of hydroxyproline in tissues and urine. Anal Biochem 1960;1:228-230.

Minimizing the untoward effects of progestin in hormonal replacement therapy

A. Kauppila, T. Raudaskoski and E. Suvanto-Luukkonen

Department of Obstetrics and Gynecology, University of Oulu, Finland

Introduction

In hormonal replacement therapy (HRT), cyclically or continuously administered progestin counteracts estrogen-induced endometrial mitotic activity and proliferation thus effectively preventing endometrial transformation to hyperplastic or malignant. The protective effect of a combination of estrogen and progestin on the endometrium has been confirmed in many studies. The cyclical combination of progestin to estrogen results in regular menstrual-like bleedings, which have been experienced as unpleasant by about 80 % of postmenopausal women (1). Most of the progestins used in the present treatment formulas are 19-nortestosteroid derivatives which may interfere with lipid and lipoprotein metabolism (2). In addition, progestin does not prevent the risk of breast cancer in women exposed to long-term estrogen treatment.

It is possible that the progestin-induced harmful side-effects associated with the conventional combination of HRT:s could be avoided using new treatment strategies. These should be aimed at keeping the endometrium quiescent while not affecting lipid metabolism. These goals in mind we planned two clinical trials which are presented briefly in this paper.

We first evaluated the clinical usefulness of a levonorgestrel (LNG) releasing intrauterine device in postmenopausal women receiving estrogen (3). The device was developed primarily for hormonal contraception and it is safe and effective in this respect (4). It is T shaped and contains a cylinder with 52 mg of LNG covered by a membrane, which controls the LNG release at a rate of 20ug/24 hours. Preliminary observations have previously shown that it can also be used during the postmenopausal years in women treated with estrogen (5).

Because natural progesterone does not alter lipid metabolism, we also wanted to evaluate its value in HRT when used continuously in micronized form with percutaneous estrogen. This combination was compared with LNG-IUD and percutaneous estrogen combination (6). The trial is still going on. Therefore the results concerning natural progesterone in HRT are predominantly from recent Belgian (7) and French (8) studies. Only preliminary observations are so far available from our trial.

Levonorgesterel releasing IUD in HRT
Forty postmenopausal women entered the trial. They were randomly allocated to be treated with either transdermal estradiol patches (Estraderm, Ciba-Geigy) and LNG-IUD (Study group) or an established regimen of a continuous oral dose of 2 mg of estradiol valerate and 1 mg of norethisterone acetate (Kliogest, Novo, Copenhagen, Denmark) daily (Control group). The LNG-IUD was inserted after a one month's pretreatment with estrogen.

Fifteen women in the study group completed the one-year trial. Two women discontinued the trial during the estrogen therapy before insertion of the IUD (one because of itching, one because of pelvic pain). In one case, cervical stenosis prevented insertion of the IUD, and two women suffering from continuous bleeding wanted the device to be be removed after 6 and 9 weeks of use. The continuation rate one year after IUD insertion was thus 88 %, which is similar to that in women using the device for contraception. Three women in the control group withdrew from the trial because of bleeding disorders (No 2) or headache (No 1).

The treatment modalities relieved climacteric symptoms effectively with no differences between the groups. Spotting was more common in the women with an IUD (14/15) than in those on oral therapy (9/17) for the first 4 months, but after this the small proportion of women with no bleeding was similar in both groups. Amenorrhoea developed sooner in the control group than in the study group. Most women with a LNG-IUD were amenorrhoeic or suffered only from slight spotting disorders at 4 months of therapy.

At ultrasonographic examination the endometrium was approximately 4.4 mm thick in the LNG-IUD group and 3.0-3.3 in the control group. The difference was due predominantly to the IUD. In cytological examination at 12 months the endometrium was atrofic in both groups, with some progestin-induced decidual changes, however, in the IUD users. No signs of hyperplacia were observed.

All 15 patients in the LNG-group wanted to continue with the present treatment after one year as the women in the control group did with their therapy. These findings indicate that the compliance of LNG-IUD is good in postmenopausal women treated with estrogen. The results also suggest that LNG-IUD provides a convenient method to counteract the endometrial side-effects of exogenous estrogen in postmenopausal women.

Simultaneous administration of natural progesterone and estrogen

Data concerning the simultaneous administration of oral natural progesterone and transcutaneous estradiol is available on a large scale from a French study (8). Ninety-two women participated in this multicentre study. Estrogen was applied daily in gel form (Estrogel, Besins Iscovesco, Paris, France) at a dose of 1.5 mg a day during the 1-25 days of each calandar month. Natural micronized progesterone (Utrogestan, Besins Iscovesco, Paris France) was given orally, 100 mg per day on the same days.

Ninety-two % of women were amenorrhoeic at the end of the 6-month trial. In accordance with clinical findings, the biopsy showed that the endometrium was thin and atrophic. However, some mitosis or mild secretory features appeared in about 30 % of the cases. Similar observations regarding clinical findings and endometrial responses were also made in the study of Foidart and coworkers (7). This combination effectively alleviated climacteric symptoms in both studies (7,8). This was also the case in our study (6) in which 13 out of 18 patients treated with percutaneous estradiol (Estrogel) and oral progesterone (Utrogestan, 100 mg a day) were amenorrhoeic after one year´s therapy, a result (72 %) which is somewhat lower than that in the French study (8). Possibly the administration of estradiol without any break in our trial explains the difference. Our preliminary observations also indicate that natural progesterone can be used as a supplement to estrogen in the hormonal replacement therapy of postmenopausal women. In this study (6), the treatment with a LNG-IUD in conjunction with coninuous percutaneous estradiol (Estrogel) resulted in amenorrhoea in 16 out of 18 women (89%). This finding further supports the clinical uselfulness of LNG-releasing IUD as a supplement to estradiol therapy in postmenopausal women.

The dissatisfaction of many women concerning the use of HRT during the postmenopausal years is caused by withdrawal bleeding. Therefore, there is a great demand for non-bleeding regimens which are being developed in many centres today. The present treatment modalities provide interesting alternatives for this purpose.

References.

1. Lind T, Cameron EC, Hunter WM, Leon C, Moran PF, Oxley A, Gerrard J, Lind UCG. A prospective controlled trial of six forms of hormone replacement therapy given to postmenopausal women. Br J Obstet Gynaecol 1979 (suppl) 86:1-29.

2. Hirvonen E, Mälkönen M, Manninen V. Effects of different progestogens on lipoproteins during postmenopausal replacement therapy. N Engl J Med 1981;304:560-

3. Raudaskoski T, Lahti E, Kauppila A, Apaja-Sarkkinen M A, Laatikainen T J. Transdermal estrogen with a levonorgestrel-releasing intrauterine device for climacteric complaints: clinicAl and endometrial responses. Amer J Obstet Gynecol. In press.

4. Nilsson CG, Johansson EDB, Luukkainen T. A d-norgestrel releasing IUD. Contraception 1975;13:503-14.

5. Andersson K, Mattson L-Å, Rybo G, Stadberg E. Intrauterine release of levonorgesterel - a new way of adding progesteron in hormone replacement therapy. Obstet Gynecol 1992;79:963-7.

6. Suvanto-Luukkonen E. Sundström H, Penttinen J, Kauppila A. Endometrial suppression by levonorgestrel-releasing IUD or oral/vaginal natural natural miccronized progesterone during percutaneous estradiol treatment in menopause. Acta Obstet Gynecol Scand. 1994, Suppl 161: 73:105.

7. Foidart JM, Dombrowicz N, Greimers R, Smet M, de Lignières B. Endometrial tolerance of long-term combined hormone replacement therapy: analysis of the cell cycle. In: Hormone replacement therapy Standardized or individually adapted doses ? Eds. B von Shoulttz, C Christiansen. The Parthenon Publishing Group, London 1994. pp 47-58.

8. Gillet J, Andre G, Faguer B, Erny R, Buvat-harbaut M, Domin M A, Kuhn J M, Hedon B, Drapier-Faure E, Barrat J, Lopes P, Magnin G, Leng J J, Bruhat M A, Philippe E. Induction of amenorrhea during hormone replacement therapy: optimal micronized progesterone dose. A multicenter study. Maturitas 1994;19:103-15.

Stimulation of prostacyclin and unaffected endothelin-1 by estradiol provides one explanation for cardiovascular protection by estrogen replacement therapy

O. Ylikorkala

Department of Obstetrics and Gynecology, Helsinki University, Helsinki, Finland

Background. Vascular endothelium regulates blood vessel tone by releasing vasoactive substances with often opposing biological effects (1). For instance, prostacyclin (PGI_2), a prostanoid, is an inhibitor of platelet aggregation and a powerful vasodilator, whereas endothelin-1 (ET-1), a 21-amino-acid peptide, is the most potent natural vasoconstrictor substance yet discovered. The balance between these factors may be important in the etiopathogenesis of many vascular disorders, such as hypertension, atherosclerosis, thrombus formation, and pre-eclampsia.

The risk of occlusive vascular disorders in women of fertile age is only approximately 20 % of the respective risk in men, but soon after the cessation of ovarian function, this risk approaches the risk in men (2); this risk can be decreased by estrogen replacement therapy (ERT)(3). The exact mechanism or mechanisms by which estrogen protects against occlusive vascular disorders are not known, but they may include favorable effects on lipid and lipoproteins, connective tissue or a direct effect on the vascular wall. The latter possibility gains strong support from data demonstrating increased blood flow in carotid arteries following ERT (4) and also from the beneficial effects of sublingual estradiol on exercise-induced myocardial ischaemia (5).

Estradiol is a primary estrogen in ERT. There are studies indicating that it stimulates PGI_2 synthesis in human umbilical vessels (6) and in piglet aortic endothelial cells (7). However, there are also studies showing that estradiol does not affect PGI_2 synthesis in human endothelial cells (8,9) and in human uterine arteries (10). We have studied the effect of estradiol on the

Material and Methods. Endothelial cells were prepared from human umbilical cord veins by a method originally described by Jaffe et al. with slight modification (11). Estradiol and tamoxifen were dissolved in ethanol and from those stock solutions they were diluted for the experiments (final ethanol concentration 0.1%0). The experiments with estradiol were also performed with 2-hydroxypropyl-ß-cyclodextrin "carrier" molecules to ensure the transport of estradiol to the cells and also to avoid the disturbing effects of ethanol. The same concentrations of ethanol or 2-hydroxypropyl-ß-cycloxtrin molecules used in experiment solutions were added to the control solutions. The effects of estradiol (0.001-1 umol/L) on PGI_2 and ET-1 productions were studied in 24-well plates by using confluent monolayers of endothelial cells.

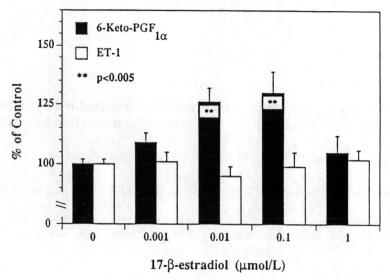

Figure 1

Effects of ethanot-predissolved (final concentration of ethanol 0.1%0 in all wells) 17ß-estradiol 6-keto-PGF$_{1\alpha}$ and ET-1 production. Confluent monolayers of human umbilical vein endothelial cells were incubated for 12 h without (control) or with the concentration indicated of 17ß-estradiol in serum free M 199. Values are means$\pm$SEM of 12 replicate determinations in three separate experiments. Statistical significances calculated against control.

The experiment medium was M 199 supplemented with 100 kU/L penicillin, 100 mg/L streptomycin, and 2 mmol/L L-glutamine. In experiments performed in serum conditions 10% pooled male AB serum was added, whereas in serum-free conditions 0.5% bovine albumin fraction V (Sigma Chemical Co.) and 2.5 mmol/L HEPES pH 7.4 (Sigma Chemical Co.) were added to this medium.

The production of PGI$_2$ was evaluated by measuring its stable hydrolysis product, 6-keto-prostaglandin F$_{1\alpha}$(6-keto-PGF$_{1\alpha}$), by radioimmunoassay (RIA)(12). The concentration of ET-1 was also measured by RIA. ET-1 antiserum was prepared in rabbits which had been immunized with ET-1 (American Peptide Co., Santa Clara, CA) coupled to KLH with glutardialdehyde. The antibody crossreacted with endothelin-2 (28%) and endothelin-3 (64%), but not with big-endothelin-1.

Results. Estradiol affected neither 6-ketoPGF$_{1\alpha}$ nor ET-1 production in HUVECs incubated with serum. However, in serum-free conditions estradiol predissolved in ethanol or in ß-cyclodextrin caused a significant stimulation in 6-keto-PGF$_{1\alpha}$ production, but ET-1 production was not affected (Figure 1 and 2). ß-cyclodextrin carrier molecules alone did not affect 6-keto-PGF$_{1\alpha}$ or ET-1 synthesis. The effect of estradiol was seen after 12 hour incubation, but not yet after 3 hour incubation. Tamoxifen prevented estradiol-induced stimulation demonstrating that the effect of estradiol on PGI$_2$ is specific.

Discussion. Our data show that estradiol stimulates the production of PGI$_2$ in human vascular endothelial cells. This effect could, however, be demonstrated only in the cells which were incubated without serum. This finding may reveal the reason for the lack of the effect of

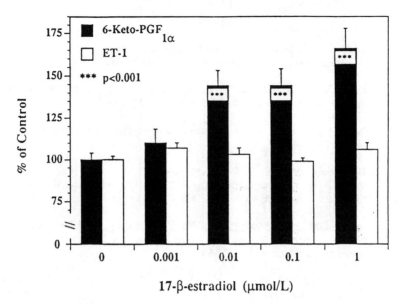

Figure 2

Effects of water soluble (dissolved in cyclodextria) 17ß 6-keto-PGF$_{1\alpha}$ and ET-1-production. Confluent monolayers of human umbilical vein endothelial cells were incubated for 12 h without (control) or with the concentration indicated of 17-ß-estradiol in serum free M 199. Values are means±SEM of 12 replicate determinations in three separate experiments. Statistical significances calculated against control.

estradiol in some earlier studies (8,9) in which serum was present. The reason of the difference on the effect in the presence and absence of serum is not known, but it may be possible that the endothelial cells may be stimulated in the presence of serum to the extent that no further stimulation by estradiol can be achieved. It is noteworthy that in vivo endothelial cells are not exposed to serum, but instead to plasma.

On the basis of the present data, estradiol seems belong to slow releasers of PGI$_2$, such as interleukin-1, tumor necrosis factor-α, tumor promoting phorbol ester and fibrin. The mechanism of the stimulation of PGI$_2$ by estradiol cannot be determined on the basis of the present data.

Estradiol did not affect ET-1 production, and this lack of effect was unrelated to the experiment conditions employed. Since PGI$_2$ and ET-1 are antagonizing regulators of blood vessel contraction (1), the PGI$_2$ dominance induced by estradiol favors vasodilatation, Since PGI$_2$ is a smooth muscle cell growth inhibitor and ET-1 a stimulator, the PGI$_2$ dominance could protect against vascular disorders. These salutary effects of estrogen could be important mechanisms in the cardiovascular protection observed in premenopausal women and in postmenopausal women receiving ERT.

References

1. Lüscher TF. 1990 Imbalance of endothelium-derived relaxing and contracting factors: A new concept in hypertension? Am J Hypertens. 3:317-30.

2. Kannel WB, Hjortland MC, McNamara PM, Gordon T. 1976 Menopause and risk of cardiovascular disease. The Framingham study. Ann Intern Med. 85:447-52.

3. Jacobs HS, Loeffler FE. 1992 Postmenopausal hormone replacement therapy. Br Med J. 305:1403-08.

4. Ganger KF, Vyas S, Whitehead M, Crook D, Meire H, Campbell S. 1991 Pulsatility index in internal carotid artery in relation to transdermal oestradiol and time since menopause. Lancet. 338:839-42.

5. Rosano GMC, Sarrel PM, Poole-Wilson PA, Collins P. 1993 Beneficial effect of oestrogen on exercise-induced myocardial ischaemia in women with coronary artery disease. Lancet. 342:133-36.

6. Mäkilä U-M, Wahlberg L, Viinikka L, Ylikorkala O. 1982 Regulation of prostacyclin and thromboxane production by human umbilical vessels: The effect of estradiol and progesterone in a superfusion model. Prostaglandins, Leukotrienes and Medicine. 8:115-124.

7. Seillan C, Ody C, Russo-Marie F, Duval D. 1983 Differential effects of sex steroids on prostaglandin synthesis by male and female cultured piglet endothelial cells. Prostaglandins. 26:3-12.

8. Muck AO, Seeger H, Korte K, Dartsch PC, Lippert TH. 1993 Natural and synthetic estrogens and prostacyclin production in human endothelial cells from umbilical cord and leg veins. Prostaglandins. 45:517-25.

9. Corvazier E, Dupuy E, Dosne AM, Maclouf J. 1984 Minimal effect of estrogens on endothelial cell growth and production of prostacyclin. Thrombosis Res. 34:303-10.

10. Steinleitner A, Stanczyk FZ, Levin JH, et al. 1989 Decreased in vitro production of 6-keto-prostaglandin F1a by uterine arteries from postmenopausal women. Am J Obstet Gynecol. 161:1677-81.

11. Ristimäki A, Renkonen R, Saijonmaa O, Ylikorkala O, Viinikka L. 1991 Human serum stimulates endothelin-1 synthesis more potently than prostacyclin production by cultured vascular endothelial cells. Life Sci. 49:603-09.

12. Mäkilä U-M, Jouppila P, Kirkinen P, Viinikka L, Ylikorkala O. 1983 Relation between umbilical prostacyclin production and blood-flow in the fetus. Lancet. 1:728-29.

Hemodynamic effects of hormonal replacement therapy in normal postmenopausal women

P.L. Montaldo, M. Tronci, M.A. Fenu, C. Montaldo, P. Soi, G. Pittau*, S. Angioni* and A. Volpe*

Università degli Studi di Cagliari, Istituto di Clinica Medica and *Istituto di Clinica Ostetrica-Ginecologica, Cagliari, Italy

Some studies suggest that plasma estrogens may be important in controlling the increase in cardiac output (CO) (1-3). Moreover, using Doppler Ecocardiography, has been showed that estrogen deprivation is associated with smaller stroke volume and flow acceleration (4). Still Amos Pines (5), using Doppler Ecocardiography on postmenopausal women in hormone replacement therapy, showed a transient vasodilatation and a long-lasting increased inotropism. Then an accurate haemodynamic study may represent an important help to know the real haemodynamic effects of estrogen replacement therapy in postmenopausal women.

PATIENTS AND METHODS

We evaluated eighteen healthy postmenopausal women aged 50 + 4.0 years (last menstruation: 12 months meanly before the start of this study). The women were randomized to receive either estrogen progesterone therapy (arm A) or placebo (arm B) (TAB.I). Estrogen: oral conjugated equine estrogens (0.625 mg daily) and progesterone: oral medrogestone (5 mg daily from 12th to 25th day of the cycle) were administrated.

The haemodynamic parameters were obtained, beat-to-beat, using Thoracic Electrical Bioimpedance (T.E.B.), that utilizes the impedance cardiograph (NCCOM3-R7; BoMed California) (Fig. 1).

ARM A		age	height	weight	BSA
	m̄	50.00	157.30	61.70	1.59
	SD	4.00	5.44	8.86	0.12
ARM B		age	height	weight	BSA
	m̄	52.40	161.80	64.40	1.66
	SD	5.37	3.27	6.35	0.09

TAB. I Anthropometric data of nine estrogen-progesterone treated postmenopausal women (ARM A) and nine placebo postmenopausal women (ARM B).

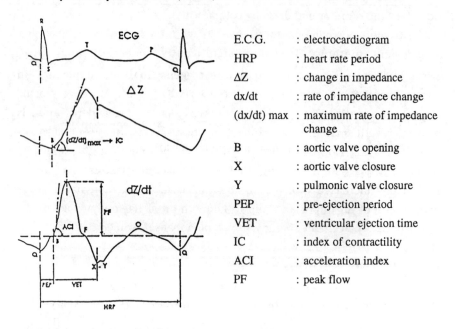

E.C.G.	: electrocardiogram
HRP	: heart rate period
ΔZ	: change in impedance
dx/dt	: rate of impedance change
(dx/dt) max	: maximum rate of impedance change
B	: aortic valve opening
X	: aortic valve closure
Y	: pulmonic valve closure
PEP	: pre-ejection period
VET	: ventricular ejection time
IC	: index of contractility
ACI	: acceleration index
PF	: peak flow

Fig. 1 Time relationship of E.C.G., impedance change (ΔZ) and rate of impedance change (dZ/dt).

EXPERIMENTAL PROTOCOL

This study was performed, at rest and in supine position, at T_0 (before any therapy), at T_1 (after three months of hormonal replacement therapy) and at T_2 (after six months of hormonal replacement therapy).

We have considered the cardiovascular impedance parameters characteristic of:
- Preload
- Heart contractility
- Cardiac performance
- Afterload

RESULTS

a) Preload

The preload is the load that stretches the muscle to its initial lenght prior to contraction. In our study it is represented by presistolic or end diastolic index ($EDI = EDV/m^2$ or end diastolic volume $/m^2$).

The treated postmenopausal women reach, at six months of hormonal replacement therapy, EDI values significantly ($p < 0.05$) higher than placebo (Fig. 2).

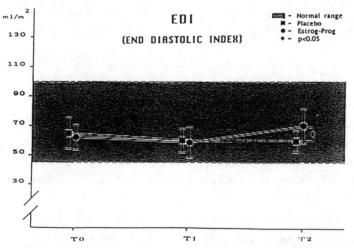

Fig. 2 End diastolic index of nine treated postmenopausal women (●) and nine placebo postmenopausal women (■) before any therapy (T_0), after three months (T_1) and after six months (T_2) of treatment.

b) Heart contractility

The heart contractility is defined as the maximum velocity of myocardial fibres shortening at zero load (V max). In our study the heart contractility is represented by acceleration index ($ACI = sec^{-2}$).

The treated postmenopausal women show a significant ($p<0.01$) increase of ACI between three (T_1) and six (T_2) months of therapy and reach, at T_2, ACI values significantly ($p<0.05$) higher than placebo (Fig.3).

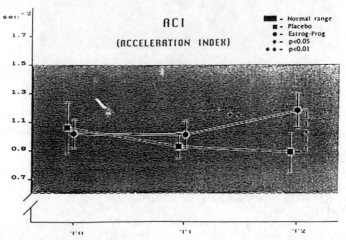

Fig. 3 Acceleration index of nine treated postmenopausal women (●) and nine placebo postmenopausal women (■) before any therapy (T_0), after three months (T_1) and after six months (T_2) of treatment.

c) Cardiac performance

The cardiac performance is defined as cardiac output (CO) and its determinants: heart rate (HR) and stroke volume (SV). In our study the cardiac performance is represented as cardiac index ($CI=CO/m^2 = L/min/m^2$), heart rate ($HR=beat/min$), and stroke index ($SI=SV/m^2 =ml/m^2$).

Cardiac index in placebo postmenopausal women remains always outside and below the normal range. In treated postmenopausal women, CI starts below the normal range, returns progressively in normality and reaches, at T_2, values significantly ($p<0.05$) higher than placebo (Fig. 4).

Heart rate remains into the normal range without significant differences between two groups.

Stroke index in treated postmenopausal women shows a significant ($p<0.01$) increase between T_1-T_2, and reaches, at T_2, values significantly ($p<0.01$) higher than placebo.

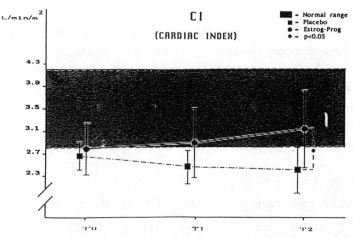

Fig. 4 Cardiac index of nine treated postmenopausal women (●)and nine placebo postmenopausal women (■) before any therapy (T_0), after three months (T_1) and after six months (T_2) of treatment.

d) Afterload

The afterload is the load that the muscle must move after it starts to contract. In our study the afterload is represented by systemic vascular resistance index ($SVRI = F.Ohm/m^2$).

SVRI in placebo postmenopausal women remains always outside and over the normal range,while in treated postmenopausal women starts over the normal range, but at six months returns in normality and reaches values significantly ($p<0.01$) lower than placebo (Fig. 5).

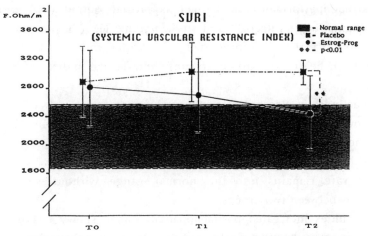

Fig. 5 Systemic vascular resistance index of nine treated postmenopausal women (●) and nine placebo postmenopausal women (■) before any therapy (T_0), after three months (T_1) and after six months (T_2) of treatment.

435

CONCLUSIONS

At the 6th month of treatment, the combined estrogen-progesterone therapy vs placebo appears capable of producing a positive haemodynamic effect in postmenopausal healthy women. We think that the observed decrease of systemic vascular resistance index (SVRI) induces an increase in cardiac output and preload. This last result may be the basis of a physiological mechanism (Frank-Starling) which produces the observed changes in the inotropic state.

REFERENCES

1. Ueland,K. and Parer,J.T. (1966). Effects of estrogens on the cardiovascular system of the ewe. *Am. J. Obstet. Gynecol.*, **96**, 400-6

2. Longo,L.D. (1983). Maternal blood volume and cardiac output during pregnancy: a hypothesis of endocrinologic control. *Am. J. Physiol.*, **245**, R720-9

3. Ueda,S., Fortune,V., Bull,B.S., Valenzuela,G.J., and Longo,L.D. (1986). Estrogen effects on plasma volume, arterial pressure, interstitial space, plasma proteins, and blood viscosity in sheep. *Am. J. Obstet. Gynecol.*, **155**, 195-201

4. Eckstein,N., Pines,A., Fisman,E.Z., Fisch,B., Limor,R., Vagman,I., Barnan,R. and Ayalon,D. (1993). The effect of the hypoestrogenic state, induced by gonadotropin-releasing hormone agonist, on Doppler-derived parameters of aortic flow. *J. Clin. Endocrinol. Metab.*, **77**, 910-2

5. Pines,A., Fisman,E.Z., Shemesh,J., Levo,Y., Ayalon,D., Kellermann,J.J., Motro,M. and Drory Y. (1992). Menopause-related changes in left ventricular function in healthy women. *Cardiology,* **80**, 413-6

Hormones and hypertension

S. Palacios, C. Menendez and A.R. Jurado

Palacios Institute of Hormones and Metabolic Research, Madrid, Spain

Introduction

Cardiovascular disease is the main cause of morbidity and mortality in industrialized societies. There are a set of risk factors present for its development such as high blood pressure, smoking and lipid and carbohydrate disorders.

It is widely known that blood pressure increases with age, both in men and in women: however, according to data from the National Center for Health Statistics, this increase is more marked in women as of menopause. Of 100 persons with high blood pressure, 60 will be women.

Menopause and Blood Pressure

Following menopause of any type, whether natural or secondary to surgery or chemotherapy, there are adverse changes to lipids, lipoproteins and, apparently, to blood pressure figures and more specifically, upon the peripheral vascular bed, which raise the risk of cardiovascular disease and, in particular, coronary heart disease.

The effects of natural or surgical menopause on blood pressure are unclear. Thus our group analyzed the possible effect of surgical menopause on blood pressure in a six-month open study of forty-one post-menopausal patients divided into two groups; twenty-one required hysterectomy with double anexectomy due to uterine myomatosis or metrorrhagia but were otherwise healthy. Their blood pressure was taken one month prior to the operation and fixed as the base, then monthly during the six months following the operation. The other twenty acted as control group, following the same design.

Systolic pressure did not alter from the base value until the sixth month, when it rose significantly ($p < 0.05$), while diastolic pressure began to rise from the fourth month, remaining high during the fifth and sixth months ($p < 0.05$) in women with surgical menopause (Fig. 1). No statistically significant variation was encountered in the control group either in blood pressure or weight (1).

The changes observed in the control group patients were of limited significance, suggesting that those observed in patients in the group undergoing hysterectomy with double annexectomy implied a direct relation between surgical menopause and the risk of high blood

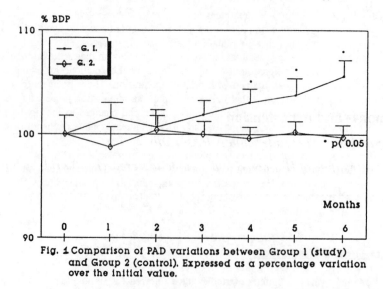

Fig. 1 Comparison of PAD variations between Group 1 (study) and Group 2 (control). Expressed as a percentage variation over the initial value.

pressure. This may be due to the sudden absence of ovarian steroids which cease acting directly or indirectly on the peripheral blood vessels.

Maintenance of the pre-menopause hormone level is thus a protection against high blood pressure and cardiovascular risk.

The mechanisms which may be responsible for this phenomenon are being examined, but some observations are available which may be useful in explaining them.

There are granules in the auricular tissue constituted by a 6-peptide polymer. This substance, known as Atrial Natriuretic Factor, acts at the level of the distal nephron and plays a major role in preventing high blood pressure. Post-menopause, there is a reduction in the production of this Factor; it may be that estrogens are a modulating element in its synthesis.

It has also been observed that the fall in estrogens is associated with reduced vascular flow, due both to increased peripheral vascular resistance caused by biochemical alterations to the vessel wall, and to prostaglandin imbalance and reduced release of the relaxant factor derived from the endothelium.

A protein has been demonstrated which is associated with the estradiol receptor in the walls of the blood vessels, suggesting that estradiol has a direct effect on the vascular bed in some areas of the body (2).

Estrogens and Blood Pressure

The most widely-accepted hypotheses for explaining the etiology of essential high blood pressure (the most common form) are the primary increase in peripheral resistances and the theory of deficient renal excretion of sodium. One of the mechanisms which might in many cases explain this increase in peripheral resistance would be the rise in angiotensin and aldosterone, due to changes to the rennin-angiotensin system.

While there is an evident relation between estrogen intake from oral contraceptives and a higher rennin substrate, it is now known that the appearance of high blood pressure is more idiosyncratic and the risk of developing this condition falls significantly with a reduction of doses (3).

Oral administration products a large quantity or "bolus" of estrogens directly released into the portal circulation, prior to the target organs as would be the case with a physiological state. This implies that hormone treatment would have a supra-physiological effect on the liver, whereas ideally the woman ought to be kept in the same metabolic conditions, and the estrogens should reach the general circulation and target organs before the liver.

It was previously suggested that the benefit of estrogens on the cardiovascular system was related to changes in lipoproteins, with increased HDLc fraction, following passage through the liver, which was attained with oral administration. There is currently evidence contrary to this supposition, now that it is known that the application of percutaneous gel, estradiol implants or transdermic estradiol induce beneficial changes to the lipidic profile, albeit more slowly; for the time being, no significant increases have been notified in the rennin substrate.

The estrogens' positive effects on blood pressure are also due to a further series of actions: of these, the most important have already been pointed out, and refer to the vessel wall, favouring dilatation by increasing prostaglandin E2, prostacyclin, changes to thesynthesis of catecholamines, vasoactive peptides, nitric oxide, etc., or preventing the formation of atheroma plate.

Progestagens and Blood Pressure

For many years, a number of studies have referred to the possible actions, to some degree antagonistic, of progesterone and its derivatives on blood pressure readings, both in normotensive women and those with prior hypertension.

It has been demonstrated that natural progesterone has an anti-hypertensive effect; at doses of 100-200 mg per day, it may cause a significant fall in blood pressure figures due to a natriuretic effect, competing as it does with aldosterone at its receptor level; also included in its anti-hypertensive action has been its effect on the adrenergic system at the level of the central nervous system, acting on vascular tone. However, progestagens (particularly OHprogesterone caproate, MPA and norethindrone acetate) may, on occasions, cause edema and weight gain, by an effect similar to that of Deoxycorti-costerone and, in predisposed subjects, may raise blood pressure.

Most studies published on the effects on blood pressure of gestagens alone used as contraceptives agree that there are no significant changes to blood pressure readings (4).

However, new formulations (lower estrogen doses, new progestagens with minimum androgenic activity - Desogestrel, Gestogene, Norgestimate) used in current oral contraceptives involve minimal metabolic disorders so that the limited incidence of hypertension in users will diminish still further.

Hormone Replacement Therapy and Blood Pressure

The effects on blood pressure of Hormone Replacement Therapy (HRT) are also unclear: some studies shown an increase in BP levels and hypertension during HRT while others however show a significant reduction in blood pressure and a clear protection of the hypertensive patient, even with the administration of natural progestagens. We shall have to wait until, in the coming years, the following two concepts, which apparently can at present be deduced, are definitively confirmed:
- Menopause, with its hypoestronism, involves a high risk of increased blood pressure.
- Hormone Replacement Therapy avoids this risk, preventing arterial hypertension.

Color Doppler analysis of ophthalmic and uterine arteries in postmenopausal patients treated with hormone replacement therapy

C. Battaglia, M.R. Sgherzi, P. Traversi*, P.G. Artini**, A.D. Genazzani and A. Volpe

Università degli Studi di Modena, Istituto di Fisiopatologia della Riproduzione Umana, Modena, *Ospedale Dalmati, Sant'Angelo Lodigiano (MI) and **Università degli Studi di Pisa, Clinica Ostetrica e Ginecologica, Pisa, Italy

INTRODUCTION

Postmenopause is characterized by high gonadotropin (Gn) and low estradiol (E2) plasma levels and is associated to typical hypoestrogenic side effects such as hot flushes, loss of libido, headache, emotional lability and fatigue (1,2). Furthermore, all organs undergo several changes which are caused by low estrogen levels (3).

Cardiovascular disease (CVD) is an age-related phenomen that seriously reduces longevity in women surpassing the rates of cancer and other diseases (4). The post-menopausal women are more vulnerable than premenopausal to CVD. Infact the incidence of coronary artery disease, wich is very low in young women, increases abruptly after menopause when endogenous production of estrogens is sharply reduced. The estrogens deficiency imparts a greater risk every year after menopause (5). However, Hormone Replacement Therapy (HRT) in postmenopausal women decreases the risk of coronary disease and cerebrovascular accidents by reducing the progression of coronary artery atherosclerosis (6,7) and the impedance to flow in all the vascular tree (8,9).

The aim of present study was to study blood flow changes on uterine and ophtalmic arteries of postmenopausal women before and after HRT.

MATERIAL AND METHODS

Sixteen healty postmenopausal women (Follicle-stimulating hormone >35 IU/mL; E2 <30 pg/ml) partecipated in the study after informed consent was obtained.

They had undergone a natural menopause at least 12 months previously. The mean menopause duration was 5.4±1.7 years (mean ± SD; range 1-10 years) and the mean age was 53.2±4.1 years (range 47-62 years).

The patients were evaluated before and after 1 month of oral estrogen therapy (0.625 mg/day) (Premarin. Wyeth, Aprilia. Italy).

All women were submitted to transvaginal ultrasonographic evaluation of pelvic organs. Endometrial thickness was also evaluated.

A color Doppler analysis of the blood flow impedance was performed at level of uterine and ophtalmic arteries.

Serum samples were collected for estradiol radioimmunoassay (Radim, Pomezia, Italy) on the same day of Doppler analysis.

Ultrasound examination of uterus and adnexa was performed by using a 6.5 MHz vaginal trasducer (Ansaldo AU 590 Asinchronous, Genova, Italy). For endometrial evaluation, multiple sagittal and trasverse planes trough the uterine fundus and lower segments were examined. Measurements included the thickest endometrial area.

Doppler flow examination of uterine arteries was performed transvaginally with a 6.5-MHz pulsed color Doppler system (Ansaldo AU 590 Asinchronous Color Doppler). A 50 Hz filter was used to eliminate low frequency signals originating from vessel wall movements. Color flow images of the ascending branches of uterine artery were sampled lateral to the cervix in a longitudinal plane. The angle of insonation was always changed to obtain maximum color intensity. When good color signals were obtained, blood flow velocity waveforms were recorded by placing the sample volume across the vessel and entering the pulsed Doppler mode (10). Doppler-flow examination of ophtalmic artery was performed by placing a 5.0-MHz convex trasducer (Ansaldo AU 590 Asinchronous Color Doppler) over a small amount of gel applied to the closed eyes of the patients. Pulsatility Index (PI), defined as the difference between peak sistolic and end-diastolic flow velocity divided by the mean flow velocity, was calculated .

Statystical analysis of the results was performed using unpaired Student's t-test . Probability <0.05 was taken as limit of staystical significance. Data are presented as mean ± standard deviation.

RESULTS

In all postmenopausal women the values of the studied parameters significantly improved after the treatment with hormone replacement therapy.

Endometrium tickness increased from 3.6±4 mm. to 5.2±3 mm (p<0.01), while plasma E_2 levels rised from 13±7 pg/ml to 46±18 pg/mL (p<0.05).

The PI of uterine artery, decreased from 3.48±0.24 to 2.24±0.18 (p<0.01) and, similarly, the PI of ophtalmic artery decreased from 1.24± 0.15 to 1.05±0.08 (p<0.01).

DISCUSSION

Postmenopausal estrogen therapy has been found to reduce the risk of coronary heart disease and stroke approximatively by 50% (8). The mechanism by which this effect operates is uncertain. The changes in lipids and lipoproteins produced by estrogen replacement therapy is not the only mechanism of cardiovascular protection. Estrogens have a direct positive action on arteries. Estrogen receptor-associated proteins have been found within the muscularis of arterial wall (11), and estrogens are known to cause the release of vasoactive substances such as prostacyclin (12,13) and endothelial derived relaxing factors.

Several studies have demonstrated that estogens administered to postmenopausal women reduce the impedance to flow in the internal carotid and uterine arteries (6,9,19,14,15). However, the Doppler-flow examination of the carotid artery is influenced by noise, ambient temperature and food intake (15). To obviate to the above interpretative difficulties we suggest to choose the ophtalmic artery for the analysis of cerebral vasculature. Ophtalmic artery is a branch of the internal carotid which reflecting the cerebral vascular system may be used to document variations in vascular cerebral resistances.

Our data showed that a decreased impedance to blood flow in uterine and ophtalmic arteries was associated to an improved estrogenic state. Since PI is believed to measure impedance to the flow downstream the point of sampling reflecting the arterial tone, the high PI value in the non-treated post-menopausal women may express elevated peripheral resistances.

Thus the estrogen replacement therapy by decreasing the central and peripheral resistences has beneficial effects on the vascular system and reduces the risk of cardiovascular diseases.

In conclusions, Color Doppler analysis of peripheral and cerebral vessels may be usefully added to the traditional endocrinologic and ultrasonographic parameters clinically used for the treatment and management of postmenopausal women.

REFERENCES

1. Jaffe, R.B. (1991). The menopause and perimenopausal period. In Yen, S.S.C, and Jaffe, R.B.(eds.). Reprod. Endocrin., 389-408 (Philadelphia: Saunder Company).

2. Battaglia, C., Artini, P.G., Bencini, S., Bianchi, R., D'Ambrogio, G., Genazzani, A.R. (1995). Doppler analysis of uterine blood flow changes in spontaneous and medically induced menopause. Gynecol.Endocrinol., 9, 1-6.

3. Luzi, G., Coata, G., Cucchia, G.C., Cosmi, E.V., Di Renzo, G.C. (1993). Doppler studies of uterine arteries in spontaneous and artificially induced menopausal women. Ultrasound Obstet. Gynecol. 3, 354-356.

4. Rogerio,A.Lobo. (1991). Cardiovascular implications of estrogen replacement therapy. Obstet. Gynecol.,75,4,18-25.

5. Kannel,W., Hjortland,M.C., McNamara,P.M., Gordon,T. (1976). Menopause and risk of cardiovascular disease: The Framingham Study. Ann.Intern:Med:,85,447-52.

6. Koudy Williams,J., Adams,M.R., Klopfenstein,H.S.(1990) Estrogen modulates responses of Atherosclerotic Coronary Arteries. Circulation,81,5.

7. Knopp, R.H. (1988) The effects of postmenopausal estrogen therapyon the incidence of arteriosclerotic vascular disease. Obstet.Gynecol.,72,235-305.

8. Gangar,K., Vyas,S., Whitehead,M.I., Crook,D., Meire,H., Campbell,S. (1992) Pulsatility index in the internal carotid artery is influenced by transdermal oestradiol and time since menopause. Lancet,338,839-42.

9. Bourne,T., Hillard,T., Crook,D., Campbell,S.(1990) Evidence for a rapid effect of oestrogens on the arterial status of postmenopausal women. Lancet,335,1470-1.

10. Padwick, M., Whitehead,M.I., Coffer,A., King,R. (1988) Demonstration of estrogen receptor related protein in female tissues. In: Studd, J.W.W., Whitehead, M.I. (eds.). The menopause. Oxford: Blackwell Scientific, 227-33.

11. Steinleitner,A., Stanczyk,F., Levin,J.M., D'Ablaing III,G., Vijod,M.A., Shahbajan, V.L. (1989). decreased in-vitro production of six-keto-prostaglandin F1 alpha on uterine arteries of postmenopausal women. AmJ.Obstet.Gynecol.,161,1677-81.

12. Gisclard,V., Millar,V., Van Houte,P. (1988) Effects of 17-beta-estradiol on endothelium dependent responses in the rabbit. Pharmacol.Exp.Ther., 244,19-22.

13. Bush,T.L., Cowan,L.D., Barrett-Connor, E.(1983) Estrogen use and all cause mortality. J.A.M.A..,249,903-6.

14. Sullivan,J.M., Vander-Zwaag,R., Lemp,G.F.(1988) Postmenopausal estrogen use and coronary atherosclerosis. Ann.Intern.Med., 108,358-63.

15. Meire,H., Campbell,S.(1991) Pulsatility index in internal carotid artery in relation to transdermal oestradiol and time since menopause. Lancet,338,5.

Hemostatic variables and estrogen substitution in postmenopausal women

U.H. Winkler

Obstetrics and Gynecology Center, University Hospital Essen, Essen, Germany

Cardiovascular disease (CVD) in women is mostly of atherothrombotic rather than atherosclerotic nature. Moreover, there is growing evidence that thromboembolic events may be the final pathway shared by both pathomechanisms. Haemostatic imbalance, i.e. the local surplus of coagulatory over fibrinolytic activity, is an essential *sine qua non* of any pathomechanism of CVD. Subsequently, high levels of fibrinogen (Fib), factor VII activity (F VIIact), von Willebrand factor (F VIIIvWF) or of the plasminogen activator inhibitor (PAI1), i.e. high coagulatory potential and low fibrinolytic activity due to high levels of the fibrinolytic inhibition have been shown to be of predictive value for an increased incidence or poor prognosis of CVD. Among the mechanisms that have unfavourable effects on these haemostatic markers there are life style factors such as smoking and diet, but also age and menopause (1).

Refined methodology allows for an assessment of intravascular fibrinolytic and coagulatory activities as well as their regulation by activators and inhibitors. The study of these haemostatic variables and their interrelationship with lipids and carbohydrates suggested that there are various mechanisms at the molecular level that may affect haemostatic function. Steroids may have effects on the synthesis of coagulation factors directly or via second messengers. However, cytokines and other second messengers are the best known mediators of the endothelial activation, the mechanism that triggers the activation of the coagulation as well as the fibrinolytic cascade. Thus, an interrelationship of the hemostatic system with lipids and carbohydrates may be based on effects on the second messenger level.

Recently, a strong correlation of the fibrinolytic system with insulin and IGF-1 levels has been shown (2) suggesting that insulin resistance is associated with an impairement of the fibrinolytic system. In fact, insulin and IGF-1 enhance PAI1 expression of HEP 2 cells and this mechanism may be involved in the poor prognosis of patients woith syndrome X.. So, PAI 1, an indicator of poor prognosis in survivors of myocardial infarction (3), may serve as an example of cytokine-induced changes of haemostatic function.

Additional haemostatic markers of CVD include substrates and zymogens of the coagulatory system such as fibrinogen, factors VII and von Willebrand factor as well as the consumption of inhibitors of coagulation such as antithrombin III (AT III). There is evidence that the synthesis of these factors is increased via direct steroidal effects on gene transcription. However, there is considerable evidence of cytokine mediated effects as well. All of these markers are acute-phase reactants and it is tempting to speculate that the common pathway of CVD at the endothelial level is inflammatory activation (4).

Estrogen substitution (ERT) was shown to be associated with a reduced incidence of CVD. It is conceivable to assume that estrogen substitution exerts beneficial effects on the endothelial level via a reduction of the chronic acute-phase reaction. Analysis of the haemostatic risk markers may serve as a best substitute to direct evaluation of endothelial function reflecting a summary of the various steroidal effects on second messengers such as cytokines and mitogens. Moreover, reaction products of actual haemostatic activity such as enzyme-inhibitor complexes or peptides cleaved from substrates by the action of activated haemostatic enzymes are indicative of the net effect of such changes on baseline function of the haemostatic system. There is growing evidence that atherothrombosis is unlikely if baseline coagulatory function is low.

We have studied these markers in 30 postmenopausal women randomly assigned to receive either transdermal estradiol (patches delivering 50 µg /day, n=16) or conjugated equine estrogens (0,625 mg oral, n=14) in combination with medrogeston (5 mg oral, day 11-21) before and at the end of a three cycle treatment period. Blood collection and handling was strictly standardized. Plasma aliquots were frozen at -8o degree Celsius and analysis was done with commercially available assays (5) in series. For statistical assessment of change to baseline student's t-test was performed with significance at $p <$ 0,05.

We found increased mean estradiol (E2) levels (transdermal E2 by 112%, CEE by 65%) and reduced FSH (transdermal E2 by 53%, CEE by 35%) in both treatment groups. The excellent reduction of typical symptoms (hot flushes) was in accord with these findings.

Unfavourable effects on haemostatic markers of CVD were not seen with both preparations except for a slight increase (16%) of the von Willebrand factor in CEE users (table 1). There is only one group that has looked at the von Willebrand factor in hormone replacement therapy (6) reporting no significant effect after 6 weeks of treatment both with CEE as with a transdermal system.

Favourable effects were observed with both preparations. A reduction of factor VII activity was only seen with the transdermal system (by 10%) while the effects on the fibrinolytic system were more pronounced with CEE. Similar results have been published recently by Kroon (6) and may be due to a differential impact of oral versus transdermal estrogens on hepatic IGF-1 synthesis (7). According to this model oral estrogens reduce IGF-1 production and thereby PAI-1 synthesis, while transdermal estrogens have only little effects on this system.

The activity of some inhibitors of coagulation (protein (Prot) S and C) was marginally reduced with both preparations but a clinical significance of these changes is unlikely due to the fact that there was no significant effect on the various reaction products of haemostatic activities. Neither reaction products indicative of thrombin activation and activity (e.g. thrombin-antithrombin III complex ,TAT) nor reaction products of plasmin activity (e.g. D-dimer fibrin-split products, D-Dimer) revealed any surplus activity. In fact, there was a slight though not significant decrease of prothrombin fragment 1+2 (F 1+2) in women on transdermal E2. This fragment is cleaved from prothrombin in the process of generating the active coagulatory enzyme thrombin and may therefore serve as an indicator of in-vivo coagulant activity. Our finding is in contrast to a recent report from Caine (8) on slight but dose dependent increasing effects of CEE on F 1+2. However, the authors of this report pointed out, that even if thrombin generation may have been slightly increased in their patients, an increased clotting activity, i.e. fibrin generation was highly unlikely: Studying several marker of fibrin generation and degradation, there was no evidence of increased fibrin turnover in these patients.D-dimer fibrin split products did not change significantly. All of these findings are confirmed by our data after three treatment cycles suggesting that there is no increase of baseline coagulation or fibrinolysis in postmenopausal women on ERT.

In summary, the effects of estrogen substitution in postmenopausal women are favourable with regard to risk factors of CVD. However, while oral CEE appear to have

Table 1: Change from pretrial assessment at the end of a three cycle treatment period with either transdermal estradiol (E2) or conjugated equine estrogens (CEE) combined with 5 mg medrogeston on day 11 to 21.

Variables	CEE	E2 transdermal	difference
Fib	n.c.	n.c.	Ø
F VII act	n.c.	-9%	p<0.05
F VIII vWF	+16%	n.c.	p<0.05
PAI 1	-39%	n.c.	p<0.05
AT III	-6%	-6%	Ø
Prot C	-7%	-10%	Ø
Prot S	-8%	-7%	Ø
F 1+2	n.c.	n.c.	Ø
TAT	n.c.	n.c.	Ø
D-Dimer	n.c.	n.c.	Ø

a more pronounced effect on the fibrinolytic system (reduction of PAI 1), transdermal E2 had more favourable effects on the coagulatory system: no increase in von Willebrand factor and reduction of factor VII activity. A differential effect on hepatic insulin-like growth factor synthesis may be responsible for these differences. However, with both preparations overall baseline activity of the haemostatic system was not increased as has been seen with ethinylestradiol in oral contraceptives (5) . Thrombogenic effects within the venous as well as in the arterial system are highly unlikely. Moreover, the observed effects of ERT are directed towards less coagulatory activity and reduced fibrinolytic inhibition and may well translate into a net benefit with regard to CVD risks.

REFERENCES

1. Winkler, U.H. (1992). Menopause, hormone replacement therapy and cardiovasascular disease: a review of haemostaseological findings. *Fibrinolysis* **6** (3), 5-10

2. Juhan-Vague, I., Alessi, M.C., Vague, P. (1991). Increased plasminogen activator inhibitor 1 levels. A possible link between insulin resistance and atherothrombosis. *Diabetologia* **34**, 457-62

3. Hamsten, A., Walldius, G., Szamosi, A., Blombäck, M., De Faire, U., Dahlen, G., Landou, C., Wimann, B. (1987). Plasminogen activator inhibitor in plasma: Risk factor for recurrent myocardial infarction. *Lancet*, July: 3-9

4. Haverkate, F. (1992). Low grade acute-phase reactions in arteriosclerosis and the consequences for haemostatic risk factors. *Fibrinolysis* **6** (3), 17-18

5. Winkler, U.H., Koslowski, S., Oberhoff, C., Schindler, E.M., Schindler, A.E. (1991). Changes of the dynamic equilibrium of hemostasis associated with the use of low dose oral contraceptives: a controlled study of cyproteroneacetate containing oral contraceptives combined with either 35 or 50 µg ethinylestradiol. *Advance. Contracept.* **7**, 273-84

6. Kroon, U.B., Silfverstolpe, G., Tengborn, L. (1994). The effects of transdermal estradiol and oral conjugated estrogens on haemostasis variables. *Thromb. Haemostas.* **71**, 420-3

7. Weissberger, A.J., Ho, K.K.Y., Lazarus, L. (1991). Contrasting effects of oral and transdermal routes of estrogen replacement therapy on 24-hour growth hormone (GH) secretion, insulin-like growth factor 1 and GH-binding protein in postmenopausal women. *J. Clin. Endocrinol. Metab.* **72**, 374-81

8. Caine, Y.G., Bauer, K.A., Barzegar, S., Ten Cate, H., Sacks, F.M., Walsh, B.W., Schiff, I., Rosenberg, R.D. (1992). Coagulation activation following estrogen administration to postmenopausal women. *Thromb. Haemostas.* **68**, 392-95

A new approach to postmenopausal hormonal treatment

N. Mercuri, P. Ardito, F. Vescio, V. Scarcella*, A. Leotta**, S.G. Lio**
and P. Vadalà

Department of Obstetrics and Gynecology, *Laboratory of Immunochemistry
and Diagnostics, Soveria Mannelli and **Laboratory of Histo-Cyto-Pathology,
AUSSL No. 6 Lamezia Terme, Italy

INTRODUCTION

The hormone replacement therapy (HRT) has proved to be very efficient in preventing osteoporosis, in reducing the risk of cardiovascular disease (CVD), in determining the disappearance of vasomotor and neurogenic disturbances and in the regression of genital-urinary atrophy. Moreover, women treated with HRT, combined with progestin, in post-menopausal age, have been seen as capable of decreasing the risk and the incidence of endometrial cancer in comparison with those women who are not treated according to this approach (1,2,3). However, oestrogen therapy also causes metabolic effects which could create problems when HRT is prescribed over a long period (4). Tibolone (Livial-ORGANON), known as Org OD 14, is a new synthetic steroid for climacteric syndrome therapy. This compound displays weak oestrogenic, weak progestogenic and very weak androgenic properties and it is particularly active on central nervous system. Moreover, Org OD 14 has a positive effect on cardiovascular system. In fact, some authors (5,6) have indicated that it lowers lipoproteins serum concentration and increases forearm blood flow, the dilator response to anoxic exercise and heart rate. Besides, several studies have shown that this compound does not influence coagulation, but it has a beneficial effect on fibrinolysis (7). In addition, recent prospective studies reported that Org OD 14 protects against post-menopausal bone mineral loss (8), with no effect on endometrial proliferation (3,9). On these bases, the aim of the present study is to evaluate the effects of short-term administration of Org OD 14 on menopausal symptoms, carbohydrate, lipid and bone metabolism, blood coagulation and endometrial histology.

MATERIAL AND METHODS

The present study involved twenty early, symptomatic, post-menopausal women (average age 56 years), who had undergone a natural menopause, with amenorrhoea of, at least, one year and a serum follicle-stimulating hormone (FSH) concentration > 30 mIU/ml.

All healthy patients enrolled had normal physical examination and no controindication for HRT. None of the women had received any hormonal treatment for at least 6 months prior to the present study. The patients were treated for 24 weeks with Org OD 14 (Livial-ORGANON) 2.5 mg in daily oral administration. FSH levels, that confirmed the menopause, were measured before the therapy, in each plasma sample, by double-antibody radioimmunoassay (RIA) using commercially available reagents (Radim, Pomezia, Italy). In each subject we evaluated, before and after the six months treatment, serum levels of total cholesterol,

453

High-Density-Lipoprotein cholesterol (HDL-c), Low-Density-Lipoprotein cholesterol (LDL-c), Triglycerides, Fibrinogen, Antitrombin III (AT III), Protrombin Time (PT), Partial Tromboplastin Time (PTT), Glycemia as well as Alkaline Phosphatase, urinary Hydroxyproline/Creatinine (OH-Pr/Cr) excretion ratio, using standard laboratory methods, while serum Bone-Gla-Protein (BGP) levels were measured by RIA technique. Menopause acute symptoms (hot flushes, sweating, depression, headache, vaginal dryness etc.) were assessed by patients using the following scoring system : 0 = absent, 1 = mild, 2 = moderate and 3 = severe; hot flushes and the other symptoms were scored weekly.

The statistical analysis of the results was performed using analysis of variance (Anova) and the Dunnet test for multiple comparison. The endometrium was assessed by taking biopsies using a Novak-type curette. Our study design included a pre-treatment biopsy (in which all patients were found to have a mainly inactive endometrium) as well as an end of study biopsy.

RESULTS

The mean (± S.E.M.) symptoms scores before and after each month of treatment, showed a significant reduction (P < 0.01) in the number of hot flushes (from > 40 per week to < 10) and associated symptoms, with a clear benefit on the vaginal mucosa. There was no significant alteration in blood pressure or weight during the study. As for the effects on lipid profile, while mean (± S.E.M.) total cholesterol level, mean (± S.E.M.) HDL-cholesterol level and mean (± S.E.M.) triglicerides level were significantly lower than those in the pre-treatment period (P < 0.01), no significant changes were seen in the mean (± S.E.M.) LDL-cholesterol level. Org OD 14 had no significant effect on Protrombin Time level and induced a negligible, unimportant increase in Partial Thromboplastin Time level. Moreover, it induced a significant fall in mean (± S.E.M.) fibrinogen levels (P <0.01) and a significant increase in mean (± S.E.M.) Antithrombin III levels (P < 0.01). Regarding the effects on fasting plasma glucose levels, we observed a slight decrease in glucose tolerance during treatment. This effect was not considered to be clinically relevant because plasma glucose levels remained within the normal range (60-110 mg%).

As for the changes on bone turn-over, Org OD 14 determined a significant reduction on mean (± S.E.M.) plasma BGP level (P< 0.01), on mean (± S.E.M.) plasma alkaline phosphatase level (P< 0.01) and in the urinary out-put mean (± S.E.M.) values of hydroxyproline (P< 0.01). Regarding the effects on endometrial activity, Org OD 14 treatment did not significantly modify endometrial histology. In fact, after therapy we observed a 75% (15 patients) of mainly inactive endometrium, a 15% (3 patients) of normal mainly-weak secretion endometrium and a 10% (2 patients) of slight proliferative endometrium. During the treatment we observed some side effects such as occasional slight vaginal bleeding (2 cases), backache (1 case), nausea (1 case). These side effects, however, have not determined the drop-out of the patients.

DISCUSSION AND CONCLUSION

The present study has clearly demonstrated that daily oral administration of 2.5 mg of Org OD 14 determined a significant reduction of hot flushes and associated symptoms in post-menopausal women. This finding is in agreement with previously published data (10). Many patients reported that relief from hot flushes was accompained by a general feeling of well being or a mood elevating effect of Org OD 14, probably in correlation with the rises in circulating ß-endorphin and ß-lipotrophin levels that have been observed (11). HRT in post-menopausal women has been associated with a protective effect against CVD (12). In the present short-term study a significant decrease both in serum total cholesterol level and serum triglyceride levels was observed with significant reduction in serum HDL-cholesterol levels. This latter phenomenon, probably related to the weak androgenic properties of the drug, was also described after 6 and 12 months of Org OD 14 treatment (8), disappearing during long-term study (13) and it is less important than Org OD 14 effect on serum triglyceride levels (14). In fact, a positive relationship between high levels of serum triglycerides and coronary heart disease risk in menopause is well known (15), but the lowering effect exerted on plasma triglycerides, by Org OD 14 therapy, may therefore be considered favourably in this regard.

It is also well known that Antithrombin III activity protects against intravascular coagulation, and a loss of this protection as measured by a low AT III level might predispose to thrombosis. In this study we observed that Org OD 14 determined, in accordance with several reports (7,16), a significant fall of fibrinogen levels along with a significant rise in AT III levels, while we did not record any significant change on both PTT and PT levels. This appears to be beneficial for post-menopausal women by an increase of fibrinolitic activity. Several studies (17) have demonstrated that the use of lower doses of oestrogen may be enough to counterbalance the adverse effect of the progestin on glucose metabolism. In our study, Org OD 14, in accordance with some reports (18), by its particular pharmacological profile did not determine any significant change in carbohydrate tolerance. Prevention of post-menopausal bone loss with oestrogen and progestogens is well established (19). While the oestrogens reduce the rate of bone resorption, the progestogens increase both periostal new bone formation and calcium contents of femur. However, the synthetic steroid hormone Org OD 14 has been found to be an effective prevention of bone loss (20). In fact, in our study, Org OD 14 significantly reduced skeletal metabolism (showed by lower both serum BGP and alkaline phosphatase levels) with a reduction of bone resorption (urinary hydroxyproline excretion decreased in all subjects) and a protective effect on post-menopausal bone mineral loss with the lowest risk of fractures. Our own findings lead us to observe that Org OD 14 clearly deserves consideration not only for the long-term prevention but also as curative treatment of post-menopausal osteoporosis. Tolerance to treatment was very good. Occasional vaginal bleeding occurred during Org OD 14 treatment; this bleeding was most probably due to the pre-treatment status of endometrium since Org OD 14 has been shown not to stimulate endometrial growth. As a matter of fact, in agreement with some reports (3,9,21), this study demonstrated the lack of any stimulatory effect on endometrium in the large majority (90%) of our study patients; only slight proliferative endometrium was seen in few cases (2 women). Of particular importance is the absence of virilization or any other androgenic side effect, for example on body weight. In conclusion, the present data demonstrate that Org OD 14, in view of its clinical and pharmacological profile, should be considered as an attractive and very safe alternative to conventional oestrogen therapy for the treatment of post-menopausal syndrome.

ACKNOWLEDGMENTS
We should like to thank Mr Domenico Mercuri for computer elaboration and Mrs Anna Rossi for the language revision.

REFERENCES

1) Schiff, I. (1982). Endometrial hyperplasia in women on cyclic or continuous regimens. Fertil. Steril. 1, 79-82

2) Whitehead, M.I. (1978). The effects of oestrogens and progestogens on the post-menopausal endometrium. Maturitas, 1, 87-98

3) Genazzani, A.R. (1991). Org OD 14 and the endometrium. Maturitas, 13, 243-251

4) Wahl, P. (1983). Effect of estrogen/progestin potency on lipid/lipoprotein cholesterol. N. Engl. J. Med., 308, 862-867

5) Kloosterboer, H.J. (1990). Long-term effects of Org OD 14 on lipid metabolism in post-menopausal women. Maturitas, 12, 37-42

6) Hardiman, P. (1991). Cardiovascular effects of Org OD 14 - a new steroidal therapy for climacteric symptoms. Maturitas, 13, 235-242

7) Cortes-Prieto, J. (1987). Coagulation and fibrinolysis in post-menopausal women treated with Org OD 14. Maturitas, suppl. 1, 67-72

8) Netelenbos, J.C. (1991). Short-term effect of Org OD 14 and 17 ß-oestradiol on bone and lipid metabolism in early post-menopausal women. Maturitas, 13, 137-149

9) Punnonen, R. (1984). Multicentre study of effects of Org OD 14 on endometrium, vaginal cytology and cervical mucus in post-menopausal and oophorectomized women. Maturitas, 5, 281-6

10) De Aloysio, D. (1987). Use of Org OD 14 for the treatment of climacteric complaints. Maturitas, suppl. 1, 49-65

11) Genazzani, A.R. (1987). Effects of Org OD 14 on pituitary and peripheral ß-endorphin in castrated rats and post-menopausal women. Maturitas, suppl.1, 35-48

12) Stampfer, M.J. (1985). A prospect study of post-menopausal oestrogen therapy and coronary heart disease. N. Engl. J. Med., 313, 1044-9

13) Benedek-Jaszmann, L.J. (1987). Long-term placebo-controlled efficacy and safety study of Org OD 14 in climacteric women. Maturitas, suppl. 1, 23-33

14) Lapidus, L. (1985). Triglycerides-main lipid risk factor for cardiovascular disease in women? Acta Med. Scand., 217, 481-9

15) Stamper, M.J. (1991). Estrogen replacement therapy and coronary heart disease: a quantitative assessment of the epidemiologic evidence. Prev. Med., 20,47-63

16) Parkin, D.E. (1987). Effects of long-term Org OD 14 admistration on blood coagulation in climacteric women. Maturitas, 9, 95-101

17) Spellacy, W. (1981). Prospective carbohydrate metabolism studies in women using a low-estrogen oral contraceptive for one year. J. Reprod. Med., 26, 295-300

18) Tax L., (1987). Clinical profile of Org OD 14. Maturitas, suppl. 1, 3-13

19) Crilly, R.G. (1981). Steroid hormones, ageing and bone. Clin. Endocrinol. Metab., 10, 115-139

20) Lindsay, R. (1980). A prospective double-blind trial of synthetic steroid (Org OD 14) for preventing post-menopausal osteoporosis. B.M.J., 280, 1207-9

21) Trevoux, R. (1983). Efficacy and safety of Org OD 14 in the treatment of climacteric complaints. Maturitas, 5, 89-96

Placebo-controlled randomized trial of melbrosia pld for the treatment of climacteric symptoms

M.O. Sator, D.M. Gruber, P. Frigo, W. Knogler and J.C. Huber

Ambulatorium MENOX, Wien, Germany

PURPOSE:

In a placebo - controlled randomized trial 67 women with a biochemically evaluated climacteric status and climacteric symptoms were treated with melbrosia or with placebo.

The benefits of a Hormone Replacement Therapy (HRT) during menopausal periode are beyond doubt and most important especially when the risk of osteoporosis and cardiovascular problems can be reduced.

There are also numerous women who do not need or who do not want to undergo hormonal therapy. They most often suffer from less severe menopausal complaints which do only concern their subjective wellbeing. For these women Royal Jelly and Pollen is an exellent alternative methode to cover these problems.

PATIENTS AND METHODS:

A total of 67 recruited women was devided into two groups. The verum group consisted of 33 women and a placebo group of 34 women.

The study was approved by the ethic comission of Menox Institute, informed consent was signed by the patients and it was carried out according to the GCP standards.

Before starting any treatment every patient had to undergo bone densitometry measurement (DEXA, Hologic Braincon Technologies), and an exact anamnesis was established.

A main exclusion criterion was low bone density. An inclusion criterion was the manifestation of climacteric complaints.
The hormonal parameters FSH, Oestradiol, Prolactin, Testosteron, TSH, T3 and T4 were measured according to present medical standards (ELISA, Boehringer Mannheim).

Treatment itself lasted three months. Blood samples were taken before therapy and monthly during treatment.
The dose of melbrosia was: three capsules per day during the first ten days, two capsules per day during the following ten days and until the end of therapy a maintenance dose of one capsule per day.

One melbrosia capsule contains 257mg pollen, 150mg bee-bread, 33mg lyophilised royal jelly equivalent to 100mg fresh royal jelly and 20mg vitaminC.
The nutritive value per 100g is 21,5g protein, 2,5g fat and 41,0g carbohydrate which is equivalent to 0,02 dietic units per capsule.

Statistical evaluation was performed by methods of student t-test.
The success of the treatment was evaluated by the patients themselves.

RESULTS:

Physical Ability:
Both groups-melbrosia and placebo-showed an improvement of the physical ability during the first month. 43% of the placebo group and 56% of the melbrosia group stated an improvement. The difference is statistically significant p<0,001.
It is remarkable that the improvement of the physical ability continued in the melbrosia group while the placebo group stopped showing progress.

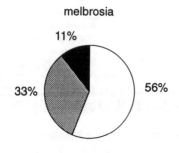

melbrosia

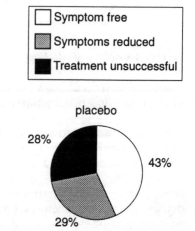

placebo

☐ Symptom free
▨ Symptoms reduced
■ Treatment unsuccessful

Headache:
Both groups showed improvements initially. However, after the first month of treatment the success of the placebo group stopped whereas women taking melbrosia improvement continued. In 70% headache had vanished while 22% of the placebo group reported an alleviation of headache.

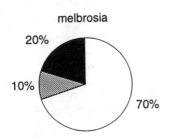

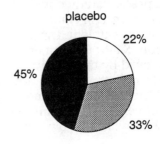

Incontinence of Urine:
Dry Vagina:
It is striking that melbrosia caused highly significant improvement compared to the placebo group in cases of incontinence of urine as well as in cases of dry vagina.
Application of melbrosia was able to eliminate a slight incontinence of urine in 40%. In the placebo group 16% showed an improvement.
A similar result was achieved in cases of dry vagina where the placebo effect was insignificant (18%).

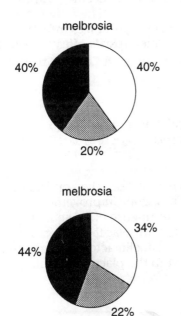

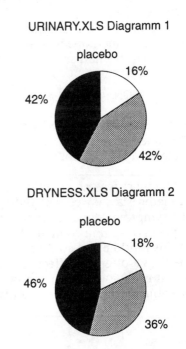

Nervousness, Insomnia, Depression, Joint and Muscle pain, Hot flushes: In these menopausal symptoms there was no difference between the verum and the placebo group.

DISCUSSION

The present study obviously demonstrates that melbrosia is able to improve certain climacteric complaints considerably compared to a placebo treatment. Especially striking was this effect in the urogenital tractus. Slight incontinence of urine and dry vagina were definitely improved by the application of melbrosia. No influence was observed concerning the serum-hormone levels. This fact leads to the conclusion that the substances contained in melbrosia are inactive in regard to steroid effects. The clinical improvement of climacteric symptoms seems to be provoked by phytohormones.

The result of this placebo controlled trial leads to the conclusion that some climacteric complaints in fact can be efficiently decreased by melbrosia and that this treatment can be offered to women who refuse a classical HRT.

Although we could not prove any activity of Prolactin and other steroidal hormones with our ELISA's it is a well hormone fact that phyto-oestrogenes are active in human organism. The correlation of phyto-oestrogenes and the incidence of prostatic hypoplasia respectively carcinoma of the prostata was described recently (Lancet 1993; vol 342).
Furthermore it is a fact that the same phytogenic substances influence paracrine functions. It is well imaginable that melbrosia's effect is based on similar mechanism.

CONCLUSION:

In a randomized trial 67 women with a biochemically evaluated climacteric status as well as climacteric complaints were treated with melbrosia or placebo.

While there was no effect on the hormonal parameters, the application of melbrosia showed a statistically significant higher improvement of the symptoms physical ability, headache, incontinence of urine and dryness of vagina compared to the treatment with placebo. The results of this randomized study showed that for certain climacteric complaints melbrosia offers an effective relief compared to the placebo treatment and it is obvious that it can be offered as an alternative to women who are reluctant to Hormonal Replacement Therapy.

Literatur

(1) Adlercreutz H. Markkanen H. Watanabe S: Plasma concentrations of phyto-oestrogens in Japanese men. Lancet 1993;342: 8881:1209-1210.

(2) Christiansen C. Christensen MS. Transbvl J: Bonemass in postmenopausal women after withdrawal of oestrogen/gestagen replacement therapy. Lancet 1981;I:459-461.

(3) De Aloysio D. Fabiani AG. Mauloni M. Bottiglione F: Analysis of the climacteric syndrome. Maturitas 1989;22:43-53.

(4) Enzelsberger H. et al: Zur Wirksamkeit einer intravaginalen Östrioltablettenapplikation bei Frauen mit Urge-Inkontinenz. Geburtsh Frauenheilk 1991;51:834-838.

(5) Foidart JM. Verliet J. Buytaert P: Efficacy of sustained-release vaginal oestriol in alleviating urogenital and systemic climacteric complaints. Maturitas 1991;13: 99-107.

(6) Gambrell RD: The menopause: benefits and risks of oestrogen-progesteron replacement therapy. Fertil Steril 1982;37: 457-474.

(7) Hanner JA. Scheider HPG: Pathogenese und Diagnostik der klimakterischen Beschwerden. Gynäkologie 1986;19:4.

(8) Huber JC: Klimakterium: Diagnose und Therapie. Berlin. Grosse. 1989.

(9) Huber JC: Substitutionstherapie in Klimakerium: Soll bei hysterektomierten Frauen auf Progesterone verzichtet werden? Geburtsh Frauenheilk 1991;51:257-261.

(10) Jazman L: Epidemiology of the climacteric syndrome. in Campell S (ed): The Management of the Menopause and the Postmenopausal years. Lancaster. MTP Press. 1976. 11-24.

(11) Lauritzen C: Kosten. Nutzen. Risiken. Analyse der Östrogenbehandlung im Klimakterium. Gynäkologe 1982;19:4.

(12) Lottge M. Spieler W. Seifert B. Hemp O: Interdisziplinares Diagnostik- und Therapiekonzept der klimakterischen Osteoporose. Zbl Gynäkol 1989;111:800-806.

(13) Oddens BJ. Boulet MJ. Lehert P. Visser AP: Has the climacteric been medicalized? A study on the use of medication for climacteric complaints in four countries. Maturitas 1992;15:117-181.

(14) Oldenhave A. Jaszmann LJ. Everaerd WT. Haspels AA: Hysterectomized women with ovarian conservation report more severe climacteric complaints than do normal climacteric women of similar age. Am J Obstet Gynecol 1993;168:765-771.

(15) Warnecke G: Psychosomatische Dysfunktionen im weiblichen Klimakterium. Klinische Wirksamkeit und Verträglichkeit von Kava-Extrakt WS 1490. Fortschr Med 1991 (4):109:119-122.

Kinetics of a new 17β-estradiol transdermal drug delivery system

U.D. Rohr, C. Nauert* and A.M. Ehrly

Center for Internal Medicine, Division of Angiology, Hospital of the J.W. Goethe University, Frankfurt and *Clinical Research, Rhône Poulenc Rorer Gmbh, Cologne, Germany

INTRODUCTION

Hormone replacement therapy in menopausal women with 17ß-Estradiol is a well established method to prevent occurrence of symptoms associated with the deficiency of natural 17ß-Estradiol[1] like hot flushes, nausea, and cardiovascular problems. Increasingly osteoporosis, disturbances of the lipid metabolism, etc. are viewed as indications for treatment with 17ß-Estradiol. In the past 10 years the transdermal route of administration of 17ß-Estradiol has gained wide spread use due to the fact

(a)   that first - pass metabolism of 17ß-Estradiol in the liver is avoided. Consequently lower doses ranging approximately 5% of the oral dose are required to suppress the symptoms associated with 17ß-Estradiol deficiency.

(b)   that patient compliance is improved, due to the convenient and every 3 - 4 day application of a patch in contrast to daily oral dosing.

An investigation of the kinetics of the leading and in most parts of the world only commercially available transdermal device showed an undesirable high initial blood concentration peak level within 8 after application, which decreased by 50% after 24 hours[1]. A second peak can be detected with this system at hour 48 and declines from there significantly[1]. The kinetics are reproducible[1]. In contrast to these findings, however, the ideal transdermal delivery mode should provide for a constant transdermal drug delivery rate leading to stable blood concentration level over the whole application period.

AIM OF THE STUDY

It is the aim of this presentation to discuss kinetic results obtained using a newly developed 17ß-Estradiol transdermal drug delivery system, with an improved stable kinetic profile, in contrast to the currently available 17ß-Estradiol transdermal formulation. The following investigations were carried out to determine the in vivo performance characteristics of the newly developed patch:

(a) In vitro transdermal flux rates

of 17ß-Estradiol through excised human skin were investigated to estimate the daily dose produced by the device.

(b) In vivo clinical pharmacokinetic study

was conducted with the newly developed 17ß-Estradiol transdermal drug delivery system to determine beneficial stable blood concentration levels.

(c) The batch to batch variability

was investigated to characterize the dosage form.

(d) In vitro/in vivo-correlation

was established as a quality control method to assess the safety of the new 17ß-Estradiol transdermal drug delivery system for later application in patients.

THEORY

Briefly a four compartment model with a side compartment to the systemic compartment is to be assumed[2] (Fig. 1). The existence of a side compartment is appropriate since 17ß-Estradiol is highly lipophilic and thus likely move into other regions of the body.

Rescigno and Segre[3] have described a simple and convenient method for writing the Laplace transform for systems consisting of compartment models. This method was implemented into a computer program. The approach is based on the fact that the Laplace transform of a compartment is divided by the inputs of the Laplace variable, s, plus the sum of the first order rate constants for the exits from the compartment. The detail of the employed method will be presented in greater detail elsewhere[2].

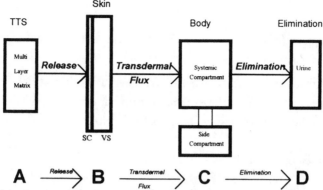

Fig. 1: 17ß-Estradiol movement from the delivery system device to the target site in transdermal systemic delivery. SC denotes stratum corneum, VS denotes viable skin.

IN VIVO AND IN VITRO METHODS

The transdermal drug delivery system consists of a matrix type system in which the drug dissolved, a backing layer, an adhesive layer which anchors the transdermal system to the skin, and a release liner. In vivo the adhesive layer assures the efficacy of the entire system by keeping the system affixed to the skin surface.

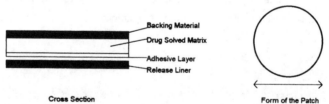

Fig. 2: Basic construction of a matrix type transdermal drug delivery system with an adhesive layer

The tested patch contained 17ß-Estradiol and was circular in shape (Fig. 2) with a skin contact area of 13.85 sq. cm. Mass balance experiments and transdermal flux experiments were conducted in vitro with a FRANZ diffusion cell (Fig. 3). 17ß-Estradiol was determined in vitro by HPLC method.

A clinical study was conducted to determine the bioavailability of ß-Estradiol provided by the newly developed transdermal drug delivery system. The test patch was identical to the above described transdermal system. The analytical method of the clinical study was a radioimmuno assay method. The lower limit of quantification was 5 pg/ml. The percent cross reaction was 0.192% with Estrone, 0.003% with Estrone sulfate, and 8.48% with 17ß-Dihydroequilenin[3].

RESULTS

(a) In vitro transdermal flux rates

of 17ß-Estradiol determined through excised human skin depicted in Fig. 4 and 5 explains the in vivo results, since an almost constant drug delivery rate of 48 µg ± 15 µ g/day per 13.85 sq.cm patch over 4 days can be detected.

(b) Blood concentration profiles

Fig. 6 depicts the blood concentration profiles of 17ß-Estradiol determined by a radioimmuno assay following application of the newly developed transdermal drug delivery system. Stable blood concentration over 84 hours after patch application can be detected, which lacks the undesirable initial peak seen in the reference transdermal drug delivery system.

(c) Batch to batch variability

No statistically significantly different transdermal flux rates of 17ß-Estradiol were detected in 3 different batches of the transdermal drug delivery system (Fig. 4). Statistical evaluations were performed with the 3-Way-Anova test on the 0.05 significance level. P values were taken as significant.

(d) In vitro/in vivo-correlation

Fig. 6 depicts calculated blood concentration levels and compares the results with clinically obtained pharmacokinetic profiles. As an input function the model uses 48 µg ß-Estradiol / day per 13.85 sq. cm patch input fluxes and a AUC (0-80h) 3799.48 (h.pg/ml) with a coefficient of variation of 31.3 %. One side compartment, depicted in Fig. 1, was included in the model calculations. The resulting agreement between calculated and experimental blood concentration profiles is excellent and fulfils Akaikes model selection criterion[4].

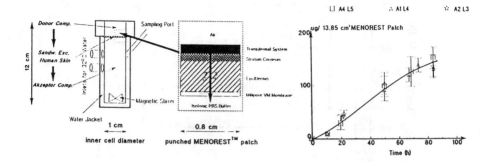

Fig. 3: in vitro FRANZ-diffusion cell

Fig. 4: in vitro transdermal fluxes of 17ß-Estradiol recorded in 3 different batches (mean and standard deviation)

in vitro Local Mass Balance of MENOREST™ Patch

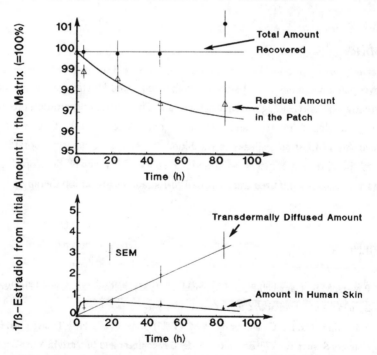

Fig. 5: in vitro local mass balance experiment (mean and standard deviation) of MENOREST™ patch

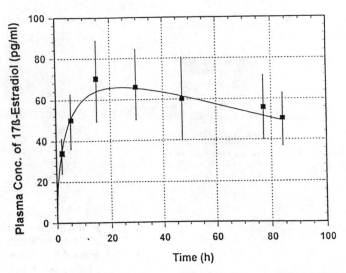

Fig. 6: Blood conc. levels of 17ß-Estradiol by transdermal delivery using MENOREST™ patch determined in a clinical trial (mean and standard deviation) and calculated (line).

SUMMARY

A novel patch containing 17ß-Estradiol exhibits improved kinetic profiles compared to the currently available leading transdermal product. The blood concentration produced by the newly developed matrix patch are stable over 3 to 4 days, thus avoiding the occurrence of 17ß-Estradiol peaks in the blood. These results are corroborated by the additional in vitro experiments as described above. This newly developed product presents a kinetically optimized transdermal 17ß-Estradiol substitution therapy.

REFERENCES

1. Powers, M.S., Campbell P., and Schenkel L. (1985). A New Transdermal Delivery System for ß-Estradiol, *J. Contr. Rel.*, **2**, 89 - 94

2. Rohr, U.D., Nauert, C., and Ehrly, A.M. (1995). Kinetics of a New Transdermal Drug Delivery System for 17ß-Estradiol: Model Development and In Vitro/In Vivo-Correlation. *Manuscript in preparation*

3. Rescigno, A. and Segre G. (1966). *Drug and Tracer Kinetics*, (Waltham MA, USA: Blaisdell Publishing Company)

4. Akaike, H. (1973). An information criterion. *Math. Sci.*, **14**, 5-9

Effect of β-estradiol therapy in menopause by transdermic means

E. Giannone, M.N.J. Abubakari, P. De Domenico, S. Bori and V. Lauro

Department of Obstetrics and Gynecology, University of Perugia, Italy

SUMMARY

A group of 65 women with age ranging from 52 to 56 years, in at least one year in menopause, were treated with a transdermic release control system containing estroprogestins. In all the women prior to the treatment, after 6 month and the end of the trial were carried out blood test, hysteroscopy with biopsy and climacteric complains (expressed in terms of presence/absence at baseline). Sweating, hot flushes, palpitations, dizziness were improved in 100%. Arthralgia, nervousness, depression, insomnia were improved in 93.75%. The endomethrium was found to be at the end of the trial in proliferative phase in 7.69%, in secretive phase in 89.23% and in simplex hyperplasia in 3.07%.

INTRODUCTION

The cessation of the ovarian activity that is observed after menopause causes important modifications in many apparatuses and systems such as the skin, mucosa, bone, cardiovascular system, nervous system, that in a great number of cases lead to effective pathologic states (1).

The estroprogestin replacement therapy therefore represents the reasonable solution (2-3).

The aim of our study is to evaluate the compliance and the therapeutic efficacy of a transdermic system (TTS), which contents 17-β-Estradiol and progestin in its noretisterone acetate form (4-5-6).

The parameters taken into consideration were principally; the evaluation of the local and systemic tolerability, the endomethrial characteristics through hysteroscopic and bioptic investigations, and the effect with regards to the general climacteric symptomatology (7-8-9). The parameters were evaluated at the beginning of the treatment, 3-6 weeks after and at the end of the treatment.

MATERIALS AND METHODS

A group of 65 patients with age ranging from 50 to 55, with at least one year in physiological menopause used a transdermic system containing estradiol, having a 50mcg/die release control every three and half days, applied to the glutei for the first 2 weeks, followed by another system containing estradiol and a 0.25mg/die release control NETA, for the successive 2 weeks, hence continuing with such rhythm for one year.

The criteria used to exclude patients were based on standard principles that contraindicate the estrogen therapies: estrogen dependent neoplasias, undefined origin genital haemorrhage, anamnestic thromboembolic events, severe arterial hypertension. These patients were evaluated 3-6 months and 1 year later. At any control, informations on collateral effects, type of bleeding, and climacteric symptomatology were acquired. Hysteroscopic and bioptic exams were carried out, at every control. The climacteric symptomatology was done through Kupperman's index, taking into consideration the most significant symptoms: hot flushes, paresthesia, insomnia, nervousness, depression, asthenia, dizziness, headache, palpitation.

RESULTS

All the patients subjected to this treatment, carried it on to the end. There was a great reduction in the climacteric symptomatology in some of these patients, a few weeks after the beginning of the treatment. Only a few number of these patients referred local allergic reactions on the site where the plaster was applied, anyhow this situation did not induce the suspension of the treatment.

At the 1°control, 3 months later, 48 (73.84%) of the 65 patients referred a neat improvement in the climacteric symptomatology, with an almost complete disappearance of the hot flushes, sweating, nervousness, insomnia, depression and headache there was an attenuation of 17/65 (26.15%) of symptoms such as arthralgia, paresthesia and asthenia. All these patients had uterine bleedings; 50/65 (76.92%) of these patients had monthly cyclic bleeding, while 15/65 (23.07%) did present irregular bleeding episodes. The endomethrial hysteroscopic exam with biopsy, revealed an endomethrium in proliferative phase in 45/65 (69.23%), 18/65 (27.69) in secretive phase and 2/65 (3.07) in atrophy.

At the 2nd control, 6 months later, the climacteric symptomatology showed clear improvement alongside with the disappearance of hot flushes, sweating, palpitation, insomnia, dizziness and depression Paresthesia, arthralgia and asthenia did persist in 8/65 (12.30%) patients. The monthly cyclic blood flow was present in 55/65 (84.61%) and remained irregular in the remaining 10/65 (25.38%). The hysteroscopic and bioptic exams revealed a proliferative phase in 12/65 (18.46%), secretive phase in 51/65 (78.46%) and a hyperplasia simplex in 2/65 (3.07%) cases.

At the end of the treatment, that is 12 months later, there was a total disappearance of the climacteric symptomatology in all patients, the paresthesia, arthralgia and asthenia persisted only in 4/65 (6.15%) patients. The hysteroscopy and biopsy of the endomethrium revealed a proliferative phase in 5/65 (7.69%), secretive phase in 58/65 (89.23%) and hyperplasia simplex in 2 cases. These 2 cases of hyperplasia simplex were different from the former cases above.

DISCUSSION

The results obtained in our study on estroprogestin transdermic therapy in menopause, do insert it in the modern and much discussed question protection roll of the hormone replacement therapy with regards to the entire symptomatology of the climacteric, preventing simultaneously the endomethrial hyperstimulation. The noretisterone acetate (NETA) is a strong progestin that substantially mimes the biological effects of progesterone. The effects of progesterone on tissues, depend on the previous stimulation of the endomethrium, activated by estrogen in the secretive phase. The progestin addition for 12 days of the cycle, to a continuos estrogen regime, prevents the endomethrial hyperstimulation, thus reducing the incidence of hyperplasia. This situation was verified only in 3,07% cases in our study. Already at the 1st control, 53.84% of these patients had secretive endomethrium, which increased to 89,23% at the 3rd control, accompanied by regular monthly cycle. At the 1st control, the menopausal symptoms were already present in 73.84% of these patients, but disappeared (100%) at the 2nd and 3rd control. Only arthralgia, paresthesia and asthenia attenuated in 26.15% at the 1st control, then reducing to 12.30% at the 2nd control and to 6.15% at the 3rd control.

CONCLUSION

The risk- benefit relation of the estroprogestin replacement therapy in menopause, to date is largely in favour of the beneficial aspects (that is, taking into consideration the global aspects of this problem).The preventive action on osteoporosis, reduction of cerebrovascular accidents, improvement of vasomotor symptoms and advantages in living qualities, with reduction in the increase of risk of carcinoma of the endomethrium associated with estrogen administration, suggesting the opportunity to establish a substitutive therapy in menopause, to be realised possibly right at the initial phases, certainly, previous to a careful selection of the patients. A hysteroscopic exam with the endomethrial hystology , permits to carry out a pharmacological action on the endomethrium, thus preventing cases of hyperplasia in its various grades, to occur. The hysteroscopic exam on our patients with age ranging from 50 to 55 years, pluripare was carried out easily in our ambulatory and without the use of anaesthesia.

REFERENCES

1) Utian W.H.: - The Climateric syndrome. - Gynecological Endocrinology - The Parthenon Publishing Group,623-33,1987.

2) Montemagno V., Affinito P., Nappi C. - Terapia sostitutiva ed endometrio. - Atti della Società Italiana di Ostetricia e Ginecologia, 111-116,1992.

3) Sismondi P. ed Al. - Terapie ormonali sostitutive in menopausa: bilancio, rischi e benefici. - In "Climaterio e menopausa: Problematiche cliniche". Med. Italia Ed.,Roncegno 1990.

4) Bologna A., Mega M., Dal Pozzo M. e Coll. - Impiego di un estroprogestinico transdermico nella terapia sostitutiva della menopausa. - Atti della Società Italiana di Ostetricia e Ginecologia - Congresso di Genova - Aprile 1992, pag. 925-26.

5) Whitehead M.I., Fraser D., Schenkel L., Crook D.,Stevenson J.C. - Somministrazione transdermica di estroprogestinici nella terapia sostitutiva ormonale. - Lancet 335: 310-12, 1990.

6) Keller P.J.- Combined transdermal hormone therapy.- Advances in Gynecological Endocrinology. - The Parthenon Publishing Group. Vol. 1, 651-57,1988.

7) Rownikar V. - Phisiology and treatment of hot flushes. - Obstet. Gynecol., 75, 4: 3-7,1990.

8) Porcelli A., Baj G., Calleri L., Priori L. and Surico N. - Transdermic estrogenic therapy with oral progesterone in postmenopause evaluation of endometrial response with a 12 months follow-up. - Current investigations in Gynecology and Obstetrics, pag 273-74,1993.

9) Leather A.T., Savvas M., Stud J.W. - Endometrial histology and bleeding patterns after 8 years of continuous combined estrogen and progestogen therapy in postmenopausal women. - Obstetr. Gynecol., Dec. 1991, 78(6), 1008-10.

Klimonorm® in postmenopausal hormonal therapy

P. Šuška, M. Borovský and D. Uherčík

1st, 2nd and 3rd Departments of Gynecology and Obstetrics, Comenius University, Bratislava, Slovakia

The necesity of hormone replacement therapy (HRT) in terms of prevention and treatment of climacteric and estrogen deficiency syndromes in postmenopausal women is generally well recognized (1,2), however the therapy remains applied in inadequate extent (3).The causes of this phenomenon are different and generally may be divided into two groups: 1. the attending physician refuse to prescribe HRT, or 2. the patient herself refuses to take HRT, mainly because of fears from side effects of applied hormones. Klimonorm[R] of the firm Jenapharm is currently the most frequent drug indicated for the purposes of HRT in Slovak Republik. Our prospective study was conducted to evaluate the effectiveness and tolerance of this drug, side effects occurence as well as patients´ attitudes toward its application.

MATERIAL AND METHODS

The study consisted of 136 patients undergoing either preventive treatment or therapy for climacteric and estrogen deficiency syndromes. Mean age of the patients was 47,1 years, 19 (14%) of the patients ranged from 20 to 40 yrs., and 117 (86%) of patients were between the age of 40 to 60 yrs. Mean age at menopause was 46,4 years. 12 (8,8%) of patients reported regular menstrual bleeding, 42 (30,8%)

of patients had irregular menstruation. In 83 (61%) of patients menstrual bleeding had stopped of whom 40 (i.e.
29,4% of the total group) have had hysterectomies.

In all patients full gynecological history was taken, risk
factors examined includes hypertension, obesity, metabolic .
disturbances, alcohol and tobacco abuse. Concurrent diseases and their treatment were also recorded. Complete gynecological examinations of patients included colposcopy,
onco- and functional cytology. Weight and blood presure of
patients were observed as well. The extent of the laboratory examinations included:blood count, cholesterol, HDL-,
LDL- and VLDL cholesterol, triglycerides, glycaemia and
hepatic tests (AST, ALT, GMT and Bi). Severity of climacteric complaints was evaluated by Kupperman index (4). Effectiveness and tolerance of the therapy were defined as
very good, good, satisfactory and bad.Following the entry
examination each patient received Klimonorm (Fig. 1) for 3
menstrual cycles and the drug was used as indicated in the
producer´s instructions (from 1st to 9th day yellow coated
tablets, then from 10th to 21st day turquoise coated
tablets and from 22nd to 28th day without therapy).

---

9 x yellow coated tablets: 2 mg estradiolvalerat

12 x turquoise coated tablets: 2 mg estradiolvalerat +
0, 15 mg levonorgestrel

Figure 1 **KLIMONORM**[R] composition

On each patient a protocol was made and patients were re-
gularly checked-up every 3 month. Therapeutic success was
assessed from the changes of the rating figures at the onset of the treatment (E_o) and during the course of treatment (E_x) - after 3 months ($E_x = E_1$), after 6 months ($E_x = E_2$)
according to the formula:

$$TS\ (\%) = 100 - \frac{100 \ x \ E_x}{E_o}$$

RESULTS AND DISCUSSION

Based on the Kupperman index values at the beginning of
the treatment, 18% of patients showed slight forms of climacteric complaints (rating below 15), mild forms (rating
15-20) were observed in 11%, 61% of patients demonstrated
moderate forms (rating 20-35) and severe forms were recorded in 10% of patients (rating over 35). A 3 month treatment program revealed the following changes: a majority of
patients (94%) had the Kupperman index values below 15,
mild form of climacteric complaints were detected in 4%
and 2% of patients disclosed moderate forms. After 6 month
of treatment, almost all patients (99%) reported only
slight or no climacteric complaints.In 1% of patients persisted mild forms of climacteric complaints (Fig. 2).

KUPPERMAN INDEX

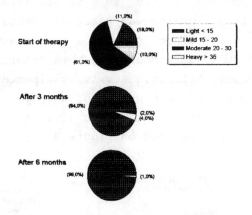

Figure 2 Changes in Kupperman index during
the treatment

Therapeutic success of climacteric syndrome treatment by
Klimonorm, calculated from the Kupperman index changes, is
presented in Table 1.

Duration of therapy	3 month	6 month
Number of patients	135	128
Patients with therapeutic succes more than 75%	69 51,1%	116 90,6%
Patients with therapeutic succes 50% - 75%	50 37,0%	10 7,8%
Patients with therapeutic succes 25% - 50%	11 8,1	1 0,8%
Patients with therapeutic succes less than 25%	4 3,0%	1 0,8%

Table 1   Therapeutic success of treatment by Klimonorm[R]

Adverse side effects included mainly intermenstrual bleeding which occurred 9x (i.e. in 6,6% of patients). In 3 patients (2,21%) migraine was recorded. In 7 patients the
therapy was discontinued (once due to aggravated hypertension, once due to bronchial asthma deterioration, twice
due to increased bilirubin levels, 3 times due to the subjective feeling of the patients than the treatment was
harmful).Changes in the body mass after the 6 month treatment program are recorded on Figure 3.

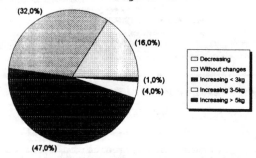

Figure 3   Changes in the body mass after
therapy by Klimonorm

476

Complete evaluation of the effectiveness and tolerance of the treatment is presented in Table 2.

Scale	Effectiveness(n = 135)	Tolerance(n = 135)
Very good	120 patients (88,9%)	116 patients (85,9%)
Good	10 patients (7,4%)	10 patients (7,4%)
Satisfactory	2 patients (1,5%)	3 patients (2,2%)
Bad	3 patients (2,2%)	6 patients (4,4%)

Table 2 General assessment of therapy by Klimonorm[R]

Our observations demonstrated that Klimonrom improved climacteric complaints in more than 95,6% of the followed-up patients. Good and very good effect was achieved in 96,3% and good and very good tolerance was recorded in 93,3% of patients. Irregular bleeding normalized in 88,1% of patients treated by Klimonorm. Regular bleeding remained uninfluenced in 88,3% of patients. In the majority (93%) of postmenopausal patients menstrual bleeding re-appeared. 22,6% of patients reported climacteric complaints of transient character during drug-free interval (i.e. days 22 to 28). The majority of patients evaluated the treatment positively. Reestablishment of menstrual bleeding was assessed negatively. More than 50% of the patients repeatedly asked about the harmfulness of HRT. The fear of cancer resulting from HRT was prevalent: these patients will most probably discontinue future treatment. Of the original set of 136 patients using HRT, 92 (67,6%) of women continued in the therapy after 6 cycles.

Current literature reflects positive attitudes towards HRT that is, unambiguous,not only due to its benefits but also because of its cost-effectiveness (5,6). As our study was of short-term character we aimed at the treatment of climacteric syndrome where the good effectiveness and tolerance of Klimonorm were observed. Its suitability in prevention of cardiovascular diseases and osteoporosis can be assumed from literature reports (7) about favourable effects its components (estradiolvalerat, levonorgestrel). The low incidence of side effects is comparable with other modern preparations. We believe along with the other authors (8), that HRT contraidications in postmenopause are the only severe forms of the diseases reported by the producers.

CONCLUSION

The results of our study demonstrate that Klimonorm^R, due to its efficacy, is a suitable HRT medication in postmenopausal women. Low incidence of side effects should remove any fears patients may have regarding HRT. In Slovakia the Klimonorm^R treatment is fully covered by national insurance.

REFERENCES

1. Jones, K. P.(ed.) (1992).Estrogen replacement therapy. Clin. Obstet. Gynecol., 35, pp. 854-935
2. Göretzlehner, G. and Lauritzen, Ch. (1992). Praktische Hormontherapie in der Gynäkologie. (Berlin, New York: Walter de Gruyter)
3. Šulc, J., Čekal, M., Velek, J. (1994). Režimy hormonální substituční léčby, teorie a praxe. Gynekolog, 3, pp. 148-153
4. Hauser, G. A. (1991). Überlegungen zu einer qualitativen und quantitativen Bemessung klimakterischer Beschwerden. In Lauritzen, Ch. (ed.) Menopause. Hormonsubstitution heute 4, pp. 70-73. (München: Informed)
5. Siddle, N. C. and Knight, M. A. (1991). Managing the Menopause. A Practical Guide to HRT. (Crawley: Novo Nordisk Pharmaceutical Ltd.)
6. Rovira, J. and Trinxet, C. (1993). Economic evaluation of hormone replacement therapy. In Cosséry, J.-M.(ed.) Medical-Economic Aspects of Hormone Replacement Therapy., pp.131-166 (Carnforth, New York: The Parthenon Publishing Group)
7. Sitruk-Ware, R. (1993). Benefits and risk of hormonal replacement therapy in postmenopausal women.In Cosséry, J.-M.(ed.) Medical-Economic Aspects of Hormone Replacement Therapy., pp. 1-16 (Carnforth, New York: The Parthenon Publishing Group)
8. Stevenson, J. C. (1994). Are some contraindications to HRT actually indications? Europ. Menopausal J., 1, p.15

Analysis of efficacy and the bleeding pattern during 6 months' treatment with sequential and continuous estrogen-progestogen therapy

T. Moskovic and S. Runic

Gynecology and Obstetrics University Hospital "Narodni Front", N. Fronta, Belgrade, Yugoslavia

INTRODUCTION

Most major complaints during the menopause period are of subjective symptoms which peak after last menstrual onset but begin to occur in women during their 40s. These are the result primarily of changes in circulating levels of estrogen and endorphin secretion mostly in hypothalamus. It is therefore natural that the frequency and severity of symptoms are subject to individual variations. It is necessary for postmenopausal women with intact uterus to take a progestin with estrogen replacement therapy, to protect the endometrium from possible neoplastic effects of unopposed Estrogens. Onset of bleeding is expected consequence of opposed hormone replacement therapy, but often undesirable specially for older postmenopausal women. Is it possible to avoid bleeding in HRT users?

AIM OF THE STUDY

Our study has been conducted to compare onset, frequency and duration of bleeding during 6 month in 87 postmenopausal women receiving sequential or continuous estrogen-progestogen therapy. The aim of the study was also to investigate is there any difference in efficasy between sequential versus continuos estrogen-progestogen therapy in the control of the vasomotor and psychological symptoms associated with natural menopause.

PATIENTS AND METHODS

A total of 88 healthy postmenopausal women (54-63 age), requiring ERT for the treatment of climacteric symptoms were enrolled in an prospectiv, comparative study lasting 6 month.

I group-sequential E-P therapy (n=40) received: 2mg oestradiol continuously + 1mg norethisterone acetate, cyclically from 13-22nd day of cycle.
II group-continuos E-P therapy (n=48) received: 2mg oestradiol + 1mg norethisterone acetate continuously.

Inclusion criteria were postmenopausal status (last menstrual period more than 12 months ago); intact uterus; at least 3 month since previous combined HRT.

The main exclusion criteria were previous unopposed estrogen therapy, undiagnosed vaginal bleeding and uncontrolled hypertension. Prior to inclusion a general medical and gynecological examination was performed. Patients were asked to complete questionnaire about onset and duration of bleeding for each of six cycles.

At the pre trial visit, after cycles 3 and cycles 6, patients were asked to complete a questionnaire with 12 questions addressing the somatic and psychological symptoms of estrogen deficiency. Efficasy was assessed of modified Kupperman index using 4-point scale: very much/always (3), rather often/rather much (2), not often/not much (1), never/not at all (0). Maximum for total inex score was 12 points.

Changes versus baseline and within treatment were analysed by paired t-test.

RESULTS

Of the 88 women enrolled, 85 completed study (528 cycles). 3 women discontinued prematurely: 1 due to irregular bleeding and 2 due to breast tenderness.

Side effect as breast tenderness occurred in 11 patients: 7 in I group and 4 in II group. Two of them discontinued due to severity symptom. One woman in the second group discontinued due irregular bleeding.

In the 85 patients who completed the study, menopausal symptoms assessed of modified Kupperman index pre trial, after 3 and after 6 cycles of sequential replacement estrogen-progestogen therapy (Figure 1) both groups. Students paired t-test shows significant improvements in the total score from baseline (pre-treatment) for cycles 3 ($p<0.001$) and cycles 6 ($p<0.001$) in both groups. Significant improvement was observed in the somatic and psychological symptoms for sequential and continuos E-P therapy.

Of a total of 240 cycles in the I group - sequential E-P therapy, 214 (89%) recorded regular bleeding, 7 (3%) irregular bleeding and 19 (8%) recorded amenorrhea. Of a total of 270 cycles in the II group - continuos E-P therapy, 81 (30%) cycles recorded regular bleeding, 19 (7%) irregular bleeding and 170 (63%) amenorrhea (Table 1).

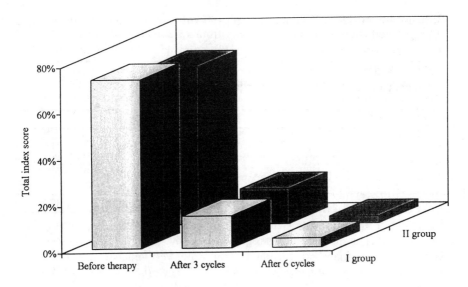

Figure 1 Total score (%) of postmenopausal symptoms in two groups. I group: sequential E-P therapy and II group: continuous E-P therapy, before therapy, after 3 and after 6 cycles.

Table 1 Bleeding pattern in 85 postmenopausal women during 6 cycles receiving sequential and continuous HRT

	HRT regime			
	I group: oestradiol continuously + norethisterone acetate/10 days (n = 40)		II group: oestradiol + norethisterone acetate continuously (n = 45)	
Bleeding pattern	N^0 of cycles	(%)	N^0 of cycles	(%)
Regular	214	89	81	30
Irregular	7	3	19	7
Amenorrhea	19	8	170	63
Total	240	100	270	100

Analysis of bleeding pattern during six cycles shows that in the I group with sequential therapy 80-94% patients have bleeding episodes in all of six treated cycles. In the II group with continuos E-P therapy percentage of patient with bleeding episodes decline from 60% in 1st cycle, to 45% in 2nd and 3rd cycle,

36% in 4th cycle. All women in 5th and 6th cycles recorded amenorrhea (Table 2).

Table 2 Women (%), with bleeding episodes during six cycles in two group postmenopausal women receiving sequential and continuous HRT

	HRT regime			
	I group: oestradiol continuously + norethisterone acetate/10 days (n = 40)		II group: oestradiol + norethisterone acetate continuously (n = 45)	
Cycles N^0	N^0 of women	(%)	N^0 of women	(%)
I	35	88	27	60
II	36	90	20	45
III	38	94	20	45
IV	38	94	16	36
V	37	93	0	0
VI	32	80	0	0

In the I group regular bleeding started on average 23 day. Bleeding lasted 1-3 days in 115 (48%) of 221 total bleeding cycles, 4 days and more in 125 (52%) of bleeding cycles (Table 3). In the II group regular bleeding started on average 16 day. Bleeding lasted 1-3 days in 83 (83%) of 100 total bleeding cycles, 4 days and more in 17 (17%) of total bleeding cycles (Table 3).

Table 3 Duration of bleeding

	HRT regime			
	I group: oestradiol continuously + norethisterone acetate/10 days (n = 40)		II group: oestradiol + norethisterone acetate continuously (n = 45)	
Duration of bleeding (days)	N^0 of cycles	(%)	N^0 of cycles	(%)
1 - 3	106	48	83	83
4 and more	115	52	17	17
Total bleeding cycles	221	100	100	100

DISCUSSION

Sequential and continuos estrogen-progestogen therapy has shown relief of vasomotor symptoms, but has also demonstrated significant improvements in both physical and psychological symptoms (1). However, previous studies (2) in postmenpausal women have shown that, although placebo effects may be pronounced during the early months, they disappear with time.

The pronounced improvement in backache and joint and limbs pain remains unclear, whether is a non specific effect due to improvement in climacteric complaints and general well-being or weather is due to specific pharmacological effects of estrogens e.g. on endorphin production.

A very few gestagen - related side effects was observed, suggesting that oral sequential estrogen-progestogen therapy is well tolerated.

In this study 86% women with sequential type of regiment have expected (3) regular bleeding . Continuos E-P therapy has been advocated by some authorities. The aim has been to induce amenorrhea, but chronic irregular bleeding is common (4). We found amenorrhea in 70% of total cycles and irregular bleeding in 8% of total cycles. Only one woman discontinued therapy due to irregular bleeding.

CONCLUSIONS

Hormonal replacement therapy is remarkably effective in the treatment of menopausal symptoms. The normal pattern of bleeding on sequential combined hormonal replacement therapy i.e. two- four day light bleed, occurs at the end of the progestogen phase of treatment. Regular bleeding is well accepted of early menopausal women. Continuous combined E-P therapy resulted in high percent of amenorrhea although in a small percentage may cause irregular bleeding. If regular, bleeding is light and short duration. Women in late menopause often not tolerate restoring of bleeding, thats why continuous E-P therapy is acceptable and well tolerated of women in late menopause.

REFERENCES

1. Bungay, G.T., Vessey, M.P., McPherson, C.K. (1980). Study of symptoms in middle life with special reference to the menopause. *Br Med. J.*, ii, 181-183.

2. Wiklund, I., Dimenas, E., Whal, E. (1990). Factor of importance when evaluating quality of life in clinical trials. *Contr. Clin Trials* ., 11, 169-179.

3. Whitehead, M.I., Hillard, T.C., Crook, D. (1990). The role and use of progestogens. *Obstetrics, and Gynecology* ., 75(suppl 4), 59S-79S.

4. Fraser, D., Whitehead, M.I., Endacott, J. et al. (1989). Are fixed-dose oestrogen-progestogen combinations ideal for all HRT users. *Brit. J of Obstet and Gynaecol.*, 96, 776-782.

Occurrence of untreated climacteric and estrogen-deficient syndrome in general medicine practice

E. Šuškova, P. Šuška, G. Kováč and A. Šoka

Department of General Medicine, Derer's Hospital, Bratislava, Slovakia

Despite existing knowledge and the well-recognized significance of hormone replacement therapy (HRT) in the prevention and treatment of climacteric and estrogen-deficiency syndrome (1,2,3),the percentage of patients treated
by HRT remains unusually low in Slovakia. Lack of suitable
preparations in the past created and sustained this
situation. Today, however,when our market is well supplied
with a variety of drugs, this situation need no longer
continue, and from the point of view of general health
care,is unacceptable. Our study was conducted to determine
the frequency and consequences of these syndromes in untreated female population as well as why women refuse
treatment.

MATERIAL AND METHODS

A general practitioner´s randomly selected group of postmenopausal women complaining of other than gynecological
problems,was examined.The occurence of climacteric syndrome was identified by establishing the Kupperman index (4).
Postmenopausal metabolic syndrome was estimated through
laboratory examinations of the blood: blood count, cholesterol, HDL-, LDL- and VLDL- cholesterols, triglycerids,

lipoproteins, glycaemia, liver tests (Bi, AST, ALT, GMT) and ionogram (Ca, P, Na, K, Cl). The occurence of osteoporosis was detected by X-raying bones of the hand. Other parameters evaluated included obesity, hypertension and ischemic heart desease. A special enquiry was conducted to determine the attitudes of those patients examined to HRT. A total set of 120 women with 92 women comprising the postmenopausal group, was examined. The group included patients who had been menopausal for at least 2 years, the control group was comprised of 28 women with regular patterns of menstrual bleeding. The characteristics of examined set are shown in table 1.

Table 1   The characteristics of examined set

	Postmenopausal patients	Premenopausal patients	Total
Number of patients	92	28	120
Mean age	58,9(48-70)yrs.	45,5(25-53)yrs.	–
Menopausal age	48,6(32-59)yrs.	–	–

RESULTS AND DISCUSSION

In the group of postmenopausal women, climacteric syndrome was found in 78% of patients, with the mean value of Kupperman index of 20 (0-41). Pathological laboratory lipid metabolism values were observed in 54%, 91% showed osteoporosis (the increase is age-related from 78-100%), obesity was recorded in 25%, hypertonic disease and ischaemic heart disease were found in 35% and 63% respectively. In the control group, climacteric syndrome was discovered in 14% of patients with mean values of Kupperman index being 8 (0-28). Pathological laboratory lipid metabolism values were observed in 35%, osteoporosis appeared in 32%, obesity in 14%, hypertonic disease in 14%. No cases of ischaemic heart disease were found in the control group. Table 2 summarizes the results of our examinations.

Table 2   Presence of pathological findings

	CS	PLT	OP	O	MH	IDC
Before menopause	14%	35%	32%	14%	14%	0%
After menopause	78%	54%	91%	35%	35%	63%
From this group:						
2- 5 years after	20(0-41)	46%	78%	34%	34%	46%
6-10 years after	21(10-30)	60%	95%	20%	20%	60%
11-34 years after	18(9-33)	57%	100%	43%	43%	77%

Explanation: CS - Climacteris syndrome
PLT- Pathological laboratory tests
OP - Osteoporosis
O - Obesitas
MH - Hypertonic disease
IDC- Ischaemic heart disease

The results of our investigation demonstrate a high incidence of climacteric and estrogen-deficiency syndromes among the female population of Slovakia. The increase in osteoporosis and cardiovascular disease induced by post-menopausal hormonal changes in our female population is reported also by orthopedists and internists (5, 6). As shown in the accessible demographic data, women in the age group 45-64 yrs, represent 23,8% of the whole female population. Expressed in absolute numbers, this accounts for more than half a million women. Data from Western sources report that 5-30% of women at risk are treated by HRT. In contrast, the percentage of women in Slovakia treated by HRT remains very low, reaching less than 1% (7). The reasons for this situation vary. Our enquiry has demonstrated that about 60% of the patients did not know about the possibilities and importance of HRT.Of patients who did know, 50% did not attribute any special significance to HRT, though they did not refuse HRT. The remaining number of the patients refused HRT, most frequently due to fears concerning cancer and obesity. The fear of possible renewal of menstrual bleeding was also a factor in their decision to refuse HRT.

CONCLUSION

The results of our investigations have confirmed that a matter of climacterium and postmenopause in Slovakia is an urgent problem and need for preventive and therapeutic HRT in Slovakia is of great concern. Improved health education through the mass media as well as intensive search for postmenopausal complaints at the general practitioner level would certainly lead to early and effective HRT initiated by our gynaecologists.

REFERENCES

1. Göretzlehner, G. and Lauritzen, Ch. (1992). Praktische Hormontherapie in der Gynäkologie. (Berlin, New York: Walter de Gruyter)
2. Riggs, B. L. (1992). Prevention and Treatment of Osteoporosis. (Seattle, Toronto, Bern, Göttingen: Hogrefe & Huber Publishers)
3. Heister, R. (1991). Herz und Kreislauf in der Postmenopause. (Berlin: Berliner Medizinische Verlagsanstalt)
4. Hauser, G. A. (1991). Überlegungen zu einer qualitativen und quantitativen Bemessung klimakterischer Beschwerden. In Lauritzen, Ch. (ed.) Menopause. Hormonsubstitution heute 4, pp.70-73.(München: Informed)
5. Murín, J. (1994). Kardiovaskulárne zmeny a komplikácie v klimaktériu. Prakt. Gynekol., 1, 17-21
6. Payer, J. (1994). Postmenopauzálna osteoporóza. Prakt. Gynekol., 1, 28-33
7. Rothe, K. (1993). Menopauseprobleme und Hormonsubstitution in den neuen Bundesländern. In Lauritzen, Ch. (ed.) Menopause. Hormonsubstitution heute 6, pp.119-22. (Basel: Aesopus Verlag GmbH)

92

Abdominal repair of small cystocele following total hysterectomy

P. Galli, P. Bellodi, R. Delli Carpini, G. Guerzoni, L. Padula, D. Tavernnari and M.A. Vezzani

Department of Obstetrics and Gynecology, Azienda USL Modena, Mirandola, Italy

---

INTRODUCTION

Moderate and functionally silent cystoceles may coexist with absolute indications to abdominal hysterectomy. Some patients may require the treatment of such cystoceles to supply at the same time of hysterectomy and straight away by abdominal access. As well, the occasion itself of the abdominal hysterectomy - even without patients request - gives the opportunity to repair small asymptomatic cystoceles.

Tovell (1) in 1978 described a trans abdominal post-hysterectomy technique usefull to repair small cystocele which we have ligthly modified (2).

SURGICAL TECHNIQUE

Removal of the uterus has been achieved and the vaginal vault is held up by four Allis clamps. The lateral angles of the vaginal vault are sutured. The bladder has been pushed down below the level of the vaginal vault. While the assistent holds back and up the bladder, the surgeon excises a triangular wedge of anterior vaginal wall.

The length of the triangle will depend to some extent to the size of the cystocele that is to be corrected (1). The two sides of the triangular wedge are sutured side to side with 2 or 3 extraflexing sutures. The vaginal vault is sutured with continuous dexon suture and reattached to the uterosacral ligaments. The vaginal vault remains opened to garantee drenage.

RESULTS

Ten patients underwent abdominal hysterectomy followed by modified Tovell colpocystopessy between 1992 and 1993. Age at time of operation was min. 46, max. 52 years. All the patients have been controlled 1, 6 and every six months after hysterectomy. Today the ten patients have an urogenital anatomic and funcional satisfactory situation and eather a regular ovarian function or a proper sostitutive hormonal treatment.

COMMENTS AND CONCLUSIONS

The natural hystory of cystoceles is rather variable: in most cases small cystoceles remain asymptomatic for a long time but may give several uro-genital anatomic and functional problems at any time of the future. For this reason we believe that when trans-abdominal hysterectomy is necessary and a moderate - even asymphomatic - cystocele is present, hysterectomy should be followed by transabdominal cystocele repair. The Tovell modified trans-abdominal cystopessy offers very fine results.

REFERENCES

1) Tovell H.M.M.: Abdominal repair of a small cystocele following a total hysterectomy. In: Tovell H.M.M. & Dank L.D: Gynecologic operation. Harper & Row Publ., N.Y., 139-147, 1978 (ISBN O-O6-142553-2).

2) Galli P., Bellodi P., Delli Carpini R., Guerzoni G., Padula L., Tavernari D., Vezzani M.A..Correzione transaddominale di cistocele dopo laparoisterectomia. In: Miniello G. e Cagnazzo G.: Urologia Ginecologica, CIC Ed. Int., 107-110, 1994 (ISBN 88-7141-174-9).

Evaluation of ovarian activity in hysterectomized women with conservation of the ovaries

E. Alba, R. Lerro, L. Corvetto, L. Nuzzo and G. Ragonesi

Università degli Studi di Torino, Istituto di Ginecologia ed Ostetricia, Cattedra B, Torino, Italy

Total hysterectomy with conservation of the ovaries (HCO) for benign uterine pathology is indicated for women in premenopausal age presenting apparent healthy ovaries. This is to avoid, or at least delay for as long as possible, the onset of a premature and therefore more problematic climacteric with all the vasomotor, psychic, osteoarticular, cardiocirculatory, urogenital troubles.

Whether HCO favours **premature onset of climacteric** as compared to non-hysterectomized women, has been differently studied with contradictory results.

Further challenge is the oncological risk of residual ovaries.

With respect to former problem we report the following results:

Beavis (1), Doyle (2) and Vuorento (3), with plasmatic and urinary samples, found that the residual ovaries maintain own activity. On the contrary, Souza (4) found, also in presence of normal endocrine activity of the ovaries, specific hystological alterations of the follicular reserve with compensatory hyperplasia of the stromal tecal cells. Menon (5) and Siddle (6) evaluated the onset of ovarian atrophy in 90 women previously subjected to HCO compared with that of 226 women in spontaneous menopause, without surgical operation. The average age of ovarian atrophy in the HCO women was calculated at 45,5 years, with respect to 49,5 years of non-operated women. This result was ascribed to vascular damage during the surgical intervention (i. e. mainly uterine artery section).

Respect the latter concern also, i. e. the **oncological risk** in women previously subjected to HCO, there are conflicting results. The rate of ovarian carcinoma resulted of 30/100.000 at New-York Cancer Registry (1984); of these the 85-90 % are ovarian tumors resulting from celomatic or mullerian epitelium and affect mainly the 50-60 years old women. From a research performed in 1989 between the english obstetricians and gynaecologists related to HCO, resulted that the 84% dont consider the ovariectomy important in ovarian cancer prevenction (7).

Bow calculated that bilateral ovariectomy for utero-ovaric benign disease reduces the rate of ovarian cancer of 12%. (8)

METHODS

We studied the residual ovarian activity in 180 women who had undergone HCO between the years 1980-1984 for benign uterine pathology (24 cases of unilateral ovariectomy) at Department of Obstetrics and Ginecology, Chair B of Turin University. The average age of women at the time of our investigation was 52 years. The research was performed through telephone questions about the most common symptomatology of climacteric (vasomotor, osteoarticular, cardiovascular,psychic, urogenital troubles). The women with uncertain answers where further evaluated by gynecological visit, thorough inverstigation and ormonal plasma samples for FSH-LH. The cut-off for the presence of climacteric was considered above 40 U/ml.

RESULTS

Of 180 women interviewed, 160 answered and where considered eligible. Of these 126 where clearly classified in climacteric and 10 not; 24 provided non clear answers and where recalled. After the following examinations and the results of ormonal samples, other 14 where classified in climacteric and 10 not. Of the 160 women investigated, 150 (93,75% with average age of 48,5 years) where in climacteric and 10 (6,25% with average age of 44 years) with good or enough ovarian activity. Analysing the 160 women in climacteric, we observed that troubles appeared on the average at 47,5 years. In previous reports, in Western Countries, the average age of climacteric is 51,4 years.(9)

The women of our research therefore presented, after HCO, a climacteric 4 years earlier, but an advantage of 5,5 years compared with age of surgical operation (average age of 42 years).Tab 1.

Table 1.   160 Women HCO   (Years 1980 - 1984)

Average age at the operation HCO...42   Years
Average age at the climacteric HCO... 47,5   Years
Average age at the climacteric in the control group............................51,4   Years
Average advantage of ovarian activity... + 5,5   Years

None of 160 women operated showed, limited to time observed (5-9 years), any case of ovarian cancer. There where only two cases of reintervention for benign ovarian pathology, although that is not statisticaly significant.

CONCLUSIONS

Our results agree with most of the Authors, i. e. global advantage for the conservation of apparent healthy ovaries in women undergoing hysterectomy for benign uterine pathology. The advantage of 5,5 years of ovarian activity by our results, with all organic and psychic benefits and poor risk of ovarian neoplasia opts for the conservation of the ovaries until 45 years.

Between 45-50 years the ovariectomy can be discussed based case by case with the woman, to informed consent upon the balanced risk-benefit.

After 50 years and in the rare cases of familiar ovarian or intestinal neoplasia (risk of secondary ovarian implant), it is not advised to conserve the ovaries.Tab 2.

Table 2. Reference proposal.

45 Years...conservation of the ovaries
50 Years...removal of the ovaries
45-50 Years...consent informed and further
                                                                prospectives researchs.

Our preliminary results will be performed by a prospectic research in that the women undergone to HCO will be recalled yearly to carry out a gynecological visit, a pelvic transvaginal sonogram and a possible FSH-LH plasma samples, to better prove the natural hystory of ovarian activity and oncological risk of a cohort of women which will be in the near future always most numericaly consistent.

REFERENCES

1) Beavis ELG, Brown JB, Smith MA.(1969). Ovarian function after hysterectomy with conservation of the ovaries in premenopausal women. *Obstet Gynaec Brit Cwlth.* , **76: 969-978.**

2) Doyle LL, Barclay DL, Duncan GW, Kirton KT. (1971). Human luteal function following hysterectomy as assessed by plasma progestin. *Amer J Obstet Gynec*, **110,1: 92-97.**

3) Vuorento T, Maenpaa J, Huhtaniemi L. (1992). Follow-up of ovarian endocrine function in premenopausal women after hysterectomy by daily measurements of salivary progesterone. Clin Endocrinol. , **36: 505-510.**

4) Souza AZ, Fonseca AM, Izzo VM, Clauzet RM, Salvatore CA. (1986). Ovarian histology and function after total abdominal histerectomy. *Obstet Gynec* **68,6: 847-849.**

5) Menon RK et al. (1987). Endocrine and metabolic effects of simple hysterectomy. *Int J Gynaecol Obstet.* **25: 459-463.**

6) Siddle N, Sarrel P, Whitehead M. (1987). The effect of hysterectomy on the age at ovarian failure: identification of a subgroup of women with premature loss of ovarian function in literature review. *Fertil Steril,* **47,1: 94-100.**

7) Jacobs I, Oram D. (1989). Prevenction of ovarian cancer: a survey of the practice of prophilactic oophorectomy by fellows and members of thr royal College of Obstetricians and Gynaecologists. *Br J Obstet Gynaecol.* **96: 510.**

8) Dowe Hl. (1984). Age-specific hysterectomy and oophorectomy prevalence rate and the risks for cancer of the reproductive system. *Am J Public Health.*74: **560-563**

9) Pescetto G, De Cecco L, Pegorari D, Ragni N. (1989). *Manuale di Ostetricia e Ginecologia.* Soc Edit Universo. Roma .

Feasability of reconstructive vaginal surgery according to Kelly-Kennedy in the treatment of genital prolapse

A. Carbonaro, R. Cantarella, V. Aidala and S. Reitano

Department of Obstetrics and Gynaecology, Santo Bambino Hospital, University of Catania, Catania, Italy

After having witnessed the growing number of "innovative" surgical techniques in the belief that improved results were linked to the different methods, today more emphasis is given to the diagnosis, in order to select cases for surgical treatment (trying to optimize the operation) or pharmacological treatment. In this view our retrospective work aims to verify the efficacy of urethroplastic surgery according to Kelly-Kennedy in correction of genital prolapse associated with urinary incontinence. This operation has often been criticised as it is considered unreliable for correction S.U.I. or in any case not suitable for prevention of its onset in case of prolapse without incontinence (1-2). However,in our opinion,careful preoperative evaluation of cases for urethroplastic surgery according to Kelly-Kennedy, adopting urodynamic tests and the Q tip test, enables this intervention to be enhanced.

METHOD AND PATIENTS

In our Obstetric and Gynaecologic Department, between September 84 and June 94, 215 women with genito-urinary prolapse underwent vaginal reconstructive surgery according to Kelly-Kennedy. The average age was 57.3 years (range 39-78),parity was 2.9 (range 0-9).
146 (80%) were in menopause and 36 (20%) menstruate (Fig.1).
Of the 215 women, 33 were lost in the follow-up. The remaining 182 were invited to undergo an anatomo-functional follow-up over a period of between 6 months and 10 years. Pre-operatively the degree of pelvic descensus was defined according to Beecham's criteria and urinary incontinence

497

TOTAL PATIENTS: 182

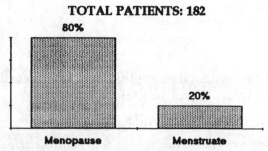

Fig.1 — Percentage of total patients correlated to their reproductive period of life.

was assessed using a protocol consisting of general and urologic history, stress test, cystometry and urethral profile and under stress according to Brown Wickam (3).
Of the 182 patients that responded, 55 (32%) suffered from 2nd degree cystocele, 69 (38%) from 3rd degree cystocele and 58 (30%) from total prolapse (Fig.2).

TOTAL PATIENTS: 182

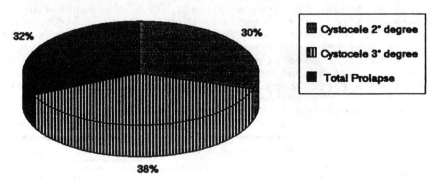

Fig.2 — Pelvic descensus grading

69 patients presented urinary incontinence. At the post-operative check-up no significant variations were observed in the urethral pressure profile. Infact in the women suffering from S.U.I. before the operation, that presented reduction in the functional length of the urethra, of the MPCU and the continence area, incontinence correction was obtained by repositioning the bladder neck in the abdominal pressure area and not due to an increase in functional length, or increased MPCU, which at the post-operative check-up both resulted reduced.

RESULTS

Pelvic descensus correction was obtained in 95% of cases, whereas 5% of patients presented a cystocele at the last follow-up visit (Fig.3).

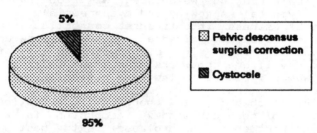

TOTAL PATIENTS: 182

Fig.3 - Surgical correction percentage

Incontinence was cured in 75% of cases whereas there was relapse in the other 25% (Fig.4).

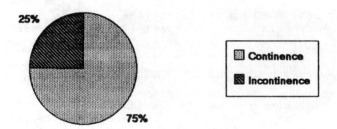

TOTAL PATIENTS: 182

Fig.4 - S.U.I. percentage after surgery

In any case, in correction of S.U.I. results depend on the different physiopathologies: in cases with low urethral pressure and dynamic sphincteral incompetence due to which stress creates a negative differential pressure between vesica and urethra, with urine escape, urethroplasty according to Kelly-Kennedy does not suffice to assure recovery. These cases would require association of a colposuspension according to Burch, aimed at repositioning the urethra in the abdomen. As regards cystocele relapses present at the last follow-up visit it must be remembered that this failure can also be correlated to progressive aging of tissue, which determines collapse of supportive means and genitourinary dystrophic alterations.

CONCLUSIONS

From our experience vaginal surgery according to Kelly-Kennedy in most cases assures good anatomic correction. Relapse of anterior vaginal hernia occurred in 5% of cases. The surgical technique we adopted was too invasive in 40% of cases (vaginal narrowing and dyspareunia).
In terms of stress incontinence correction the Kelly-Kennedy technique determined a long term follow-up recovery rate equal to 75%. In our opinion this figure is satisfactory if one considers the high number of obese and old age women included in the case histories.
We are certain that, with carefull selection of cases (exclusion of obesity, low surgical risk patients etc.), association of cervicocystopexy according to Burch with vaginal correction of the prolapse, is the best solution to functional outcome of this surgery, respecting in vaginal reconstruction, the objective of safeguarding the sex life of the patient.

BIBLIOGRAFY

1 STANTON S.L., CARDOZO L. 1979.   A comparison of vaginal and suprapubic surgery in the correction of incontinence due to urethral sfincter incompetence.
   Br. J. Urol. 51:479

2 DONADIO, GNEO 1991. Correzione vaginale del cistocele. Incontinenza urinaria femminile e prolasso genitale – dalla diagnosi alla terapia. Atti 2° Corso monotematico SIUD. Ed. Clas International

3 MILANI R., COLOMBO M., VITOBELLO D., SCALAMBRINO S. 1994. La chirurgia ricostruttiva vaginale con uretrocistopessi sec.   Kelly-Kennedy nel prolasso genitourinario severo.   Urologia ginecologica. IV congresso naz. AIUG. CIC' Ed. Internazionali

Medical therapy in the prevention of recurrent dysfunctional uterine bleeding

S. Dessole, E. Coccollone, G. Ambrosini, N. Vargiu, A. Scapinelli and P.L. Cherchi

Institute of Obstetrics and Gynecology, University of Sassari, Sassari, Italy

Dysfunctional uterine bleeding (DUB) is one of the most common gynaecological problems and it indicates every uterine bleeding not related to pathological disorders. This condition is clinically important because, in addition to the notable discomfort for women, it represents 10-20% of the outpatient gynaecological pathologies (1,2). In more than 50% of the cases, this condition occurs in the premenopausal period and in 90% of the cases the menstrual cycle is anovulatory (3). In most cases a relative hyperestrogenism plays an important role. The medical treatment is considered as a first option, but a recurrence occurs in 30-50% of the cases within 6-12 months from the suspension of the therapy. The medical treatment for recurrent DUB is focused on preventing the recurrence and the complications related to the hyperestrogenism, like atypical hyperplasia and endometrial carcinoma.

A vast array of substances is used for medical treatment: progestogens, oral contraceptives, Danazol and GnRH analogues, antifibrinolytic drugs, prostaglandin inhibitors, ovulation inductors (4). These different treatments must be personalised with respect to the patient's age, the presence of contraindications for several drugs and the pregnancy desire.

(A) Goserelin (GnRHa) for three month (1 vial/28 days)

(B) Goserelin (GnRHa) for three month followed by MAP (1 tablet/day for 12 days for three months)

(C) MAP (1 tablet/day for 12 days for three months)

(D) MAP (1 tablet/day for 12 days for three months)

in the prevention of DUB in the advanced fertile period.

MATERIAL AND METHOD

The study involved 28 patients, aged from 38 to 50 years, suffering from DUB (at least 3 episodes in the last 12 months) and treated in the acute phase of the latest episode with estroprogestogens (EE 50 mg + LNG 20 mg) (2 cp./day until the end of the hematic loss, then 1 tablet/day for two weeks). The first day of the menstrual flow after the treatment suspension was considered the first day of the cycle.

The patients were randomized in two groups: the Group A consisting of 15 patients, treated with Goserelin (GnRHa) from the first day of the cycle for three cycles. This group was then subdivided into two subgroups, A1 and A2. The subgroup A1, consisting of 8 patients, treated with Medrossiprogesterone acetate (MAP) for three cycles. The subgroup A2, consisting of 7 patients, who did not undergo further treatment.

Group B, consisting of 13 patients treated with MAP for three cycles. This group was also subdivided into two subgroups, B1 and B2. The subgroup B1 consisting of 6 patients, who continued the treatment with MAP for three additional cycles; the subgroup B2, consisting of 7 patients, who did not undergo any additional treatment.

We evaluated:

-the variation of the blood loss, on the basis of records completed by the patients using a pictorial chart (5).

-variations in the haemoglobin and iron blood level

-the variation in the lipid profile (cholesterol, HDL, LDL)

-the variation in the hepatic profile (GOT, GPT, Bilirubin)

-the variation in the bone mineral density, measured with 2 determinations at the distal extremity of the forearm

- the incidence of side effects

- the incidence of recurrence in the 12 months following the suspension of treatment.

The statistical analysis was performed using the t-Student.

RESULTS

The variation in the patient blood loss is reported in Table 1. In the 15 patients of Group A, after the third administration of Goserelin (GnRHa), there were 14 cases (93%) of amenorrhoea and one case (6%) of blood loss reduction. The patients in Group B showed a reduction in the menstrual blood loss in 10 cases (77%), no change in 2 cases (15.3 %), and an increase in one case (7.6%).

Table 1. Variations of blood loss.

	N.		N	%	N	%	N	%
GROUP A		Increase	2	(13,3)	-	-	-	-
	1	No change	4	(26,6)	-	-	-	-
GnRHa	5	Decrease	9	(60,0)	6	(40,0)	1	(6,0)
		Absent	0	-	9	(60,0)	14	(93,3)
GROUP B		Increase	3	(23,0)	-	-	1	(7,6)
	1	No change	3	(23,0)	3	(23,0)	2	(15,3)
MAP	3	Decrease	7	(53,0)	10	(76,0)	10	(77,0)
		Absent	0	-	0	-	0	0
				1		2	3	months

The variation in the blood loss for the successive three cycles is reported in Table 2. Into the subgroup A1 (GnRHa), normal menstrual flows occurred in 6 cases (75%), reduced blood loss in 2 (25%) cases. Into the subgroup A2, an abundant blood loss occurred in 2 cases (28.5%), a normal in 4 cases (57.1%) and a reduced one in 1 case (14.2%). Into the subgroup B1, an abundant blood loss occurred in 1 case (6.6%), a normal in 4 cases (66.6%) and a litle one in 1 (16,6%). Into the subgroup B2, an abundant blood loss occurred in 2 cases (28.5%) and a normal one in 5 cases (71.4%).

In Table 3, are reported the variation in the Hb and iron blood levels for every subgroup. The subgroup A1 showed, a significant increase in the Hb and iron blood levels was measured at the end of the treatment.

Table 2. Variations of blood loss into the subgroup during the 3 cycles

	N.		N	%	N	%	N	%
GROUP A1		Abundant	-	-	-	-	-	-
GnRHa and	8	Normal	5	(62.5)	6	(75.0)	6	(75.0)
MAP		Reduced	3	(37.5)	2	(25.0)	2	(25.0)
GROUP A2		Abundant		-		-	2	(28.5)
GnRHa and	7	Normal	3	(42.8)	5	(71.4)	4	(57.1)
observation		Reduced	4	(57.1)	2	(28.5)	1	(14.2)
GROUP B1		Abundant		-		-	1	(16.6
MAP	6	Normal	5	(83.3)	6	(100)	4	(66.6)
N.6		Reduced	1	(16.7)	-	-	1	(16.6)
GROUP B2		Abundant		-	1	(14.2)	2	(28.5)
MAP and	7	Normal	5	(71.5)	5	(71.4)	5	(71.4)
observation		Reduced	7	(28.5)	1	(14.2)	-	-
			1		2		3	months

Table 3. Variation of blood crasis.

	N.		BASAL	3	6 months	P
GROUP A1	8	Hb	11.2	12.4	13.6	>0.05
GnRHa and MAP		IRON	45	53	102	>0.05
GROUP A2	7	Hb	11.0	12.1	12.8	NS
GnRHa-observation		IRON	41	50	64	NS
GROUP B1	6	Hb	11.4	11.8	12.1	NS
MAP		IRON	47	52	55	NS
GROUP B2	7	Hb	11.1	11.7	11.5	NS
MAP-observation		IRON	40	48	43	NS

Table 4. Hepatic assessment

	N.		1	3	6 months	P
GROUP A1	8	GOT	16	16.5	16.8	NS
GnRHa and		GPT	20.4	22.2	21.8	NS
MAP		Bilirubin	0.72	0.76	0.68	NS
GROUP A2	7	GOT	17.7	20.8	23.5	NS
GnRHa and		GPT	19.2	25.4	24.8	NS
observation		Bilirubin	0.66	0.66	0.69	NS
GROUP B1	6	GOT	20.2	19.4	22,4	NS
MAP		GPT	21	25.6	25.2	NS
		Bilirubin	0.64	0.68	0.71	NS
GROUP B2	7	GOT	17.1	19.6	21.2	NS
MAP and		GPT	20.4	22.4	23	NS
observation		Bilirubin	0.78	0.76	0.82	NS

There were no significant modifications in the hepatic or lipid profiles (Tables 4 and 5) for all the four treatment groups.

Table 5. Lipid assessment

	N		1	3	6 months	P
GROUP A1	8	CHOLESTEROL	198,6	200,2	200,4	NS
GnRHa-MAP		HDL	56,4	57,2	57,6	NS
N.8		LDL	155	156,3	160,3	NS
GROUP A2	7	CHOLESTEROL	206,4	216,7	222,9	NS
GnRHa -		HDL	55,4	56,5	57,8	NS
observation		LDL	156,2	159,4	159,6	NS
GROUP B1	6	CHOLESTEROL	196,7	198,4	204,8	NS
MAP		HDL	54,4	55,4	58,7	NS
		LDL	161	164,3	167	NS
GROUP B2	7	CHOLESTEROL	190,7	199,8	194,6	NS
MAP -		HDL	58,3	59,4	60,2	NS
observation		LDL	152,6	156,7	155,9	NS

The bone density values, performed at the distal extremity of the forearm are reported in Table 6. No significant variations were observed.

Table 6.

	N.		Basal	3	6 months	P
GROUP A1	8	BD-UDST	424.2	424	420	NS
GnRHa-MAP		BD-MDST	730.8	726	722	NS
GROUP A2	7	BD-UDST	404.4	398.6	395.4	NS
GnRHa-observation		BD-MDST	724.2	708.8	707.6	NS
GROUP B1	6	BD-UDST	436.2	430.8	432.8	NS
MAP		BD-MDST	734.6	736.2	732.6	NS
GROUP B2	7	BD-UDST	428.8	430.2	426.8	NS
MAP-observation		BD-MDST	726.6	720.8	722.2	NS

The incidence of side effects was more present in the GnRH-a patient group. We did not suspend the treatment in any case.
The follow-up, performed 12 months after the suspension of treatment showed a recurrence percentage of 12% into the subgroup A1 and 42.8% in subgroup B2 (Figure 1).

Fig.1. 12 Months follow-up.

Recurrence after end of therapy.

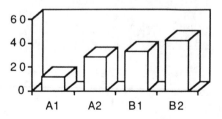

CONCLUSIONS

The treatment with Goserelin followed by MAP proved a better effectiveness than either Goserelin or MAP used alone in reducing the quantity of menstrual blood loss and favouring a more rapid restoration of the hematic crasis. The hepatic and lipid profile and the bone mineral density did not demonstrate variations in the treatments with different therapeutic schemes. The incidence of side effects was higher in the group treated with Goserelin, but it was not necessary to stop treatment in any case. Furthermore, there was a lower incidence of recurrence in the group treated with both Goserelin and MAP. We believe that such treatment can be usesful widely utilised in the prevention of recurrent DUB in the advanced fertile period.

REFERENCES

1.Milson, J, Anderson, K et al. (1991) : A comparison of flurbiprofen, tranexamic acid, and levonorgestrel-releasing intrauterine contraceptive device in the treatment of idiopathic menorrhagia. Am J Obstet Gynecol **164**: 879

2.Laufer, MR, Rein, MS (1993):,Treatment of abnormal Uterine Bleeding with Gonadotropin-Releasing Hormone Analogues. Clin Obstet Gynecol **36**:668,

3.Ferraris, DT, Colombatto, S, Re A, Bellino, R, Gordini, G, Lanza, A,(1989): Il metabolismo glicidico e delle poliamine nell'endometrio disfunzionale In Vadora: Le Metrorragie Disfunzionali" Roma CIC Edizioni internazionali,pp 17-26,

4.Shaw, RW (1994): Assessment of medical treatment for menorrhagia: Br J Obstet Gynaecol **101**,Supp 11,15-18

5.Higham, J M, O'Brien, PM, Shaw, RW (1990): Assessment of menstrual blood loss using a pictorial chart. Br J Obstet Gynaec **97**:734-739

MAP and LHRH agonists combination in the treatment of simple endometrial hyperplasia

P. Galli, P. Bellodi, R. Delli Carpini, G. Guerzoni, L. Padula, D. Tavernari and M.A. Vezzani

Department of Obstetrics and Gynecology, Azienda USL Modena, Mirandola, Italy

INTRODUCTION

We found very few references which would support our idea that long acting GnRH agonist could be used in the management of perimenopausal endometrial hyperplasia (1,2,3). Long acting GnRH agonists induce a reversible suppression of pituitary-ovarian function over a period of a month; in pre-menopausal women lasting GnRH administration may lead to menopause. Because endometrial hyperplasia can be considered as a hormon dependent lesion, we decided to monitor patients affected by Simple Cystic Endometrial Hyperplasia (SCEH) treated with medrossi-acetate-progesterone (MAP) and GnRH agonists.

Nevertheless, being such treatment extrimely expensive, we reserved it only to those patients at very high risk of progestinic long term treatment and to those anemic patient resistent to medical treatment and who refused hysterectomy. For this reason we collected very few patients in three years.

MATERIAL AND METHOD

During years 1992-94 nine patients between 47 and 58 years of age affected by abnormal uterine bleeding were assessed by endometrial citology, hysteroscopy and endometrial byopsy. All the patients resulted affected by simple cistic endometrial hyperplasia (SCEH) and were treated as follows. 20 mg/day of MAP were assumed per os between the 5th and 25th day of the cycle. Beginning from the following withdrawing bleeding, 3.75 mg of triptoreline were administered every 28 days for at least 6 times. At the end of the treatment and 6 months later, endometrial citology and byopsy had been repeated for controlls.

RESULTS

Six patients became asympthomatic and no SCEH was found at the controlls. One patient has barely stopped triptorelin and only one endometrial controll has been made. Two patients had abnormal bleeding after three GnRH administrations and asked for hysterectomy: areas of irregular endometrial growth were found without evidence of endometrial hyperplasia.

COMMENT AND CONCLUSIONS

We found very few references regarding GnRH analogous in the treatment of abnormal bleeding due to SCEH nevertheless the results concerning the management of SCEH are very encouraging being the almost totality of treated cases cured (1,2,3). We only have a very limited experience which moreover differs from literature because of the pretreatment with MAP.

In agreement with the literature regarding GNRH treatment of SCEH, our limited experience shows some indications that MAP pretreatment and GnRH treatment of SCEH may even reserve interesting developments in the prevention of more important perimenopausal endometrial abnormalities different from simple cystic hyperplasia and ensuing to it.

Because the GNRH agonists long term treatment is very expensive if compared to other medical treatments of SCEH, we conclude that maight be reserved to those patients at high risk of progestinic or surgical treatment of sympthomatic endometrial hyperplasia.

REFERENCES

1) Garozzo G., La greca M., Lomeo E., Panella M.: Goserelin treatment in glandular hyperplasia. Clin.Exp.Obst.Gyn., XX,4,268-272, 1993.

2) Colacurci N., de Placido G., Galasso M., Ruocco M., Perino A., Cittadini E.: Long acting GnRh agonist, goserelin,in the management of perimenopausal abnormal bleeding. 13th World FIGO Congress, Singapore, Int.J.Gynec. Obstet., Abstr. 0503, 148, 1991.

3) Oliva G.C., Sonsini C., Fratoni A.: An open non-comparativee study of the effects of "zoladex" (goserelin) 3.6 mg depot in the treatment of endometrial hyperplasia. 13th World FIGO Congress, Singapore, Int.J.Gynec.Obstet., Abstr.0825, 251,1991.

Hysteroscopic diagnosis in women with abnormal uterine bleeding

V. Benedetto, V. Palmara, G. Zona, E. Crea, M. Rigano, J. Leonardi and M. Micalizzi

Department of Gynecology, University of Messina, Italy

INTRODUCTION

In patients with abnormal uterine bleeding in peri or post - menopause, hysteroscopy with endometrial sampling has definite advantages over conventional investigative methods to make an accurate diagnosis or to guide therapy; a thorough inspection of the uterine cavity allows to detect or to exclude an uterine pathology that could explain the bleeding, thus avoiding often repeated and unnecessary dilatation and currettage under anaesthesia. Here we report the isteroscopic findings in 1112 women with abnormal uterine bleeding (AUB). (1, 2, 3, 4, 5, 6, 7, 8, 9, 10, 11, 12, 13)

MATERIAL AND METHODS

In our hysteroscopy out patients clinic 2456 hysteroscpies have been performed from January 1990 to Decenber 1994.

Hysteroscpy was performed using a Storz 4 mm rigid hysteroscope, in the proliferative phase of premenopausal women and at any time in post - menopausal women (or in emergencies).

The uterine cavity was dilatated by CO_2 insufflation (30/50 ml/mm) at an average pressure of 40 mmhg (never more than 80 mmhg).

The patients received 10 mg diazepam and 0,5 mg atropine i.m. 30 minutes before the examination. (14, 15)

RESULTS

A total of 1112 women with abnormal uterine bleeding was included in this study, the youngest being 38 and the oldest 83 years of age.

420 patients were pre or perimenopausal, 692 were post - menopausal. (Tab. I)

Cytological examination was performed in all the patients; biopsy and hystological examination was performed in patients with abnormal hysteroscopic finding.

Of the 1112 women examined the finding were: 472 (42,44%) were found to have normal and functional endometrium, 144 (12,94%) had atrophic endometrium, 22 (1,97%) had disfunctional endometrium, 14 (1,25%) had endometritis, 108 (9,71%) had fibroids, 110 (9,89%) had polyps, 144 (12,94%) had low risk hyperplasia, 10 (0,89%) had high risk hyperplasia, 4 (0,35%) had haematometra, 6 (0,53%) had pyometra, 78 (7,01%) had adenocarcinoma. (Tab. II)

The uterine cavity could be inspected adeguately in all the patients, but a second examination was performed in 98 patints: in 42 women because of active bleeding obscuring the view during the first examination, in 56 women under general anaesthesia because of cervical stenosis, intolerable pain or inadeguate view of uterine cavity during the first examination. (Tab. III)

No complication attributable to the procedure occurred and no patients required admission after hysteroscopy.

CONCLUSION

In 108 patients we founded a submucosus fibroid and 110 patients had polyps: these pathologycal alteration could have not been founded using convetional investigative methods. (Tab. II)

The resections by curette was enough to remove small fibroids (38 patients) and small endometrial polyps (77 patients); the eiectric resector was used under general anesthesia for removing larger fibroids and polyps.

Endometrial sample was taken by curette or Novak cannula in all the patients, and there was always enough material for a correct cytological examination even in patients with atrophic endometrium (144 patients). (Tab. II)

With the histologycal examination, performed in all the patients with abnormal uterine finding, 78 cases of adenocarcinoma and 10 cases of high risk of hyperplasia have been diagnosed. (Tab. II)

The large majority of patients considered as tolereble the pain occurred during the examination, similar to pain occurring during painfull menstruations.

No complication attributable to the procedure occurred.

The pre-medication with diazepam and atropine i.m. has been used successfully in this study and it provides a valid alternative paracervical block anesthesia and general anesthesia. (14 ,15)

Our results confirm the value of diagnostic hysteroscopy with direct endometrial sample or biopsy in AUB, as it gives informations on uterine cavity and endometrial pathology, it allows an aimed biopsy and it cost much less than conventional curettage and general anesthesia.

<table>
<tr><td colspan="2">Tab. I: Total patients examined</td><td colspan="2">Tab. II: hysteroscopy result of 1112 patients</td></tr>
<tr><td></td><td></td><td></td><td></td></tr>
<tr><td>n. patients 1112 (years >38 <83)</td><td></td><td>472 normal /functional endometrium</td><td>42,44%</td></tr>
<tr><td>pre- or peri-menopausal</td><td>420</td><td>144 atrophic endometrium</td><td>12,95%</td></tr>
<tr><td>post-menopausal</td><td>692</td><td>22 disfunctional endometrium</td><td>1,97%</td></tr>
<tr><td></td><td></td><td>14 endometritis</td><td>1,25%</td></tr>
<tr><td></td><td></td><td>108 fibroids</td><td>9,71%</td></tr>
<tr><td></td><td></td><td>110 polyps</td><td>9,89%</td></tr>
<tr><td></td><td></td><td>144 low risk hyperplasia</td><td>12,94%</td></tr>
<tr><td>Tab.III: second examination</td><td></td><td>10 high risk hyperplasia</td><td>0,89%</td></tr>
<tr><td></td><td></td><td>4 haematometra</td><td>0,35%</td></tr>
<tr><td>severe bleeding</td><td>42</td><td>6 pyometra</td><td>0,53%</td></tr>
<tr><td>general anesthesia</td><td>56</td><td>78 adenocarcinoma</td><td>7,01%</td></tr>
<tr><td>total</td><td>98</td><td></td><td></td></tr>
</table>

REFERENCE

1 Hamou J. (1984): Hysteroscopie et microcolpohysteroscopie. Atlas et Traité. Palermo, COFESE Publisher .

2 Mencaglia L., Perino A., Giannone E., Gilardi G. (1987). Nuove prospettive nella diagnosi della iperplasia e del carcinoma dell'endometrio. Oncol Ginecol 6: 153.

3 Deutschmann C., Lueken R.P., Lindemann H.J. (1983). Hysteroscopic findings in post-menopausal bleeding in " Histeroscopic. Principies and Practice ". Edited by A.M. Siegler, H. J., Lindemann, Philadelphia. Lippincott Publisher.

4 Dexeus S., Labastida R., Galera L. (1982). Oncological indications of hysteroscopy. Eur. J. Gynecol. Oncol. 2:61.

5 Isaacs J.H., Ross F.H. (1978). Cytologic evaluation of the endometrium in women with postmenopausal bleeding. Amer. J. Obst. Gyn. 131: 410.

6 Koss L.G., Schreiber K., Moussouris H., Oberlander S.G. (1982). Endometrial carcinoma and
   its precursors: detectin and screening. Clin. Obst. Gyn. 25: 49.

7 Mencaglia L., Scarselli G.F., Tantini C. (1984). Hysteroscopic evaluetion of endometrial cancer. J. Reprod. Med. 29: 701.

8 Mencaglia L., Scarselli G.F. (1985). Etats precanceroux de l'endometre in Hysteroscopie et Microcolpohysteroscopie. Edited by J. Hamou. Palermo, COFESE Publisher, p.143.

9 Mencaglia L., Perino A. (1987). Hysteroscopy in peri- menopausal and post - menopausal women with abnormal uetrine bleeding. J. Reprod. Med. 32: 577.

10 Benedetto V., Zona G. (1990). Hysteroscopic diagnosis of endometrial carcinoma. Human Reprod. II Joint Meeting 74: 240.

11 Benedetto V., Zona G. (1991). Hysteroscopic with abnormal uterine bleeding in peri-menopause and post- menopause. Second international Cours of diagnostic and operative gynecological endoscopy. Rome April.

12 Cittadini E., Allegra A., Perino A. (1983). L'endoscopia ginecologica. Palermo, COFESE Publisher.

13 Hajnes P.J., et al (1979). Treatment of menstrual blood loss in patients with menorrhagia. Br. J. Obst. Gyn. 84: 763.

14 De Jong P., Doel F., Falconer A. (1990). Outpatient diagnostic hysteroscopy. Br. J. Obst. Gynaec. 97, 299- 303.

15 Loffer F.D. (1989). Hysteroscopy with selective endometrial sampling compared with D&C for abnormal uterine bleeding: the value of negative hysteroscopic view. Obst. Gyn. 73,

Hysterectomy in Finland

E.-M. Rutanen and R. Luoto

Department of Obstetrics and Gynecology, Helsinki University Central Hospital and Department of Public Health, University of Helsinki, Finland

The occurrence, indications and trends of hysterectomy have been extensively studied in many countries. Before 1986, the probable incidence of hysterectomy in Finland could be studied only indirectly through incidences of hospitalizations for gynecologic symptoms and diseases. Since 1987 national data on surgical procedures are included in the hospital discharge register, making it possible to get out directly the annual number and indications as well as the method of hysterectomies in the whole country.

In 1987-1989, the total number of hysterectomies in Finland was 27 000, giving an annual incidence of 390/100 000 women. The prevalence among the age-group 45 - 64 year-old women was 19 %. The incidence of hysterectomy is higher in Finland than in other Scandinavian countries, but still much lower than in the United States, where every third over 60-year-old women have undergone this operation. The trend in the rate in Finland is moving upward during the recent years. There are wide regional variation in the occurence of hysterectomy also in national settings. In Finland, the regional incidence varies over three-fold. Reasons for variations at international as well as national levels are multiple, including sociodemographic factors, changes in gynecological morbidity, use of contraceptive methods and hormone replacement therapy, as well as availability of health services.

The most common age at the time of hysterectomy is the same in different countries, being between 40 to 49. In Finland the mean age at the time of operation varies between 43-45 years. As hysterectomy can be performed only once, the 'population at risk' differs from that for many other surgical procedures. Correction of rates by using only women with intact uteri - the true 'at risk' population - produces higher rates of hysterectomy, especially in older age-groups. In the United States for example, the 'uterus at risk' - corrected rate of hysterectomies in 1984 for women aged 30-34 was 6.5 % higher than the uncorrected rate.

In the age-group 70-74 years, the difference between uncorrected and corrected rates was even larger, being 56 % (NCHC 1987). Hysterectomy also has an impact in the incidence of uterine cancer. In Finland, the age-adjusted annual incidence of endometrial cancer was 14/100 000 in 1991 (Cancer Register 1994). This incidence , however, rises in total by 26 %, if corrected 'for uterus at risk' population. The incidence of the cancer of the cervix uteri increases by 16 %.

The two most common indications for hysterectomy were leiomyoma and endometriosis, and myomas and other benign neoplasms comprised nearly half of the indications for hysterectomy Finnish disharge register. This is in keeping with the statistics from other countries. Generally, myomas and bleeding disorders together appear to cover about the same part of indications in different countries. Interestingly, malignancy was the reason for hysterectomy in less than 10 % of cases in Finland, and the numbers are similar in countries where statistics are available.

The two main types of traditional hysterectomy are abdominal and vaginal. In Finnish study, the relative proportions of the types of hysterectomy varied by indication. The most common type of operation was total abdominal hysterectomy (63 %), and vaginal hysterectomy was performed in 15 % only. The percentages, and also indications of vaginal and abdominal hysterectomies show large variation in different countries. The major indication for vaginal hysterectomy in Finland was uterine prolapse. In leiomyoma and bleeding disorders, hysterectomy for women aged 50-54 was most often accompanied by bilateral oophorectomy. The attitude towards bilateral oophorectomy appears to be most liberal in the United States, in Finland the percentage is about 25 %. The frequency of subtotal hysterectomy (20 %) is much higher in Finland than, for example, in Great Britain where it is less than 1 % (Vessey et al. 1992). The proportion of subtotal hysterectomy has remarkably increased also in Sweden during 1980's.

First laparoscopic hysterectomies in Finland were performed in 1992. According to the National Register of laparoscopic hysterectomies, the number of operations was 350 in 1993 and in 1994 the number is predicted to be more than 1000 (J. Sjöberg, personal communication). Laparoscopic operations were started at our five University Hospitals, but this technique is now widely used even in small hospitals throughout the country. Courses and workshops have been organized by Finnish Gynecological Association, and all operations are listed in the National Register for further evaluation.

Studies on the occurrence, indications and methods of traditional hysterectomy are appropriate especially now, when less invasive laparoscopic and hysteroscopic techniques are gradually replacing traditional abdominal hysterectomy, and when the effectiveness of different operative techniques and alternative treatment methods need to be compared. Most recent reports comparing the effectiveness of alternative methods and hysterectomy have concluded that hysterectoimy remains an important procedure when conservative treatment has failed. The major question to be answered is, what type of hysterectomy is the most beneficial in each case. The short-term outcome and complications of hysterectomy are well known, but studies on long-term consequences regarding especially new techniques are still lacking.

REFERENCES:

Carlson KJ et al: Indications for hysterectomy. N Engl J Med 1993; 328:856-860.

Luoto R: Hysterectomy in Finland - occurrence, indications and association with cardiovascular morbidity. Academic dissertation, University of Helsinki, 1995.

Vessey MP et al. The epidemiology of hysterectomy: findings in a large cohort study. Br J Obstet Gynecol 1992; 99; 402-407.

Wilcox LS et al. Hysterectomy in the United States, 1988-1990. Obstet gynecol 1994;83:549-545.

Menopausal profile: proposal of a synthetic index on menopausal state

G. Fiorentino, A. Celona*, L. Barbaro** and C. Pullè*

Division of Gynecology, Papardo Hospital, *Institute of Gynecology, University of Messina and **Family Counselling Unit, Messina, Italy

Menopause Centers of MESSINA suggest the possibility to have an easy identification of the most rational and personal way to resolve disorders typical of this age, for every woman.

To attain this working with a large number of women, we recommend to divide the sample in homogeneus groups, identify the type of woman, and send the single woman to related group.

We think that a good way to make this, is the MENOPAUSAL PROFILE.

We define this as a simple tools that allow us to incorporate the women, at the moment of acceptance, into one of 4 therapeutical groups identifited.

The function of Acceptance becomes with the Reservation for first interview.

In the course of <u>First Interview</u> we use the following steps:

1. hearing the patient;
2. application of acceptance criteria;
3. informations about menopausal problems, solutions and proceedings of the Center;
4. informed consensus by patient;
5. enlistment;
6. prescribe the Basal Check-up for starting assessment.

We accept the women whom have at least one of the following items <u>(ACCEPTANCE CRITERIA)</u> :

1. Women > 40 - 65 < years old
2. Menstrual Troubles ≥ 6 months
3. Climateric Symptoms

Combining theese factors it's possible to obtain 3 patient-type groups for acceptance :

GROUP A: women > 40 aged, with or without Climateric Symptoms, with Menstrual Troubles > 6 months;

GROUP B: women < 65 aged in post-menopause, with Amenorrhea > 1 year, with or without Climateric Symptoms;

GROUP C: women < 40 aged, with assured Praecox Menopause, or like observers (Clinic-Epidemiologic Observatory = C.E.O.).

(SPECIAL GROUP : not talking about in this work)

519

After checking of the results, in a second appointment with the patient, we fill in the forms of MENOPAUSAL SCORE [M.S.].

This tools results from combination between Menstrual Score and Symptomatologic Score [Kupperman Score modified].

The MENSTRUAL SCORE assigns a score increasing with the gravity of symptomatogy :

1. > FSH	1 point	
2. < Pg	1 "	
3. Polimenorrhea	1 "	
4. Polypus and/or fibroma	2 points	
5. Endometrial hyperplasia (E.H.)	2 "	
6. Spotting and/or Hypermenorrhea	2 "	
7. Oligomenorrhea	3 points	
8. Menstrual rhythm ON/OFF	3 "	
9. Amenorrhea ≥ 6 months	3 "	

To compute the Menopausal Score, we assign an Low (L) value when the menstrual score is ≤ 3 points; Medium (M) value > 4- 9 < points; High (H) value > 10 points.

The same by the Symptomatologic Score : (L) < 10 points; (M) > 10 - 20 < points; (H) > 20 points.

An (L) value is 1 point for the Menopausal Score, an (M) value is 2 points, an (H) value is 3 points.

We obtain the following values :

(L) when the M.S. is < 2 points;
(M) when the M.S. is > 2-4 < points;
(H) when the M.S. is > 4 points.

Combining the value of Menstrual, Symptomatologic and Menopausal Scores is possible remark four patient-type frames :

	Menstrual Score	Symptomatologic Score	Menopausal Score	Name
FRAME 1 :	(L)	(L)	(L)	Observer
FRAME 2 :	(L)	(L) or (M)	(M)	Psychosomatic
FRAME 3 :	(M)	(L)	(M)	Pregnancy-risk
FRAME 4 :	(H)	(M) or (H)	(H)	Menopause

Every frame corresponds to a following MENOPAUSAL PROFILE:

PROFILE 1: - OBSERVERS - Women > 40 aged that have no menstrual troubles and no climateric symptoms. These patients
(L-L-L) don't need any particular therapy, so that they are able to enter in our Clinical and Epidemiological Observatory (C.E.O.).

PROFILE 2 : - PSYCHOSOMATIC - Women that have few flushes but not important menstrual alterations (not very frequent
(L-L/M-M) condition). In these cases patients resolutely ask a specific treatment : together with psychological help, we give Veralipride as first choise and inscript them into C.E.O.. Bromocriptina, Clonidina or α-metil-DOPA can also be use, expecially if hypertension exists.

PROFILE 3: -PREGNANCY-RISK   -   Women   that   refer   menstrual
           alterations whith oligo-polymenorrhea, absence of some
(M-L-M)   cycle, without hot-flushes and sweating. In these cases
           treatment should be the followinig:

    a) if woman has no flushes, is still in fertile age and
has no wish of conceptions, oral contraceptive regularizes
menstrual cycle and gives to her the advantages of
Hormonal Replacement Therapy (HRT).
    b) if woman doesn't accept contraception,progestagens can
be administred in second half of menstrual cycle, in order
to test estrogenic state of woman (Progesterone Challenge
Test - PCT) and balance endogenous pool of estrogens,
until PCT becomes negative. In this case, the preventive
value of HRT must be considered from phisician and
purpose to patient.

PROFILE 4:-MENOPAUSE - Women that have menstrual alterations and
          climateric symptoms. These patients find in HRT the
(H-M/H-H) best preventive and therapeutical approach in relation
          to climateric syndrome.
          The ways of administration for HRT are:
          a) oral , b) transdermal and c) transvaginal.

    a) The oral way is able to modify lipidic balance
in antiaterogenetic way, because it rises HDL levels
and decreases LDL levels (at the same time, estrogens
seem to be able to decrease hypertension events and to
rise, at central and perypherical level, substances
causing vasodilatation, as opiate peptydes). This route
is suitable, therefore, in those conditions that need
to reset a dishomogeneous lipidic metabolism.

    b) The transdermal way extends indications of this
type of therapy to all women which are suffering from
gall-stones   or   hepatopathy   or   high-risk   for
thrombophilic   accidents.   A   severe   follow-up   is
indicated in all cases.

c) The transvaginal way is preferred in all situations
in which uro-genital problems are most important . If
we want to have a more strong topycal effect (in
special way if exists some controindication to systemic
therapy), Promestriene has been used. Estriolo can be
used in those situations with bad compliance to the
HRT.

    In conclusion, we hope that the application into a routine
of Menopausal Profile for patients acceptance, make easy you too
to assign a rational therapy to every patient.

SUMMARY

It is well Known that therapeutic approach to climateric syndrome must be extremely individualized;therefore,the right indication to a determinate treatment depends upon symtoms complained from women,upon medical and diagnostic investigations and upon the way by which women live this phase of their life.

The Authors suggest a decisional algorithm with a low level of precision to obtain a global vision of total deductive process.After admittance to Menopause Center,women,by some key-aspects of menopausal state,are automatically sent to different and personal protocol.

To obtain a greater easiness in reading of algorithm,detailed explanations of investga= tions carried out have beensuppressed,making,therefore,this pattern utilizable also from single workers which use different diagnostic tests.The Authors,in fact,suggest to throw proposal of a multicentric control of such a pattern to those who are interested in menopausal problems and find constructive such an exchange of experiences.

BIBLIOGRAPHY.

1. Ballinger S. : Psychosocial Stress and Symptoms of Menopause: Comparative study of menopause Clinic patients and non-patiens. Maturitas, 7,315,1985

2. Buvet J., Buvet M. : La menopause. Revue Française de Gynecologie et d'Obstetrique, 79, 1, 1984

3. Celona A., Fiorentino G., Barbaro L., Barbaro C., Pullè C. : Therapeuthic decisional patterns in menopause. Acta of Foundation Congress of the European Society for Gynecologic and Obstetric Investigation - Madonna di Campiglio - February 7-14, 1993.

4. De Aloysio D., Bottiglioni F., Mauloni F. : Aspetti sintomatologici del climaterio femminile. Atti Soc. Ital. di Ost. e Gin. Vol. LVII, Monduzzi Ed. Bologna, 1983, pag.21 -81

5. Greenblatt R.B.,Teran A.Z.:Advice to post-menopausal women,in The Climateric and beyond, a cura di Zichella L.,Whitehead M., van Keep P.A., New Jersey, USA, Partenon Publishing Group Inc., 1988

100

Intrafascial vaginal hysterectomy, an alternative to traditional surgery: indications

S. Maffei, A. Di Gregorio, G. Sarpa, A. Re, L. Leo, A. Venuti, G. Gordini*,
R. Bellino, M. Tessarolo, G. Visca, G. Osnengo**, T. Wierdis and A. Lanza

*Department B of Gynecology and Obstetrics Institute, University of Turin,
*Department of Pathology and **Department B of Obstetrics and Gynecology,
S. Anna Hospital, Turin, Italy*

INTRODUCTION

Laparoscopic hystectomy was first described by Reich in 1989 (1). Since then a lot of studies appeared with the description of laparoscopic hysterectomies (2,3), laparoscopically assisted vaginal hysterectomy (4,5,6,), pelviscopic intrafascial hysterectomy without colpotomy (7,8). In 1993 Semm described the intrafascial vaginal hysterectomy with or without pelviscopic assistance (9). Our type of operation is the same described by Semm without pelviscopic assistance (9) with anterior precipitation of the uterus. Cardinal and utero - sacral ligaments, uterine arteries main trunk, and vagina are not sectioned. Therefore, with this surgical procedure we have the preservation of pelvic floor integrity and its blood supply. Pelvic sympathetic and parasympathetic nerves form Frankenhauser's plexus around the cervix and vaginal superior third. At this level vescical and rectal sensations arrive from the organs and go to them.

Surgical removal of the cervix results in the loss of numerous ganglia leading to a possible dysfunction of bladder and rectum. Preserving the cervix, those dysfunctions can be avoided. Finally, vaginal orgasm is due to stimulation of vaginal - uterine plexus that closely surrounds the cervix and upper vagina. Then cervical removal may also lead to sexual arousal and orgasm dysfunctions. Since our first operation with this technique that preserves the cervix, we have worried about removing all the potential sources of cancer.

It is well known the old convinction that patients who underwent subtotal hysterectomy were at greater risk of cervical cancer.

In reality we have to differentiate coincidental cancer, that appears within two years from operation and seems to be due to an improper pre - surgical screening, from true cancer that arises from the cervical strump and has the same incidence as that of women with the whole uterus (10 - 17).

In 1994 Lütteges et al (18) published a study about pathological aspects in Semm's supracervical hysterectomy (7). They discovered that in all cases the resection edge was over the exocervical transformation zone and mild dysplasia areas; in two cases there were retenction cysts in the edge of resection, but cancer never was found in the depth of a cyst. All endocervical mucosa was removed.

The purpose of our study is to valuate in the first 10 cases the epithelization of the cervical stump, the ovarian function after 1 and 10 months from operation, and the complete removal endocervical epithelium.

MATERIAL and METHODS

One year ago we began intrafascial vaginal hysterectomy without pelviscopic assistance in Department B of Institute of Obstetriscs and Gynecology, University of Turin. Since than we have treated 10 patients.

Indications to this kind of intervention were: endometriosis, uterine fibroids, pharmacological treatable methrorrhagias, endometrial hyperplasia (even with atypia), and cervical intraepithelial neoplasia grade I. Preoperative management of the patients is very important. The patients have colposcopy and microcolpohysteroscopy perfomed in order to define the height of squamous - columnar junction, the extent of trasformation zone, and the grade and extention of an intraepithelial lesion. If there is an HPV infection, the virus is typized by PCR in our Laboratory of Molecular Biology.

Women at risk require a continuos cytologic surveillance transvaginal sonography in order to define the length of the cervix and the thickness of endocervical mucosa.

On the basis of these data we choose a calibrated uterine resection tool (CURT) of appropiate diameter. Transvaginal sonography can also be useful in the detection of ovarian functionality in order to decide a removal or a retention of the adnexa.

We perform this type of hysterectomy only in patients with normal pelvic floor. We studied the accuracy of the removal of tissues, from which a cancer may develop, reviewing pathological specimens (extent of transformation zone, resection edges, characteristics of endocervical mucosa till the internal uterine os).

We also controlled 10 uteruses removed from other patients who underwent total hysterectomy for benign diseases, using the CURT on those pieces in order to evaluate the endocervical tissue and the remnants on the cervix.

With microcolpohysteroscopy we evaluated cervical stump epithelization. Ovarian function was studied one and twelve months after surgery with estradiol values and transvaginal sonography.

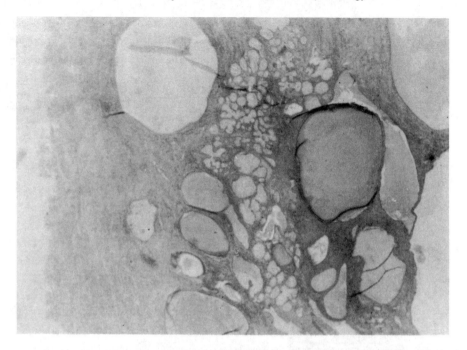

Figure 1 A longitudinal view of the segment removed with the C.U.R.T.. In spite of a glandular adenosis with cystic transformation the removal of endocervical glands was complete. Left: surgical edge.

RESULTS and DISCUSSION

In the first ten cases who underwent intrafascial vaginal hysterectomy, the endocervical segment, removed with C.U.R.T., was complete of glandes. In the ten uteruses removed with the traditional technique, the endocervical segment sperimentally removed with C.U.R.T. is complete of endocervical glands in 8 cases and the residual tissue does not have any of them. In 2 cases the cervical stump after removal of the endocervical canal with C.U.R.T. still had glands. In another case there was a retention cyst lined by simple stratified epithelium. In all the 20 cases the squamous-columner line and the transformation zone were in the removed endocervical segment.

Microcolpohysteroscopy showed cervical stumps without transformation zone or squamous-columner line in all the patients during follow-up.

The same exam showed an earlier closure of the residual cavity of cervical stump due to adhesion of the walls. The study of ovarian functionality (follow-up 2-10 months) with Estradiol, FSH, and LH plasma levels showed a regular production of estradiol (167.8 ± 94.6 pg/ml) while FSH and LH were of menopausal values in 2 patients (53 and 56 years old). In the same two cases estradiol had the lowest values. Transvaginal sonography evidenced ovarian follicles in only 2 cases. In the others ovaries had a compact aspect.

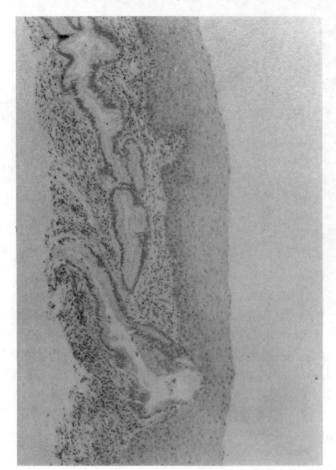

Figure 2 Glandular remuants in the cervical stump after C.U.R.T.. The glands were neither connected with the endocervical lumen nor with cervical surface. Left: surgical edge.

The problem of cervical stump cancer (12-17) according to Lüttges et als (18) work and our preliminary data is not related to this kind of operation.

The transformation zone from which cancer arises in 99 % of the cases (19) is always completely removed by C.U.R.T.. According to Lüttges et als (18) this operation is therapeutical also in case of mild dysplasia. When a large transformation zone is found on exocervix, Semm (7) advices a conization before the intrafascial hysterectomy.

Retention cysts lined by simple stratifical epithelium are not at risk of malignant degeneration. It has never been described a cancer arose from those cysts (18).

Endocervical glandes a branching that have been found in cervical stumps will become retention cysts within the atrophied stump. The glandular epithelium is not in close contact with external noxious stimuli and, even though this tissue is not screened during cytology, it should not transform into cancer.

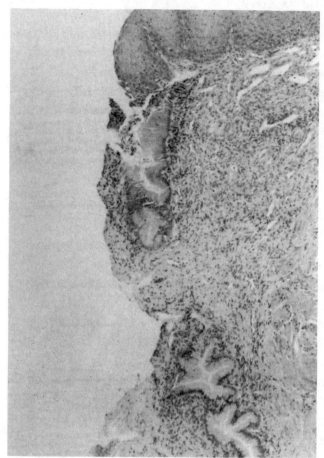

Figure 3 Surgical stump after C.U.R.T. with residual glandular " cul de sac ". The healing process will entrap them into the scar avoiding external connection. Left: surgical edge.

In fact cancer of the cervical stump is almost always an epidermoid one. According to Wolff et als (13) the majority of adenocarcinomas are due to neoplastic inclusions not detected before subtotal hysterectomy.

Despite our few data and the short follow-up, it seems useful the retention of the ovaries in women below 45-47 years of age.

Acknowledgment: the authors thank Pharmacia / Farmitalia Carlo Erba

REFERENCES

1. Reich, H., DeCaprio, J., McGlynn, F.. (1989). Laparoscopic hysterectomy. *J. Gynecol.Surg.*, **5**, 213

2. Liu, C. Y.. (1992). Laparoscopic hysterectomy: A review of 72 cases. *J. Reprod. Med.*, **37**, 351

3. Langebrekke A., Skar, O. J., Urnes, A.. (1992). *Acta Obstet. Gynecol. Scand.*, **71**, 226

4. Padial, J. G., Sotolongo, J., Casey, M. J., et al. (1992). Laparoscopically-assisted vaginal hysterectomy: Report of 75 consecutive cases. *J. Gynecol. Surg.*, **8**, 81

5. Maher, P. J., Wood, E. C., Hill, D. J., et al.. (1992). Laparoscopically assisted hysterectomy. *Med. J. Aust.*, **156**, 316

6. Nezhat, F., Nezhat, C., Gordon, S., et al. (1992). *J. Reprod. Med.*, **37**, 247

7. Semm, K..(1991). Hysterectomy via laparotomy or pelviscopy: A new CASH method without colpotomy. *Geburtshilfe Frauenheilkd*, **51**, 996

8. Vietz, P. F., Ahn, T. S. (1994). A new approach to hysterectomy without colpotomy: Pelviscopic intrafascial hysterectomy. *Am. J. Obstet. Gynecol.*, **170**, 609-13

9. Semm, K. (1993). Intrafasziale vaginale Hysterektomie (IVH) mit oder ohne pelviskopisher *Assistenz. Geburtsh. u. Frauenheilk.*, **53**, 873-878

10. Hasson, H. M.. (1993). Cervical Removal at hysterectomy for Benign Disease Risks and Benefits. *Journal of Reproductive Medicine*, **38**, 781

11. Mikuta, J.. (1969). Cervical stump cancer. *Am. J. Obstet. Gynecol.*, **105**, 490

12. Decker, D. G., Hunt, A. B., Fricke, R. E., et al. (1957). Carcinoma of the cervical stump. *Am. J. Obstet. Gynecol.*, **73**, 974

13. Wolff, J. P., Lacoru, J., Chassagne, D., et al. (1972). Cancer of the cervical stump: A study of 173 patients. *Obstet. Gynecol.*, **39**, 10

14. Lachmann, A.. (1950). Cancer of the cervical stump. *Acta Obstet. gynecol. Scand.*, **30**, 169

15. Caulk, R. M. (1954). Transvaginal Roentgen therapy in cancer of the cervical stump. *Am. J. Roentgenol*, **72**, 469

16. Storm, H. H., Clemmensen, I. H., Manders, T., et al. (1992). Supravaginal uterine amputation in Denmark 1978- 1988 and risk of cancer. *Gynecol. Oncol.*, **45**, 198

17. Kovalic, J.J., Grigsby, P.W., Perez, C.A., et al. (1991). Cervical stump carcinoma. *Int. J. Radiat. Oncol. Biol. Phys.*, **20**, 933.

18. Lüttges, J.E., Lehmann-Willenbrook, E., Semm, K. (1994). Histopathological aspects of pelviscopic hysterectomy. *Gynecol. Obstet. Invest.*, **37**, 118-122.

19. Richard, R.M. (1973). Cervical intraepithelial neoplasia. *Pathology Annual*. New York, Appleton Century Crofts. Pp. 301-328.

Hormone replacement therapy or intact ovaries in radical surgery for cervical cancer in young women

S. Maffei, R. Bellino, A. Re, M. Tessarolo, L. Leo, A. Venuti, G. Sarpa, T. Wierdis, G. Visca and A. Lanza

Department B of Gynecology and Obstetrics Institute, University of Turin, Turin, Italy

INTRODUCTION

It has always been an unsolved question and an open dilemme, whether the ovaries must be removed during radical surgery for cervical cancer in young patients. Many are the problems a gynecologist has to face before, during, and after surgery.

The age of the patient and the compliance for the use of hormonal replacement therapy are important features. Furthermore, radical surgery may affect ovarian blood supply with an early ovarian failure and subsequent menopause.

Another factor we have to consider is the possibility of ovarian metastasis from cervical cancer; a rare but present event.

From Literature we assume that it is not very common to find ovarian metastases either in squamous cancer or adenocarcinoma. (1 - 12).

In Stage II and III cancers the patients receive post - surgical radiotherapy, but at a dosage of 1,000 rad. or less, which means less that the normalquantity given in advanced tumors, we have castration. That implies a transposition of grossly normal ovaries during radical surgery if we know or assume that cancer has already spread to lymphonodes or parametria or vagina.

It has been proposed a prophilactic ovariectomy either in benign or malignant diseases of the uterus especially in women at great risk of ovarian cancer (13 - 14). Ovariectomy reduces the chances of ovarian neoplasm by 11-12%(14),

but the concern is always the compliance of the patients with hormone replacement therapy.

In this study we reviewed our cases of cervical cancer and the incidence of ovarian metastases in order to evaluate the flasibility of ovarian retention during radical surgery.

MATERIAL AND METHODS

From January 1977 to December 1992, 252 cervical cancer patients (Stage I A_1 - IV) were surgically treated at Department B of the Institute of Obstetrics and Gynecology, University of Turin.

The mean age of our patients was $49.62 \pm$ S.D. 11.15 (median 50; range 22 - 74).

There were 76 lymphonodal metastases (30.16 %) among our patients.

Women with and an age ≤ 40 years were 58, 10 of whom were 30 years old or less (17.24 %), while patients with an age between 41 and 45 were 35. On the whole, 93 cases (36.99 %) were premenopausal women. Among these 93 cases there were: 77 squamous cancers (12 with microinvasion; 7 I A_1 and 5 I A_2), 14 adenocarcinomas (2 I A_2), and 2 neuroendocrine tumors (one small-cell cancer and an indifferentiated one).

529

The clinical stage was: 61 stage I, 25 stage II, 4 stage III, and 3 stage IV.

All, but 5 of these patients underwent Wertheim's radical hysterectomy with bilateral salpingo-oophorectomy in spite of the age of the patients, with pelvic and paraaortic lymphadenectomy according to Valle's technique. The other 5 had an exploratory laparatomy because of the spread of the tumor to paraaortic lymphonodes, parametrium, or other organs.

All the cases with lymphonodal, parametrial, and vaginal invasion and external third of cervical stromal invasion and capillary like space embolism received post surgical radiotherapy.

RESULTS

We did not find microscopic ovarian metastates in none of the 93 patients. In only a 42 - years - old woman there were tubaric metastases and peritoneal diffusion of the tumor. She had G2 epidermoid cancer with parametrial, corpus uteri,and paraaortic lymphonodes involvements.

Among the other ≥ 46 - years - old patients only one woman with a G1 endocervical adenocarcinoma had a microscopic spread to the ovaries with clinical involvement of peritoneum and other pelvic organs.

There were also 23 cases (24.7 %) with of lymphonodal metastases, with a median of 3 positive lymphonodes (mean 4.04, range 1 - 24), 1 7 parametrial involvements (18.3 %), and 9 vaginal spread (9.6%).(Table1).

DISCUSSION

Various studies illustrated that the ovarian metastases from cervical carcinoma are rare, being present just in a small percentage of cases.

In our retrospective study on 252 patients with cervical carcinoma we had only 1 patient with ovarian metastasis, with an incidence of 0,39 %. This result matches with those obtained by other Authors in the past years.

Combining the available data we can find that, regardless the histological type, on a total of 3345 patients studied, 22 had been affected by ovarian metastases, with a total incidence of 0,73 %. (Table2). The incidence changes however if the histological type is considered, being higher for the adenocarcinoma. (Table 3).

This low risk of ovarian metastases is the major ratio for the preservation of the adnexa in the younger women with cervical carcinoma in order to avoid the complications of estrogen deficiency due to castration. (15 - 16 - 17).

For some Authors this turns into a reduced safety of the ovarian preservation in case of adenocarcinoma (10 - 12), while for others is reasonable to conserve ovaries which appear normal during laparatomy. (9 - 11).

However, other objections had been raised in the past years regarding the real utility, in terms of function and safety, of the ovarian preservation in premenopausal women.

The loss of hormonal function of the ovaries seems to be faster in women who have hysterectomy if compared to those who dont's, being the average age of menopause respectively of 44 and 51 (18).

This could be due to the decline in blood irroration caused by the surgical manipulation and particulary to the abolition of the uterus-ovarian arteries which alone provide the two-third of the ovarian blood flow. (18). Only 68 % of the patients who had hysterectomy between the ages of 40 and 55 has normal hormonal production (19).

Secondly the postoperative radiotherapy (RT) received by the patients with lymphonodal metastases, leads to the cessation of the ovarian function and to an increased risk of ovarian cancer. Only 26 out of 93 women with less than 45 years in our study, didn't receive pelvic radiation.

In order to avoid these problems, the lateral ovarian transposition (LOT) can be performed.

Many Authors however do not consider LOT useful in preserving ovarian cysts which might require reoperation. (18).

Finally a Residual Ovary Syndrome may develop in these patients, with pelvic pain, pelvic mass and dyspaureunia (20) in a percentage of cases which ranges from 1,8 to 5,2 %. (18) and which might lead to further surgery.

Parker estimated that 20 % of the patients with ovarian preservation will undergo a premature menopause, 5-8 % will need reoperation for benign ovarian disease, 1,4 % may develop a ovarian carcinoma. (21).

In consideration of:

- the premature decline of the ovarian function after hystyerectomy,
- the effects of pelvic radiation on the adnexa and the little utility of the LOT,
- the possible development of a Residual Ovary Syndrome,
- the risk of an autonomous ovarian cancer,

we decided to treat our patients with bilateral salpingo-oophorectomy (BSO) plus Hormonal Replacement Therapy.

Even under an economical point of view the BSO plus HRT can be considered convenient for the social expence for HRT is similar to the costs of the potential ovarian disease therapy. (21).

Acknowledgment: the autors thank Pharmacia / Farmitalia Carlo Erba

Table 1 Histological characteristics of patients with cervical carcinoma with age ≤ 45 years

	P+	V+	C+	C.C.+	1/3 EXT+	CLS+
N+ 23	11	4	11	9	16	10
(24,73 %)	47,815	17,39 %	47,81 %	39,13 %	69,56	43,47 %
N- 70	6	5	6	16	22	13
(75,26 %)	8,57 %	7,14 %	8,57 %	22,85 %	31,41 %	18,57 %

N = lymphonodes; P = paranmetrium; V = vagina; C = corpus uteri; C.C. = endometrial canal; 1/3 EXT = stroma external third; CLS = capillary-like spaces

Table 2 Incidence of ovarian metastasis in patients with cancer of the uterine cervix

Author and date	Total n° of cases of cervical cancer	n° of cases with ovarian metastases	Stage of cervical cancer
Ketcham et al (1971)	84	3	I to III
Baltzer et al (1981)	749	4	IB to II
Shingleton and Orr (1982)	258	1	
Kjorstad and Bond (1984)	149	2	IB
Kaminski and Norris (1984)	161	1	I
Tabata et al. (1987)	26	2	I
Hopkins et al (1988)	32	0	I
Owens et al. (1989)	99	0	IB
Browen et al. (1990)	25	1	I
Toki et al. (1990)	597	3	IB to IIIB
Sutton et al. (1991)	990	6	IB
(This study)	252	1	IA to IV
TOTAL	3422	25 (0,73 %)	

Table 3 Incidence of ovarian metastasis in cervical cancer patients by histologic type

	Epidermoid carcinoma		Adenocarcinoma	
	Cases	Ovarian mts	Cases	Ovarian mts
10 Toki (1991)	524	1 (0,19 %)	36	2 (5,5 %)
11 Sutton (1991)	770	4 (0,5 %)	121	2 (1,7 %)

REFERENCES

1. Ketcham, A.S., Hoye, R. C., Taylor, P. T., Deckers, L. J., Thomas, L. B., Chretien, P. B. (1971). Radical Hysterectomy and pelvic lynphadenectomy for carcinoma of the uterine cervix. *Cancer*, **28**, 1272-1277
2. Baltzer, J., Lohe, K. J., Kopcke, W., Zander, J.. (1981) Metastatischer befall der ovarien beim operierte plattenepithelial karzinom der zervix. *Geburtshilfe Frauenheilkd*, **41**, 672-3
3. Shingleton, H. M., Orr, J. W.. (1983). Cancer of the cervix. *New York: Churchill Livingston*, **132**
4. Kiorstad, K. E., Bond, B.. (1984) Stage I B adenocarcinoma of the cervix: metastatic potential and patterns of disseminatiuon. *Am. J. Obstet. Gynecol*, **150**, 197-9
5. Kaminsky, P. F., Norris, H. J.. (1984). Coexistence of ovarian neoplasms and endocervical adenocarcinoma.Obstet. Gynecol, **64**, 553-6
6. Tabata, M., Ichnoe, K., Sakuragi, N.,Shiima, Y., Yamaguchi, T., Mabuchi Y.. (1986).. Incidence of ovarian metastasis in patients with cancer of the uterine cervix. *Gynecol Oncol*, **28**, 255-61
7. Hopkins, M. P., Schmidt, R. W., Roberts, J. A.,and Morley, G. W.. (1988). The prognosis and treatment of stage I adenocarcinoma of the cervix. *Obstet. Gynecol.*, **72**, 915-921
8. Owens, S., Roberts W. S., Fiorica J. V., Hoffman, M. S., LaPolla, J. P., Cavanagh, D.(1989). Ovarian Management at the Time of Radical Hysterectomy for Cancer of the Cervix. *Gynecologic Oncology*, **35**, 349-351.
9. Brown, J. V., Fu, Y. S., Bereck, J. S..(1990). Ovarian Metastases Are Rare in Stage I Adenocarcinoma of the Cervix. *Obstetrics & Gynecology*, vol. **76**, 623-626
10. Toki, N., Tsukamoto, N., Kaku, T., Toh, N., Saito, T., Kamura, T., Matsukuma, K., and Nakano, H.. (1991). Microscopic Ovarian Metastasis of the Uterine Cervical Cancer. *Gynecologic Oncology*, **41**, 46-51
11. Sutton, G. P., Bundy, B. N., Delgrado, G., Sevin, B.u., Creasman, W. T., Major, F. J., Zaino, R.(1991). Ovarian metastases in stage IB carcinoma of the cervix: A gynecologic oncology Group study. *Am. J Obstet. Gynecol*, vol. **166**, 50-53
12. Mann, W., Chumas, J., Amalfitano, T., Westermann, C., Patsner, B.. (1987). Ovarian Metastases From Stage I B Adenocarcinoma of the Cervix. *Cancer*, **60**, 1123-1126
13. Giai, M., Ponzone, r., Roagna, R., Biglia, N., Sgro, L., Sismondi, P.. (1994). The Uncertain Fate of Ovaries at the Time of Hysterectomy. *It. J. Gynaecol. Obstet.*, **4**, 75-85
14. NIH Consensus Conference, April 5-7, 1994. Ovarian Cancer: Screening, Treatment and Follow up. pp. 1-15
15. McCall, M. L., Keaty, E. C., Thompson, J. D.. (1958). Conservation of ovarian tissue in the treatment of carcinoma of the cervix with radical surgery. *Am. J. Obstet. Gynecol.*, **75**, 590-605
16. Yagi, H..(1955). Extendet abdominal hysterectomy with pelvic lymphadenectomy for carcinoma of the cervix. Am. J. Obstet. Gynecol., **69**, 33-47
17. Webb, G. A., F.A.C.O.G., F.A.C.S.. (1974). The role of ovarian conservation in the treatment of carcinoma of the cervix with radical surgery. *Am. J. Obstet. Gynecol.*, **122**, 476-484
18. Chambers, S. K., Chambers, J. T., Holm, C., Peschel, R. E., Schwartz, P. E.. (1990). Sequelae of Lateral Ovarian Transposition in Unirradiated Carvical Cancer POatients. *Gynecologic Oncology*, **39**, 155-159
19. Anderson, J., La Polla, D., Turner, G., Chapman,., Buller, R. (1993). Ovarian Transposition in Cervical Cancer. *Gynecologic Oncology*, **49**, 206-214
20. Ellsworth, H. H., Allen, J. A., Nisher. (1993). Ovarian function after radicsal hysterectomy for Stage I B Carcinoma of cervix. *Am. J. Obstet. Gynecol.*, **145**, 185
21. Parker, M., Bosscher, J., Barnhill, D., Park, R..(1993). Ovarian Managment During Radical Hysterectomy in the Premenopausal Patient. *Obstetrics & Gynecology*, **82**, 187-190

SECTION 4

Obstetric Care – Prenatal Medicine

First-trimester serum screening for Down syndrome

K.J. Powell and J.G. Grudzinskas

Academic Unit of Obstetrics and Gynecology, The Royal London Hospital, London, UK

Because of the high cost to society and the family of supporting individuals affected by Down syndrome (DS), most European governments have fostered programmes of antenatal screening. Screening by maternal age and second trimester maternal serum screening are well established, respectively offering theoretical detection rates of 30% and 65% for a 5% false positive rate (1).

This article will review recent developments in the field of first trimester serum screening for pregnancies affected by DS.

ALPHA FETO-PROTEIN (AFP)

Since the first observation of depressed AFP in association with DS in the second trimester (2), a number of studies have confirmed the median of AFP in affected pregnancies as around 0.75 multiples of the median (MOM) of normal pregnancies. In the first trimester the situation is very similar: median AFP in DS is 0.7 to 0.8 times the MOM for normal pregnancies (Table 1). AFP is widely used in combination biochemical screening tests in the second trimester, but it is not yet clear if it can be expected to perform a similar role in the first trimester.

PREGNANCY ASSOCIATED PLASMA PROTEIN A (PAPP-A)

Low levels of maternal serum PAPP-A in the first trimester are associated with DS. The difference is greater at early gestations and is no longer evident by the second trimester (3). It has been suggested that by using measurements of PAPP-A in association with maternal age one would be able to detect 71% of cases of trisomy for a false positive rate of 5%(4,5). (Table 2).

Assays vary in their ability to distinguishing between affected and unaffected pregnancies because of variation in the antibody used and cross reactions with non–specific components of serum. Further investigations are warranted to decide which assays will provide the most efficient quick measurements.

HUMAN CHORIONIC GONADOTROPHIN

In the second trimester total hCG is raised in association with DS (6). The free beta subunit (which constitutes about 4% of circulating hCG), is increased to a greater extent, making it the single most efficient biochemical marker of DS in the second trimester (7). It is currently used in almost all second trimester serum screening tests.

Levels of total hCG in pregnancies affected by trisomy 21 in the first trimester are very similar to levels in normal pregnancies: levels of the free beta subunit are elevated in the first trimester, although the magnitude of the difference between normal and abnormal pregnancies is much less than in the second trimester (Table 3). HCG or free beta hCG may be useful components of screening tests in the first trimester, but would need to be applied in combination with more powerful indicators.

OESTRIOL

In the first and second trimesters maternal serum levels of unconjugated oestriol (uE3) are reduced in pregnancies associated with DS, and the magnitude of the reduction is very similar (median in affected pregnancies 0.74 MOM of normal pregnancies). Concerns exist because uE3 may be significantly correlated with AFP in DS pregnancies (8), and because the assay imprecision of uE3 lends imprecision to the final risk estimate (9).

OTHER BIOCHEMICAL MARKERS

SP1 has been found to be decreased in DS the first trimester to (10). Some of the observed reduction may be due to selection of samples from failing pregnancies

Comparison of a number of other potential markers, including placental alkaline phosphatase, cancer antigen 125 (CA 125), and inhibin, have failed to show any useful differences between normal and DS pregnancies. (11,12)

MARKERS OF DS IN THE FIRST TRIMESTER

Table 1   Serum Alpha Feto-protein

Study	no. of DS	MoM	Gestation (weeks)
Crandall et al 1991 (14)	10	0.75	9-12
Johnson et al 1991 (15)	9	0.71	8-12
Furhman et al 1993 (16)	19	0.97	9-12
Aitken et al 1993 (17)	17	0.65	7-14
Crandall et al 1993 (18)	11	0.74	11-14
van Lith et al 1994 (19)	32	0.83	8-12

Table 2   Serum PAPP-A
Diagnosis made at term or at CVS.

Study	No. Cases	TERM/CVS	MoM	Gestation (weeks)
Wald et 1992 (20)	19	Term	0.23	9-12
Brambati et al 1993 (4)	24	CVS	0.31	8-12
Muller et al (21)	17	Term	0.42	9-14
Hurley et al 1993 (22)	7	CVS	0.33	9-11
Aitken et al 1993 (23)	21		0.63	7-14
van Lith et al 1995 (24)	20	CVS	0.24	8-12
Brambati et al 1994 (13)	45	CVS	0.36	6-12

Table 3   hCG and free beta hCG

Study	No of DS	MoM	Gestation (weeks)
hCG			
Johnson et al 1991 (15)	11	0.91	9-12
Kratzer et al 1991 (25)	17	1.2	9-12
van Lith et al 1992 (26)	24	1.19	8-12
Aitken et al 1993 (17)	16	0.97	7-14
Crandall et al 1993 (18)	11	1.73	11-14
Free beta hCG			
Spencer et al 1992 (7)	13	1.85	9-13
Macri et al 1993 (27)	38	2.2	9-13
Aitken et al 1993 (17)	16	1.96	7-14
Brambati et al 1994 (13)	45	1.2	6-12

CONCLUSION

There are now a number of first trimester markers which carry great promise. PAPP-A appears to be the most promising and free beta hCG may be useful too, although with a lower sensitivity than that seen in the second trimester. Brambati et al have estimated that in the first trimester with a fixed 5% false positive rate one would detect 22% of DS using maternal age, as compared with 71% using maternal age and serum PAPP-A, 33% using age and serum hCG or 78 to 90% using all three (13).

REFERENCES

1.   Wald NJ, Cuckle HS, Densem JW, et al. (1988) Maternal serum screening for Down Syndrome in early pregnancy. Br. Med. J., 297, 883-7

2.   Chard T, Lowings C, Kitau MJ. (1984) Alpha feto-protein and chorionic gonadotrophin in relation to Down's Syndrome. Lancet 983, 750.

3. Aitken DA, McKinnon D, Crossley JA et al (1993). Changes in maternal serum concentrations of PAPP-A and SP-1 in down syndrome pregnancies between the first and second trimesters. In Proc of the Ass. Clin. Biochemists National Meeting. Ed SM Martin, Halloran SP, Green AJE. p72. London. Ass. Clin. Biochemists.

4.   Brambati B, Macintosh MCM, Teisner et al (1993a) Low maternal serum levels of pregnancy associated plasma protein A in the first trimester in association with abnormal fetal karyotype. B J Obstet Gynaecol 100:324-6.

5.   Brambati B, Tului L, Bonnachi I, Shrimanker K, Suzuki Y, Grudzinskas JG, (1993b) Serum PAPP-A and free beta hCG are first trimester screening markers for Down Syndrome (Abstract) Hum Reprod 8(Suppl 1):183.

7.   Spencer K, Macri JN, Aitken DA, Connor JM 1992. Free beta human chorionic gonadotrophin is a first trimester marker for fetal trisomy. Lancet 339, 1480.

8.   Davis CJ, Selby C, Spencer K (1991). Multicentre retrospective clinical trial for the prenatal detection of Down Syndrome. Clin. Chem., 37, 943.

9.   Reynolds T, John R. (1992). A comparison of unconjugated oestriol assay kits shows that expression of results as multiples of the median causes unacceptable variation in calculated Down syndrome risk factors. Clin Chem. 38:1888-93.

10. Macintosh MCM, Brambati B, Chard T, Grudzinskas JG (1993). First trimester maternal serum Schwangerschafts protein 1 (SP1) in pregnancies associated with chromosomal anomalies. Prenatal Diagn. 13. 563–8.

11. van Lith JMM, Mantingh JR, Beekhuis JR, de Bruijn HWA, (1991) First trimester CA125 levels and Down syndrome. Br J Obstet Gynaecol 98:493–4.

12. van Lith JMM, Mantingh A, Pratt JJ. (1994) First trimester maternal serum inhibin levels in chromosomally normal and abnormal pregnancies. Obstet. Gynaecol. 83(5):661–664.

13. Brambati B, Tului L, Bonnachi I, Suzuki Y, Shrimanker K, Grudzinskas JG, (1994) Biochemical screening for Down syndrome in the first trimester. In "Screening for Down Syndrome", eds JG Grudzinskas et al. pp285–94. Cambridge. Cambridge University Press.

14. Crandall BF, Golbus MS, Goldberg JD, Matsumoto M. (1991). First trimester maternal serum unconjugated oestriol and alpha–fetoprotein in fetal Down syndrome. Prenatal Diagn., 11:377–80.

15. Johnson A, Cowchock FS, Darby M, Wapner R, Jackson LG. (1991). First trimester maternal serum alph–fetoprotein and chorionic gonadotrophin in aneuploid pregnancies. Prenatal Diagn., 11, 443–50.

16. Fuhrmann W, Altland K, Jovanovic V et al (1993) First trimester alpha–fetoprotein screening for Down syndrome. Prenatal Diagn 13:215–8.

17. Aitken DA, McCaw G, Crossley JA et al 1993 First trimester biochemical screening for fetal chromosome abnormalities and neural tube defects. Prenatal Diagn., 13, 68–9.

18. Crandall BF, Hansen FW, Keener MS, Matsumo BS, Miller W. (1993) Maternal serum screening for alpha–fetoprotein, unconjugated oestriol and human chorionic gonadotrophin between 11 and 15 weeks of pregnancy to detect fetal chromosome abnormalities. Am J Obstet Gynaecol. 168:1864–9.

19. van Lith JMM. (1994). First trimester maternal serum alpha feto–protein as a marker for chromosomal disorders. Prenatal Diagnosis 14: 233–4

20. Wald NJ, Cuckle HS, Grudzinskas JG et al (1992) First trimester concentrations of pregnancy associated plasma protein A and placental protein 14 in Down syndrome. Br Med J 305:28.

21. Muller F, Cuckle HS, Teisner B, Grudzinskas JG. (1993) Serum PAPP-A levels are depressed in women with fetal Down syndrome in early pregnancy. Prenatal Diagn 13:633-6.

22. Hurley PA, Ward RHT, Teisner B, Iles RK, Lucas M, Grudzinskas JG. (1993). Serum PAPP-A measurements in first trimester screening for Down syndrome. Prenatal Diagn 12:505-12.

23. Aitken DA, Spencer K, Macri JN, Anderson R, Connor JM. (1993) PAPP-A as a marker of trisomy 21 in the first trimester. Clin Chem 39:1993

25. Krazer PG, Globus MS, Monroe SE Finklestein DE, Taylor RN. (1991). First trimester aneuploidy screening using serum human chorionic gonadotrophin, free alpha hCG and progesterone. Prenatal Diagn. 11:751-65.

26. van Lith JM. (1992). First trimester maternal serum human chorionic gonadotrophin as a marker for fetal chromosomal disorders, The Dutch Working Party on Prenatal Diagnosis. Prenatal Diag. 12:495-504.

27. Macri JN, Spencer K, Aitken D, Garver K, Buchanan PD, Muller F, Boue A. (1993) First trimester free beta hCG screening for Down Syndrome. Prenatal Diagn 13:557-62.

Chromosome mosaicism in prenatal diagnosis

S. Agosti, G. Nocera, P. Ilardi, C. Bombelli, N. Cotrozzi, F. Gramellini, D. Coviello and L. Dalprà*

V Clinic and *I Clinic of Obstetrics and Gynecology, University of Milan, Italy

INTRODUCTION

One of the major diagnostic problems in genetic counseling concerns chromosome mosaicism in prenatal diagnosis.

The incidence of chromosome mosaicism, very low at birth (0.02%) (1), is higher in selected populations submitted to prenatal diagnosis for chromosome anomalies. The incidence of chromosome mosaicism in CVS, confirmed on control fetal tissues, results as 0.3% (2, 3). The same incidence was reported for amniotic fluid cell cultures (0.1-0.3%) (4, 5, 6).

In the majority of cases it is difficult to evaluate the influence of a pathological cell line on the phenotype at birth and on child development. However the follow-up of babies submitted in utero to prenatal diagnosis is mandatory for a correct genetic counseling about karyotypes difficult to evaluate.

PATIENTS AND METHODS

In a ten years period (1983-1993) at our Prenatal Diagnosis Unit 1462 CVS and 3141 amniocenteses for fetal karyotyping were performed.

Amniocentesis

The incidence of unbalanced chromosome anomalies was 2.13% (67/3141). Of these cases 17 were mosaics (25.3%): 4 level II mosaics (several colonies in the same culture), and 13 level III mosaics (several colonies in different cultures).

CVS

The incidence of unbalanced chromosome anomalies was 3.8% (56/1462). Of these cases, 24 were mosaics (42%). In 9 of these the cell line anomaly was identified on spontaneous mitoses of cytotrophoblasts (direct analysis), in 8 on long term cultures, in 5 on both methods. In the 2 remaining cases a placental mosaicism was suspected because the direct analysis was in disagreement with the villi cultures.

RESULTS AND DISCUSSION

On amniotic fluid cell cultures 17 chromosome mosaics were found: 12 of them were related to heterosomes, 4 to autosomes. In one case a chromosome chimerism (46,XX and a 46,XY cell line) was found. A cytogenetic control on fetal tissues was performed in all cases except in 3 (46,XX/46,XXq-; 45,X/46,XY; 45,X/47,XXX). Seven chromosome mosaicisms were confirmed, while the chimerism has been confirmed on the second amniotic fluid sample, but not on chorion villus sample.

On CVS 24 chromosome mosaics were found: 4 involving heterosomes, 14 autosomes and 3 with structural anomalies. In the remaining 3 cases a diploid/tetraploid karyotype was observed. In three of these cases mosaicism has been confirmed.

The outcome of pregnancy was: 13 legal terminations (6 after amniocentesis and 7 after CVS), one fetal death at 28th week of pregnancy, one drop out at follow-up and 26 livebirths.

In tables 1 and 2 are reported outcomes and long-term evaluations. The follow-up included growth, psychomotor development, general health status and hospitalizations.

In all checked cases (time interval: 2 months-9 years) there were no developmental anomalies and general health conditions were normal.

As reported (7), a higher frequency of heterosome mosaicisms on amniotic cells cultures was observed as a demonstration of a greater viability, when compared to autosome mosaics. The mosaicism frequencies reported in the present study (0.4%) are in agreement with literature (0.1 - 0.3%) (4, 5, 6).

In CVS 14 out of 24 mosaicisms involved autosomes and 4 heterosomes, in opposition to the 2nd trimester data. Consequently it can be suggested that a confined placental mosaicism does not play a role in the evolution of pregnancy and in the fetus. None of the 8 autosome mosaicisms

Table 1   Amniocentesis: follow-up

	control	outcome	follow-up
45,X/46,XX	AF=46,XX	liveborn 37th 2950g	missing
45,X/46,XX	FB=46,XX	liveborn 40th 3300g	missing
45,X/47,XXX	not performed	liveborn 38th 3000g	82 months 28kg - 131,5cm
45,X/46,XY/47,XYY*	CV, AF=46,XY	liveborn 38th 2160g	79 months 23kg - 90cm
46,XX/47,XXX**	AF=46,XX/47,XXX** PB=46,XX	liveborn 40th 2900g - 45cm Peters' anomaly	2 months 4050g
46,XY/47,XXY	PB=46,XY/47,XXY	liveborn 39th 3130g - 51cm	2 months 5400g - 58cm
46,XX/46,XXq-	not performed	liveborn 3060g	missing
46,XY/46,X,+mar	AF, FB=46,XY/46,X,+mar	liveborn 40th 3840g - 52cm	3 months 7kg - 62cm
46/47,+2	AF=46,XY	liveborn 41th 2870g - 48cm	16 months 9,7kg - 78cm
46/47,+3	AF, FB=46,XX	liveborn 39th 3620g - 50cm	24 months 12,5kg - 87cm
46/47,+9***	FB=46/47,+9	intrauterine death 28th week	==

AF	= amniotic fluid; FB = fetal blood;
CV	= chorionic villus; PB = peripheral blood
*	= twin gestation, 2nd twin karyotype: 46,XY
**	= 1 colony
***	= twin gestation, 2nd twin karyotype: 46,XY (liveborn, 36th week)

pregnancies was complicated by miscarriage. Confirmed mosaicisms in the present study was 0.2%, as previously reported (2, 3).

Follow-up included 22 cases. None of them had growth nor psychomotor anomalies. Nevertheless most of heterosome mosaicisms could show clinical complications at the puberty.

Table 2   CVS : follow-up

	control	outcome	follow-up
46/47,+2	AF=46/47,+2* FB, AF=46,XX	liveborn 39th 3100g - 50cm	16 months 10kg - 80cm
46/47,+3	AF=46,XX	liveborn 42nd 3010g - 51cm	3 months 4800g - 57cm
46/47,+6	AF=46,XY	liveborn 39th 3610g - 52cm	48 months 17kg - 105cm
46/47,+7	AF=46,XX	liveborn 40th 3400g	missing
46/47,+9	AF=46,XY	liveborn 39th 2850g - 49cm	8 months 9kg - 76cm
46/47,+10	AF, CV=46,XX	liveborn 35th 2200g	missing
46/47,+14	AF=46,XY	liveborn 40th 2650g - 49cm hereditary spherocitosis	24 months 11,6kg - 88,5cm
46/47,+16	AF, CV=46,XX	liveborn 38th 2700g	36 months 13kg - 95cm
46,XY/92,XXYY	AF=46,XY	liveborn 40th 3150g - 49cm	27 months 15kg - 89cm
46,XX/92,XXXX	AF=46,XX	liveborn 39th 3200g	56 months 15kg - 110cm
46,XY/92,XXYY	AF=46,XY	liveborn 39th 3550g - 50cm	62 months 21kg - 120cm bowel stenosis
46/46,1p+	AF=46,XY	liveborn 37th 2680g - 47cm	86 months 23kg - 123cm
46/46,-22,+mar	AF=46,XY	liveborn 41th 3070g - 51cm	35 months 15kg - 95cm
46/46,t(2q;8q)	AF=46,XY	liveborn 40th 3050g	24 months 11,5kg - 84cm
45,X/46,XY	AF=46,XY	liveborn 38th 3050g PB=46,XY	116 months 30kg - 132cm
45,X/46,XY	AF, FB=45,X/46,XY	liveborn 32nd 1400g - 41,5cm	18 months 11,5kg - 78cm
45,X/46,X,t(X;X)	AF=46,XX	liveborn 28th 960g - 37cm	3 months 2430g 85cm PB=45,X/46,XX/46,X,t(X;X) (3.5%, 93.8%, 2.7%) 27 months 11kg - 85cm PB2=45,X/46,XX (3%,97%)

AF   = amniotic fluid; FB = fetal blood;
CV   = chorionic villus; PB = peripheral blood; PB2 = 2nd peripheral blood
         (age 12 months)
    * = 1 colony

REFERENCES

1 Jacobs P.A. and Hassold T.J. (1987). Chromosome abnormalities: origin and etiology in abortion and livebirths. In *Human Genetics* edited by F.Vogel and K. Sperling, 233-244

2 Nocera G., Dalprà L., Tibiletti M.G., Martinoli E., Ilardi P., Tessa E., Agosti S., Gramellini F., Oldrini A., Brambati B. (1989). Prenatal chromosome mosaicism in the first trimester. In *Chorionic Villus Sampling and Early Prenatal Diagnosis* edited by A. Antsaklis and C. Metaxotou, 181-182

3 Pittalis M.C., Dalprà L., Torricelli F., Rizzo N., Nocera G., Cariati E., Santarini L., Tibiletti M.G., Agosti S., Bovicelli L., Forabosco A. (1994). The predictive value of cytogenetic diagnosis after CVS based on 4860 cases with both direct and culture methods. *Prenat Diagn*, **14**, 267-278

4 Hsu L.Y.F., Perlis T. (1984). United States Survey on Chromosome Mosaicism and Pseudomosaicism in Prenatal Diagnosis. *Prenat. Diagn (Special Issue)*, **4**, 97-130

5 Bui T.H., Iselius L., Lindsten J. (1984). European Collaborative Study on Prenatal Diagnosis: mosaicism, pseudomosaicism and single abnormal cell in amniotic fluid cell cultures. *Prenat. Diagn. (Special Issue)*, **4**, 145-162

6 Worton R.G., Stern R. (1984). A Canadian Collaborative Study of mosaicism in amniotic fluid cell cultures. *Prenat. Diagn. (Special Issue)*, **4**, 131-144

7 Hsu L.Y.F. (1992). In *Genetic Disorders and The Fetus*, 3d ed., edited by A. Milunsky

This work was supported by C.N.R., project "Prevention and Control of Disease Factors" subproject 7, No 91.00.134.PF41.115.19572

545

Hemoglobin, glucose, α-fetoprotein and endocrine changes during normal pregnancy

F.R. Pérez-López, J. Hergueta, J. Robert, M.D. Abós and V. Peg

Departments of Obstetrics and Gynecology, and Nuclear Medicine, University of Zaragoza Hospital Clínico, and Ambulatorio 'San José', Zaragoza, Spain

INTRODUCTION

During human pregnancy there are multiple systemic changes in the maternal physiology and new hormones are present in blood. These metabolic and endocrinologic readjustments in the maternal organism are necessary for the development of the fetus. The synthesis of steroid hormones requires the integration of fetal organs and the placenta, which Diczfalusy described as the "fetoplacental unit" concept. The desgin of diagnostical and therapeutical actions based on the alterations in different fetoplacentary parametres with respect to the normal curves has been attempted for a long time. However, the initial optimism and hopes have not been recompensed with simple and effective clinical action schemes. Below, we present the results of a study carried out many years ago, on the physiological changes in the levels of hemoglobin, glucose, alphafetoprotein and different fetoplacentary hormones in child bearing women who until then had experienced regular menstrual cycles and whose last date in which the date of menstruation was well documented.

MATERIAL AND METHODS

Women without pathological history whose pregnancies had been controlled from

547

very early on participated voluntarily in the study. There was no doubt about the date of the last menstruation, their menstrual cycles were regular every 28-30 days, and during pregnancy no pathology of any type had been detected. The obstetric controls carried out at regular intervals were normal, the samples taken at gestational ages ± 1 day are indicated in the figures and tables, and delivery took place between 36 and 43 weeks counted from the last menstruation, giving birth to healthy fetuses whose weights oscilated between 2,501 and 4,000 grammes.

After 12 weeks of gestation, they received a multivitamin supplement containing 150 mg of ferrous sulphate and 600 mg of calcium carbonate (Matrabec®). The child bearing women with serum values of hemoglobin lower than 11 g/dL received 1-2 tablets of a preparations containing 270 mg of ferrous sulphate and 80 mg of mucoprotease (Tardyferon®) and one capsule of 10 mg of folic acid (Aspol®).

The determination of serum hemoglobin was carried out with a Coulter hematological analyser. Glucose levels were determined with a Hitachi 705 autoanalyser following the hexoquinase/glucose-6-fosphate deshidrogenase technique. The determinations of ß-HCG, alphafetoprotein, estriol, progesterone, and placental lactogen were carried out using radioimmunoassay methods validated previously (Pérez-López et al. 1982).

The statistical comparisons were carried out using Duncan-Kramer's the multiple range test, considering significant differences for $P < 0.05$.

RESULTS AND COMMENTS

Figures 1-7 and tables 1-7 present the median values ± standard error of the mean, gestational age, number of samples studied for each gestational period and statistical comparison with its grade of significance.

The changes in the hemoglobin levels during pregnancy could be related to the hemodynamic changes experienced during pregnancy and the the fetus's need for iron. The glucose levels are lower than those found in a non child bearing women. The plasmatic changes in alphafetoprotein and in the different hormones studied are compatible with studies published previously, resulting from the functional placentary activity or of the fetoplacentary integration.

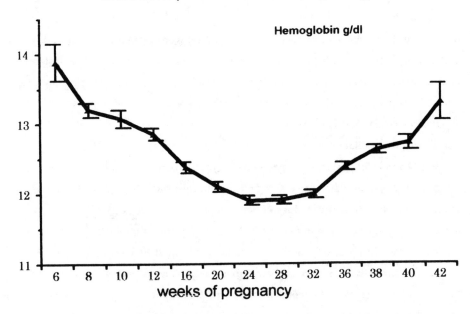

Figure 1 Mean ± SEM hemoglobin levels in normal pregnant women. The number of samples is indicated in table 1.

Table 1 Groups, weeks of pregnancy, number of samples and statistical significance among the different groups of pregnant women in which hemoglobin was studied. 0 = NS; + $p<0.05$; * $p<0.01$

Group number	n	2	3	4	5	6	7	8	9	10	11	12	13
1 = 6 weeks	9	+	+	*	*	*	*	*	*	*	*	*	0
2 = 8 weeks	49		0	+	*	*	*	*	*	*	*	*	0
3 = 10 weeks	52			0	*	*	*	*	*	*	*	+	0
4 = 12 weeks	77				*	*	*	*	*	*	0	0	0
5 = 16 weeks	103					*	*	*	*	0	+	*	+
6 = 20 weeks	125						0	0	0	*	*	*	*
7 = 24 weeks	153							0	0	*	*	*	*
8 = 28 weeks	166								0	*	*	*	*
9 = 32 weeks	169									*	*	*	*
10 = 36 weeks	183										*	*	+
11 = 38 weeks	165											0	0
12 = 40 weeks	79												0
13 = 42 weeks	7												

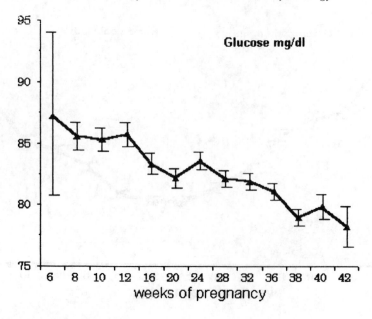

Figure 2 Mean ± SEM glucose levels in normal pregnant women. The number of samples is indicated in table 2.

Table 2 Groups, weeks of pregnancy, number of samples and statistical significance among the different groups of pregnant women in which glucose was studied. 0 = NS; + p<0.05; * p<0.01

Group number	n	2	3	4	5	6	7	8	9	10	11	12	13
1 = 6 weeks	7	0	0	0	0	0	0	0	0	0	+	0	0
2 = 8 weeks	49		0	0	0	+	0	+	+	*	*	*	0
3 = 10 weeks	52			0	0	+	0	+	+	*	*	*	0
4 = 12 weeks	76				0	+	0	*	*	*	*	*	0
5 = 16 weeks	104					0	0	0	0	0	*	+	0
6 = 20 weeks	125						0	0	0	0	*	0	0
7 = 24 weeks	155							0	0	+	*	*	0
8 = 28 weeks	167								0	0	*	0	0
9 = 32 weeks	172									0	*	0	0
10 = 36 weeks	184										+	0	0
11 = 38 weeks	164											0	0
12 = 40 weeks	79												0
13 = 42 weeks	7												

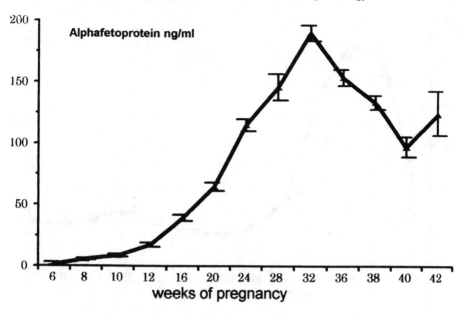

Figure 3   Mean ± SEM α-fetoprotein levels in normal pregnant women.   The number of samples is indicated in table 3.

Table 3   Groups, weeks of pregnancy, number of samples and statistical significance among the different groups of pregnant women in which α-fetoprotein was studied. 0 = NS; + p<0.05; * p<0.01

Group number	n	2	3	4	5	6	7	8	9	10	11	12	13
1 = 6 weeks	5	*	*	*	*	*	*	*	*	*	*	*	*
2 = 8 weeks	30		*	*	*	*	*	*	*	*	*	*	*
3 = 10 weeks	42			*	*	*	*	*	*	*	*	*	*
4 = 12 weeks	56				*	*	*	*	*	*	*	*	*
5 = 16 weeks	80					*	*	*	*	*	*	*	*
6 = 20 weeks	101						*	*	*	*	*	*	*
7 = 24 weeks	125							*	*	*	0	0	0
8 = 28 weeks	127								*	0	0	*	0
9 = 32 weeks	146									*	*	*	0
10 = 36 weeks	159										0	*	0
11 = 38 weeks	140											*	0
12 = 40 weeks	71												0
13 = 42 weeks	7												

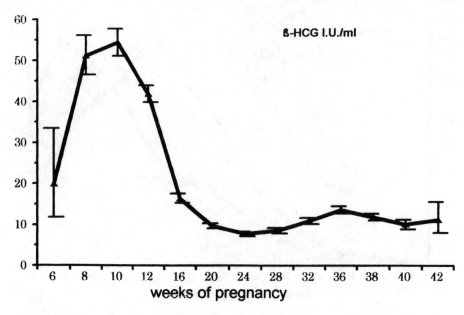

Figure 4 Mean ± SEM ß-HCG levels in normal pregnant women. The number of samples is indicated in table 4.

Table 4 Groups, weeks of pregnancy, number of samples and statistical significance among the different groups of pregnant women in which ß-HCG was studied. 0 = NS; + $p<0.05$; * $p<0.01$

Group number	n	2	3	4	5	6	7	8	9	10	11	12	13
1 = 6 weeks	5	+	*	+	0	0	+	+	0	0	0	0	0
2 = 8 weeks	33		0	0	*	*	*	*	*	*	*	*	*
3 = 10 weeks	42			0	*	*	*	*	*	*	*	*	*
4 = 12 weeks	56				*	*	*	*	*	*	*	*	*
5 = 16 weeks	79					*	*	*	*	0	*	*	0
6 = 20 weeks	101						+	0	0	*	0	0	0
7 = 24 weeks	127							0	*	*	*	+	0
8 = 28 weeks	128								+	*	*	0	0
9 = 32 weeks	148									+	0	0	0
10 = 36 weeks	159										0	+	0
11 = 38 weeks	139											0	0
12 = 40 weeks	71												0
13 = 42 weeks	7												

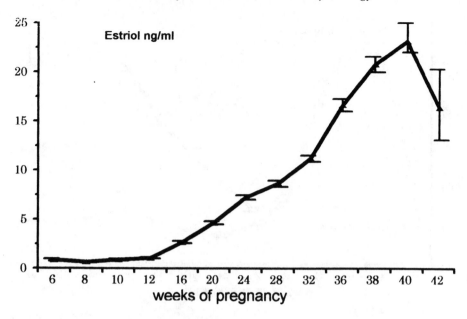

Figure 5   Mean ± SEM estriol levels in normal pregnant women. The number of samples is indicated in table 5.

Table 5   Groups, weeks of pregnancy, number of samples and   statistical significance among the different groups of pregnant women in which estriol was studied. 0 = NS; + p<0.05; * p<0.01

Group number	n	2	3	4	5	6	7	8	9	10	11	12	13
1 = 6 weeks	2	0	0	0	+	*	*	*	*	*	*	*	*
2 = 8 weeks	27		0	*	*	*	*	*	*	*	*	*	*
3 = 10 weeks	39			0	*	*	*	*	*	*	*	*	*
4 = 12 weeks	56				*	*	*	*	*	*	*	*	*
5 = 16 weeks	80					*	*	*	*	*	*	*	*
6 = 20 weeks	101						*	*	*	*	*	*	*
7 = 24 weeks	127							*	*	*	*	*	*
8 = 28 weeks	128								*	*	*	*	*
9 = 32 weeks	148									*	*	*	+
10 = 36 weeks	158										*	*	0
11 = 38 weeks	140											+	0
12 = 40 weeks	72												+
13 = 42 weeks	7												

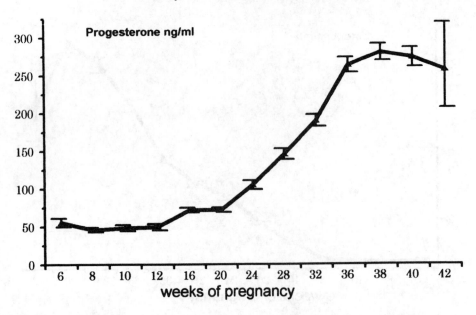

Figure 6   Mean ± SEM progesterone levels in normal pregnant women.   The number of samples is indicated in table 6.

Table 6   Groups, weeks of pregnancy, number of samples and   statistical significance among the different groups of pregnant women in which progesterone was studied. 0 = NS; + p<0.05; * p<0.01

Group number	n	2	3	4	5	6	7	8	9	10	11	12	13
1 = 6 weeks	5	0	0	0	0	0	*	*	*	*	*	*	*
2 = 8 weeks	33		0	0	*	*	*	*	*	*	*	*	*
3 = 10 weeks	42			0	*	*	*	*	*	*	*	*	*
4 = 12 weeks	56				*	*	*	*	*	*	*	*	*
5 = 16 weeks	80					0	*	*	*	*	*	*	*
6 = 20 weeks	101						*	*	*	*	*	*	*
7 = 24 weeks	126							*	*	*	*	*	*
8 = 28 weeks	128								*	*	*	*	*
9 = 32 weeks	148									*	*	*	0
10 = 36 weeks	159										0	0	0
11 = 38 weeks	139											0	0
12 = 40 weeks	72												0
13 = 42 weeks	7												

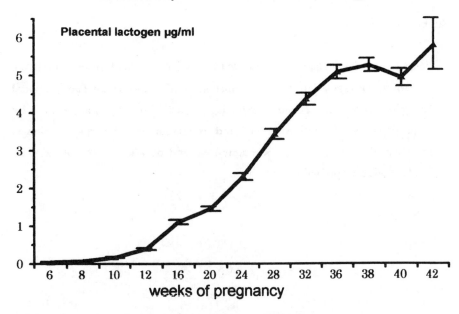

Figure 7   Mean ± SEM placental lactogen levels in normal pregnant women. The number of samples is indicated in table 7.

Table 7   Groups, weeks of pregnancy, number of samples and   statistical significance among the different groups of pregnant women in which placental lactogen was studied. 0 = NS; + p<0.05; * p<0.01

Group	n	2	3	4	5	6	7	8	9	10	11	12	13
1 = 6 weeks	3	0	0	0	*	*	*	*	*	*	*	*	*
2 = 8 weeks	32		0	*	*	*	*	*	*	*	*	*	*
3 = 10 weeks	42			*	*	*	*	*	*	*	*	*	*
4 = 12 weeks	56				*	*	*	*	*	*	*	*	*
5 = 16 weeks	80					*	*	*	*	*	*	*	*
6 = 20 weeks	100						*	*	*	*	*	*	*
7 = 24 weeks	126							*	*	*	*	*	*
8 = 28 weeks	126								*	*	*	*	*
9 = 32 weeks	147									*	*	+	0
10 = 36 weeks	158										0	0	0
11 = 38 weeks	139											0	0
12 = 40 weeks	72												0
13 = 42 weeks	7												

REFERENCE

1. Pérez-López, F.R., Tierz, J.A., Abós, M.D., Pellejero, S. and Teijeiro, J. (1982). Dopaminergic regulation of human prolactin, ACTH, aldosterone, TSH, placental lactogen, chorionic gonadotropin and estriol during pregnancy. In: Neuropeptides, meurotransmitters and regulation of endocrine processes, Endröczi, E. , Angelucci, U., Scapagnini, U. and de Wied, E. eds. Akadémiai Kiadó: Budapest pp. 459-66

Pregnancy and diabetes

R. Navalesi, G. Di Cianni, L. Volpe, P. Orsini and L. Benzi

Department of Metabolic Diseases, University of Pisa, Pisa, Italy

INTRODUCTION

Carbohydrate intolerance during gestation can be grouped into two categories: 1) Type 1 Diabetes (IDDM), Type 2 Diabetes (NIDDM) or Impaired Glucose Tolerance (IGT) already present before pregnancy; 2) Gestational Diabetes (GDM) and Impaired Gestational Glucose tolerance (IGGT) detected for the first time during pregnancy. Both categories heavily influence the pregnancy outcome being associated with an increased risk of maternal morbidity and perinatal morbility and mortality.

Improved control of hyperglycemia during pregnancy has greatly decreased perinatal mortality in offspring of diabetic pregnants. Nevertheless, congenital malformations are still found in 4-5% of newborns of diabetic women. This value is higher than that of normal nondiabetic women but it is markedly decreased throught the last years. Advances in understanding fetal physiology and in application of perinatology techniques have reduced the frequency and severity of neonatal morbidity, but fetal macrosomia, cesarean section and preterm delivery still result elevated in respect to non diabetic population (1-2).

EFFECTS OF DIABETES ON PREGNANCY

Malformations and neonatal morbility

The impaired metabolic maternal milieu has been generally considered as the most acceptable explanation for the increased incidence of fetal malformation. In IDDM, these metabolic derangements exist before pregnancy and their influence on the organogenesis leads to important malformations often life threathening.

Several studies have shown a strong increase in malformations when a good metabolic control is not obtained during prepregancy and early postconception. Moreover an increase of maternal HbA1c at the end of the first quarter has been correlated with an higher incidence of the principal congenital malformations: anencephalus, encephalocele, regression caudal syndrome, vertebral agenesis, transposition of great vessel, vasculopaties (3).

Diabetic embryopathy appears to be multifactorial. At present the more probable hypothesis to explain its pathogenesis is linked to fetal hyperinsulinemia in response to the transplacental passagge of the aberrant fuels and fuel related components of the diabetic state (high glucose, ketones, aminoacids, free fat acids, osmolality, somatomedin inhibitors, etc.). Insulin is secreted by fetal pancreatic islets starting from twelvth week of gestation, and represents an important growth factor for placenta and fetus. Increased insulin levels in fetal blood are probably responsible for macrosomia and fetal organomegalia. On the other hand hyperinsulinemia determines villi's hypertrophy and consequently, intervillar spaces and blood flow reduction. The decreased transplacental blood flow causes hypossia and microsomia. Moreover fetal hyperinsulinemia is implicated in neonatal hypoglicaemia, respiratory distress syndrom (RDS), hyperbilirubinemia, polycytemia (4).

Medical and obstetric complications

Diabetic pregnancies can be associated with every known obstetric complication. Because even trivial problems upset diabetic control and pose greater hazards for the mother and fetus, every effort is made to ensure early recognition and treatment of untoward events.Prevention of most medical problems in diabetic pregnancies is possible with preconception counseling that includes diabetes reeducation.

In pregnant women with diabetes, the tre most common problems that adversely affect metabolic control are emotional stress, infection (viral illnesses, urinary tract infections) and hypoglycemia. The most common causes of hypoglycemia are overinsulinization (by a zelous patient or her physician in the attempt to achieve "perfect control"), abnormal counterregulatory responses, anti-insulin antibodies and impaired subcutaneous absorption of insulin. During pregnancy, frequent and severe episodies of hypoglycemia are a serios risk for both mother and fetus. Also ketoacidosis is frequent in pregnant women with IDDM. Infection with a concomitant deficiency of insulin is the most common precipitating factor for this metabolic emercency.

Maternal obstetrical complications often present in diabetic pregancy include: preeclampsia-eclampsia, preterm labor, premature rupture of membranes, hydramnios. Fetal obstetrical complications are: spontaneous abortion, fetal death and preterm birth. The firs condition occour in association with fetal chromosomal or structural anomalies with the cause of the ramainder unknown; fetal hyperglycemia in poorly controlled diabetic women can lead to progressive fetal hypoxemia, acidosis and, eventually,death; early delivery of infant of diabetic mothers remain a problem in diabetic pregnancies, probably due to maternal complications.

EFFECT OF PREGNANCY ON DIABETIC COMPLICATIONS

Considerable progress has been made in our knowdlege of the effects of pregnancy on the progression of diabetic chronic complications and on the strategies to prevent their worsening.

Retinopathy

Several clinical epidemiology studies have described the impact of pregnancy on retinal changes (5-6). Diabetic retinopathy may worsen during pregnancy, particularly if advanced non-proliferative or proliferative lesions are present prior to conception. In IDDM the unfavorable progression of both retinopathy stadies are correlated with a longer duration of diabetes, older age at examination, higher concentrations of glycosilated hemoglobin.

Laser photocoagulation can be administered to patients with advanced retynopathy prior to conception to limit the chance of worsening during pregnancy and can also be used to treat advancing retinopathy during gestation. Thus, management of retinopathy should include a preconceptional eye's exam and a carefull follow up during pregnancy. Non proliferative changes that arise during pregnancy often regress after delivery.

Nephropathy

Diabetic nephropathy in pregnancy (7-8) has been traditionally diagnosed on the basis of urinary protein excretion before 20 weeks gestation. Overt nephropathy (excretion of 300 mg/day) is frequently (30-50% of cases) associated with elevated blood pressure and increased proteinuria during the latter half of gestation. The clinical picture is difficult to distinguish from pre-eclampsia and preterm delivery is often necessary. Intrauterine growth retardation is also a risk with overt nephropathy. However, total protein excretion > 190 mg/dl before 20 weeks gestation has been associated with an increased risk of pre-eclampsia that is similar to the risk in overt nephropathy. The impact of pregnancy on maternal renal function is not clear, although most evidence does not support a decline in renal function as result of pregnancy. Patients who become pregnant with overt nephropathy often develop renal failure after pregnancy, a fact that should be considered during preconceptional or early pregnancy counseling. Every mounthly fundus oculi and renal function could be evaluated.

DIABETES TREATMENT IN PREGNANCY

Dietary and insulin therapy are the keystone of both GDM and IDDM. During pregnancy it is recommeded an additional 300 kcal/day in the 2th and 3rd trimester to obtain a weight gain of 11-12 Kg for a full-term gestation. Several authors suggest that an underweight (BMI<20 Kg/m^2) pregnant can have a weight gain of 16-18 Kg while 7-8 Kg increase is the target for an obese woman (BMI>30 Kg/m^2). Althought it has has been demostrated very clearly that weight reduction ameliorates insulin resistance and lowers fasting plasma levels of glucose, insulin and lipid in nonpregnant obese diabetic women, a strong weight reduction during pregnancy is not recommended. Infact it is associated with FFA mobilization and production of ketones which are very dangerous to fetal cerebral growth. Diet could be composed by 50% carbohydrate, 20% protein, 30% lipid expecially monoinsatur. It is a good law to take several small lunches during the day to obtain a better glycemic control (9).

During gestation ideal value of fastin plasma glucose glycemia is 90-95 mg/dl at fast and 120-130 mg/dl two hours after lunch. To obtain this aim the insulin therapy must be "intensive", with four administrations/daily: regular insulin before breackfast, lunch and dinner, intermediate insulin at "bed time". After the initial insulin calculation, the dose is adjusted for each women until blood glucose levels obtained before and after each meal are close to the normal valuee. Six or more self blood glucose measurements each day are required to optimize insulin therapy (10).

DIABETIC CONTROL BEFORE CONCEPTION

Several studies have shown a marked decrease in malformations when prepregnancy and early postconception metabolic control is very good (HbA1c < 7%). All women with IDDM or NIDDM should be urged to have preconception counseling and become aware of the role that good control of diabetes plays in the prevention of congenital malformation (11). Counselors generally request that both the patient and her partner partecipate. The importance of diabetic control before conception must be stressed and each women is advised to have a comprehensive medical assessment, instruction in blood glucose monitoring, a retinal examination, renal evaluation and nutrition counseling. Frequent supervisory appointments every few weeks at a diabetes center are essential to achieve and mantain diabetic control. Once the plasma glucose is stabilized and is well maintained for another 3 to 4 months, pregnancy can safely be undertaken.

BLOOD GLUCOSE CONTROL IN PREGNANCY

Pregnant with IDDM or NIDDM since the preconception to the end of gestation we must obtain a really strong glicemic balance. Women have to determine their glucose values by destrosticks and frequent ambulatorial visits. It is not appropriate to monitor glycemia through glycosuria because of its physiological increase in pregnancy. Every 3-4 weeks it's necessary to check her HbAlc and fruttosamine. Both blood glucose monitoring and insulin therapy continue till the delivery (38-40 weeks). With the onset of active labor insulin requirements decrease to zero and glucose demands are relatively consistent at 2.5 mg/Kg/min. From these data, a protocol for supplying the glucose needs of labor has been developed (12). The goal is to mantain a blood glucose of 70 to 90 mg/dl. With onset of active spontaneous labor, insulin is withheld, and an intravenous dextrose infusion is begun at a rate of 2.5 mg/Kg/min. If labor is latent, normal saline is usually sufficient to mantain normoglycemia. Blood glucose is then monitored hourly, and if belove <60 mg%, the infusion rate is doubled for the subsequent hour. If blood glucose rises to > 140 mg/dl 4-6 I.U. rapid acting insulin are given subcutaneously each hour until the blood glucose is 70 to 80 mg/dl.

When elective cesarean sections are planned the insulin bedtime is given and on the day of surgery we determine fasting glycemia and start intravenous infusions of 5% dextrose then monitoring blood glucose hourly with meter at bedside. For glucose levels > 110 mg/dl add 5 UI regular insulin to 500 ml Dw5 and continue infusion rate of 125 ml/h (1.25 U insulin/h). We have to keep infusion rate constant. Insulin adjustments are made hourly if necessary by doubling or halving the insulin concentration to mantain blood glucose at 70-120 mg/dl.

Maternal insulin requirements usually decrease for 48-96 hours postpartum; insulin requirements should be recalculated at 0,6 IU/kg based on postpartum weight and should be started almost an hour after the delivery and when plasma glucose is above 150 mg/dl to evoid severe hypoglycemia. The postpartum caloric requirements are 25 kcal/kg/day, based on postpartum weight. Normoglycemia especially should be mantained in nursing diabetic women, because hyperglycemia elevates milk glucose levels.

Women with previous GDM run a much increased risk of developing IGT or NIDDM later in life. For this reason it's important to repeat un oral glucose tollerance test 3 months after delivery and each year.

REFERENCES

1) Ramos Arroyo, M.A., Pinilla, D. (1992). Maternal Diabetes: the risk for specific birth defect. *Eur J Epidemiol* **8** : 503-508.

2) Miodnovick, M., Minouni, F. (1988). Maior malformations in newborn infants of IDDM women. *Diabetes Care* **11** : 713-718.

3) Greene, M.F., Hare, J. W.(1989). First trimester hemoglobin A1 and risk for major malformation and spontaneous abortion in diabetic pregnancy. *Teratology* **39**: 225-231.

4) Persson, B., Hanson, U. (1992). Diabetes Mellitus and pregnancy. In Alberti, K.G.M.M., De Fronzo,(eds) *International Textbook of Diabetes Mellitus*, 1085-1101.(New York, J. Wiley and Sons).

5) Elman, K.D., Welch, R.A. (1990). Diabetic Retinopathy in pregnancy: a review. *Obstet Gynecol*, **75**, 119-127.

6) Rosenn, B., Miodonovik, M.(1992). Progression of diabetic retinopathy in pregnancy: association with hypertension in pregnancy. *Am J Obstet Gynecol,* **4,** 1214-1218.

7) Buchanan, T. (1994) Diabetic micronagiopathy in pregnancy. In 15th *International Diabetes Federation Congress,* Abstracts, 64.

8) Combs, C.A., Kitzmiller L.M.B., Greene, M.F.(1992). First trimester urinary albumin excretion predicts birth weight in diabetic pregnancies. *Diabetes,* **4** (Suppl.1), 133A.

9) Jovanovic-Peterson, L., Peterson, C.M. (1992). Pregnancy in the diabetic woman: guidelines for a successful outcome. *Endocrinol Metab Clin North Am* **21,** 2: 433-455.

10) Kitzmiller, J.L. (1993). Sweet success with diabetes: development of insulin therapy and glycemic control for pregnancy. *Diabetes Care* **16,** 107-121.

11) Mills, J.L., Knopp, R.H. (1988). Lack of relation of increased malformation rates in Infants of diabetic mothers to glycemic control during organogenesis. *N Engl J Med* **318,** 671-676.

12) Moore, T.R. (1992). Management of diabetes during labor and delivery. In Hollingsworth, D.R. (eds.) *Pregnancy, Diabetes and Birth,* 233-237 (Baltimora, Williams & Wilkins)

Hypertension in pregnancy and insulin-resistant syndrome

O. Ylikorkala

Department of Obstetrics and Gynecology, Helsinki University, Helsinki, Finland

Background. Hyperinsulinemia and insulin resistance are common findings in hypertensive individuals (1). Patients with hypertension and insulin resistance often have elevated serum triglycerides and decreased high-density lipoprotein (HDL) cholesterol levels. It has been suggested that insulin resistance might be the common etiologic factor causing hyperinsulinemia, hypertension, hypertriglyceridemia, and low serum HDL cholesterol- acluster of risk fators for coronary artery disease also designated "syndrome X or" insulin resistnat syndrome" (1). An interesting analogy can be observed in pregnancy-induced hypertension. The condition occurs more frequently in women with impaired glucose tolerance (2) and is characterized by elevated serum triglyceride levels (3). We have studied serum insulin, lipids, lipoproteins, and thestable urinary metabolites of prostacyclin (PGI2) and thromboxane (A2) in hypertensive and normotensive pregnancies.

Patients and Methods. Thirty-one pregnant women (23 nulliparous and eight multiparous) were admitted to the hospital because pregnancy-induced hypertension, defined as a rise in blood pressure above 140/90 mmHg (measured at least twice more than 6 hours apart) after 20 weeks of pregnancy, which resolved completely within 4 weeks post postpartum. These women, none of whom smoked, were healthy before pregnancy and their mean (+- SD) body mass index (MBI) was 24.5 (3.8) kg/m2. In eight women, proteinuria exceeded 0.5 g/day (proteinuric, pre-eclamptic group) and in 23, no macroproteinuria (less than 0.5 g/day) was found (nonproteinuric group). The subjects were studied between 30-39 weeks' gestation (mean 35) before the start of antihypertensive medication. Twenty-one (14 nulliparous, seven parous) healthy, nonsmoking, pregnant, normotensive controls, with a similar parity and BMI (22.8 +- 4.1 kg/m2) were studied a comparable gestational ages. No patient had a history of pre-existing hypertension, hyperlipidemia, or carbohydrate intolerance.

Blood samples were drawn after overnight fasting for insulin, lipid, and lipoprotein determinations. Spot urine samples for prostanoid metabolites were also collected from all subjects, but 27 samples had to be excluded because of the occasional use of aspirin or other nonsteroidal anti-inflammatory drugs during the 2 weeks preceding the sampling. Urinary prostanoid metabolites could be measured in 17 patients with pregnancy-induced hypertension (five proteinuric) and in eight controls.

Total and lipoprotein cholesterol concentrations as well as insulin and uric acid levels were measured with established methods. Urine samples were assayed for the stable degradation products of PGI2, 6-keto-prostaglandin (PG) F1a and 2-3-dinor-6-keto- PGF1a and those of TxA2, thromboxane B2 (TxB2) and 2,3-dinor TxB2, by high-pressure- liquid chromatography followed by radioimmunoassay (4).To circumvent differing hydration levels, the urinary excretion of prostanoid metabolites was expressed in relation to creatinine excretion.

Results. Women with pregnancy-induced hypertension exhibited 18 % lower mean serum HDL2 cholesterol levels and 65 % higher mean triglyceride levels compared to controls, whereas other serum lipid and apolipoprotein values showed no significant differences (Table 1). The levels of insulin and uric

Table 1. Blood Pressure, Cholesterol, Triglyceride, Apolipoproteins A1 and B, Insulin, and Uric Acid Concentrations.

	Hypertensive women			Controls
	Proteinuric	Nonproteinuric	All	
N	8	23	31	21
Blood pressure (mmHg)				
-systolic	151(10)**	157(15)**	155(13)**	128(11)
-diastolic	94(13)*	99(19)*	97(17)*	81(8)
Total cholesterol (mmol/L)	7.0(1.6)	7.2(1.1)	7.1(1.3)	6.8(1.1)
HDL$_2$-cholesterol (mmol/L)	0.8(0.1)*	0.9(0.2)*	0.9(0.2)*	1.1(0.1)
LDL-cholesterol (mmol/L)	3.2(1.0)	4.4(0.9)	4.2(0.9)	3.9(0.9)
Apolipoprotein A$_1$ (mg/mL)	1.7(0.2)	1.8(0.2)	1.7(0.2)	1.7(0.2)
Apolipoprotein B (mg/mL)	1.1(0.2)	1.4(0.3)	1.3(0.3)	1.4(0.4)
Triglyceride (mmol/L)	3.7(1.4)*	3.1(1.0)*	3.3(1.2)*	2.0(0.7)
Insulin (mU/L)	13.8(8.2)**	13.2(6.3)**	13.3(6.6)**	6.5(2.4)
Uric acid (umol/L)	371.3(87.8)**	325.9(69.7)**	339.7(77.6)**	231.2(29.8)

*p<0.05 compared to controls
**p<0.01 compared to controls
Values are mean (standard deviation)
HDL = high density lipoprotein
LDL = low density lipoprotein

Table 2. Urinary Prostanoid Excretion

	Hypertensive women			Controls
	Proteinuric	Nonproteinuric	All	
N	5	12	17	8
6-keto-PGF$_{1a}$	23.8(9.7)*	25.5(9.6)*	25.0(9.3)*	39.1(15.5)
2,3-dinor-6-keto-PGF$_{1a}$	16.3(8.1)*	18.9(8.9)*	18.1(7.0)*	33.2(14.9)
TxB$_2$	7.4(2.7)	9.9(7.0)	9.2(6.1)	10.5(6.0)
2,3-dinor-TxB$_2$	50.1(20.9)	63.2(43.3)	59.3(38.0)	63.9(28.1)

*P<0.05 compared to control
Values are mean (standard deviation)[ng/mmol creatinine]

acid were significantly higher in pregnancy-induced hypertensive women than in the controls. The urinary excretion of PGI2 metabolites was reduced in hypertensive patients, whereas the excretion of TxA2 metabolites was normal (Table 2).

For studying the relationships among lipids, insulin, and prostanoid output, the data from 17 subjects with pregnancy- induced hypertension and eight controls were pooled. Serum HDL-2- cholesterol concentrations correlated positively with urinary excretion of 2,3-dinor-6-keto-PGF1a (R2 = 0.36, p< 0.001). Serum triglyceride concentrations correlated positively with urinary excretion of 2,3-dinor- TxB2 (R2 = 0.19, p< 0.027). Inverse correlations were observed between serum HDL2-cholesterol and serum insulin (R2 =-0.18, p= 0.002) in all women. Positive correlations existed between serum insulin and triglyceride (r2 = 0.20, p = 0.0009).

Discussion. The hypertensive pregnant women exhibited high triglyceride and insulin levels, and low HDL_2 cholesterol levels, findings resembling the key characteristics of the "insulin resistance syndrome" (1). Our data were not affected by the presence of proteinuria. Hyperuricemia, characteristic of hypertensive pregnancies, and also seen in our patients, has been linked recently with insulin resistance in nonpregnant, nondiabetic subjects (5). It is known that there is insulin resistance in normal pregnancy and that there is an association between the degree of insulin elevation and hypertension during the third trimester of pregnancy. Thus, our findings could be explained by an augmented insulin peripheral resistance as described originally by Ferrannini et al. (1) in nonpregnant subjects with essential hypertension. To prove a true insulin resistance, studies using euglycemic clamp technique would be necessary. The elevated serum triglyceride levels could be explained by overproduction of very low density lipoproteins (VLDL) in the liver due to hyperinsulinemia. In addition, resistance of lipoprotein lipase to insulin action in peripheral tissues could impair VLDL catabolism. Either way, the inverse relationship between VLDL and HDL_2 concentrations would result in decreased HDL_2 cholesterol levels.

There is abundant evidence of endothelial cell dysfunction in preeclampsia, but it has remained unclear whether or not it is a primary - and then a possible cause of preeclampsia - or just a secondary change. Recent data suggest that maternal lipids could contribute to endothelial dysfunction. Lorentzen et al (6) showed that the content of triglyceride in cultured human endothelial cells was increased three-fold if the cells were cultured in the presence of sera of preeclamptic women. This led to an 80% reduction in PGI_2 synthesis by the same cells. The same group then demonstrated that sera of preeclamptic women were characterized by high availability of free fatty acids and that these sera stimulated the synthesis of triglycerides by the endothelial cells (7). Our data showing high triglyceride levels and low PGI_2 output are in accordance with these notions. Hyperinsulinemia present in pregancy-induced hypertension may also be a factor because insulin can reduce PGI_2 production in several animal models. Low HDL_2 cholesterol, which was seen in pregnancy-induced hypertension, could also contribute to PGI_2 suppression because HDL deficiency reduces PGI_2 synthesis in in vitro experiments. Further support for the HDL and PGI_2 connection has been obtained from healthy nonpregnant premenopausal (8) and postmenopausal (9) women as well. The weak but statistically significant positive correlation observed between TxA_2 metabolite excretion and serum triglyceride levels, as well as possible metabolic links existing between thromboxane A_2 and lipoproteins, remain to be confirmed in other studies.

REFERENCES

1) Ferrannini E, Buzzigoli G, Bonadonna R, et al. Insulin resistance in essential hypertension. N Engl J Med 1987;317:350-7.

2) Suhonen L, Teramo K. Hypertension and preeclampsia in women with gestational glucose intolerance. Acta Obstet Gynecol Scand 1993;72:269-72.

3) Potter MF, Nestel PJ. The hyperlipidemia of pregnancy in normal and complicated pregnancies. Am J Obstet Gynecol 1979; 133:165-70.

4) Tulppala M, Viinikka L, Ylikorkala O. Thromboxane dominance and prostacyclin deficiency in habitual abortion. Lancet 1991; 337:879-81.

5) Vuorinen-Markkola H, Yki-Jarvinen H. Hyperuricemia and insulin resistance. J Clin Endocrinol Metab 1994; 78: 25-9.

6) Lorentzen B, Endresen MJ, Haug E, Henriksen T. Sera from preeclamptic women increase the content of triglycerides and reduce the release of prostacyclin in cultured endothelial cells. Thromb Res 1991;63:363-72.

7) Endresen MJ, Lorentzen B, HenriksenT. Increased lipolytic activity and high ratio of free fatty acids to albumin in sera from women with preeclampsia leads to triglyceride accumulation in cultured endothelial cells. Am J Obstet Gynecol 1992;167:440-7.

8) Ylikorkala O, Kuusi T, Tikkanen M, Viinikka L. Desogestrel- and levonorgestrel-containing oral contraceptives have different effects on urinary excretion of prostacyclin metabolites and serum high density lipoproteins. J Clin Endocrinol Metab 1987;65:1238-42.

9) Foidart JM, Dombrowics N, de Lignières B. Urinary excretion of prostacyclin and thromboxane metabolites in postmenopausal women treated with percutaneous estradiol (Oestrogel) or conjugated estrogens (Premarin). In: Dusitsin N, Notelovitz M, eds. Physiological hormone replacement therapy. London: Parthenon Publishing, 1990:99-107.

Hypoplastic left heart syndrome: implications of the prenatal diagnosis

P. Bogatti, G. Maso, S. Alberico, R. Pinzano and S. Guaschino

Obstetric and Gynecological Clinic, University of Trieste, Trieste, Italy

ABSTRACT

In this article we analyze the ethiopathogenesis of the hypoplastic left heart

syndrome (HLHS) reporting on our observation of five cases by means of fetal

echocardiography. We observed two cases of isolated HLHS with normal karyotype.

Chromosomal aberrations were present in two cases (40%) with other associated

anomalies in a picture typical of trisomy 13. A further case was affected by

diaphragmatic hernia with a lung malformation without chromosomal disorders.

We conclude that the risk of occurrence of HLHS may be related either to a

chromosomal disorder or extracardiac malformations if associated.

INTRODUCTION

The hypoplastic left heart syndrome (HLHS) is characterized by a series of

anomalies, including a diminutive left ventricle with hypoplasia or atresia of the

aortic valve, aortic arch and mitral valve. Varying degrees of severity are usually

seen, ranging from critical aortic stenosis with nearly normal left ventricular and mitral valve dimensions to aortic and mitral valve atresia and the absence or underdevelopment of the left ventricle [1,2] .

In its most severe form the aortic root can end blindly within the cardiac muscle, just below the coronary arteries , without the formation of the valve.

In cases of mitral valve atresia the left ventricular chamber can only be a slit-like pouch within the myocardium, depicting one form of univentricular heart with the atrio-ventricular connections absent.

The prenatal diagnosis of HLHS implies counseling the parents and managing the present and future pregnancies. In this work we present our experience in diagnosing and managing pregnancies with HLHS detected in utero.

MATERIALS AND METHODS

All the fetal echocardiograms performed at our institution between March 1992 and June 1993 were reviewed. These included 1220 routine examinations carried out on the normal obstetrical population as apart of the screening programs and 49 examinations performed on cases referred because of fetal malformations.

All these examinations werew performed on cases transabdominally using a multifrequency (3,5-5 MHz) sector probe (Acuson 128 XP 10) with pulsed and color Doppler facilities. All the cases that met the ultrasonic criteria for HLHS were selected.

The clinical and autopsy data were accurately recorded as well as the results of the chromosomal analysis that was carried out in each case. associated anomalies were also recorded.

The parents were immediately informed of the ultrasound findings and offered pregnancy continuation, with either neonatal cardiac transplantation or staged palliative surgery, or termination , when the gestational age was less than 25 weeks.

RESULTS

During the oeriod of observation we diagnosed HLHS in 5 cases. 3 of these were detected during rolutine screening for malformations with an incidence of 0,23% among the population not at risk. Two more cases were referred to us becauise of an abnormal four chambre view of the heart.

The diagnosis was made on the basis of the observation of a diminutive left ventricle and aortic root with possibly enlarged right chambers

The pathological and chromosomal characteristics of the affected cases are shown in Table 1.

Gestational age at the time of diagnosis ranged between 19 and 23 weeks. The absence of blood flow into the left ventricle with mitral valve atresia was evident in 1 case, wich was also characterized by extreme hypoplasia of thr left ventricle, atrium and aortic   root wich resembled an atrio-ventricular canal with right predominance.

The mitral valve was not considered grossly abnormal in the remaining 4 cases, in wich the aortic valve was stenotic (3 cases) or atretic (1 case).

Concomitant hypoplasia of the atrium was evident in only 3 cases. Chromosomal aberrations were present in 2 cases (40%) with associated anomalies in a picture suggestive of trisomy 13.

Table 1: Pathological findings and karyotype

Case		Anomalies	Karyotype
1	CV	Hypoplastic left ventricle	46XY
		Aortic valve stenosis	
2	CV	Hypoplastic left atrium	47XX + 13
		Hypoplastic left ventricle	
		Aortic valve stenosis	
		Aortic arch hypoplasia	
	CF	Hypotelorism	
	CNS	Partial agenesis of the cerebellar vermis	
3	CV	D I A	47XX + 13
		Hypoplastic left ventricle	
		Aortic valve stenosis	
	CF	Cleft lip	
		Cleft palate	
	CNS	Agenesis of the corpus callosum	
4	CV	D I A, D I V	46 XX
		Hypoplastic left atrium	
		Hypoplastic left ventricle	
		Aortic valve atresia	
		Enlarged pulmonary valve	
5	CV	Complete common A-V canal	46XY
		Aortic valve hypoplasia	
		Aortic arch hypoplasia	
	RESP	Abnormal lobation of lungs	
	GI	Diaphragmatic hernia	
	other	Two vassel cord	

*Abbreviations: CV=cardiovascular; CNS=central nervous system;

CF=craniofacial; RESP=respiratory.

A further case was affected by diaphragmatic hernia and lung malformations with normal karyotype.

All the families chose to terminate the pregnancy.

DISCUSSION

HLHS is a rare defect at birth, accounting for less than 1% of all cyanotic

congenital heart disease [4]. The birth prevalence of this cardiopathy is estimated to

be about 0,016% of live births [4,5], but it accounts for 15% of all neonatal

congenital heart defect deaths in the first month of life.

Since the introduction of echocardiography in clinical pravtice, in either screening

programs or referral cases, prenatal diagnosis of HLHS has continously improved [3]

and is now one of the most common prenatal diagnoses. In our population,

undergoing prenatal screening for malformations, its incidence data is caused by

the high rate of intrauterine demise of the fetuses affected [6] wich can often escape

accurate pathologicl examination and hence diagnosis.

As far as the ethiopathogenesis of this malformation is concerned, hypoplasia of the

fourth left arch and with it hypoplasia of the aortic portion of the truncus may be

present [7]. Alternatively some factors interfering with blood flow into the left cardiac

chambers may be involved.

We know, in fact, that a reduce blood flow trough the left side of the heart and

aorta can lead to inderdevelopment of the miocardium.

The pattern of genetic inheritance of HLHS is unclear. The possibility of a rare

mode of autosomal recessive inheritance was not excluded due to the occurence of

this defect in elder siblings of affected infants [8,9]. Nevertheless, a multifactorial

inheritance with a 2-4 % of reccurence risk [10] seems to be more common.

The association with chromosomal anomalies (40 % in our population) is described

in literature [2,4]. The real incidence may be understimated due to the phenotipic variability of some chromosomal anomaly rather than that of the cardiac

mlformation itself.

Congenital malformations are also associated with HLHS in 12-37% of the cases,

but the data in literature is biased by the lack of searches for all extracardiac

anomalies , as well as the accurate definition of single locus disorders, idiopatic

malformation complexes and teratogenic exposure.

Finally, a malformation sequence can be put forward in cases of compressed

ascending aorta by a primitive malformation [11] which increases the resistence to the

left sided blood flow and causes the cardiac defect.

This hypothesis may be supported by the observed increased frequency of HLHS in

the Turner Syndrome with a webbed nech which can lead to thoracic duct

distension and heart compression. This pathogenesis may be advocated for our case

affected by diaphragmatic hernia, which can eventually have a risk of occurrence

related only to that of the gastrointestinal malformation.

REFERENCES

1.   Blake, D.M., Copel, J.A. and Kleinman, C.S. (1991). Hypoplastic left heart
     syndrome: Prenatal diagnosis, clinical profile and management. Am. J.
     Obstet. Gynecol., **165**, 529-34.

2.   Natowicz, M., Chatten, J., Clancy, R. (1988). Genetic disorders and major
     extracardiac anomalies associated with the hypoplastic left heart syndrome.
     Pediatrics, **82** , 698-706.

3.   Allan, L.D., Cook, A., Sullivan, I., Sharland, G.K. (1991). Hypoplastic left heart syndrome: effects of fetal echocardiography on birth prevalence. <u>Lancet</u> **337,** 959-61.

4.   Morris, D. M., Outcalt, J., Menashe, V.D., (1990).Hypoplastic left heart syndrome: Natural history in a geographically defined population. <u>Pediatrics,</u> **85,**977-83.

5.   Copel, J.A., Cullen, M., Green, J.J., (1988). The frequency of aneuploidy in prenatally diagnosed congenital heart disease: an indication for fetal karyotyping. <u>Am. J. Obstet. Gynecol.,</u> **158,** 409-13.

6.   Crawford, D.C., Chita ,S.K., Allan, L.D. (1988). Prenatal detection of congenital heart disease: factors affecting obstetric management and survival. <u>Am. J. Obstet. Gynecol.,</u> **159,** 352-6.

7.   Lev, M., (1952). Pathologic Anatomy and   interrelationship of hypoplasia of the aortic tract complexes. <u>Lab. Invest.,</u> **1,** 61-70.

8.   Brownell, L.G., Shokeir, M.H.K., (1976). Inheritance of hypoplastic left heart syndrome (HLHS): furter observations. <u>Cit. Genet.,</u> **9,** 245-9.

9.   Boughman, J.A., Berg, K.A., Astemborski, J.A., (1987). Familiar risks of congenital heart defect assessed in a population-based epidemiologic study. <u>Am. J. Med: Genet.,</u> **26,** 839-49.

10.   Nora, J.J., Nora, A.H., (1978). <u>Genetics and Genetic Counseling in cardiovascular diseases</u> (Springfield, I.L., Chas. C. Thomas).

11.   Clark, E.B., (1984). Neck web and congenital heart defects: A pathogenic association in 45,X0 Turner Syndrome?. <u>Teratology,</u> **29,** 355-61.

Intrauterine growth retardation and antiphospholipid antibody syndrome

S. Reitano, V. Aidala, R. Platania, R. Cantarella and A. Carbonaro

Department of Gynecology and Obstetrics, University of Catania, Catania, Italy

INTRODUCTION

The antiphospholipid antibody syndrome (AAS) is commonly diagnosed by the presence of antiphospholipid antibodies (ACA, LAC) associated with fetal loss, artery or vein thrombosis and autoimmune thrombocytopenia. The combination of the antibodies with one or more clinical factors (fetal loss etc.) characterizes the entity of the syndrome. The LAC and ACA are IgG or IgM immunoglobulins that bind to membrane phopholipids. LAC, thus named as primarily observed in LES (lupus erythematosus) patients, in vitro causes a prolonged phospholipid-related coagulation time (such as activated PTT), and moreover causes syphilis false-positive serologic reaction due to phospholipids and interferes with thrombin activation. In recent years numerous Researchers have observed that cytotrophoblastic hyperplasia of the basal membrane, together with placental hemorrhage infarction, are common in pregnancies complicated by vascular disorders in the mother and in the IUGR[1-2].

Cytotrophoblastic hyperplasia, although reproduced in vitro with low oxygen pressure, which could demonstrate its ischemic genesis, could have an immunitary explanation. The same Researchers (Brunsens, Evans, Garite, Ott, Trudinberg) correlate obstructive arterio-necrosis to thrombosis and acute atheroma that can be present in local ischemia of the villi (IUGR and preeclampsia) with the presence of antiphospholipid antibodies in pregnant women.

The purpose of the present research was to verify benefits of early therapeutic treatment in women with AAS to avoid onset of IUGR.

MATERIALS and METHODS

From 1988 to 1991 we selected a sample of 21 women (9 primigravidas, 12 multigravidas, between 20 and 34 years old) (<u>Group A</u>) with a clinical or obstetric history of systemic lupus erythematosus (1), events of thrombosis or thromboembolism (in previous pregnancies or postpartum, or concurring with contraceptive estro-progestagen therapy after parturition) (4), transient ischemic attacks (2), thrombocytopenia (2), chronic hypertension (11) and other autoimmune diseases. The anatomo-pathological aspect of previous pregnancies presented extensive infarction, demonstrating abnormal utero-placental vascularization, represented by fibrinoid necrosis, acute atheroma and intraluminal thrombosis of arterial spirals of the basal plate.

Another sample of 34 pregnant women was recruited (control <u>Group B</u>), consisting of 18 primigravidas and 16 multigravidas, aged between 19 and 32; 21 with PROM (premature rupture of membranes) and 13 with preterm labour.

Positive antibody was diagnosed adopting the following selective criteria according to Harris[3]:

- positive lupus anticoagulant(LAC) or
- positive IgG ACA or
- positive IgM ACA and positive (LAC).

Diagnosis of positive lupus anticoagulant (LAC) can be made by:

- Kaolin clotting test
- activated partial thromboplastin time (aPTT)
- diluted aPTT
- Viper Russel Venom test (VPVT)

Diagnosis of positivity for anticardiolipin antibodies can be made using the ELISA method in the solid stage:

- ACA IgG titre > 15 GPL
- ACA IgM titre > 15 MPL

From 1991 to 1994 we administered:

- immunoglobulins I.V. (0.5 g per Kg. bodyweight) alone;
- low-dose aspirin (60-100 mg die) plus heparin (10,000 U/die);
- nifedipine (20-40 mg/die) or isradipine (5 mg/die) plus heparan-sulphate (100-200 mg/die) as alternative therapeutic protocols to group A on their new pregnancy.

In the period between the 14th and 35th week an ultrasound scan investigation was performed every 4 weeks with real-time scanner Au 920 or Au 450 with a convex transducer and ultrasound velocity of 1540 m/sec. We also measured the BPD, DFO, HC, HA, DTA, DAPA, AC, AA, HC/AC ratio, CTD, femor and homerus length. Centile range of single ultrasound parameters previously obtained in our Department were used as reference. Neonatal weight has been referred to centiles for the normal population.

RESULTS and CONCLUSIONS

Group A resulted in 26 pregnancies between 1991 and 1994. The relationship between neonatal weight and gestational age is reported in fig.1.

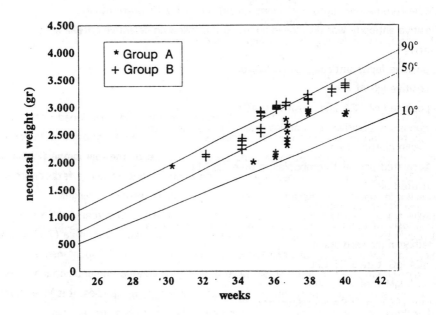

Figure 1 Relationship betwen neonatal weight and gestational age trough 10°, 50°, 90° percentile analysis.

The mean gestational age was 35 weeks (range 30-40)(three fetuses were delivered at the 40th week, 7 at the 38th, 10 at the 37th, 3 at the 36th, 2 at the 35th and 1 at the 30th). The mean gestational age in group B was 36.1 weeks (range 35.1-37.2).

The mean weight of surviving newborns was 2455± 468g for group A and 2850±587g for group B.

Fetal weight at birth was significantly lower in patients with anticardiolipin antibodies.

J.Henk underlines that fetal weight at birth is significantly lower in patients with an obstetric history of fetal death (2765 g after one fetal death, 2610 g after two or more, 1870 g after treatment with high prednisone doses, for a mean gestational age of 36.9 weeks in the sample).

The mean weight in patients treated with:

1) only high-dose immunoglobulins;

2) low-dose aspirin plus heparin;

3) nifedipine or Isradipine plus heparan-sulphate

was   1) = 2525 ± 0.69

2) = 2571 ± 189

3) = 2605 ± 315

Case n.7, a neonate weighing 1050 g, born to a mother that developed gestational diabetes during the second trimester, with subsequent modest gestational hypertension from the 28th week and preterm rupture of the membrane (PROM) in the 30th week (operative delivery: Cesarean Sections due to acute fetal distress), was not included in our data to avoid distortion of mean results on weight.

Delivery was spontaneous in 18 cases, operative in 8 (4 Cesarean Sections and 4 Vacuum Extractor) in group A. In group B 11 deliveries were operative (7 Cesarean Sections, 3 V.E. applications and 1 V.E. plus manuduction) and 23 spontaneous.

In accord with Romanini[4] et al. we believe that intravenous immunoglobulins (IVIG) efficacy is probably due to the presence of antiidiotype antibodies. It is well known that these antibodies manipulate the immune system in at least three ways.

First, they can neutralize an autoantibody by forming an idiotype-antiidiotype dimer; secondly, antiidiotypic antibodies may bind and down regulate the B-cell receptor for antigen decreasing autoantibody production; third regulatory T-cells may recognize antiidiotypic antibody or a complex of antiidiotypic antibodies and a critical concentration of idiotype-antiidiotype dimers may be required to activate binding and subsequent suppression by lymphokines from these regulatory T cells.

Our decision to use calcium antagonists (isradipine or nifedipine) derived from encouraging results in previous research on repeated abortion presented at the VI th FRESERH in Brussels[5].

This previous initial idea, jointing a beta stimulant to a calcium antagonist according to Fleckenstein's hypothesis, afterwords was modificated associating tho the calcium antagonist drug heparan-sulphate (mucopolysaccharidic copolymeric, structure characterized by repetitive units containing glycuronic acid and N-acetylate and N-sulphatase glucosamina).

The results of this association which is new to present literature, and results of the traditional association of heparin and low-dose acetylsalycidic acid seem to provide real hope.

REFERENCES

1- Polzin W.J., Kopelman J.N., Robinson R.D., Read J.A., Brady K. (1991). The association of antiphospholipid antibodies with pregnancies complicated by fetal growth restriction. Obstet. Gynecol 78: 1108-11

2- Out H.J., Bruinsen H.W., Cristiaens G., Van Vilet M., De Groot P., Nieuwenhuis H.K., Derksen R. (1992). A prospective, controlled multicenter study on the obstetric risks of pregnant women with antiphospholipid antibodies. AM. J. Obstet. Gyencol; 167:26-32

3- Harris N.F. (1990). Antiphospholipid antibodies. Br. J. Haematol. 74, 1-9

4- Valensise H., Vaquero E., De Carolis C., Miriello D., Arduini D., Romanini C. (1993). Fetal growth and intravenous gammaglobulin (IVIG) treatment in antiphospholipid syndrome: a preliminary report. Proceedings of 2nd World congress of perinatal medicine. Rome and Florence, Vol. 1, 393-396

5- Boemi P., Reitano S. (1982). Therapeutic aspects of calcium-antagonists in obstetrics in "Uterine contractility" VI th FRESERH, International Symposium. Brussels. MASSON pub. U.S.A., inc. 465-474.

Antiphospholipid antibodies and pre-eclamptic disorders

S. Reitano, V. Aidala, R. Cantarella and A. Carbonaro

Department of Gynecology and Obstetrics, University of Catania, Catania, Italy

INTRODUCTION

The risk of gestational loss in women presenting autoimmune antiphopholipid antibodies[1-2] capable of cross-reacting with certain trophoblast antigens is linked to the production of auto-antibodies of the LAC or ACA type. These could interfere with the conversion process of the arachidonic acid into prostaglandins and thromboxans, through enzymatic or metabolic blockage of prostanoids leading to a reduction in prostacyclin and a relative or absolute increase in thromboxans (that would explain generalized vasospasm and finally the reduction in blood intake in the placental intervillous spaces). Moreover, the fundamental characteristic on which preeclamptic predisposition is based is said to be placental hypoperfusion caused by an abnormal placentation, immunologic interaction, by a microcirculatory system pathology or by too large a placenta. It is hence evident that the hypoperfused feto-placental unit is the true cause of vasoactive agent production capable of influencing the vascular endothelium, both in AAS and in preeclampsia.

The purpose of the present research is to establish any correlation between the antiphospholipid antibody syndrome (AAS) and hypertensive disorders of a preeclamptic nature.

MATERIALS and METHODS

In accord with Rote, Branch[3], Brown and Harris diagnosis of positive antibody can be made through the following selective criteria:

- positive lupus anticoagulant (LAC) or

- positive IgG ACA or

- positive IgM ACA and positive (LAC).

Diagnosis of positive lupus anticoagulant (LAC) can be made by performing:

- Kaolin clotting test

- activated partial thromboplastin time (aPTT)

- diluted aPTT

- Viper Russel Venom test (VPVT).

Diagnosis of positive anticardiolipin antibody can be performed using the ELISA method in the solid phase:

- ACA IgG titre > 15 GPL

- ACA IgM titre > 15 MPL

From 1988 to 1991 we selected 21 women with a clinical and/or obstetric history of systemic lupus erythematosus (1), thrombosis or thromboembolism (in previous pregnancy or postpartum, or concurring to contraceptive estroprogestagen therapy after parturition) (4), transient ischemic attacks (2), thrombocytopenia (2), chronic hypertensive disorders (11), other autoimmune disorders (1).

The sample was LAC positive in 94% of cases, positive to IgG ACA > 20 GPL U/ml in 86% of cases, LAC and ACA positive in 100% of cases and false-positive serology in 61% of cases.

As concerns the anatamo-pathological aspect the placenta presented signs of extensive infarction involving over 10% of placental substantia. This extensive infarction demonstrated abnormal utero-placental vascularization as the cause, manifesting itself in fibrinoid necrosis, acute atheroma and intraluminal thrombosis of the arterial spirals of the basal plate.

Under microscopic examination the villi appear massed together with obliteration of placental blood spaces.

A section of the basal plate reveals some spiral arteries with modifications normal to the gravid condition, whereas most of the decidual vasa did not manifest these physiological events.

Vasculopathy of the efferent utero-placental artery was associated to this picture.

From 1991 to 1994, on new gravidic events, the sample was administered:

- immunoglobulins I.V.(0.5 g per Kg bodyweight);

- aspirin low-dose (60-100 mg/die);

- heparin (10,000 U/die);

- heparan-sulphate (100-200 mg/die), alone or in association plus:

- nifedipine(20-40 mg/die);

- isradipine (5 mg/die).

RESULTS

Between 1991-1994 there were 26 pregnancies in the sample of women selected: nineteen women were pregnant once, two were pregnant twice and one three times. The gestational outcome was: 78% (20) live birth, 18% (5) spontaneous abortions, 4% (1) neonatal death. The mean gestational age and the mean weight of live newborns at birth is showen in tab.1.

Table 1 Mean gestational age (MGA) and mean weight of newborns (MWN)

MGA   was 35 weeks (range 30-40 weeks)
- 3 fetuses were born in the 40th wk.;
- 7 "   "   "   " " 38th " ;
- 10 "   "   "   " " 37th " ;
- 3 "   "   "   " " 36th " ;
- 2 "   "   "   " " 35th " ;
- 1 "   "   "   " " 30th " .
MWN at birth was 2567±711 g.

Only one case of neonatal death arose (4%). This outcome was attributed to pulmonary complications (a hiatus hernia was also diagnosed).

The neonatal survival percentage corresponding to therapeutic treatment with I.V. high-dose immunoglobulins alone, associations of heparin plus low-dose aspirin, nifedipine or isradipine plus heparan-sulphate, was 96%.

In accord with D.W. Branch we calculated the therapeutic efficacy comparing outcome in untreated first pregnancies to the first treated pregnancy. The newborn survival rate was 28 and 96% respectively (P< 0.001).

The correlation between the different treatments and clinical history (LES, false-positive syphilis test, IgG anticardiolipin levels etc.) was not significant (P>0.05).

However, we are convinced that the three therapeutic protocols were highly effective (we are unable to rank them as the sample was too small).

As regards complications, one patient developed gestational diabetes during the second trimester with subsequent modest gestational hypertension from the 28th week, and premature rupture of the membranes (PROM) in the 30th week: delivery was operative (Cesarean Section) due to fetal distress and neonate weight was 1050 g. The newborn later died due to pulmonary complications linked to prematurity.

Acute fetal distress was observed in 2 cases, chronic distress in 4 and PROM in six gravidae.

Only one case of amaurosis fugax was observed. Delivery was spontaneous in 18 cases and operative in 8 (4 Cesarean Sections, 4 Vacuum Extractor).

CONCLUSIONS

Branch[4] observed that the risk of subsequent gestational loss in women with antiphospholipid antibodies was unknown but probably over 60%.

Even if fetal death would seem to be the worst event specifically related to SAA we observed only one case, reported above, which was in any case complicated by gestational diabetes.

The lack of control group could be interpreted as an incorrect methodological approach. However, we believe that a more deontological conduct would be to compare untreated with treated pregnancies in the same patient, rather than adopt a sample of untreated AAS women as a reference.

As regards therapy, success was not related to the specific type of therapy.

Contrary to other Authors we did not consider administration of prednisone necessary, due to the risk of bone decalcification with a predisposition to fractures and malformation.

Our data contrast to Branch's who, due to preeclampsia or fetal distress, only obtained 37% successful pregnancies at or before the 32nd week.

The causal link interacting between the antiphospholipid antibody system on the one hand, and preeclampsia on the other, demonstrates that the feto-placental unit is the target of a series of events aimed at unbalancing vascular tone and circulating mass, underlining the incapacity of the vascular tree to adapt to blood mass increase determined by the pregnancy[5-6]. Endothelial dysfunction, in turn, causes an increase in vascular sensitivity to vasopressor agents in circulation, with serious vasospasms and multiorganic hypoperfusion. The decreased anticoagulant function of the endothelium and the increased procoagulant activity bring about a knock-on effect in coagulation.

In consideration of the above, we conclude that very early medical treatment at the beginning of pregnancy to combat unbalancing, in any of the above forms, can constitute the key to long-term fetal outcome.

REFERENCES

1- Harris N.F. (1990). Antiphospholipid antibodies. Br. J. Haematol. 74; 1-9

2- Brown H.L. (1991). Antiphospholipid antibodies and recurrent pregnancy loss Clin. Obstet. Gynecol 34; 1: 17-26

3- Branch D. W., Andres R., Digre B.K., Rote S.N., Scott R.J. (1989). The association of antiphospholipid antibodies with severe preeclampsia. Obstet. Gynecol; 73: 541-545

4- Branch D.W., Silver R.M., Blackwell J.L., Reading J.C., Scott J.R. (1992). Outcome of treated pregnancies in women with antiphospholipid syndrome: an update of the Utah experience. Obstet. Gynecol; 80: 614-20

5- Walsh S.W. (1985). Preclampsia. An imbalance in placental prostacyclin and tromboxane production. Am. J. Obstet. Gynecol; 152: 335-40

6- Branch D.W., Andres R., Digre K.B., Rote N.S., Scott J.R. (1990). The association of antiphospholipid antibodies with severe preeclampsia. Obstet. Gynecol; 73: 541-5.

Activin A, parturition and preterm labor

F. Petraglia, P. Florio*, A. Gallinelli, D. De Vita, P. Scida*, M. Simonelli*, C. Salvestroni*, M. Lombardo* and A.R. Genazzani*

Departments of Obstetrics and Gynecology, University of Modena, Modena and *University of Pisa, Pisa, Italy*

A growing number of studies provided strong evidences that human placenta may play a role in the physiology of pregnancy. As endocrine organ it is source of several steroid or peptide hormones, as well as target of this hormonal productions throughout paracrine autocrine mechanisms. To date, human placenta produces brain, pituitary, gonadal, and adrenocortical hormones chemically identical and as biologically active as their counterparts. In particular, hypophyseotropic releasing or inhibiting factors have been found in human placenta, and some aspects of the control of hormonal secretion can be compared to the organization like hypothalamus-pituitary-target organ axes (1). In addition, interactions among the intrauterine tissues (placenta, amnion-chorion leave and maternal decidua) occurs, playing a role during pregnancy from implantation to the timing of parturition.

Among the hormones produced by intrauterine tissues, activin A (ßA/ßA) is a dimeric protein synthesized by human trophoblast, decidua and fetal membranes which stimulates the release of hCG and progesterone from cultured placental cells, and of prostaglandin from amnion cells (2-4). Among the three forms of activin (activin A, B, AB) since now recognized, activin A is only one measurable in maternal circulation, while activin B is undetectable and no specific assay for activin AB have been developed. In healthy pregnant women maternal serum and amniotic fluid activin A levels increase with advancing gestational age, reaching the highest concentrations at term (5). Activin A levels decrease after delivery suggesting a placental or fetal origin of the circulating maternal activin A. Maternal decidua is also a possible source of maternal activin A, as supported by the expression of βA subunit mRNA.

The measurement of activin A levels at delivery revealed that the highest concentration of activin A is found in women after spontaneous labor; between the early stage of labor and vaginal delivery a further release of activin A occurs in maternal circulation. The lack of changes of activin A concentrations in women undergoing to elective cesarean section suggests a possible partecipation of activin A to the stress-related events of parturition (6). The labor-dependent difference has been also shown in amniotic fluid activin A concentration. In fact, women delivering at term after spontaneous labor have higher amniotic concentrations than women out of labor.

Maternal serum activin A levels in patients with preterm labor (gestational age between 26 and 35 weeks) have been compared to those of healthy pregnant women at term not in labor (gestational age 38-40 weeks). The evidence that activin A concentration in women with preterm labor is higher than in pregnant women at term not in labor (Figure 1), indicates that parturition is associated with an increase in maternal serum activin A, regardless of gestational age. This is further supported by the evidence of the highest maternal serum activin A concentration found in pregnant women with preterm labor who later delivered <48 hours. An increased activin A release in preterm labor is also observed in fetal compartement. In fact, in contrast to the healthy control patients, activin A was measurable in cord blood of patients with preterm labor, suggesting an increased release of the protein in this compartment. However, the concentration did not correlate with the time of delivery. A possible role for activin A in modulating the hormonal response to the stress of labor is supported by the evidence that oxytocin or ACTH secretion is augmented in rats following activin administration.

Fetal membranes (amnion, chorion) play a role in the mechanisms of human parturition. Their embryological origin is from mesoderm and represent the anatomical interface between the uterus and the fetus. In the last decade, several studies demonstrated that fetal membranes produce a large number of hormones and regulatory substances, also expressing receptors for various factos. In amniotic fluid changes of activin A at labor have also been studied. In fact, delivery show high values of activin A concentration in amniotic fluid. Amnion cells are known to express ßA subunit mRNA, supporting that the high levels of activin A in women at term may be due to an increased synthesis of activin A. In fact, the fetus may secrete activin A into the amniotic compartment, from fetal urine or lung secretions, and expression of activin A ßA subunit mRNA has been described in fetal gonads and adrenals (5). However, a fetal or placental contribution to activin A in amniotic fluid cannot be excluded.

Recently, two types of activin receptors have been cloned, type II and type IIB receptors, 70 kDa molecular weight membrane proteins (7, 8), the first transmembrane serine/threonine kinase receptors (9). Human placenta and fetal-maternal intrauterine membranes express activin receptors (10). In particular, the evidence that in syncytiotrophoblasts the expression of ActRIIB is higher than that of

ActRII suggests that this type of receptors is mainly involved in the regulation of hCG and progesterone release (2, 11). The presence of mRNA for activin receptors in amnion, chorion and maternal decidua has been shown (10), thus suggesting that activin A may stimulate the release of prostaglandins acting on its amnion-chorion receptors.

These findings support the possible role of amniotic activin A in the events of the labor. In fact, activin A, trasforming growth factor α, and epidermal growth factor, increase PG release from amniotic cells in culture, indicating that growth factors may be included among the factors patrecipating to the biochemical events of human parturition, thus suggesting a local paracrine/autocrine role. The factors that stimulate activin A synthesis and/or secretion in preterm labor and gestational diabetes (12) are not known. Increased placental synthesis and/or release of activin A or a decreased rate of the protein in these pathophysiological conditions are possible. Supporting this hypothesis, several reports indicate a hypersecretion of placental hormones in women with preterm labor (13-15) or gestational diabetes (16-17). Studies performed on cultured placental cells have not shown no changes in activin A secretion after incubation with relaxin or forskolin (18).

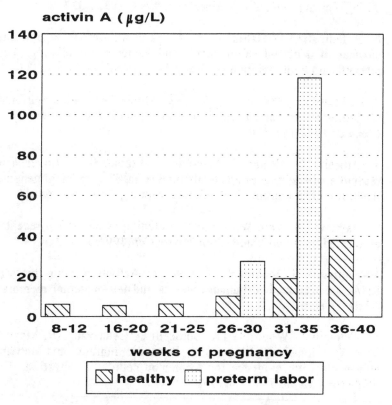

Figure 1. Mean levels of circulating maternal activin A.

References

1- F. Petraglia, A.Volpe, A.R.Genazzani et al. Neuroendocrinology of the Human Placenta. *Front Neuroendo.* 1990; 11 (1): 6-37

2- F. Petraglia, J. Vaughan, W. Vale: Inhibin and activin modulate the release of Gn-RH, hCG and progestrone from cultured human placental cells. *Proc Natl Acad Sci USA* 1989; 86: 5114-7

3- F. Petraglia, L. Calza', G.C. Garuti, et al.: Presence of syntesis of inhibin subunits in human decidua. *J Clin Endocrinol Metab.* 1990; 71: 487-492

4- F. Petraglia, M.M. Anceschi, L. Calza', et al.: Inhibin and activin in human fetal membranes: evidence for a local effect on prostaglandin release. *J Clin Endocrinol Metab.* 77: 542-548

5- F. Petraglia, S. Garg, P. Florio et al. Activin A and Activin B measured in maternal serum, cord blood serum and amniotic fluid during human pregnancy. *Endocrine J.* 1993, 1: 323-327

6- F. Petraglia, A. Gallinelli, K. Lewis et al. Activin at parturition: changes of maternal serum levels and evidence for binding sites in placenta and fetal membranes. *Obstetric Gynecol. 1994, 84: 278-282.*

7- Donaldson C, Mathews L, Vale W. Molecular cloning and binding properties of the human type II activin receptor. *Biochem Biophys Res Commun 1992;184:310.*

8- Attisano L, Wrana J, Cheifetz S, Massague J. Novel activin receptors: distinct genes and alternative mRNA splicing generate a repertoire of serine/threonine kinase receptors. *Cell 1992; 68:97*

9- Mathews LS, Vale W. Expression cloning of an activin receptor, a predicated transmembrane serine kinase *Cell 1991;65:973*

10- Petraglia F, Mathews LS, Vale W. Activin receptor messenger RNAs are localized in human placenta and feto-maternal membranes. *Obstet Gynecol*

11- Petraglia F, Woodruff TK, Botticelli G, Genazzani AR, Mayo KE, Vale W. Gonadotropin-releasing hormone, inhibin, and activin in human placenta: evidence for a common cellular localization. *J Clin Endocrinol Metab 1992;74:1184.*

12- F. Petraglia, D. De Vita, A. Gallinelli, et al.: Abnormal concentration of maternal serum activin-A in gestational diseases. *J Clin Endocrinol Metab. 1995, 80: 558-561.*

13- M. McLean, W.A.W. Walters, R. Smith. Prediction and early diagnosis of preterm labor: a critical review. *Obstet. Gynecol. Surv. 1993, 48:209-225.*

14- R. Romero, M. Mazor. Infection and preterm labor. *Clin. Obstet. Gynecol. 1988, 31: 554-584.*

15- L.K. Petersen, K. Skajaa, N. Uldbjerg. Serum relaxin as a potential marker for preterm labour. *Br. J Obstet. Gynecol. 1992, 99: 292-295.*

16- J. Larinkari, L. Laatikainen, T. Ranta, P. Moronen, K. Pesonen, T. Laatikainen. Metabolic control and serum hormone levels in relation to retinopathy in diabetic pregnancy. *Diabetologia. 1982, 22:327-332.*

17- H.A. Selenkow, K. Varma, D. Younger, P. White, K. Emerson. Patterns of serum immunoreactive human placental lactogen (IR-HPL) and chorionic gonadotropin (IR-HCG) in diabetic pregnancy. *Diabetes. 20:696-706.*

18- J. Rabinovici, P.C. Goldsmith, C.L. Librach, R.B. Jaffe. Localization and regulation of the activin-A dimer in human placental cells. J. Clin. Endocrinol. Metab. 1992, 75:571-576.

Neurotransmitters in the myometrium

N.-O. Sjöberg and M. Stjernquist

Department of Obstetrics and Gynecology, Malmö University Hospital, Malmö, Sweden

For more than a century it has been known that the uterus receives an extensive nerve supply. During the last decade of the 19th century Langley and Anderson described the autonomic innervation of the uterus. They found the sympathetic nerves to originate in the 3rd-5th lumbar segments of the spinal cord, and then enter the 4th-6th lumbar ganglia of the sympathetic chain to continue, via the inferior mesenteric ganglia, in the two hypogastric nerves. The parasympathetic or pelvic nerves have their origin in the first 3 to 4 sacral roots and, after forming the two pelvic nerves, meet the sympathetic nerves in the paracervical tissue, giving the impression of a ganglion formation, which has been given the name of Frankenhäuser's plexus or ganglion. The active ganglia are found very close to the utero-vaginal junction, and are also located within the vaginal wall. These peripheral ganglia are a relay not only for the parasympathetic nerves but also for a considerable proportion of the sympathetic nerves, as shown in denervation experiments. These findings conflict with the classic concept of the organization of the autonomic nervous system, in which the sympathetic post-ganglionic nerve fibres are supposed to derive from cell bodies located at a considerable distance from the effector organ. The post-ganglionic nerve fibres originating in cell bodies at the utero-vaginal junction have been termed 'short adrenergic neurons' and seem to be a feature unique to the genital organs.

The adrenergic nerves of the uterus are uniquely sensitive to the action of ovarian sex steroids. Through these effects and additional mechanical effects exerted by the growing conceptus, the uterus undergoes a complete — and entirely physiological — adrenergic denervation in the course of pregnancy, with a slow and incomplete restitution post-partum. This reflects a particularly high degree of plasticity in the myometrial autonomic

595

nerve plexus. The changes may be functionally associated with the maintenance of pregnancy, initiation of labour, and expulsion of the fetus during parturition.

The division of the autonomic nervous system into two parts, the sympathetic (adrenergic) and parasympathetic (cholinergic), is incomplete from a functional and morphological point of view. Thus, the presence of so-called 'non-adrenergic, non-cholinergic' (NANC) neuronal mechanisms has been demonstrated in miscellaneous organ preparations. The development of immunocytochemical techniques has made it possible to demonstrate several peptides in nervous tissue. These have been termed 'neuropeptides', and 'peptidergic' nerves have been encountered in various organs including the uterus. Both *in vivo* and *in vitro* several of these neruopeptides exert biological effects and thus seem to possess regulatory properties.

The major motor innervation of the uterine cervix appears to be cholinergic in nature, to be subject to axo-axonal cross-talk from adjacent adrenergic fibres, and to be modulated by both VIP and NPY. Substance P is present in primary sensory nerves, extending branches into vascular as well as non-vascular smooth musculature of the uterus, and distributing among the neurons forming the peripheral autonomic ganglia. In this way, both smooth muscle contractility and ganglionic transmission may be modulated by the nociceptive transmitter, substance P. Numerous other peptides have been identified in the uterine nerves: enkephalins, CGRP, PHI, GRP, and galanin. These peptides exert both direct and indirect effects on the smooth musculature in different parts of the reproductive tract.

Hence, when discussing the innervation of the myometrium we have to consider not only the adrenergic and cholinergic, but also the peptidergic nerves. In view of the specialized neurobiological and functional properties of the autonomic innervation of the female reproductive tract, and on the basis of the peculiar sensitivity of these adrenergic, cholinergic, and peptidergic nerves to the effect of humoral interactions, it would seem reasonable to view this part of the autonomic nervous system as a peripheral neuro-endocrine mechanism, regulating smooth muscle functions in the myometrium.

REFERENCES

1. Langley, J. N. and Anderson, H. K. (1985). The innervation of the pelvic and adjoining viscera. Part 4. The international generative organs. *J. Physiol. (London)*, **19,** 122-30

2. Sjöberg, N-O. (1967). The adrenergic transmitter of the female reproductive tract: distribution and functional changes. *Acta Physiol. Scand.,* **65,** Suppl 257, 1-82

3. Alm, P., Owman, Ch., Sjöberg, N-O., Stjernquist , M. and Sundler, F. (1986). Histochemical demonstration of a concomitant reduction in neuronal vasoactive intestinal polypeptide (VIP), acetylcholinesterase and noradrenaline of cat uterus during pregnancy. *Neuroscience,* **18,** 713-26

4. Owman, Ch., Stjernquist, M., Helm, G., Kannisto, P., Sjöberg, N-O. and Sundler, F. (1986). Comparative histochemical distribution of nerve fibers storing noradrenaline and neuropeptide Y (NPY) in human ovary, Fallopian tube, and uterus. *Med. Biol.,* **64,** 57-65

5. Ottesen, B., Söndergaard, F. and Fahrenkrug, J. (1983). Neuropeptides in the regulation of female genital smooth muscle contractility. *Acta Obstet. Gynecol. Scand.,* **62,** 591-2

6. Stjernquist, M. and Sjöberg, N-O. (1994). Neurotransmitter in the myometrium. In Chard, T. and Grunzinskas, J.C. (eds.) *The Utero*, pp. 193-229. (Cambridge series in human reproduction)

Biological changes preceding onset of labor

A. Skret

Department of Obstetrics and Gynecology, Rzeszów, Poland

INTRODUCTION

The active labor is preceded by interval of uterine preparedness for labor when functional changes which are required for labor are implemented.

In this phase, the cascade of biomolecular and physiological processes takes place, which brings the gestational uterine contractive unresponsiveness suspended. Although original signal triggering this cascade is unknown, many biochemical factors involved are identified/2/.

Parturation is, to some extend, analogoues but reversal to early gestational development process. In the latter, the hormonal and biomolecular changes accompanied by some biophysical alterations, including those induced by vasodilatation, are videly reported.

In contrary, parturation until now has been studied only in hormonal and biomolecular aspects. The aim of this study is to assess prelabor daily changes in some biophysical parameters i.e.: Doppler flows in umbilical artery and in fetal vessels and amniotic fluid volume(AFV).

PATIENTS AND METHODS

Total of 380 patients in advanced high risk pregnancies were prospectively taken into a scope. All of them were under biophysical monitoring including Doppler measurements: umbilical artery(UA) flow, middle cerebral artery(MCA), descending aorta(DA) flow and sonographic assessment of amniotic fluid index(AFI). Only 200 patients who entered the spontaneus labor and had no evidence of fetal and neonatal morbidity /including intrauterine growth retardation(IUGR), prematurity and postmaturity/, were retrospectively enrolled in further study.

Flowmetric measurements were performed with Aloca SSD 280, Hitachi EUB 565 and Dornier AI 5200.

In the study group Doppler waveform measurements were performed in UA - 787 measurements, MCA - 235 measurements and DA - 243 measurements. AFI was assessed 462 times. In each of 200 patients, placenta was evaluated according to Granumm scale.

Similarly as in our previous studies we compared longitudinal values of systolic/diastolic(S/D) ratio and AFI to their values on the third or fourth day before labor respectively, using Wilcoxon signed-rank test. Correlation between examined parameters and days before labor were assessed with correlation coefficient.

RESULTS

When we related flowmetric values to prelabor scale we found that in last 8 days before spontaneous labor the S/D ratio decreased, reaching its minimal value on the third day. This

Days to spontaneous labor

	8	7	6	5	4	3	2	1	0
AFI (cm)	12.3 (8.6-19.0)	12.5 (8.0-17.9)	13.0 (6.6-18.0)	13.3 (6.7-17.5)	* 13.9 (8.0-20.0)	12.6 (5.9-22.6)	11.7 (5.7-19.4)	11.1 (6.0-19.0)	↓ 10.2 (5.2-18.2)
S/D ratio in UA	↑ 2.32 (1.60-3.00)	↑ 2.25 (1.51-3.35)	↑ 2.27 (1.57-3.44)	↑ 2.17 (1.68-3.44)	↑ 2.19 (1.49-2.83)	* 2.08 (1.51-2.79)	2.15 (1.57-2.87)	↑ 2.25 (1.45-2.89)	↑ 2.34 (1.61-3.54)
S/D ratio in MCA	2.68 (1.92-4.25)	2.54 (2.01-4.43)	2.45 (1.86-4.60)	2.71 (1.89-3.08)	2.79 (1.85-4.58)	2.45 (1.89-3.77)	2.93 (1.52-4.70)	3.06 (2.14-4.89)	2.36 (1.82-3.75)
S/D ratio in DA	4.76 (3.98-5.65)	4.72 (2.95-5.40)	4.69 (3.72-5.47)	4.24 (2.48-5.80)	3.98 (3.11-5.27)	4.03 (2.57-4.97)	4.79 (2.73-5.81)	4.40 (2.39-5.63)	3.44 (2.07-4.57)

↑/↓ - significantly higher or lower than on the day signed by asterisk * (Wilcoxon signed-rank test, $p < 0.005$)

Table 1.
Prelabor daily values /medians and ranges/ of AFI and S/D ratio in umbilical artery/UA/, middle cerebral artery/MCA/ and descending aorta/DA/ in 200 women with uneventful pregnancies and spontaneous onset of labor.

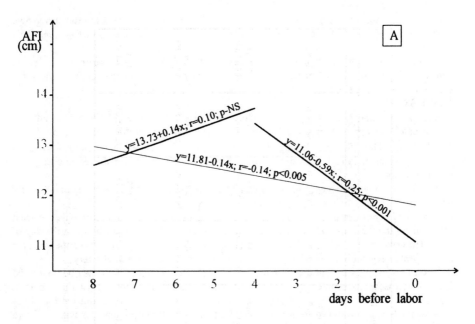

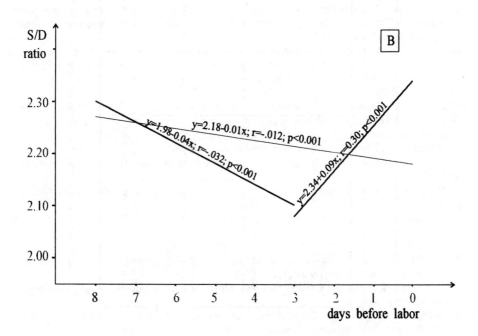

Figure 1.
Correlation between AFI /A/ and S/D ratio in umbilical artery /B/ and time to spontaneous labor in group of 200 women.

decrease was statistically significant (r=-0.32; p<0.001). Since then, the S/D ratio has grown up to the day of labor. That phenomenon appeared both in pregnancies with G-II and G-III placenta.

We could not find similar changes in fetal vessels(MCA, DA). Their values remained stable before labor. When we analyzed prelabor changes in AFI we found its significant decrease since the fourth day before labor (r=-0.25; p<0.001).

DISCUSSION

The studies of biophysical changes preceding onset of labor are few and have been conducted in post-date/1/ and premature rupture of membranes(PROM) complicated pregnancies/ 3/.

The lack of wider literature dealing with that problem may be explained by authoritative statement, presented in early flowmetric study /4/, that Doppler indices remained unchanged in prelabor period.

In contrary to above statement, we previously found characteristic changes in umbilical artery flow in group of uncomplicated pregnancies/5/.

Present study confirmed the gestational decrease of S/D ratio in umbilical artery which reached the nadir on the third day before labor, and since that day it started to grow up to the day of labor. However, in this study we found additionally that this pattern of S/D ratio appeared only in umbilical artery but not in fetal vessels (descending aorta, middle cerebral artery).

Previously we suggested that the changes in umbilical artery Doppler flow may be connected with an increased cotyledon component of total umbilical artery resistance. Trying to explain it we assessed simultaneusly AFI and placenta according to Granumm' scale and we found the same characteristic prelabor pattern of umbilical artery S/D ratio in pregnancies with G-II and G-III sonographic type of placenta. Thus, the increase in S/D ratio in umbilical artery does not seem to be related to cotyledon component.

The prelabor changes in umbilical artery S/D ratio were accompanied by a decrease of AFI starting on the 4th day before onset of labor. This finding may support the hypothesis that diminished AFV may evoke partial cord compression and this way increase venous component of total umbilical artery resistance.

Another explanation of those prelabor UA flow changes is presence of some vasoactive substances in amniotic fluid (for example endothelin) which may effect contractility of umbilical vessels and this way change their resistance.

CONCLUSIONS

Our results indicate that labor is preceded by some changes in umbilical but not in fetal vessels flow. Prelabor changes in umbilical artery flow seem to be connected with elevated tone of umbilical vessels but not with increased cotyledons component of resistance.

Alterations in umbilical vasculature tone may result from prelabor decrease of amniotic fluid volume. The tone of umbilical vessels may be also affected by vasoactive agents present in amniotic fluid.

Further studies on biophysical prelabor events may help to elucidate the mechanism of parturation.

REFERENCES

1.Battaglia C.,Larocca E.,Lanzani A.,Coukos G.,Genazzani A.R.(1991)*Doppler velocimetry in prolonged pregnancy*. Obstet.Gynecol.,77,213-215.

2.Cunningham F.G. et all. (1993). *Williams Obstetrics*. 19th Edition. Appleton&Lange, Norwalk,Connecticut.

3.Fleming A.D.,Salafia C.M.,Vintzileos A.M.,Rodis J.F.,Campbell W.A., Bantham K.F.(1991)*The relationship among umbilical artery velocimetry, fetal biophysical profile, and placental inflammation in preterm premature rupture of membranes*. Am.J.Obstet.Gynecol.,164,38-41.

4. Skręt A.,Klimek R.,Cebulak K.,Dorski A.,Janeczko J.,Klimek M.,Palczak R., Lassota L. (1993)*Flowmetric biological scale in advanced pregnancy.* Int.J.Prenatal and Perinatal Psychology and Medicine,Vol.5,Nr 2,135-141.
5. Trudinger B.J.,Giles W.B.,Cook C.M.,Bombardieri J.,Collins L.(1985) *Fetal umbilical artery flow velocity waveforms and placental resistance:clinical significance.* Br.J.Obstet. Gynaecol.,1985,92,23-30.

Endogenous oxytocin at term and preterm parturition: the intrauterine pattern

A. Mauri, C. Ticconi* and E. Piccione*

"B.B. Brodie" Department of Neuroscience of the University Of Cagliari and *Department of Surgery, Division of Gynecological Endocrinology of "Tor Vergata" University of Rome, Italy

INTRODUCTION

The mechanism leading to the onset and maintenance of spontaneous labor in the human is still unknown. However, the neurohypophyseal hormone oxytocin (OT) seems to have a pivotal role in this phenomenon. Indeed, OT is the most powerful uterotonic agent known so far (1) and its specific receptors are present in the myometrium at highest level during early labor (2). Moreover, the administration of the hormone in the sensitized uterus generates an uterine activity identical to that occurring in the spontaneous labor. Nevertheless, both the onset and the maintenance of the parturitional process may not depend on changes in maternal OT, due to the little or no evidence of increased plasma hormone immediately before or during labor and to the paucity of investigations reporting fluctuations of its levels throughout the phenomenon. Recently, both OT mRNA and immunoreactive (I.R.) OT have been detected in animal and human amniochorion and decidua at term gestation (3-5). These findings suggest that OT may be not only synthesized but also released by these tissues to act on the pregnant uterus as a local mediator. Aimed at ascertaining whether differences in the peptide concentrations are demonstrable in gestational tissues in relation to the time of parturition we have measured the I.R.OT content in human placental decidua and fetal membranes obtained after term and preterm delivery. The study has been corredated by the examination of I.R.OT levels in umbilical plasma and amniotic fluid.

METHODS

Briefly, tissue processing included repeated mincing and rinsing with ice cold saline of the specimens, their boiling in 2N acetic acid solution, homogenization, ultracentrifugation, concentration under vacuum and resuspension in 0.1% trifluoroacetic acid (TFA) for following passage through Sep-Pak c_{18} cartridge.

The peptidic content was eluted with acetonitrile, concentrated and resuspended in phosphate buffer for RIA which was performed by using a very sensitive antibody showing a negligible cross-reactivity with Arg-Vasopressin and Vasotocin. After collection, umbilical blood and amniotic fluid were centrifuged and the plasma and the supernatant, respectively, were concentrated , resuspended in 0.1% TFA and passed through Sep-Pak c_{18} cartridge. The following phases of extraction and detection of OT are identical to those already described for tissues.

RESULTS

As reported in the figure both amniochorion and decidua contained low but detectable amounts (pg/g of wet tissue) of I.R.OT. Moreover, the peptide content at term gestation did not differ in relation to labor in both tissues. Preterm parturition was instead associated with marked changes in I.R.OT concentrations with higher and lower hormonal content in fetal membranes and decidua respectively, in comparison to term delivery . With regard to fetal fluids, I.R.OT levels were greater in umbilical artery after preterm spontaneous parturition than after both term vaginal and cesarean delivery, whereas the peptide content was more elevated in amniotic fluid during preterm and term spontaneous labor in respect to term cesarean section.

DISCUSSION

The present investigation provides evidence that both human fetal membranes and decidua contain detectable levels of OT. However, the observation that spontaneous labor at term is not associated with changes in tissutal OT content would argue against a role for the locally

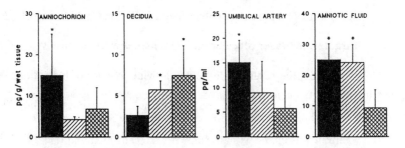

Figure: OT concentrations in amniochorion, decidua, umbilical artery blood and amniotic fluid of preterm (■) and term (◲)spontaneous parturition and term (⊠) cesarean delivery. Data are expressed as mean ⁺/. SD. ✳ :p<0.05; *:p<0.01. See also the text for explanations.

synthesized substance in the parturitional process. Nevertheless, the higher OT mRNA found by other authors (4) in these tissues after labor might equally be consistent with an increased release also in the absence of an altered content. In contrast preterm labor was associated with marked variations in tissutal OT concentrations. In this regard, we can only speculate that the relevant decrease of decidual OT coupled with the increase of the peptide in the fetal membranes are sustained by alterations in the local OT enzymatic degradation. OT was shown to be raised in the amniotic fluid either during term or preterm spontaneous labor. Although a greater part of the hormone present in amniotic fluid seems to be of fetal origin, the fetal membranes might also represent a source of OT in this fluid. Concerning the mechanism of action, the "in utero" synthesized OT could induce and/or maintain labor through the direct stimulation of muscular contractility. The myometrium could be reached by diffusion through the fetal membranes. Alternatively, OT may elicit indirectly uterine activity by stimulating in a paracrine/autocrine manner prostaglandins synthesis by

intrauterine tissues (decidua and fetal membranes) themselves (2,6). In

conclusion, the results of this study provide a series of indications that,

considered on the whole, can sustain a role for intrauterine OT in

human parturition: 1) OT is contained in both fetal membranes and

decidua, 2) OT levels do not change in these tissues in relation to labor

at term but are markedly modified in case of preterm parturition, 3)

OT rises in the amniotic compartment either during term or preterm

spontaneous labor.

REFERENCES

1. Fuchs, F. (1985). Role of maternal and fetal oxytocin in human parturition. In Amico J.A., Robinson A.G. (Eds). Oxytocin: Clinical and Laboratory Studies. pp. 236-56 (Amsterdam: Elsevier).

2. Fuchs A.R., Fuchs, F., Husslein, P. and Soloff, M.S. (1984). Oxytocin receptors in the human uterus during pregnancy and parturition. Am. J. Obstet. Gynecol., 150, 734-41.

3. Lefebvre, D.L., Lariviere, R. and Zingg, H.H. (1993). Rat amnion: a novel site of oxytocin production. Biol. Reprod., 48, 632-8.

4. Miller, F.D., Chibbar, R., and Mitchell B.F. (1993). Synthesis of oxytocin in amnion, chorion and decidua: a potential paracrine role for oxytocin in the onset of human parturition. Regul. Pept., 45, 247-51.

5. Mauri, A., Argiolas, A., Ticconi, C. and Piccione, E. Oxytocin in human intrauterine tissues at parturition. Reprod. Fert. Develop. In Print.

6. Moore, J.J., Dubyak, G.R., Moore, R.M. and Van der Kooy, D. (1988). Oxytocin activates the inositol-phospholipid protein kinase C system and stimulates prostaglandin production in human amnion cells. Endocrinology, 123, 1771-7.

The influence of non-clinical factors on the decision for vaginal delivery after prior Caesarean section

E. Alba, R. Lerro, M. Fenocchio and G. Visca

Università degli Studi di Torino, Istituto di Ginecologia ed Ostetricia, Cattedra B, Torino, Italy

The rate of cesarean section (CS) performed in western countries has dramatically increased during the past 20 years. (1) The highest rates are seen in United States (4,5% in 1965 to 24,7% in 1988); the rise has been slower in Scotland, Norway, Ungary, Czechoslovakia, Slovenia, Japan; The Netherlands have the lowest rates (about 6-7%) among the developed countries. (2)

The developing countries also have been on the rise. In India the CS rate rose gradualy from 1% in 1950 to 10% of 1992. In Brazil the actual rate is of 27,9%; in Nigeria of 6,9-19,8%; in Zaria, Kuwait, Egypt, South East Asia the rate vary from 10 to 20%. (3)

In Italy the national data indicate a rise from 4,2% in 1970 to 24,3% in 1990. (4)(5)(6) In the U.K. the the CS rates for 1990 are reported as 12-14%. In Ireland, by contrast,the rate at the Maternity Hospital of Dublin was almost constant at about 4-5% from 1965 to 1990.

In the increasing rate of CS, a particular focus has been repeat CS, which account for 35-40% of all CS. (7) Despite the demonstrated safety of vaginal birth after cesarean (VBAC) and recommendation that obstetricians adopt VBAC as a standard of practice, only 10-12% women, with previous CS, in the World adopt the vaginal birth. Several investigations suggest that, with increasing clinical indications for the first CS, there is a consistent burden of non clinical factors influencing the decision on repeat CS, (hospital teaching status, privatly or publicaly insurance, hospital size, socioeconomic status, the presence of a neonatal intensive care unit). (8) Furthermore in Italy other important factors are involved, i. e. the overestimation of the risk of uterine scar rupture during vaginal delivery, the obstetrician's and assistent personal's convenience, the patient's request to undergo a second CS, given the decreased parity and decreased morbility related to CS, fear of legal proceedings in case of maternal and fetal complications related to vaginal delivery attempts and, lastly, the lack of an official protocol agreed upon by italian gynecologists.

METHODS

We analise 7880 hospital births in the Department of Obstetrics and Gynecology, Chair B, Turin, between the years 1990-1994; of these the global rate of CS were 1844 (23,4%), particularly **(tab 1):**

Table 1.	total births	CS	%
1990	1584	332	20,9
1991	1602	374	23,3
1992	1592	368	23,1
1993	1542	368	23,8
1994	1560	402	25,7
	7880	1844	23,4

The rates of repeated CS were, on the whole, 36-40% of all CS approximately, with a slight reduction in the last two years, when we passed from an almost total repetition of CS in the early years to a gradual introduction of labor trial in 60% of prior CS, with a recent 12% vaginal delivery success rate.

In the past years we began to evaluate, during initial labor, the thickness of uterine scar of prior CS with transvaginal echography, in the perspective of VBAC. The results are that measurement of uterine scars are important , but the final criterion is the global clinical judgment upon the labor course. (8)

RESULTS AND CONCLUSIONS

In our experience the non clinical factors mainly influencing the decision of repeat CS are not the socioeconomic status of women, neither the modality of payment. In our hospital we have a very performed theaching level, a large number of total births with high level equipments of diagnosis and cure, the presence of a neonatal intensive unit, the prevalent (nearly total) public insurance. In Italy and in our Department the most important non clinical factors orienting toward a repeat CS, are, on the contrary, the lack of official protocol upon the management of labor trial of prior CS and, of course, the fear of the medicolegal implications. Although we have seen recently a modest rise in VBAC, there are in Italy, and in our hospital, important differences among various obstetricians, various hours of day and night, ferial and week-end.

The increased health care costs associated with still too elevated rates of CS and the lack of clinical justifications for not reducing the repeated CS (as well the first CS), make it critical in Italy to evaluate the influence of the financing and organization of health care services.

REFERENCES

1) Gordon H. (1994). The appropriate role of Caesarean section in modern obstetric practice; breech an multiple pregnancy. In *'Women's Health Today'* Edited Popkin-Peddle, Montreal, **71-74**

2) Bhasker Rao K. (1994). Global aspects of a rising Caesarean section rate. In *'Women's Health Today'* Edited Popkin-Peddle, Montreal, **59-63.**

3) Signorelli C, Elliot P, Cattaruzza MS, Osborn J. (1991). Trends in Caesarean section in Italy. *Int J Epidemiol.* **20: 712-716.**

4) Parazzini F, Pirotta N, Vecchia C, Fedele L. (1992). Determinants of Ceasarean section rates in Italy. *Br J Obstet Gynaecol.* **99: 203-206.**

5) Bertollini R, Dilallo D, Spadia T, Perucci C. (1992). Caesarean rates in Italy by hospital payment mode. *Am J Public Health.* **82: 257-261.**

6) Stronge JM. (1994). Strategies for reducing the Caesarean section rate. In *'Women's Health Today'* Edited Popkin-Peddle, Montreal, **55-58.**

7) Paul RH. (1994). Once a section, always a scar! Vaginal birth after Caesarean section. In *'Women's Health Today'* Edited Popkin-Peddle, Montreal, *75-80.*

8) Randall S, Stafford PhD. (1991). The impact of non clinical factors on repeat Cesarean section. *JAMA* **265,1: 59-63.**

Comparison of Ondansetron versus acupuncture to preserve postoperative nausea and vomiting in Caesarean section: is it always a useful preventive therapeutic intervention?

F. Capone, V. Cozzolino, C. D'Auria*, E. Desiderio, F. Lollo, G. D'Aniello, C. Pagano, M. Piscopo, R. Molaro, A. Castaldo, G. Lubrano and G. Vairo

Department of Anaesthesia, Intensive Care Unit and *Department of Obstetrics and Gynecology, "Mauro Scarlato" Hospital, Scafati (Salerno), Italy

SUMMARY.

The Authors in their research compared the effects of no-pharmacological treatments (Acupuncture) versus pharmacological treatments (Ondansetron) to prevent nausea and vomiting in patients who had to undergo caesarean section in general anaesthesia.
The analysis of results did not show statistically significant differences between the two groups of patients, in connection with the forecast aim of the study.
Key words : Acupuncture, Ondansetron, P.O.N.V., Prevention

INTRODUCTION.

Post-operative nausea and vomiting represent "historical" problems characteristic of anaesthesia, as a matter of fact they are originated from anaesthesia itself; from the first descriptions, with a frequency near to about 80 % in anaesthesia administred with N2O, ether, chloroform and cyclo-propane, the incidence has strongly reduced by the introduction of intravenous anaesthetic drugs and of inhalant anaesthetics in clinic practice (between 11 % and 21% according a study carried out in various centres by Cohen in 1990).
Nevertheless in some surgical sectors the frequency of P. O.N.V. can concern up to about the 83% of patients as in gynaecological-obstetrical surgery, thus remaining a present problem. In clinic practice the most important matter which anaesthetists have to face is the following :
- what have anaesthetists to prefer: prevention or treatement of P.O.N.V. in progress ? -
In theory it seems logical to prefer prevention: the aim of the present study is precisely to test the efficacy of

613

new antiemetic drugs, more endurable and efficacious than
the ones used up to this moment, which were characterized
by important collateral effects.
Moreover in consideration of recent researches it has been
thought useful to reconsider the role which is proper of
no-pharmacological techniques as for example acupuncture.
This study compares the incidence of P.O.N.V. during a period of 24 hours after a surgical operation of caesarean
section made with general anaesthesia, in Ondansetron (a
selective 5-HT3 serotoninergic receptor antagonist) treated
patients versus acupuncture treated patients.

MATERIAL AND METHODS .

Emetic symptoms, particularly frequent in obstetrics and
during anaesthesia for caesarean section, besides increasing mother's post-operative illness contribute to limit
mother-newborn relationship, thus giving rise to important
clinical and psychological implications.
The present research has been carried out on a group of 51
women, who had to undergo a caesarean section owing to mother and fetal problems.
The above 51 patients were between seventeen and thirty-se
ven years of age; 38-40 week pregnant; A.S.A. phisical status I-II . All patients studied for this research were previously informed about the aims of the same and gave their
consent to partecipate in it.
Patients were divided at random in two different groups: A
and O , which characteristics are reported on Table 1.

Table 1   Parameters af studied groups.

Parameters	A GROUP (25 patients)	O GROUP (26 patients)
AGE (years)	26.4 + 4.5	25.6 + 3
WEIGHT (kg)	61 + 3	64 + 4.5
PRIMIPARAE	10	12
MULTIPARAE	15	14
URGENT C.S.	---	8
PROGRAMMED C.S.	25	18
ASA I	20	19
ASA II	5	7
PREGNANCY WK	38-40	

Patients affected with diseases (as reported on Table 2)
were excluded from the study. O/group patients were given
Ondansetron 4 mg i.v. 10 min prior to anaesthetic induction; while A/group on the contrary 30 min prior to anaesthetic induction were submitted to acupuncture by penetration of a needle in point No.6 (Neiguan) of blood vessels meridian, bilaterally, and the needles were electri-
cally stimulated with "chinese" wawe for 20 min by means
of a proper apparatus.

Table 2   Exclusion criteria.

Diabetes mellitus
Ketoacidosis
Gastroparesis
Obesity
Haematologic Abnormalities
Hepatic   "
Renal   "
Nasogastric tube
Antiemetic drugs °

° Taken in the 24 hours prior to surgical operation.

Both for group A and group O , anaesthetical process was
the following :
-Premedication : Atropine-sulphate 0,005 mg/kg^{-1} i.v.
-Induction   : Pentothal-sodium 3,5/4,0 mg/kg-1 i.v.
-Management   : Atracurium-besilato 0,6 mg/kg-1 i.v.
                  O.T.I.
                  $N_2O + O_2$ (3:1 proportion)
                  Fentanyl 0,005 mg/kg^{-1} i.v. (successi-
                  vely to the extraction)
-Monitoring   : Control of arterial pressure and E.C.G.
                  in progress

The occurrence of nausea and vomiting was valued in a period of 24 hours after surgical operation, by dividing the
above mentioned period in the following times:
T0 (awaking), T1 (30 min), T2 (120 min), T3 (8 hours), T4
(24 hours) .
Prior to surgical operation and after 24 hours were carri-
ed out on each patient admitted to the study the following
clinical laboratory tests:
AST, ALT, ALP, LDH, RBC, WBC, PTL, Hct, Hb, MCV, MCH,
MCHC, Bilirubinemia, Creatininemia, Albuminemia, Blood-
proteins-electrophoresis, Uremia, Glycemia.
Moreover eventual collateral effects were checked both on
awaking and after a period of 24 hours:
Headache, Itch, Urticaria, Sedation, Muscolar Stiffness,
Chest pain(non specific), Bronchospasm, Laryngospasm.
Finally it was valued in the new-born the Apgar score at
1, 5 and 10 minutes.

RESULTS .

In the whole group submitted to the study, symptomatic patients to nausea and vomiting resulted to be 10 (19,6%);
symptomatic patients to nausea resulted to be 4 (7,8%);
while patients symptomatic to vomiting were 6 (11,7%).
In A/group 2 patients (8%) showed nausea during T2 time
(120 min) and 3 patients (12%) showed vomiting during T3
time (8 hours) .
In O/group 2 patients (7,7%) showed nausea and 3 patients

(11,5%) showed vomiting; all of them during T3 time (8 hours).
The Apgar score did not show any significant difference between two groups.

CONCLUSIONS.

The comparative analysis of Ondansetron and Acupuncture to prevent post-operative nausea and vomiting in patients undergone to surgical operation of caesarean section under general anaesthesia didn't show a substantial difference, statistically significant, between no-pharmacological techniques treated patients and patients pharmacologically treated, even if nausea manifested itself earlier in A/group patients than O/group ones.
There weren't significant differences in clinical laboratory tests prior and after 24 hours from surgical operation.
Nor the neonatologists noted any difference in Apgar score.
It is useful to show how being able to warrant a confortable post-operative period can be beneficial not only from clinical point of view, but also from psychological point of view.
Therefore preventing the occurrence of P.O.N.V. also means to cut down hospital charges.
Moreover the unimportant difference shown by results obtained with the two different techniques utilized, persuaded us to reconsider the role which is proper of other no-pharmacological techniques in the treatment of this non secondary post-operative complication, as the latter are a simple means, not expensive and quite reliable to correct potential emetic situations, in a pre-operative phase and to select high risk patients to be submitted on the contrary to invading prophylaxis both pharmacological and no-pharmacological. The above no-pharmacological techniques can be pointed out into the correct valuation and eventual treatment of emetic factors relevant to physiopathological characteristics of each patient and to his age, relevant to anaesthesia and to anaesthetists'experience and finally relevant to surgical operation and post-surgical factors.
The Authors of theis research hope to devote a future study to the valuation and to the eventual treatment of the afore-mentioned emetic factors.

REFERENCES.

1) Blackwell,CP, Harding, SM,(1989). The clinical pharmacology of Ondansetron. Eur.J.Cancer and Clinical Oncology, Suppl.1, 821-4 .
2) Clarke,RST, (1984) . Nausea and Vomiting. B.J.Anaesth., 56, 19 .
3) Cohen,MM, Camerun,CB, Duncan,PG, (1990). Pediatric anesthesia morbidity and mortality in the perioperative period. Anesth.Analg. 70, 160-7 .
4) Fassoulaki,A, Papilas,K, Sarantopoulos,C, Zotou,M,(1993) Transcutaneous electrical nerve stimulation reduces the

incidence of vomiting after hysterectomy. Anesth.Analg., 76, 1012-4 .

5) Lermann,J, (1992).Surgical and patients factors involved in postoperative nausea and vomiting. B.J.Anaesth., 69 (Suppl.1), 24S-32S .

6) Merciai,V, Batacchi,S, Bucciardini,L, Linden,M, (1994). Il controllo della nausea e del vomito postoperatorio nelle diverse specialità chirurgiche. Min.Anest.,60(Suppl.1), 15-33 .

7) Nimmo,WS, (1992). Nausea and vomiting in obstetrics. J. Obstet.Gynecol.,83, 121 .

8) Rabey,PG, Smith,G, (1992). Anaesthetic factors contributing to postoperative nausea and vomiting. Br.J.Anaesth., 69 (Suppl.1), 405-55 .

9) Watcha,MF, Whithe,PF, (1992). Postoperative nausea and vomiting; its etiology, treatment and prevention. Anesthesiology,77, 162-84 .

10) Zilletti,L, (1994). Note di fisiofarmacologia dell'emesi.Min.Anest.,60(Suppl.1), 11-4 .

We thank, for their essential cooperation in the drawing up of the present research, Mrs Cinzia BUONANNO, Matron by I.C.U. of the "Mauro Scarlato" Hospital .

Intensive care during pregnancy: our experience

F. Lollo, F. Capone, E. Desiderio, P. De Luca, A. Castaldo Tuccillo and G. Vairo

Intensive Care Unit, M. Scarlato Hospital, Scafati, Italy

INTRODUCTION

The number of patients needing intensive care during pregnancy, delivery and post-delivery is unexpectedly high. This critic case that happens to gravid women has become more probable for various reasons:

a) the prosecution of working and social activity during pregnancy that exposes women to traumas and accidents frequently;

b) the best quality of care allows women with invalidating patologies (like respiratory, metabolic and neurologic diseases) to reach the fertil age and to face pregnancy;

c) the increase of incidence of cesarean sections and so of the risks connected with the anaesthesia and surgical operations.

REASON OF THE ADMISSION TO THE INTENSIVE CARE UNIT

1) Non connected with pregnancy (traumas, poisonings)

2) Connected with pregnancy   a) indirect

b) direct

a) (indirect) pre-existing pathologies made worse by pregnancy:

cardiopaties, diabetes, myasthenia.

b) (direct) pathologies which occurred during pregnancy:

preeclampsia, uterine hemorrhage.

3) Iatrogenic injuries (surgical and anaesthetic accidents).

MATERIAL AND METHODS

In a retrospective study of obstetric admission to the Intensive Care Unit (ICU) from january 1981 to august 1994 we have analysed:

a) the reasons of the admission to ICU

b) the state of health at the admission

c) the length of permanence in ICU

d) the outcome at the dismission.

In the examinated period the patients admitted have been 94 out of 12,665 deliveries (0.74%).

The most frequent cause of the admission is represented by obstetric pathology which accounted for 73.4%:

DIC.....................4

hellp syndrome.........3

eclampsia.............33

hemorrhagic shock.....20

pulmunar embolism......2

PIH....................7

Anaesthetic complications accounted for 15.9%:

hipoxia by difficult intubation............2

cardiac arrhytmias........................1

```
respiratory depression.....................3
aspiration pneumonitis....................1
anaphylactic shock........................1
cardiac arrest............................1
bronchispasm..............................3
laryngospasm..............................3
```

Medical complications accounted for 7.4%:

```
                cardiopathy.............2
                myasthenia..............1
                liver cirrhosis.........1
                asthma..................2
                diabetic ketoacidosis...1
```

Poisonings accounted for 3.1% by:

```
                parasiticide..........1
                bleach................2
```

The average lenght of permanence in ICU has been of 4.39 days.

The major part of admission has occurred in the post-partum (78.8%), above all after cesarean section; in the second four mounth there have been 14.8% of the admissions while in the first four mounths 6.3%.

The incidence of maternal death is 0.047%; the causes of the death:

```
                CID...................................1
                hypossia by difficult intubation......1
                hemorragic schock.....................3
                liver cirrhosis.......................1
```

The most frequent cause of death is the HAEMORRHAGE in the post-partum; the most frequent cause od admission is ECLAMPSIA.

In our study the valuation of the state of health at the moment of the admission has been carried out with the "Semplified Acute Physiology

Score for Obstetrics" (SAPSO) (Margaria et al. 1994).

The general prognostic scoring systems, habitually used to value the seriousness of the intensive care patients (APACHE II, SAPS, MPM) are not usefull for obstetric patients.

In these patients we propose to value and to treat conditions of risk precociously rather than to check critical situations.

In the SAPSO, unlike the SAPS, is considered diastolic pressure that is an early sign of pathology induced by pregnancy.

The parameters age, glucose and electrolitics are disregarded.

Creatinine, platelets and enzyms liver are considered to make early diagnosis and therapy of most involving complications of PIH; the

D-Dimero as a sign of DIC and pulmonary embolism.

Pulse oximetry has been inserted instead of ventilation and respiratory rate to easily detect maternal hypoxia.

Algic symptoms and recurrent nausea and vomiting play an important role in disclosing specific or superimposed pathologies.

In all the cases the low score revealed at the moment of the admission considering the 16 parameters of SAPSO is predicting of a short period of permanence and of a good prognosis.

CONCLUSIONS

We think that it is possible to recognise from this retrospective research a disposition to widen the reasons, for these patients, for the admission to the Intensive Care Unit and chiefly aiming to use a careful and instrumental monitoring turned to safe the maternal and fetal prognosis.

REFERENCES

-Crawford J.S.: Principles and practice of obstetric anaesthesia. Blackwell, Oxford; 1984

-Le GAll et Al.: A simplified acute physiology score for ICU pt. Critical Care Medicine, 12,11: 975-77; 1984

-Margaria E. el Al.: SAPS modified for obstetric pt. (SAPSO). Atti Società Europea di Algoanestesia Ostetrica. Firenze 1994

-Pachi A.: Mortalità materna e perinatale. In Zichella e Coll.: Ginecologia ed Ostetricia. Monduzzi Ed. Bologna 1982

-Rosen M.: Deaths associated with anaesthesia for obstetrics. Anaesthesia 36: 145-146; 1981

-Shnider S.M., Levinson G.: Anesthesia for obstetrics. Williams & Wilkins Ed. 1993

P.S.

We thank, for their essential cooperation in the drawing up of the present research, Mrs Cinzia BUONANNO, Matron by I.C.U. of the "Mauro Scarlato" Hospital .

Spinal block in emergency Caesarean section: our experience

E. Desiderio, G. Lubrano, F. Lollo, R. Molaro, M. Piscopo, M. Grieco, C. D'Auria* and G. Vairo

Department of Anesthesia, Intensive Care Unit and *Department of Obstetrics and Gynecology, Scarlato Hospital, Scafati, Italy

INTRODUCTION

The aim of this work is to assess the spinal block in emergency Cesarean section.

The peculiar conditions of the pregnant patients and the side effects connected with spinal block were the factors which for the past, made prefer in the emergency the general anesthesia (Fig. 1).

On the other hand the general anesthesia in patients considered to "full stomach" isn't risk-free, without considering the other frustrating conditions which don't allow to be present at an event so important as the birth of a own son.

These physiological and psycological factors with a more attentive knowledge of the phisiopathology of spinal block increased the interest for this anesthesiological techique.

The supports of a corret spinal block could be summed up in

625

the following points:

- To prevent hypotension : often a consequence of the
  spinal block.

- To prevent nausea and vomiting.

- To prevent post dural puncture headache (PDPH).

MATERIALS and METHODS

We studied, previous consensus, 40 patients belonged to the classes ASA I and ASA II, subjected to emergency Cesarean section through spinal block (Fig. 2).

The range of age was 20-28 years, the range of weight was 60-75 kg, and the patients were between 38°-40° week of pregnancy.

The exclusion criteria were: the patients'refusal, patologies connected with pregnancy (placenta previa,eclampsia etc.), coagulopathy, neurological diseases, positive anamnesis for headache, spinal cord diseases, local infections. Patients were premedicated with Atropine 0.01 mg/kg and Metoclopramide 10 mg I.M. 20 minutes before the operation.

All patients were subjected to preoperative administration of 15 ml/kg cristalloid solution.

The spinal block were executed with the patient in sitting position, at the level of L2-L3,using atraumatic needle (ATRAUCAN tm) 26 G, administering 10-12 mg hyperbaric bupivacaina to 1%.

Once the spinal block was executed the patient was placed, suddenly, in supine position to avoid a hard descend of the local anesthetic and it was arranged for moving the utherus

toward left to prevent aorto-caval compression syndrome.
They were evalued the maternal hypotension (intended as a
reduction of 20 mmhg of the basal values), nausea, vomiting and postspinal headache incidence.

In different times from 0 to 240 minutes, it was evalued
the post operative analgesia trough a score arbitrary scale
where 0=no pain, 1=light pain, 2=moderate pain, 3=severe
pain, 4= strong pain.

RESULTS

The result were very comforting.

The spinal block succeeded in all the patients.

Haemodinamic stability was very good.

The hypotension, however moderate, developed in only 3
patients and treated with infusion of low dosing vasopressor agents (Dimetofrina tm).

No vomiting, and nausea involved only 2 patients may be
referred to the temporary hypotension.

The analgesia 4 hours after operation was still good and
PDPH no occur.

DISCUSSION

The symphatetic blockade produces postarteriolar pooling of
blood which decreases effective circulating blood volume.

When a large area of the vascular bed is denervated in this
manner, the venous return to the heart can be reduced.

In addition, in the pregnant patient the vascular tone
depends more on sympathetic control.

These factors connected with the possible aorto-cava compression make the pregnant more susceptible to the effects following the sympathetic blockade.

In addition, the pregnant presents an hypersensivity to the local anesthetic due to two factors:

1) the compensated alkalemia induced by hyperventilation increases the persistence in the compartiment of injection of the local anesthetic.

2) the increased concentration of plasmatic progesterone causes a vasodilatation which is expressed at the level of the subarachnoid and epidural vessels too, increasing, in this way, the expansion of the anesthetic solution; the slowed meningeal capillary circulation retards the absortion of the drug, prologing the duration of the analgesia.

Recent works have, moreover, showed as the blood pressure decrement is connected with the level of the spinal anesthesia.

The more severe hypotension matches, in fact, when they are interested T5 levels and up,causing the block of the cardiac symphatetic nerve.

This is the rationale for preoperative hydratation intended to increase the venous return to the heart, and for the low dosing of local anesthetic used by us in comparison with international literature.

Nausea and vomiting are symptoms which appear frequently during Cesarean section made in spinal block and they depend on different factors connected in part with the pregnance and in part with the level of the block, bradycardia, hypotension (causing cerebral ipoxia), surgical stimulations and the administration of drugs, like oppiates, oxitocin and hergotamine.

Moreover all the measures to prevent the maternal hypotension (pre-hydratation, dislocation toward left of the uterus) reduce the incidence of nausea and vomiting.

We believe that the preoperative administration of Metoclopramide contributes to the reduction of nausea and vomiting, favouring the gastro-duodeno motility and the gastric emptying.

The absence of PDPH can be attribuited to the use of small gauge atraumatic needles.

The good postoperating analgesia characterized our work was attribuited to the major permanence of the local anesthetic in the point of injection.

CONCLUSION

In the international literature and in our results, the spinal block seems a method of choice in emergency Cesarean section in not complicated patients.

The knowledge of pregnant phisiology and also a deep knowledge of physiopathologic alterations which happen in this type of periferic block, seem the fundamental presuppositions for a current execution of this easy and rapid thecnic.

REFERENCES

1) Brorvik K; Larsen RG; Rolfseng OK; Olseth E;

   TDSSKR NOR LAEGEFOREN (Norway) Nov 30 1992 112/29 (3662-

   4) Regional Anesthesia in emergency Cesarean section.

   Quality of epidural and spinal anesthesia.

2) Cam FY; Broome IJ; Mathews P.

   Anesthesiology 49/1 (65-67) 1994

   A comparison of postoperative analgesia following spinal

   or epidural anaesthesia for Cesarean section.

3) Juhani TP; Hannele H.

   Reg. Anesth (USA) Mar-Apr 1993 18/2 (128-131)

   Complications during spinal anesthesia for Cesarean

   delivery: a clinical report of one year's' experience

4) Matta BF; Magele P.

   Can. J. Anesth. (Canada) dec 1992 39/10 (1067-8)

   Wenckeback type heart block following spinal anesthesia

   for Cesarean section.

5) Rout CC; Rocke DA.

   Int-Anesthesiol. Clin. 32/2 (117-135) 1994.

   Prevention of hypotension following spinal anesthesia

   for   Cesarean section.

6) Scott et al.

   Reg. Anaesth. 1993 18 (213-217).

   Atraucan: a new needle for spinal anesthesia.

7) Shiroyama K; Nakagawa I; Izumi H; Korokawa H; Kuroda M;

   JPN J Anesthesiol. 43/5 (697-701) 1994.

   Cause of Hypotension during spinal anesthesia. The

   relation between the level of anesthesia and the hypo-

   tention.

Incidence of ectopic pregnancy: preliminary results of a population-based register in Lithuania

G. Bogdanskiene, I. Dirsaite and *J.G. Grudzinskas

Vilnius University Hospital, Vilnius, Lithuania and *Academic Unit of Obstetrics and Gynaecology, Royal London Hospital, London, UK

INTRODUCTION

In 1994, a register of ectopic pregnancy (EP) was established in five Vilnius hospitals. The primary target was to calculate the incidence of ectopic pregnancy in an urban Lithuanian population and to compare it those reported in other countries. Secondary aims included, determination of fertility in the year following treatment for ectopic pregnancy in women in Vilnius City, and the examination of the subsequent fertility in these women in relation to sociodemographic factors, operative findings and treatment of the ectopic pregnancy.

We describe here an ectopic pregnancy register and fertility in women after ectopic pregnancy during the year 1993 in the population of Vilnius, Lithuania.

MATERIALS AND METHODS

The register is population-based and covers female residents of Vilnius City which had 592,000 inhabitants in 1993.

For calculation of the incidence of ectopic pregnancy, we ascertained the number of women of reproductive age, annual numbers of live births and legally induced abortions. These data were obtained from the national population register and health statistics of the Ministry of Health of Lithuania.

The method of case record retrieval was used. We have examined operating theatre registers, case records and discharge diagnosis files. For fertility assessment, we have used postal and telephone contact.

STATISTICAL METHODS

Rates of ectopic pregnancy have been calculated per 1000 live births, 1000 reported pregnancies (reported pregnancies being defined as the sum of live births, legally induced abortions and ectopic pregnancies) and 10,000 women of reproductive age (15-44 years). Statistical significance of the differences observed between subgroup rates were tested with the Chi-square test for homogeneity.

RESULTS

A total of 145 women were treated for ectopic pregnancy in five of six Vilnius hospitals in 1993. We have been able to follow up 100 women to date.

The numbers of ectopic pregnancy cases, live births, legally induced abortions and women of reproductive age are summarised in Table 1.

TABLE I - Number of reported pregnancies in relation to women of reproductive age in 1993[a]

Geographical area	No of EP	No of induced abortions	No of live births	No of women aged 15-44
Vilnius	145	4,920	7,662	142,799

[a]   Data obtained from Ministry of Health statistics

Number of legally induced abortions does not include "menstrual regulation" i.e. vacuum aspiration of uterus before six weeks amenorrhoea. The percentage of menstrual regulation in Lithuanian women undergoing legally induced abortions is estimated to be 57%.

TABLE II - Rates of ectopic pregnancy in Vilnius in 1993

Geographical area	Rates expressed as promiles of:-		
	Live births(a)	Reported pregnancies(b)	Women aged 15-44(c)
Vilnius	18.9	11.2	10.1

[a] Per 1000 live births
[b] Per 1000 live-born infants, legally induced abortions and ectopic pregnancy
[c] Per 10,000 women aged 15-44 years

The rates of ectopic pregnancy in Vilnius in 1993 were: 18.9 per 1000 live births, 11.2 per 1000 reported pregnancies and 10.1 per 10,000 women of reproductive age. Table II, III, IV and V summarise the rates of ectopic pregnancy by age group, comparative rates of ectopic pregnancy in France, Finland, USA and Lithuania and comparative rates of ectopic pregnancy and births by age group in Lithuania and France. There was a highly significant increase in the incidence of EP with respect to maternal age in Lithuania (Table III).

Table III - Rates of ectopic pregnancy by age group in the Vilnius population
Chi Square - 93.15, p<0.0001)

Age group (years)	No of EP	No of live births	Rate per 1000 live births	Rate per 10,000 women of repro- ductive age	No of women aged 15-44
< 25	28	3,468	8.01	6.34	44,169
25-29	38	2,253	16.87	16.07	23,648
30-34	39	1,319	29.57	14.18	27,513
35-44	40	622	64.31	8.43	47,469

Table IV - Comparative rates of ectopic pregnancy in France, Finland, USA and Lithuania

Ectopic Pregnancy rate	France(1992)	Finland(1991)	USA(1989)	Lithuania(1993)
Per 1000 live births	20.2	28.0	22.0	18.9
Per 1000 reported pregnancies	15.8	21.0	16.1	11.2
Per 10,000 women of reproductive age	9.5	16.3	15.5	10.1

Table V - Comparative rates of ectopic pregnancy and births by age group in Lithuania and France

	Lithuania (1993)		France (1992)	
	Ectopic pregnancy rate	Birth rate	Ectopic pregnancy rate	Birth rate
<25	6.34	7.86	3.9	3.4
25-29	16.07	9.53	14.0	11.99
30-34	14.18	4.79	17.6	7.66
35-44	8.43	1.31	9.1	1.58

The ectopic pregnancy rates per 1000 live births are similar in all countries. The rate per 1000 reported pregnancies (11.2) is similar to one in France (15.8) but significantly lower than in Finland (21.0). The rate per 10,000 women of reproductive age (10.1) is similar to the rate in France (9.5) but significantly lower than in Finland (16.3) and USA (15.5).

We are examining our findings in relation to sociodemographic factors, operative findings and treatment in the 145 women treated for EP in Vilnius in 1993 (in preparation). Of the 100 women followed up at the time of writing, 31 wished to conceive and 15 became pregnant.

CONCLUSION

We have established a register for EP based on a survey of the Vilnius population in 1993 based on the study of Coste et al (1994). The rate of EP in relation to due births appears to be equivalent to that in the other countries studies, but lower than the rates seen in some countries when analysed with respect to reported pregnancies and the proportion of women of reproductive age. Follow up in the year subsequent to treatment for EP has led to a high ascertainment rate by mail and telephone contact.

Further analysis will include an examination of the patient's characteristics and her treatment with respect to subsequent pregnancy outcome.

REFERENCES

1.   Coste J, Job-Spira N, Aublet-Cuvelier B, Germain E, Glowaczower E, Fernandez H, Pouly JL (1994). Incidence of ectopic pregnancy. First results of a population-based register in France. <u>Hum Reprod</u> 9,4:742-745

Blood lead levels in pregnant women: a study conducted in Pisa and surrounding areas

G. Guazzelli, M.A. Celano, E. Neri, M.C. Papa, S. Masoni, C. Salvestroni and C. De Punzio

Department of Gynecology and Obstetrics, University of Pisa, Pisa, Italy

INTRODUCTION

High blood lead levels in people is a sign of pollution linked to local industry, traffic or to the workplace.(1) Dust, water and paint chips are still major sources of lead but lead from folk remedies cosmetics, food supplements, food preparation utensils, and improperly prepared infant formula has caused severe lead toxicity.(2) Lead toxicity causes hematological gastrointestinal and neurological dysfunctions in adults and children.(2) Severe or prolonged exposure may also cause chronic nephropathy, hypertension and reproductive impairment.(1)(2) When lead blood levels increase by 100 micrograms, blood pressure increases by 3 mm/Hg.(1) Lead inhibits some enzymes, so that it can alter cellular calcium metabolism, stimulate synthesis of binding proteins in kidney, brain and bone and slow down nerve conduction.(6) Bone lead may be a significant source of target organ exposure under certain conditions such as pregnancy, kidney disease and menopause. The accumulation of lead in bone cells may have toxic consequences for bone status and some of the mechanisms by which lead could affect bone mineral metabolism may also play a role in other target organ effects of lead.(1)(6) High blood lead levels in women can cause infertility, miscarriage, increased incidence of spontaneous abortion, premature rupture of the membranes, pre-eclampsia, pregnancy hypertension and preterm delivery, while a possible teratogen effect is still to be demonstrated.(5)(10)(11) Manifestations in the fetus and in newborn include prematurity, fetal hypotrophy, low birth weight in infants and malformations, Intelligence Quotient (IQ) deficits, behavior disorders, slowed growth and impaired hearing.(1)(7)(8)(9) The placental barrier is permeable to free serum lead, and levels in cord blood reach 5-10% of the maternal blood level. In addition, lead may be released from maternal bone reserves during pregnancy and thus become a source of intoxication for the fetus. Lead content in fetal organs increases with gestational age and may affect the nervous system and calcium dependent organs.(1)

METHODS

The study group was made up of 79 pregnant women, randomly chosen from those attending our Department for routine pregnancy screening from June 1993 to March 1994.

Each woman was adequately informed and gave 4 cc of blood, which was collected in a tube with EDTA in order to determine blood lead levels.

For blood lead level measurements, the laboratory used atomic absorption spectrometry with electrothermal atomization. Personal information on each population group and geographical area was collected by administering a standardized questionnaire.

In order to evaluate statistical significance, the pregnant women were divided into two groups, depending on whether they lived in urban or rural centers.

Then another statistical test was done according to neonatal birth weight.

Statistical evaluation was done by factorial Anova and total χ square.

RESULTS

The group of urban dwellers was represented by 41 pregnant women, while 38 women lived in rural areas.

The groups were homogeneous according to age (mean age 29,8 yrs. in the former and 29,7 yrs. in the latter) and working conditions.

No significant difference was seen concerning cigarette smoking in the two groups (14,5% vs. 9,5%).

Blood lead levels were respectively 7,6±2,7 µg/dl (range 3-18) and 7,3±4,0 µg/dl (range 4-27), thus the difference was not significant ($p > 0,05$).

One woman had a miscarriage sine causa and her blood lead level was 3,6 µg/dl. Another had preterm delivery at 30th week and her blood lead level was 7 µg/dl.

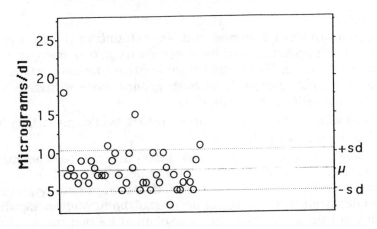

Distribution of blood lead levels in women living
in URBAN zones

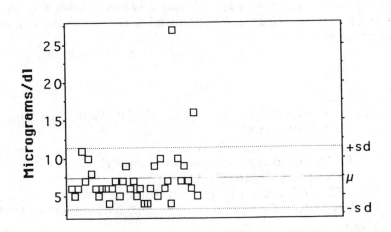

Distribution of blood lead levels in women living
in RURAL zones

All the others delivered a normal weight infant at term, except for
one, who delivered a baby with a weight lower than 2500 gr and an
Apgar score lower than 7. Blood lead levels in this woman were 7
µg/dl.

DISCUSSION

The comparative evaluation of lead levels found in women living in high and low population density zones shows that in our geographic area there is no significant difference between the two groups.

Moreover, blood lead levels in both groups were included in the normality range (i.e. <35 µg/dl).(12)

Only one woman had a value of 27 µg/dl, while the others were even lower than18 µg/dl.

This woman, however, had no risk factors in her own anamnesis; none woman had a job connected to lead pollution.(1)(13)

Contrary to other studies (12), we found that in our study group the few women who had a smoking or alcohol habit had no significant increase in lead levels. This can be explained by their reduced daily consumption due to their pregnancy .

We can conclude that the low lead levels found in our study indicate that it is not necessary to routinely screen pregnant women for elevated lead levels in our geographic area.

In consideration of the danger of lead on many maternal and fetal organs (1)(2)(6), we think it is advisable a careful surveillance of the pregnant women in case of real exposure risk due to the profession (paints, glass, ceramic industries etc.) or to the residence in pollution area.

REFERENCES

1)   KLEIN M, KAMINSKY P, BARBE' F, DUC M: "Saturnisme au cours de la grossesse".
     La Presse Mèdicale 1994: 23:576-9

2)   LOCKITCH G.: "Perspectives on lead toxicity".
     Clin.Biochem. 1993:26:371-81

3)   MULLER L e DIETER HH: "Lead in drinking water: determination of a new limit value and the problem of lead pipes
     Gesundheitswesen 1993:55:514-20

4)   ZIMMERMANN L, PAGES N, ANTEBI H, HAFI A, BOUDENE C, ALCINDOR LG: "Lead effect on the oxydation resistance of erythrocyte membrane in rat triton induced hyperlipidemia".
     Biol.Trace.Flem.Res. 1993:38:311-8

5)   WINDER C: "Lead, reproduction and development".
     Neurotoxicology 1993:14:303-17

6)   SILBERGELD EK, SAUK J, SOMERMAN M, TODD A, Mc NEILL F, FOWLER B, FONTAINE A, VAN BUREN J: "Lead in bone: storage site, exposure source and target organ".
     Neurotoxicology 1993:14:225-36

7) COMMITTEE ON ENVIRONMENTAL HEALTH : "Lead poisoning: from screening to primary prevention".
    Pediatrics 1993:92:176-83

8) BELLINGER D, SLOMAN J, LEVITON A, RABINOWITZ M, NEEDLEMAN HL, WATERNAUX C: "Low level lead exposure and children's cognitive function in the preschool years".
    Pediatrics 1991:87:219-27

9) CARRINGTON CD, SHEEHAN DM, BOLGER PM: "Hazard assessment of lead".
    Food Addit.Contam. 1993:10:325-35

10) GERONIMUS AT, HILLEMEIER MM: "Patterns of blood lead levels in U.S. black and white women of childbearing age"
    Ethn.Dis. 1992:2:222-31

11) HUELL G, TUBERT P, FRERY N, MOREAU T, DREYFUS J: "Joint effect of gestational age and maternal lead exposure on psychomotor development of the child at six years".
    Neurotoxicology 1992:13:249-54

12) MORRISI G, PATRIARCA M, CARRIERI MP, FONDI G., TAGGI F.: "Lead exposure: assessment of the risk for the general italian population".
    Ann.Ist.Super.Sanità 1989:25:423-36

13) CORDIER S, GOUJARD J : "Occupational exposure to chemical substances and congenital anomalies: state of the art."
    Rev.Epidemiol.Sante Publique 1994:42:144-59

Early transvaginal ecocardiography

M.A. Vezzani, R. Guidetti, A. Carani, A. Colombo, R. Fiozzi and P. Galli

Department of Obstetrics and Gynecology, Azienda USL Modena, Mirandola, Italy

INTRODUCTION

Congenital cardiopathy, isolated or associated with a pattern of polymalformation, represents the majority of congenital malformations with an estimated occurrance of around 9%° of births. Therefore prenatal diagnosis, above all for its timeliness, is a fondamental support in the accurate supervision of the pregnancy, with a range of possibilities from voluntary interruption of the pregnancy to programmed birth in a sanitary environment suitable for neonatal cardio-surgical treatment.

Compared with an adult, the traditional fetal echo-cardiography, i.e. Trans-Abdominal Echo-Cardiography (TAFEC), on the one hand is aggravated by unsurmountable obstacles presented by the reduced size of the heart and movement of the fetus, and on the other hand is facilitated by pulmunary collapse and by the presence of amniotic fluid (1).

In practice, provided that the maternal fat, the anterior placental implant or perhaps an oligohydramnios do not complicate the TAFEC, we must continuously adapt to the equally continuously changig position of the fetus during the execution of the examination. If we then, with the fetus in a longitudinal dorsal back position, manage to reach all the scanning levels (4 chambers, long axis, short axis, venous returns, arch of aorta), with a lateral dorsal or dorsal front position the examination posibilities are reduced.

Recently the clinical application of high-frequency (6.5 MHz) endovaginal probes have allowed avoiding some of the above mentioned problems, so that we set ourselves the target to investigate the minimum useful pregnancy age in which sufficient results may be obtained to allow an adequate examination of the fetal heart through the use of vaginal probes (Trans-Vaginal Fetal Eco-Cardiography: TVFEC).

MATERIAL AND METHOD

In the two-year period 1992-93 pregnant patients, who during the first trimester had came to our department, were proposed to undergo fetal eco-cardiographic examination using the trans-vaginal probe (TVFEC) (ESAOTE BIOMEDICA AU 450) at 14-16 weeks, repeated at 20-24 weeks using the trans-abdominal probe (TAFEC) and finally, in the first postnatal days before discarge.

Considering the fetal heart as a structure divisible in threeparts, i.e. the atria, the ventricles, and the large arteries and veins, we examined this organ according to the following outline: 1) interatrial, interventicular septum and structural symmetry between atria and ventricules; 2) connection between atria and ventricles by examining the mitral and tricuspid valves; 3) connection between ventricles and arteries, venous returns to the atria, mobility of the aortic and pulmonary valves and arch of the aorta.

Both TAFEC and TVFEC were, therefore, carried out in a logical sequence: 1) projection of 4 chambers, 2) long axis for left ventricle and ascending aorta, 3) long axis for right ventricle and pulmonary artery, 4) short axis for right ventricle, pulmonary artery and Botallo's duct, 5) longitudinal scanning for venous returns to right atrium, inferior and superior vena cava and 6) arch of the aorta and brachicephalous branches.

RESULTS AND CONCLUSIONS

In the two-year period 1992-93, 247 fetuses of as many single pregnancies were subjected to TAFEC, TVFEC and neonatal diagnosis.

In 65% of the caes, TVFEC allowed all levels of scanning; in 35% of the cases it was only possible to obtain three projections. With respect to the already mentined technical difficulties relative to TAFEC, also TVFEC poses some difficulties caused by the reduced mobility of the trans-vaginal probe and the fetal position and presentation being the longitudinal breech the most unfavourable.

In none of the 247 fetuses congenital heart anomalies were encountered and in all cases at leastthe early neonatal diagnosis cofirmed the prenatal diagnosis.

Our experience leads us to maintain that TVFEC may supply extensive and sufficient information on the anatomy of the fetal heart, already at 14-16 weeks of pregnancy (2,3,4) and thus earlier than TAFEC. Certainly the ecocardiography of the second trimester has its limits, mainly connected with the fact that some cardiopathies always appear later, or because the structural defects is too small and, therefore, cannot be ecographically demonstrated (i.e. the coercion of the aorta) or because thE display is connected with the functional damage resulting froM it, and which only manifests itself proporcionally as the pregnancy progresses (i.e. the cardiomiopathies).

Although no cardiac malformations were found in our examinations with TVFEC, but were later confirmed with TAFEC and/or at birth, we can in any case assume that TVFEC coul make an earlier identification than with TAFEC possible, at least for some important cardiac defects, as, for example, a ventricular atrium chennel, the hypoplasie of the left heart, the many defects of the intraventricular septum and the transposition of the great arteries.

Although we agree that the global morphological examination of the fetus is preferable because optimal only after the twentieth week, and some cardiac malformations might be recognized much later, and than sometimes only because of the effect of secondary functional alterations in the malformations themselves, we maintain that, following our experience, because it can be carried out earlier and with equal qualitative results, would be preferable to TAFEC or at least desirable in cases of cardiac malformation risks.

In conclusion, we maintain in particular that certain cardiac malformation risk conditions, of which on the maternal side hereditary cardiopathy, exposure to teratogenic insults, also generic, maternal diabetes and maternal autoimmune diseases, represent absolute indications to resort to TVFEC.

REFERENCES

1) Bovicelli L., Baccarani G., Picchio F.M., Pilu G.L.
Prenatal diagnosis and treatment of congenital cardiopathy. Masson, Milan, 1985.

2) D'Amelio R., Giorlandino C. et alii.
Fetal Echocardiography using trans-vaginal and trans-abdominal probes during the first period of pregnancy. Prenatal Diagnosis, 11, 69-75, 1991.

3) Gembruch U., Knopfle G. et alii
First trimester diagnosis of fetal congenital heart disease by trans-vaginal two-dimensional and doppler echocardiography. Obstet. Gynaecol., 75:3, 496-498,1990.

4) Brohnstein M., Blumenfeld Z. et alii
Detection of fetal cardiac malformation by trans-vaginal sonography in the first and early second trimester. In: 1st World Congress of Ultrasound in Obstetrics and Gynaecology, Parthenon Publ., London, 6-10, 1991.

Diagnostic approach to urinary incontinence in pregnancy

A. Carbonaro, R. Cantarella, V. Aidala and S. Reitano

Department of Obstetrics and Gynaecology, Santo Bambino Hospital, University of Catania, Catania, Italy

It has been proved that natural childbirth phenomena play an important role in the origin of prolapse and incontinence. In fact during delivery the perineo is hyperdistensive, often beyond its physiological capacity, and is subject to lacerations, microlesions and reparative fibrosis with a resulting reduction in contractile tone and capacity. This is confirmed by the fact that women with true S.U.I. have an abnormal conduction in the perineal crus of the pudendal nerve that innervates the striate periurethral muscle (Snooks et al. 1985) (2).
Hence it is important to identify women with S.U.I. during their first pregnancy whether transient or permanent even after delivery.

MATERIALS AND METHODS

From January 94 to October 94 we invited 110 pregnant women visiting our Department of Gynaecologic and Obstetric Pathology, University of Catania, to answer a self-assessment questionnaire (draw up P. Di Benedetto e coll.) (3). The purpose was to focus attention on a problem often neglected as is urinary incontinence in pregnancy. Pregnant women suffering from stress incontinence were evaluated from a urogynaecological point of view through physical examination, PC test and urodynamic tests. Of the 110 women examinated, 88 (80%) were nulliparous and 22 (20%) pluriparous (Fig. 1).

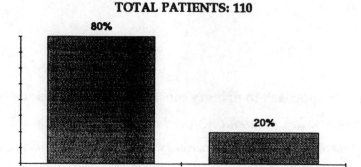

Fig.1

The average age was 28.5 years (range 18-36). The outcome of the present pregnancy was physiological for all. 77 gravidae (70%) were continent, whereas 33 (30%), of which 10 pluriparous and 23 nulliparous, suffered from stress incontinence that had arisen in most cases during the 3rd trimester of pregnancy (Fig.2).

TOTAL PATIENTS: 110

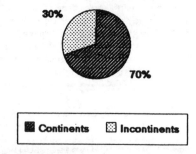

Fig.2 - S.U.I. Percentage

Two pluriparous women were suffering from incontinence before the pregnancy and during the present pregnancy it had worsened. Of the 10 pluriparous women suffering from S.U.I. 6 (60%) had undergone operative deliveries (2 with forceps operation and 4 with vacuum extractor) (Fig.3).

TOTAL PATIENTS: 10

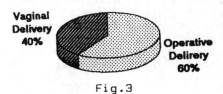

Fig.3

In the pluriparous incontinent women there were 6 macrosome fetuses (60%) (Fig.4).

TOTAL PATIENTS: 10

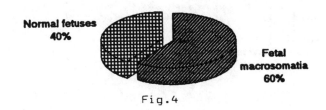

Fig.4

RESULTS

Involuntary escape of urine occurred weekly in 8 of 10 pluriparous women (80%), and daily on 2 out of 10 cases (20%). Whereas in nulliparous cases incontinence occurred weekly in 19 out of 23 (83%), and daily in the other 4 cases (17%) (Tab. 1).

Tab.1   S.U.I.

		Nulliparous	Pluriparous
Weekly	frequence	19	8
Daily	frequence	4	2
Total		23	10

All incontinent gravidae reported urinary escape only under

stress (coughing, sneezing), and in upright position. The disorder in clinostatism is less manifest. In any cases escape was limited to a few drops. Only two pluriparous cases (with an anamnesis of operative delivery with macrosome fetus), report a spurt of urine under stress. All women complaining of this disorder presented a typical urodynamic picture of true stress incontinence, while perineal muscle planes presented a reduced contractile capacity associated to a degree of hypotone. The PC test gave low values (1-2) in all incontinent women, whereas in 26 out of 33 patients (79%) there was inversion of the command (Fig.5).

TOTAL PATIENTS: 33

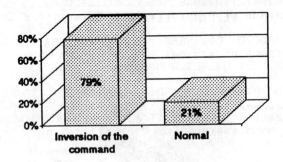

Fig.5

In 30 out of 33 cases perineal contraction was associated with contraction of the gluteus, adductor and abdomenal muscles. All women were advised to carry out a cycle of rehabilitative therapy 4-5 months after giving birth.

CONCLUSIONS

The onset of S.U.I., even in the 23 of the 88 nulliparous cases (26.1%), underlines a problem that to date has been somewhat neglected, both in terms of prevention and diagnostically. During prenatal visits the gravidae must be made aware of their perineo and the anatomy and continence mechanisms must be explained. Moreover, diagnosis of a S.U.I. in pregnancy obliges monitoring after delivery in order to verify persistence of incontinence and its relation to delivery type and weight of the neonate. Indeed a prolonged vaginal delivery and the resulting stay in the birth canal, compromise the sphincteral and supportive sistem, hence women that give birth to macrosome fetuses following prolonged vaginal delivery would seem at " higher risk". This observation is confirmed by our data (6 out of 10 incontinent pluriparous cases gave birth to macrosomes). In view of above it is our duty to invite all women, from the very first pregnancy, to answer some simple questions on the problem of incontinence and assess them from a urogynaecological point of a view, to determine cases requiring rehabilitative treatment capable of assuring continence, of preserving pelvic statics and maintaining a satisfactory sex life (1).

BIBLIOGRAFY

1 SPREAFICO L. 1990. Gravidanza-parto-puerperio: quale prevenzione pre il prolasso genitale e l'incontinenza urinaria? RIABILITAZIONE NEUROUROGINECOLOGICA p.175 Ed. Associazione di Riabilitazione Triestina 2^Ediz.

2 TAPP A., CARDOZO L., VERSI E., MONTGOMERY J., STUDD I. 1988. The effect of vaginal delivery on the urethral sphincter BR. J. OBSTET.GYNAECOL. 95 142

3 DI BENEDETTO P., FABIANI C., MOSETTI S., TAUZZI M.L. 1990. La valutazione fisiatrica perineale "preriabilitativa". RIABILITAZIONE NEUROUROGINECOLOGICA p.190. Ed. Associazione di Riabilitazione Triestina 2^Ediz.

Laparoscopic treatment of ectopic pregnancy

D. Cirillo, A. Tolino, E. Sole, A. Petrone, P. Ferrara, E. Parente, C. Rapicano and C. Nappi

Faculty of Medicine and Surgery, Obstetrics and Gynecology, University of Naples "Federico II", Naples, Italy

Introduction

Laparoscopy for the treatment of ectopic pregnancy pathologies is a primary tool for the diagnosis, since ultrasounds and the ß-HCG (1) plasma level assay alone cannot guarantee a sure diagnosis.

The evolution of laparoscopic (9) procedures both for diagnostic and therapeutic (2-8) purposes made us consider the use of laparoscopy for the surgical treatment of the extrauterine (12) pregnancy as an alternative to the traditional laparoscopic surgery.

Materials and Methods

Between March 1992 and July 1994 we treated 37 patients with ectopic pregnancy .
Out of our group of 37 patients 31 underwent a laparoscopic treatment (4) .
As concerns the other 6 patients, in three cases it was necessary to resort to emergency laparotomic surgeries because of the unstable hemodynamic conditions of the patients when we first saw them. They were in a state of shock due to the rupture of tubes and to the consequent hemoperitoneum. In all these three cases the patients for different reasons had not yet undergone an echography or a plasma ß-HCG assay, but had done only a urine pregnancy test.
As concerns the other three women, in one case the patient had amenorrhea for 12 weeks, showed a large left adnexal mass of about 5 cm and an empty uterus at the echography, her ß-HCG level was of 12,000 mIU/dl, she had blood discharge from the external genitals and pain in the left ileac fossa. Also in this case we deemed

necessary to use traditional surgery. After the laparoscopic examination revealed that the pregnancy was in the ovary and in the homolateral tube, we performed an ovariosalpingectomy.

In the other two case we did try a laparoscopic approach, but the inspection in both cases showed an irreversibly damaged tube, and we encountered serious difficulties in the maneuvers to mobilize the affected organs. As a consequence we preferred to continue by means of a laparotomy so as to avoid the risk of unnecessary bleeding.

Three different surgical techniques were used for the 31 patients treated by laparoscopy (7) .

In four cases (12.9%) the patients underwent tubal expression for the removal of the conceptus of pregnancy. To do this we increased the tubal internal pressure by means of an Aquapurator so as to detach the trophoblast from the tubal mucosa. We could use this technique in the cases of small ectopic pregnancies (no larger than 2 cm) at no later than 7 weeks of pregnancy, of course if the tube was not ruptured, if there was no bleeding and if the affected site was the infundibulum and/or the ampulla.

In 13 cases (41.9%) we performed an incision on the antimesenteric side of the tube (10). Also in these cases we produced an increase in the tubal pressure by means of an Aquapurator, then the conceptus of pregnancy was aspirated. The salpinx was left open, and we did not suture it but rather coagulated the bleeding points by means of a monopolar, thin-pointed electrocoagulator. This technique was applied to those cases whose pregnancy was slightly larger than 2 cm, with bleeding of the distal portion of the tube, which however was not ruptured.

In the other 14 cases (45.2% of the patients) we had to perform total or partial salpingectomies (8). The radical surgery was necessary for several reasons: first of all when the tube appeared ruptured at the laparoscopic inspection, even if it was only partially ruptured; in a single patient who had previously undergone tubal ligation; in those cases where, although the tube was not ruptured, during the surgical maneuvers we had abundant bleeding, which could not be otherwise controlled; and in those patients who had already undergone conservative surgery for a previous ectopic pregnancy in the same tube. We also used this technique on patients who had an history of salpingitis or who had already undergone microsurgery on the affected tube, as well as on patients who did not desire to become pregnant again.

In all salpingectomies we used a forceps applied to a bipolar electrocoagulator and a pair of scissors. We coagulated and cut the tube and the mesosalpinx, upon application of a Roeder's double snare so as to reduce the blood supply and as a consequence the bleeding as well.

Results:

All treated patients have been followed for a period of 40 - 50 days. The follow-up consisted of serial assays of plasma ß-HCG and an echography every 6 days (5 - 6).

Only one case treated by means of the tubal expression technique showed persistent levels of ß-HCG. Since we did not obtain any result from the pharmacological treatment with metotrexate , the patient underwent a partial salpingectomy, by laparoscopy again, six weeks after the first surgery.

Mainly thanks to the most accurate selection of the patients at the time of hospitalization, among our 31 patients operated on with laparoscopy we did not observe any intraoperative and/or postoperative complications such as to require laparotomy.

The average duration of laparoscopic surgeries was of about 90 minutes (range 40 - 120 min.), and not significantly different from that of laparotomic surgeries.

The hospitalization lasted 36 hours in the average, and reached 48 hours only in 7 cases, against the 5 - 7 days necessary to discharge patients treated by laparotomy. Moreover all patients treated by laparoscopy went back to work within 10 - 15 days from surgery, while patients treated by abdominal operation needed a period of convalescence of at least one month .

Discussion

Laparoscopy has been used for both the diagnosis and the treatment of many pathologies for many years now.
Today the endoscopic examination allows to dispel diagnostic doubts without submitting the patient to useless surgeries. The instruments we have available today such as the vaginal ultrasonographic imaging of the uterus and of the adnexa together with the radioimmunoassay (RIA) for the detection of the B subunit of the human chorionic gonadotropin made the early diagnosis of an ectopic pregnancy viable (3 - 5 - 6). It is possible to have a high degree of accuracy (more than 90%) in the detection of an extrauterine pregnancy at a stage where this has not yet caused damages to the tube which thus does not need to be ablated.

It is therefore preferable to diagnose an ectopic pregnancy as soon as possible, so as to have not only the possibility to preserve the tube but also to perform the surgery by endoscopic route and reduce the risk to jeopardize the future fertility of the patients treated (13). In our experience we preferred to resort to laparotomic surgery in up to 6 out of the 37 cases which came to our observation. This was because, unlike other authors (14), when the patients are in unstable hemodynamic conditions we prefer the laparotomic approach so as to avoid loosing more time. The time for the preliminary preparation required by laparoscopy (i.e. creation of a pneumoperitoneum, insertion of a trocar for the passage of instruments necessary for the surgery) could be precious to save the lives of patients who are already in a state of shock. Beyond the risks related to emergency cases, laparoscopic surgery for the treatment of ectopic pregnancy is undoubtedly becoming more and more valuable, not only to preserve the future fertility of the patients treated, but also to use a treatment for the ectopic pregnancy which costs less than the traditional surgery, and this is due to the shorter hospitalization and convalescence (11) .

Bibliography

1) Tolino A.: "Gravidanza ectopica." in "Endocrinologia Ostetrica" Ed. Ghedini, Milano - 1993

2) Churgay CA et all.: "Ectopic Pregnancy. An update on technology advances in diagnosis and treatment". Prim. Care - 1993 - Sep. 20 (3) - 629-38 (29 ref.)

3) Weckstein LN., Boucher AR., Tucker H., Gipson D., Retenmaier MA,: "Accurate diagnosis of early ectopic pregnancy." Obstes. Gynecol. 1985; 65: 393-397

4) Marchbanks PA., Annegers JF., Coulam CB., Strathy JH., Kurland LT.: "Risk factors for ectopic pregnancy: A population-based study." JAMA 1988, 259: 1823-1827

5) Kadar N., DeVore G., Romerom R.: "Discriminatory LCGzone. Its use in sonographic evaluation for ectopic pregnancy." Obstet. Gynecol. 1981; 58: 156

6) Soussis I. et all.: "Diagnosis of ectopic pregnancy by vaginal ultrasonography in combination with a discriminatory serum HCG level of 1000 IU/l" Br. J. Obstet. Gynaecol. 1991. Feb; 98(3): 233

7) Chapron C., Querleu D., Crepin G.: "Laparoscopic treatment of ectopic pregnancies: a one hundred case study." Eur. J. Obstet. Gynecol. Repr. Biol. 41 (1991): 187 - 190

8) Reich H., Johns A. D., De Caprio J., McGlynn F., Reich E.: Laparoscopic treatment of 109 consecutive ectopic pregnancies." J. Reprod. Med. 1988; 33: 885-890

9) Semm K.: "Advances in pelviscopic surgery." Curr. Probl. Obstet. Gynecol. 5:7, 1982

10) Vermesh M., Silvia P.D., Rosen G.F., Stein A.L, Fossum G.J., Sauer M.V.: "Management of unruptured ectopic gestation by linear salpingostomy: A

prospective randomized clinical trial of laparoscopy versus laparotomy." Obstet. Gynecol. 73(3) part 1. Mar. 1989: 400-404

11) Erny R., Campion-Budar M.P.: "Advantageséconomiques du traitment coelioscopique de la grossesse extra-utérine." J. Gynecol. Obstet. Biol. Reprod. 1989 - 18: 930- 932

12) Silvia P.D.: " A laparoscopi approach can be applied to most cases of ectopic pregnancy." Obstet. Gynecol 72(6) Dec. 1988

13) Meyer W.R., Decherney A.H., Diamond M.P.: "Tubal ectopic pregnancy: contemporary diagnosis, treatment and reproductive potential." J. Gynecol. Surg. 1989, 5: 343- 352

14) Soderstrom R.M.: " Physiologic considerations during anesthesia for laparoscopy." in Operative Laparoscopy Ed. Raven Press - New York.

Operative hysteroscopy and pregnancies

V. Benedetto, V. Palmara, M. Rigano, G. Zona, F.V. Ardita, J. Leonardi and R. Leonardi

Department of Gynecology, University of Messina, Italy

INTRODUCTION

The use of operative hysteroscopy has cosiderably increased during the last years.

This is due essentially to the technological improvement of instruments that has permitted to carry out a lot more operation with fewer risks. (1, 2, 3)

Hysteroscopic investigation carried out on patients with amenorrhea or secondary oligo-amenorrhea, recurrent abortion, or unexplained infertility have evidenced the frequent presence of adhesions, that were not detected by other means of investigation especially when they were of little extension and not very dense.

Various authors considered that 20% of positive false diagnosis and 35% of negative false diagnosis can be ascribed to hysterosalpingography. Without doubts, synechialisis, as in the Ascherman's syndrome, metroplastic for uterus septum, myomectomy and polypectomy have bettered fertility.

MATERIALS AND METHODS

These are the data collected between January 1988 and July 1994 at the department of hysteroscopy of the Institute of Ginecology of the University of Messina.

During that period 572 patients, aged betweeen 20 and 38 yaers, underwent hysteroscopic investigation because they were affected with sterility or infertility. (Tab. I)

The patients that had operative hysteroscopy done were 109, of these we had 27 uterine sinechiae (8 endometrial and 19 myometrial), 25 intracavitary myomas, 25 endometrial polyps, 9 complete uterus septum and 23 uterus subseptum (tab. II), 43 patients had had at leats one spontaneous miscarriage, 66 were never pregnant. (Tab. III)

We used the same surgical method described by other authors; all patients were treated by general anesthesia (13). CO_2 was used for the distension of the uterine cavity during brief operations, such as synechiae and polyps, and urologic solution (sorbitol-mannitol) for septum and myoma resections (3, 14).

An Hamou hysteroscope, of 7.5 mm., and a semi-rigid scissors were used for synechialysis and polyps; a Storz resectoscope was instead used for incomplete septum and myomectomies.

Tab.I: Total HSS

Tab. II: OPERATIVE HYSTEROSCOPY

572 patients
age >20 <38

endometrial synechiae	8
miometrial synechiae	19
intracavitary myomas	25
endometrial polyps	25
complete uterus septum	9
uterus subseptum	23
total	109

Tab.III: PREVIOUS PREGNANCIES IN 109 WOMEN SUBMITTED TO OPERATIVE HS

43 > 1 miscarriage
66   0 pregnancies

POST-OPERATIVE FOLLOW UP

Different authors have a different therapeutic treatment during the pre- and post-operative period; some recommend antibiotic treatment (15), others a cycle therapy with Danazol or with LH-RH agonist (16) or substitive hormone therapy with conjugate extrogens and medrossiprogesterone, others apply an intra-uterine device. (10, 15, 17)

We preferred the prescription of antibiotic therapy for a brief period, a hysteroscopic folow up a month after operation and a hysterosalpingography if there had been septum-lysis.

OBSTETRIC HYSTORY

The results obtained were encouraging; after synechialisis, we had 16 pregnancies with a 50.25 % conception rate, 10 pregnancies with alive and vital fetuses (of these 8 at term, 1 at 36 weeks an 1 at 34 weeks), that is 37 % of the treated cases. (Tab. IV)

After the treatment of myomas and polyps, we had 29 pregancies with a 58 % conception rate, 20 pregancies with alive and vital fetuses (of these 16 at term, 2 at 36 weeks, 1 at 34 weeks and 1 a 33 weeks), that is 40 % of the treated cases. (Tab. V)

The case treated for incomplete septum were 23 and we had 9 pregancies with a 39 % conception rate, 5 pregnancies with alive and vital fetuses, that is 21.74 % (of these 3 at term, 1 at 35 weeks and 1 at 33 weeks). (Tab. VI)

We had 3 pregnancies among the women with complete septum, that is 33 % conception rate, with 2 alive and vital births, that is 22.2 % of the treated cases (of these 1 at 34 weeks and 1 at 33 weeks). (Tab. VII)

CONCLUSIONS

Hysteroscopy should be without doubt considered preferible to traditional surgery in laparotomy, considering that during the last years, the technological improvements have been remarkable and have thus transformed it from a simply diagnostic technique into a therapeutic method.

The data that we find in literature and our own experience show that the treatment in hysteroscopy gives very good results, above all in those cases chosen for their patology correlated with infertility-sterility.

Tab. IV: <u>PREGNANCIES IN 27 WOMEN AFTER HYSTEROSCOPY SYECHIAE LYSIS</u>

16 pregnancies = 59,26 %
    * 6 miscarriage
    *10 alive and vital fetuses = 37 % of treated cases
        - 8 at term
        - 1 at 36 weeks
        - 1 at 34 weeks

Tab. V: <u>PREGNANCIES IN 50 WOMEN AFTER MYOMECTOMY AND POLYPECTOMY HYSTEROSCOPIC RESECTIONS</u>

myomectomy 25
              } 29 pregnancies = 58 %
polypectomy 25
  * 9 miscarriage
  * 20 alive and vital fetuses = 40 % of treated cases
        - 16 at term
        - 2 at 36 weeks
        - 1 at 34 weeks
        - 1 at 33 weeks

Tab. VI: <u>PREGNANCIES IN 23 WOMEN AFTER INCOMPLETE SEPTUM RESECTION</u>

pregnancies 9 = 39 %
* 4 miscarriage
* 5 alive and vital fetuses = 21,74 % of treated cases
        - 4 at term
        - 1 at 35 weeks
        - 1 at 33 weeks

Tab. VII: <u>PREGNANCIES IN 9 WOMEN AFTER COMPLETE SEPTUM RESECTION</u>

pregnancies 3 = 33,3 %
* 1 miscarriage
* 2 alive and vital fetuses = 22,2 % of treated cases
        - 1 at 34 weeks
        - 1 at 33 weeks

REFERENCES

1 Edstrom K. (1974): Intrauterine surgical procedures during hystreroscopy. Endoscopy 6: 175,
2 Gallinat A. (1984): Hysteroscopy as a diagnostic and therapeutic procedure in "Hysteroscopy: principles and practice", Edited by AM Siegler, HJ Lindemann, Philadelphia, Lilpinccott publisher, p. 180.
3 Hamou J.E.: Mencaglia L., Perino A., Gilardi G.(1988): L'electroresection en hysteroscopie et microcolpohysteroscopie operatoire. In "Isteroscopia operativa e laser chirurgia in ginecologia", Edited by E.Cittadini, G. Scarselli, L. Mencaglia, A. Perino, Roma, CIC Edizioni Intmazionali Publisher, p. 31.
4 Hamou J., Salat-Baroux J., Siegler AM. (1983): Diagnosis and treatment of intrauterine adhesions by microcolhysteroscopy. Fertilm Steril 39: 231.
5 March C.M., Israel R. (1987): Hysteroscopic management of recurrent abortion caused by septate uterus. Amer J Obstet Gynecol 156: 834.

6 Rock J.A., Jones H.W. jr (1977): The clinical management of the double uterus. Fertil Steril 28: 798,
7 Neuwrth R.S (1983): Hysteroscopic management of symptomatic submucosus fibroids. Obstet Gynecol 62: 509.
8 Mencaglia L., Tantini C., Bucci L., Noci I., Chelo E., Scarselli G. (1983): Correlazione tra dati isterosalpingografici ed isteroscopici in un gruppo selezionato di pazienti infertili. In "Fertilità e sterilità ", edited by P.G. Grossignani, Bologna, Monduzzi Publisher, p. 15.
9 Siegler A.M. (1977): Hysterography and hysteroscopy in the infertile patients. J reprod Med 18: 143.
10 Mencaglia L., Tantini C., Bargelli G., Noci I., Scarselli G. (1983): Trattamento e follow up delle sinechie uterine per via isteroscopica. In "Fertilità e sterilita" , edited by P.G. Grossignani, Bologna, Monduzzi Publisher, p. 491.
11 Hamou J., Mencaglia L., Perino A., Catinella E., Pertronio M., Tommasino ML. (1987):Diagnosi e trattamento isteroscopico delle sinechie intrauterine. In "atti del II corso di aggiornamento di Microcolpoisterocopia". Edited by G. De Placido, A Perino, N. Colacurci, L. Mencaglia, Palermo COFESE Publisher, p. 53.
12 De Cherney A.H., Russel J.B., Graeb R.A., Polan L.M. (1986): Resectoscopic management of mullerian fusion defects. Fertil Steril 45: 726.
13 Valle R.F., Sciarra J.J. (1986: Hysteroscopic treatment of the septed uterus. Obst. Gynecol 67: 253.
14 Chevernak F.A., Neuwirth R.S. (1981): Hysteroscopic resection of the uterine sptum. Amer. J. Obst. Gyn. 141:35.
15 Rock J.A., Murphy A.A., Cooper W.H. (1987): Resectoscopy tecniques for the lysis of a class V complete uterine septum. Fertil Steril 48: 495, 1987.
16 Corson S.L., Batzer F.R. (1986): CO_2 uterin distenzion for hysteroscopic septal incision. J. Reprod Med 31: 710.
17 Daly D., Mayer D. (1987): One to six yaer follow up of hysteroscopic metroplasy. Presented at the Forthy-Third Annual Meeting of the American fertility Society, Reno, Amer Fertil Soc Programm Supplement, p. 13.

Microalbuminuria and PIH

G. Menato, M. Anzivino, P. Petruzzelli, B. Masturzo, M. Massobrio and Q. Carta*

Università degli Studi di Torino, Clinica Ostetrica e Ginecologica, Ospedale Mauriziano "Umberto I" and *Divisione di Diabetologia, Ospedale Maggiore "S. Giovanni Battista", Turin, Italy

INTRODUCTION

Microalbuminuria may be defined as the persistent subclinical elevation of urinary albumin excretion, below that of dipstick detection but above that of the normal range (30 - 300 mg/24 hours) (1).

Proteinuria is a late sign of the development of preeclampsia, but it is one of its characteristic features. With the recent development of a radioimmunoassay for the detection of albuminuria, it is now possible to detect minimal elevations in albumin excretion that would have gone unnoticed in the past. These methods have proven useful in the early diagnosis of nephrological changes, and microalbuminuria has been shown to be predictive of clinical nephropathy in insulin-dependent diabetics (1).

It has been strongly suggested that pregnant women destined to develop hypertension may show an elevation of albumin excretion before the clinical manifestations, although few studies have fully examined the significance of the microalbuminuria as a predictor of pregnancy induced hypertension (PIH) (2, 3, 4, 5).

The purpose of this study was to investigate whether the presence of microalbuminuria in normotensive pregnant women at risk for hypertension could predict the subsequent development of PIH.

MATERIAL AND METHODS

We studied longitudinally 32 normotensive pregnant women comparable for alimentary habits. The samples were taken between 10 and 12 weeks, 20 and 30 weeks, and finally 31 and 41 weeks of gestation. No woman was given either antihypertensive drugs or preventive treatment (calcium, magnesium, ASA).

All women were at risk for PIH according to the following criteria: 13 nulliparous, 8 women more than 35 years old, 5 obeses, 2 with twin pregnancies, 4 with familiar history for hypertension.

The patients were submitted to several analyses: plasma concentration of urea, creatinine and uric acid, blood creatinine and urea clearances and finally urine concentration of albumin. The hematochemical parameters were evaluated through colorimetric method.

The urinary samples for the evaluation of microalbuminuria were collected with the "overnight method" during three following nights. Urine was collected in special box containing 1 gr. of sodioazide as antifermentative agent.

Week-end nights were avoided in order to better standardize the urinary collection, expecially in relation to body exercise and nutrition. The women were requested to report the evening time of the start and the morning time of the end of urine collection.

All the urinary samples were tested with albustix to exclude the presence of clinical proteinuria and submitted to white blood cell count to exclude urinary infections. The urinary albumin excretion was measured using an antibody radioimmunoassay technique (R.I.A.), using the "Pharmacia Albumin , RIA 100" kit. The urinary albumin excretion was measured as Albumin Excretion Rate (AER) in $\mu g/min$.

All the pregnant women were submitted to 24 hours blood pressure monitoring, using Beta-Pressing, 203 Y MII machine. The blood pressure values were elaborated through the population mean cosinor method.

Statistical analyses was performed by the impaired Student's t test and the receiver operator curve of microalbuminuria was calculated.

RESULTS

Eleven out of the 32 examined pregnant women developed PIH without clinical proteinuria. During the third trimester the systolic blood pressure mesor was 96.2 ± 4 mmHg in 21 normotensive pregnant women, while in the pregnant women who developed PIH it was 121.5 ± 2 mmHg The dyastolic blood pressure mesor was 64.9 ± 2 mmHg in normotensive pregnant women and 85.5 ± 1.3 mmHg in the PIH patients. There was a significant difference ($p<0.001$) for systolic and dyastolic mesor in the two groups of patients. The table 1 presents the data about renal function between the 20 -30 weeks of gestation in the two groups. The figure 1 and the table 2 report the mean and standard deviation values of the microalbuminuria during the three trimesters of pregnancy in healty pregnant women and in the patients in whom PIH developed, while the single values of AER are shown in figure 2. The microalbuminuria values in patients developing PIH were significantly higher, already during the first and even more in the second and third trimester of pregnancy, when compared to those of healty pregnant women (tab. 2). On the other hand microalbuminuria rised significantly during pregnancy within each group (fig. 1). With the use of the receiver operator curve, four different threshold values of microalbuminuria (3, 4, 5, 6 ug/min) as predictive for the subsequent development of PIH were chosen (fig. 3). Then sensitivity and specificity for each of these cut-off is shown in figure 3.

DISCUSSION

Several reports indicate that the increased albumin excretion in the normal pregnancy is due to a raise of glomerular filtration (6, 7). According to others the increase in protein excretion is due to the reduction in the tubular reabsorbtive capacity (8, 9).

Preeclampsia can cause changes in virtually all organs, most notably the cardiovascular, renal, hematologic and immunologic systems. Some of these changes are present before the clinical diagnosis of preeclampsia (10). Proteinuria is a common feature of varius forms of hypertension and renal disorders. Minimally increased excretion of albumin is not generally measurable by the dipstick method, which is the test ordinarily used to screen for proteinuria. Such sligthly increased excretion of albumin has

	Diuresis	BCC	BUC	creat.	urea	uricemia
	cc.	ml/min	ml/min	mg/dl	mg/dl	mg/dl
Normotensive (n=21)	1600 ± 425	135.1 ± 18	60.2 ± 15	0.5 ± 0.18	15 ± 6.4	3.6 ± 1.3
PIH (n=11)	1400 ± 460	125.3 ± 13	58.1 ± 18	0.8 ± 0.11	30 ± 8.2	5.7 ± 2.1
					p < 0.02	p < 0.01

Tab. 1 : Renal function parameters between 20-30 weeks of gestation in normal pregnancy and PIH

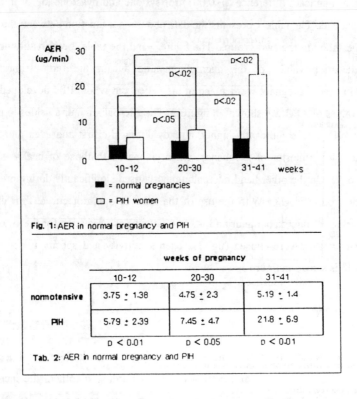

Fig. 1: AER in normal pregnancy and PIH

	weeks of pregnancy		
	10-12	20-30	31-41
normotensive	3.75 ± 1.38	4.75 ± 2.3	5.19 ± 1.4
PIH	5.79 ± 2.39	7.45 ± 4.7	21.8 ± 6.9
	p < 0.01	p < 0.05	p < 0.01

Tab. 2: AER in normal pregnancy and PIH

been shown to be predictive for the subsequent development of clinical nephropathy in insulin-dependent diabetic patients (2).

Some studies failed to pointed out a significant difference in the urinary excretion between PIH patients and normal pregnant women (2, 3); other authors, in accordance to our results, indicated a significative increase in AER of women who will develope PIH (11, 4).

We observed a significant raise of the microalbuminuria mean levels during the three trimesters of pregnancy in both the healty pregnant women and in the PIH patients,

668

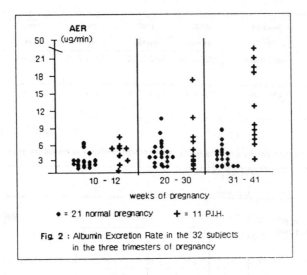

Fig. 2 : Albumin Excretion Rate in the 32 subjects
in the three trimesters of pregnancy

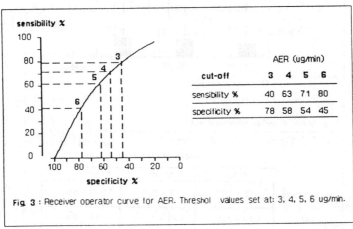

Fig. 3 : Receiver operator curve for AER. Threshol values set at: 3, 4, 5, 6 ug/min.

although these values always remained in the normal range for women out of pregnancy (AER= 20-200 µg/min).

Rodriguez observed an urine albumin concentration ≥ 11 µg/ml in 5 of out 10 patients in whom preeclampsia developed, but the sensitivity of the test was only 50% and specificity 82% (2).

In our study a significant difference in AER between normal pregnant women and women developing PIH already in the first trimester was observed. It confirms that changes in renal function are present in some otherwise symptom-free patients in whom PIH will develop. Unfortunately, due to the great variability of AER values in both normal pregnancy and PIH, our results didn't evidence a cut-off value of AER able to clearly discriminate the women destined to develop PIH before the clinical signs appear. However our data suggest that AER may be used as a quantitative and objective parameter for monitoring therapy or control of PIH.

REFERENCES

1. Viberti G. et al. (1988). Aetiology and prognostic significance of albuminuria in diabetes. *Diabetes Care*, **11**, 840.

2. Rodriguez M.H., Masaki D.I., Mestman J., Kumar D., Rude R. (1988). Calcium/creatinine ratio and microalbuminuria in the prediction of preeclampsia. *Am. J. Obstet. Gynaecol*, **159**, 1452.

3. Konstantin-Hansen K.F., Hesseldahl H. and Pedersen S.M. (1992). Microalbuminuria as a predictor of preeclampsia. *Acta Obstet. Gynecol. Scand*, **71**, 343.

4. Nakamura T,, Yoshimura M.I., Mabe K. and Okamura H. (1992). Usefulness of the urinary microalbumin/creatinine ratio in predicting pregnancy-induced hypertension. *Int. J. Gynecol. Obstet.*, **37**, 99.

5. Wright A., Steel P., Bennett J. R., Watts G., Polak A. (1987). The urinary excretion of albumin in normal pregnancy. *British J. of Obstetrics and Gynaecology*, **94**, 408.

6. McCance D.R., Traub A.I. et al. (1989). Urinary albumin excretion in diabetic pregnancy. *Diabetologia*, **32**, 236.

7. Biesenbach G., Zazgornik J. (1989). Incidence of transient nephrotic syndrom during pregnancy in diabetic women with and without pre-exsisting microalbuminuria. *Br. Med. J.*, **299**, 366.

8. Beetham R. et al. (1988). Urinary excretion of albumin and retinol binding protein during normal pregnancy. *J. Clin. Pathol.*, **41**, 1089.

9. Gero G., Anthony F., Rowe D.J.F., Dennis K.J. (1986). Increased urinary excretion of retinol- binding protein during normal pregnancies. *Clin. Chem.*, **32**, 916.

10. Gant N.F., Daley G.L., Chand S., Whalley P.J., MacDonald P.C. (1973). A study of angiotensin II pressor response throughout primigravid pregnancy. *J. Clin. Invest.*, **52**, 2682.

11. Misiani R., Marchesi D., Tiraboschi G., Gualandris L., Pagni R., Goglio G., Amuso G., Muratore D., Bertuletti P., Massazza M. (1991). Urinary albumin excretion in normal pregnancy and pregnancy-induced hypertension. *Nephron*, **59**, 416.

Obstetric management of PROM

F. Polatti, F. Perotti, C. Belloni*, U. Maccarini, N. Filippa, M. Ciccarese and A. Catinella

Institute of Obstetrics and Gynecology and *Neonatal Intensive Care "S. Matteo" Hospital, IRCCS, Pavia, Italy

INTRODUCTION

Premature rupture of the membranes (PROM) is clearly associated with perinatal morbidity and mortality. Maternal risks are in relation with the degree of infection (amnionitis, post-partum infections), fetal and neonatal ones include preterm delivery, anoxia, respiratory distress syndrome (RDS), polmonary hypoplasia, skeletal deformities, umbilical cord prolapse and anomalous presentations.

PROM percentage varies from 3 to 18.5% of all deliveries, in relation to heterogeneity of casistics, imprecision of some diagnostic methods and doubs about the definition of PROM.

Aethiology of PROM is unknown, but many factors have been related to this disease: cervico-vaginal infections, multiple gestations, polyhydramnios, traumas, cervical incontinence, previous PROM, repeated vaginal explorations, anomalous presentations, ascorbic acid deficit and low socio-economic level.

In 80-90% of pregnant women at term uterine contractions arise within 24 hours from PROM: PROM-Delivery latency period tends to rise in early gestational age and in nulliparous women.

PROM exposes fetus to three types of complications: those related with prematurity (with RDS risk in those cases that take place before 35th week of gestational age), with bacteriological infections (especially when PROM-Delivery latency period is higher than 24 hours) and with olygohydramnios (because of compression of umbilical cord or polmonary hypoplasia).

In all cases of PROM, treatment will have to consider on one hand the possible consquences of prematurity, on the other hand the potential infectious risks, performing a conservative treatment before 35 weeks of gestational age (period of complete pulmonar maturation) and an interventionist one after this period

MATERIALS AND METHODS

In the period 1990-1994 we studied 99 patients with PROM between 23 and 35 weeks of gestation, subdivided in three groups according to their gestational age:

GROUP A (35 Pts): 23 <= wks <= 29
GROUP B (28 Pts): 30 <= wks <= 32
GROUP C (36 Pts): 33 <= wks <= 35
All patients received careful in-hospital surveillance and underwent to:
- vaginal exploration and evaluation of Bishop's Score
- vaginal swab + ABG (every 2 days)
- WC + LF, ESV and RCP (every 2 days)
- maternal temperature
- CTG monitoring (every 12 hours for 20 minutes)
- foetal biometry and evaluation of Amniotic Fluid Index (once a week)
- fluximetry (twice a week).
Whenever possible we used an expectant mangement with use of antibiotics (specific therapy in case of vaginal colture positive for Group B Streptococcus, Klebsiella, Pseudomonas and E.Coli, antibiotic prophylaxis with Ampicillin 1gr x3/day for 7 days in the other cases), tocolytic treatment with Beta-mimethic (Ritodrine 5 ml iv. in physiological solution 250 cc. every 8 h.) and RDS prophylaxis (Betamethasone 12 mg im. every 24 h. in 2 administrations every 10 days).
An active management (cesarean section) was adopted only for obstetric indication (twin pregnancy, breech presentation, malformed foetuses) or in presence of at least two of the following pathological findings: anidramnios, decelerations at CTG, maternal fever and leucocytosis, pathological fluximetry.

RESULTS AND DISCUSSION

Table 1 shows the latency period PROM-Delivery in every group of patients, related to type of delivery (eutocic or cesarean section). All Group C patients delivered within 48 hours from PROM.

Group A: 35 Pts with PROM between 23 and 29 wks

Time (hours)	T <=48	48 <= T <= 96	T > 96*
# Pts	15	4	16
Eutocic	26.6%	75%	56.2%
Cesarean Section (obst. indication)	73.3% (27.2%)	25% (100%)	43.7% (71%)

*T = 17.3 +/- 13.4 days

Group B: 30 Pts with PROM between 30 and 32 wks

Time (hours)	<=48	48 <= T <= 96	T > 96*
# Pts	18	3	7
Eutocic	27.7%	25%	28.5%
Cesarean Section (obst. indication)	72.2% (53%)	75% (100%)	71% (60%)

*T = 19.2 +/- 9.0 days

Group C: 36 Pts with PROM between 33 and 35 wks

Latency	T <= 48 hours
Eutocic	78.7%
Cesarean	30.3%

Tab. 1

Table 2 correlates the incidence of neonatal RDS with maternal corticosteroid prophylaxis which we considered "complete" only when delivery followed within 24 hours from the 2nd corticosteroid administration.

	"Complete"Corticosteroid Prophylaxis	RDS
Group A (35 Pts)	20 Pts (57.1%)	35%
Group B (28 Pts)	10 Pts (35.7%)	--
Group C (36 Pts)	--	--

Tab.2

Correlations between the number of positive vaginal swabs, latency period and gestational age are showed in table 3: it's evident a positive relation between percentage of vaginal colonization and increase of latency period.

Group A: 35 Pts between 23 and 29 wks

# + Vaginal Swabs	#1	#2	#3	%	% + at delivery
T <= 48 h.	4	1	0	26.3%	100%
T > 48 h.	6	3	3 (+ at delivery)	75%	25%

Group B: 28 Pts between 30 and 32 wks

# + Vaginal Swabs	#1	#2	#3	%	% + at delivery
T <= 48 h.	7	0	0	33.3%	100%
T > 48 h.	0	4	2	85.7%	0%

Group C: 36 Pts between 33 and 35 wks

# + Vaginal Swabs	#1	#2	#3	%	% + at delivery
T <= 48 h.	10	0	0	27.7%	100%

Tab. 3

The cut-off used for evaluation of neonatal Apgar Score (at 5th minute) was 7: table 4 illustrates its correlations with maternal gestational age of PROM.

Group A

Apgar Score (5th. min.)	<= 7	>7
# Pts.	12	23
X +/- S.D.	6.0 +/- 1.2	8.9 +/- 0.79

Group B

Apgar Score (5th. min.)	<= 7	>7
# Pts.	1	27
X +/- S.D.	6.0	8.42 +/- 0.5

Group C

Apgar Score (5th. min.)	<= 7	>7
# Pts.	1	35
X +/- S.D.	7.0	9.42 +/- 0.6

Tab. 4

Premature rupture of membranes prior to 35 weeks of gestation is associated with a high risk of perinatal mortality and morbidity. The main risk for the fetus is related to prematurity.

The aim of the study was to prolong the latency period PROM-Delivery, in order to decrease the risk of neonatal RDS. Consequently, it was necessary to prevent onset of vaginal infections and accurately evaluate all the paramethers useful for early identification of fetal well-being alterations (CTG, amniotic fluid index, fluximetry).

The results of the study (good perinatal outcome), in agreement with most of the recent investigations, confirm the validity of expectant management for the treatment of PROM: systematic use of tocolysis, corticosteroid prophylaxis (especially between 30 and 35 weeks) and antibiotics has strongly decreased the risks of neonatal RDS and feto-maternal infections.

REFERENCES

Christmas J.T., Cox S.M., Andrews W. et al.
Expectant management of preterm ruptured membranes: effects of antimicrobial therapy.
Obstet. Gynecol., 1992; 80: 759-762.

Crowley P., Chalmers I., Keirse M.J.
The effect of corticosteroid administration before preterm delivery: an overwiew of the evidence from controlled trials.
Br. J. Obstet. Gynecol., 1990; 97: 11-25.

Dowd J., Sci B.M., Permezel M.
Pregnancy outcome following preterm premature rupture of the membranes at less than 26 weeks' gestation.
Aust. N. Z. J. Obstet. Gynecol., 1992; 32, 2: 120-24.

Egan D., O'Herlihy C.
Expectant management of spontaneous rupture of the membranes at term.
J. Obstet. Gynecol., 1988; 243-247.

Guise J.M., Duff P., Christian J.S.
Mangement of term patients with premature rupture of membranes and an unfavorable cervix.
Am. J. Perinatol., 1992; 9, 1: 56-60.

Higby K., Xenakis E., Pauerstein C.J.
Do tocolytic agents stop preterm labour? A critical and cprehensive rewiew of efficacy and safety.
Am. J. Obstet. Gynecol., 1993; 168: 1247-59.

Kurky T., Hallman M., Zilliacus R. et al.
Premature rupture of the membranes: effect of penicillin prophylaxis and long term outcome of the children.
Am. J. Perinatol., 1992; 1: 11-16.

Joinston M., Sanchez-Ramos L. et al.
Antibiotic therapy in preterm premature rupture of membranes: a randomized, prospective, double blind trial.
Am. J. Obstet. Gynecol., 1990; 163: 743-747.

Morales W.J., Angel J.L., O'Brien W.F. et al.
Use of ampicillin and corticosteroids in premature rupture of membranes: a randomized study.
Obstet. Gynecol., 1989; 73: 721-726.

Ohlsson A.
Treatment of preterm premature rupture of the membranes: a meta-analysis.
Am. J. Obstet. Gynecol., 1989; 160: 890-906.

Vintzileos A., Bors-Koefoed R. et al.
The use of fetal biophysical profile improves pregnancy outcome in premature rupture of the membranes.
Am. J. Obstet. Gynecol., 1987; 157: 236-240.

Infections of the
Lower Genital Tract

Sexually transmitted diseases and infertility: a global perspective

G. Benagiano and P. Rowe

UNDP/UNFPA/WHO/World Bank Special Programme of Research Development and Research Training in Human Reproduction, Geneva, Switzerland

Current estimates evaluate infertility worldwide as affecting between 20 and 40 million couples. The WHO standardized investigation of the infertile couple, which involved more than 10,000 couples in 33 centres in 25 countries, has shown that in women hormonal causes of infertility account for about one third of all cases, infertility resulting from pelvic infection another third, whereas in the remaining third no cause for infertility can be found.

With regard to infertility caused by infection, when the small number of women with pelvic tuberculosis are excluded, the remainder have acquired their condition from infection by a sexually transmitted organism. In most cases, the organisms are the *Gonococcus* or *Chlamydia*. Thus, the relationship between sexually transmitted diseases (STDs) and infertility is well established and widely recognized. What is less known is the extent of the problem and its major consequences in the developing countries of the world.

Indeed, four-fifths of the world's couples have no possibility to accede to Assisted Reproduction Technologies (ART), which means that tubal obstruction in the female partner, or post-infection testicular, vasal or accessory gland damage in the male represent, for all practical purposes, untreatable causes of infertility for them.

679

Since many cases of infertility are preventable, and infertility in general is a condition that requires sophisticated - and hence expensive - facilities for diagnosis and treatment, a cost-effective intervention must concentrate on prevention. For this reason, information regarding prevalence, diagnosis, and treatment of female genital tract infections is vital to any strategy wishing to decrease the burden of infertility worldwide. Concurrently, it is also important to know the prevalence of infertility in different populations and establish the link with prevalence of STDs in the same communities.

The situation is very serious in certain parts of the world: in sub-Saharan Africa, for instance, up to two thirds of women who have never been pregnant can ascribe their infertility to previous pelvic infections.

Both *Chlamydia trachomatis* and *Neisseria gonorrhoea* cause salpingitis and pelvic infection resulting in tubal occlusion, pelvic adhesions, infertility and chronic pelvic pain, but *Chlamydia* apparently causes more severe subclinical inflammation and subsequent tubal damage than other agents. There have only been twelve studies in developing countries on chlamydial antibody detection and these suggest that the relative contributions of chlamydial and gonococcal infection to tubal disease are probably different from industrialized countries, with a higher proportion of past gonococcal disease.

Chlamydia and *Neisseria* are not the sole causative organisms in acute salpingitis. In a study involving 50 women with acute PID, *Neisseria gonorrhoea* was isolated in 12%, *Chlamydia trachomatis* in 4%, and other pathogens in 20%. Many of these other pathogens are also implicated in bacterial vaginosis and to date there is very little information available on the prevalence of this condition in developing countries. Further research is needed to establish its role in upper genital tract infection as well as the risk markers for lower genital tract infection.

The probability of tubal blockage resulting from infection increases from approximately 17% after one episode to more than 60% with three episodes even if they are treated. In an ongoing study of subsequent fertility of women admitted to hospital with clinically suspected pelvic infection, 244 cases have been recruited and are being followed up for up to five years after their hospitalization. Initial results suggest that fertility, up to 24 months after the original hospitalization, is adversely affected to a degree which is proportional to the severity of the disease.

These data indicate that, to prevent infertility, it is essential to decrease the prevalence and severity of STDs. Unfortunately, the clinical diagnosis of salpingitis is not easy and the diagnosis of chlamydial salpingitis requires direct visual inspection of the internal pelvic organs through laparoscopy and the positive culture of the chlamydial organism. Moreover, to culture *Chlamydia* is difficult even under well controlled laboratory conditions.

A new, simple, diagnostic blood test, which will greatly simplify the diagnosis of acute chlamydial infection of the female genital tract and a similar urinary test for men are being developed. Their widespread utilization will help in the prevention of the infection that is considered today as the major cause of obstructive infertility.

Molecular applications in the diagnosis of sexually transmitted diseases

M. Comar*,** and S. Guaschino**

*I.C.G.E.B. and **Clinica Ostetrica e Ginecolgica, I.R.C.C.S. 'Burlo Garofolo', Trieste, Italy

Sexually transmitted disease (STD) are the most frequently reported bacterial infection.

In 1990 slightly more than 700000 cases of gonococcal disease were reported to the centres for disease control and the estimated annual incidence of chlamydial infections is 3 to 4 million .

Thanks to effective control measures gonorrhea, syphilis, and chancroid are all decreasing in the industrialzed countries.

In contrast, there has not been any decrease in these three bacterial STDs in the third world.

With improved control of gonorrhea, genital chlamydial infections have emerged as the major bacterial STD in the developed countries and recent studies have found an incresed risk of premature delivery in pregnant women with chlamydial infections.

It seems certain that failure to control chlamydial infections has been due mainly to problems with case finding.

Diagnostic testing and screening by isolation of the organism in tissue culture are not widely available, or are too expensive where available, and tracing of contacts of patients with clinical evidence of chlamydial infection has had a low priority.

However, with the advent of technically simpler immunodiagnostic and molecular methods for diagnosis of chlamidial infection, the prospect for better control of these infections is good.

Sexually trasmitted infections with viruses such as herpes simplex virus (HSV), human papilloma virusses (HPV), hepatitis B virus (HBV), and human immunodeficiency virus (HIV-1) are incresing in incidence and importance and are becaming more common than the traditional bacterial STDs in developed countries.

The late sequelae of STDs include ectopic pregnancy, infertility, and a variety of cancers, probably related to genital infections with HPV; hepatocellular carcinoma due to HBV; Kaposi's sarcoma and B cell lymphomas related to AIDS. As these complications arise at various and prolonged time following acquisation of infection, an effective, accurate and sensitive diagnosis is required.

Many of the new methods of biotechnology have been applied very early to the diagnosis of STDs.

Monoclonal antibodies and/or DNA probes have already been developed and tested for diagnosis of infections due to a varayety of STD pathogens including HIV-1/2 and other retroviruses such as HTLV1-2.

Morover, molecular techniques have been used to enhance serologic techniques by use of cloned proteins and recombinant antigens.

The application of recombinant DNA methods for diagnosis of infectious disease has been most extensively explored for viral and some bacterial infectious where current methods are cumbersome and results are delayed and at least, they can replace current microbial growth methods if cost-effectiveness, speed, and precision requirements can be met.

Filter in situ hybridization, which had been used for detection of acute and chronic herpes infection in tissues or cultered cells and for HPV detection in fresh and formaline fixed tissues , is now thought to be non specific and insensitive.

Dot-blot Dna hybridization assay suffer to low sensitivity and also Southern blot DNA hybridization has demostrated poor reproducibility of results and has a variable sensitivity that is highly dependet on the adequacy of the cervical cell samples.

In this regard, the capability of enzymatically amplifying specific pathogen DNA sequences using PCR may prove useful.

In fact, the ability of an infectious disease diagnostic test to detect very small amounts of pathogen in clinical sample is crucial in determining clinical sensitivity.

The use of short oligonucleotides based on conserved regions to prime amplification of as-yet uncharacterized sequences related to known groups of viruses, as well the ability to ampify and detect rare pathogen sequences in the present of a vast excess of host nucleic acids, illustrates the broad potential of PCR for clinical diagnosis.

By incorporating molecular amplification, the sensitivity for detecting sexually trasmitted infections has become markedly enhanced, and organism that were difficult or impossible to cultivate, such as human papillomavirus or Treponema pallidum can now be detected and monitored.

PCR has rapidly became established as one of the most widely used techniques of molecular biology, and with good reason; it is a rapid, inexpensive, and simple means of producing microgram amounts of DNA from minute quantities of source material and is relatively tolerant of poor quality template .

PCR shows sensitivity and specificity of 100% if comparable to other enymatic or hybridization techniques and, due to its high sensitivity level, it is possible to detect one molecule in very low concentration of nucleic acids extracted from biologicol samples.

This methodology can be used not only to detect the presence of a specific target sequence, but also to provide a quantitative evaluation of the number of copies present in the sample.(Competitive PCR).

The competitive PCR technique involves the coamplification of the sample with a reference template (competitor) sharing most of the sequence with the target and differing in site.

Since the amount of competitor added is know the amount of target can be easily derived.

This approach permitting the absolute quantification of DNA and RNA species , may be useful to a better understanding of the pathogenic steps of most viral disease and for a precise monitoring of patients treated with current therapy.

The detection of tnfectious disease pathogens has been revolutionized by the use of specific nucleic acid hybridization probes. In particular, PCR has helped realize the potential of clinical DNA based diagnosis by producing enough of the target sequence so that a powerful methods for pathogen's detection and identification can be employed also for retrospective molecular studies.

DNA technology and its molecular tools allow important clinical applications, better diagnose, treat, and more effectively control of sexually trasmitted disease spread .

Cervicitis and vaginitis in elderly women diagnosed by the Papanicolaou smear

V.G. Gandulfo, J.B. Silva and N.R. Pereira

Divisão de Endocrinologia Ginecológica e Climatério, Departamento de Ginecologia e Ostetrícia e Departamento de Patologia, Universidade de Brasília, Brasil

Cervicitis and vaginitis are common problems aflicting women of all ages and are the main reason for visits to gynecologists (1). The vaginal microecology consists on a delicate equilibrium sustained by the interaction between host (as represented by the vaginal epithelial wall and secretions) and flora. Slight shifts may stand for the difference from a physiologic to a diseased state (2-3). Frequent agents found to be responsible for cervicitis and vaginitis are yeasts (4-5), *Trichomonas vaginalis* (6), *Gardnerella vaginalis* (7), human papillomavirus (8), *Chlamydia trachomatis* (9), and nonspecific bacteria (7,10).

An endogenous factor that has profound effects on the vaginal equilibrium is ovarian failure, which results in reduction in the production of glycogen and in the lactobacilli population, epithelial atrophy and rising of the vaginal pH (2,10). It is known that, as a consequence, the vagina tends to become colonized by bacteria of fecal type (10). On the other hand, little has been determined about the influence of the shift from a pre to a post-menopausal state on the incidence of the agents previously presented.

This retrospective study, based on the Papanicolaou smear as the screening method, was designed to evaluate the relationship between increasing age and those infectious agents.

MATERIAL AND METHODS

The results of 24830 Papanicolaou smears collected from women 35 to 59 years old, attending gynecologic visits at the Hospital Universitário de Brasília, during a ten year period (1984 - 1993), were revised.

The cytologic criteria for diagnosis of infections were: identification of pseudo-hyphae (yeasts); identification of "clue" cells (*Gardnerella vaginalis*); identification of tricomonads (*Trichomonas vaginalis*); presence of transformed lymphocytes and increased histiocytes, and/or identification of metaplastic or endocervical cells bearing cytoplasmic inclusions (*Chlamydia trachomatis*); coilocytosis, dysceratosis

(HPV); identification of cocci bacteria and inflammation, in the absence of specific agents (nonspecific bacteria).

Smears collected as post-treatment controls were excluded.

Patientes were divided into groups according to age: G1 = 35 - 39 (8601 patients); G2 = 40 - 44 (6546 patients); G3 = 45 - 49 (4935 patients); G4 = 50 - 54 (3065 patients); G5 = 55 - 59 (1683 patients).

Statistical analysis was carried out with the Chi-square test.

RESULTS

Among the 24830 Pap smears, nonspecific bacteria was found in 30.2%, *Trichomonas vaginalis* in 12.4%, *Candida albicans* in 7.2%, *Gardnerella vaginalis* in 7.0%, *Chlamydia trachomatis* in 1.9%, and human papillomavirus in 1.0% (Table 1).

Table 1 Cumulative prevalence of infectious agents (1984 - 1993)

AGENTS	PREVALENCE	
	n	%
Nonspecific bacteria	7518	30.2
Trichomonas	3097	12.4
Candida	1806	7.2
Gardnerella	1746	7.0
Chlamydia	474	1.9
HPV	265	1.0

n, number of patients; HPV, human papillomavirus.

In all age groups, infections occurred over more than 50% of the studied population, and had a positive correlation with age. There were no statistical significance among proportion of infections between G1, G2 and G3. The comparison of G3 and G4 showed $p < 0.001$, and of G4 and G5 showed $p < 0.05$ (Figure 1).

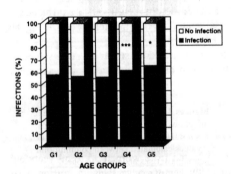

Figure 1. Frequency of vaginitis and cervicitis according to age.
$* = p < 0.05$; $** = p < 0.01$; $*** = p < 0.001$. p values calculated between column bearing asterisks and previous one.

The annual prevalence curves showed a progressive fall for yeasts, *C. trachomatis* and *T. vaginalis,* and a progressive rise for *G. vaginalis,* HPV and nonspecific infections (Figures 2A and 2B).

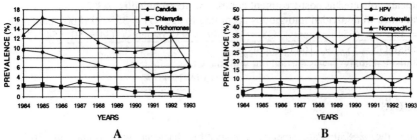

Figures 2A and 2B. Annual curves for infectious agents with declining and ascending prevalences, respectively.

There was no correlation between age and prevalence of HPV and *T. vaginalis* (Figure 3A). A negative correlation was found between age and prevalence of yeasts and *G. vaginalis* (Figure 3B). For yeasts, there was a progressive significant fall in prevalence: from G1 to G2 ($p < 0.001$), G2 to G3 ($p < 0.05$), and G3 to G4 ($p < 0.001$). For *G. vaginalis*, the fall occurred in older groups: G3 to G4 ($p < 0.001$) and G4 to G5 ($p < 0.05$). Finally, a positive correlation was found between age and prevalence of *C. trachomatis* and nonspecific bacteria (Figure 3C). For *C. trachomatis*, a statistically significant rise was determined between the groups G1, G2 and G3, and the older G4 and G5 ($p < 0.01$). For nonspecific bacteria, the significant rise occurred for older groups: G3 to G4 ($p < 0.001$), and G4 to G5 ($p < 0.001$).

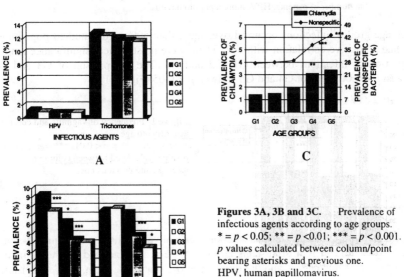

Figures 3A, 3B and 3C. Prevalence of infectious agents according to age groups. * $= p < 0.05$; ** $= p < 0.01$; *** $= p < 0.001$. *p* values calculated between column/point bearing asterisks and previous one. HPV, human papillomavirus.

Specific agents were identified in 7388 smears, and in 625 (8.4%), two or three agents were associated. The agents most frequently associated were HPV and *G. vaginalis* (Table 2): of all the diagnosys of HPV and *G. vaginalis*, 23.7% and 11.0%, respectively, showed associations.

Table 2 Frequency of diagnosys of specific agent in associated condition

AGENT	ASSOCIATIONS (%)
HPV	23.7
Gardnerella	11.0
Chlamydia	10.1
Trichomonas	7.8
Candida	4.3

HPV, human papillomavirus.

The most frequent associations were between *T. vaginalis* and *G. vaginalis* (47.2%), *T. vaginalis* and yeasts (14.4%), and *T. vaginalis* and *C. trachomatis* (11.6%) (Table 3).

Table 3 Types of associations of specific agents (present in 7388 smears)

ASSOCIATIONS	FREQUENCY	
	n	%
Trichomonas + Gardnerella	147	47.2
Trichomonas + Candida	45	14.4
Trichomonas + Chlamydia	35	11.6
HPV + Gardnerella	28	9.0
Candida + Gardnerella	15	4.8
HPV + Trichomonas	14	4.5
HPV + Candida	13	4.2
HPV + Chlamydia	5	1.6
Candida + Chlamydia	3	0.9
Chlamydia + Gardnerella	3	0.9
HPV + Candida + Trichomonas	1	0.3
HPV + Candida + Chlamydia	1	0.3
HPV + Trichomonas + Chlamydia	1	0.3
TOTAL	625	100.0

n, number of patients; HPV, human papillomavirus.

CONCLUSIONS

The vaginal microecology consists of a complex and yet fragile equilibrium between a host and its flora. The host sustains an environment characterized by the epithelial lining of vagina and cervix, and the fluid secretions that bathe them, thus establishing conditions that select its colonizing flora. This equilibrium is susceptible to common shifts caused by a variety of endogenous and exogenous factors (2). As a result, cervicitis and vaginitis are very frequent problems regarding women of all ages (1), and such fact was confirmed by our results, in which over 50% of the studied population, aged 35 to 59 years, was diagnosed at least one infectious agent.

An endogenous factor known to modify the physiology of the vaginal microecology is ovarian failure. With the onset of declining estrogen production, the vaginal and cervical epithelium undergo atrophy and the glycogen content in its cells is reduced. Responding to those changes, the lactobacilli population decreases, the vaginal pH increases, and these conditions are favorable to colonization by bacteria of fecal type (10). Importantly, in our study a positive correlation was verified between age and prevalence of infectious agents, thus suggesting that older women are at higher risk for lower genital tract infections of diverse etiology, specially nonspecific bacteria. Although it was not a purpose of this study to identify the post-menopausal women, data from brazilian literature mention that menopause occurs at the age of 47 - 48 years (11), suggesting that our older groups, G4 and G5, were composed mainly by post-menopausal patients.

Analysis of the cumulative prevalence results showed that nonspecific bacteria were the most prevalent infectious agents, and that the most prevalent specific agents were *T. vaginalis*, yeasts, and *G. vaginalis*. Over the ten-year period studied (1984 - 1993), the prevalence of yeasts, *C. trachomatis* and *T. vaginalis* have decreased, while the prevalence of *G. vaginalis*, HPV and nonspecific bacteria have increased. There are no data in the available literature to allow comparison of the prevalence and annual prevalence curves of these infectious agents, for patients in the studied age group. According to Kent (1), these specific agents predominate in younger patients as well.

A negative correlation was found between age and prevalence of yeasts and *G. vaginalis*. For yeasts, an explanation for these results relies in its characteristic development under low pH, glycogen-rich environments, and in its estrogen-dependent replication, conditions not related to older women (3-5). *G. vaginalis* also seems to be influenced and dependent on estrogen, and this would explain its decrease in older patients (3).

A positive correlation was found between age and prevalence of nonspecific bacteria and *C. trachomatis*. The mechanisms involved in facilitated vaginal colonization of older women by nonspecific bacteria were discussed previously. For *C. trachomatis*, an ATP-dependent microrganism, although known that such bacteria do not show tropism towards squamous cells (9), the exposure of basal cells (with intense metabolism and high ATP production) in post-menopausal women due to epithelial atrophy may facilitate genital infection.

No correlation was verified between age and prevalence of HPV and *T. vaginalis*. Such results for *T. vaginalis* are in agreement with Kent (1), while differing from Ford et al. (12), who detected the presence of estrogen receptors in the protozoan, and from Stein and Cope (13), who suggested a possible role for estrogen as a multiplication modulator.

Specific agents were found to be associated in 625 smears (8.4% among smears of specific agents). The agent most frequently associated was HPV (23.7% of the diagnosis). The most frequent association was between *T. vaginalis* and *G. vaginalis* (47.2% of all associations). This association can be explained by the similar habitat conditions found in the presence of infection by either agent (homogenous discharge, pH > 4.5, anaerobic flora replacing lactobacilli, presence of nitrosamines), so that sharing of the same habitat is viable (14).

REFERENCES

1. Kent, H. L. (1991). Epidemiology of vaginitis. *Am. J. Obstet. Gynecol.*, **165**, 1168-76.
2. Larsen, B. (1993). Vaginal flora in health and disease. *Clin. Obstet. Gynecol.*, **36**, 107-21.
3. Mardh, P-A. (1991). The vaginal ecosystem. *Am. J. Obstet. Gynecol.*, **165**, 1163-8.
4. Drake, T. E. and Maibach, H. I. (1985). Candida and candidiasis. 1. Cultural conditions, epidemiology and pathogenesis. *Postgrad. Med.*, **53**, 83-7.
5. Horowitz, B. J. (1991). Mycotic vulvovaginitis: a broad overview. *Am. J. Obstet. Gynecol.*, **165**, 1188-92.
6. Thomason, J. L. and Gelbart, S. M. (1989). Trichomonas vaginalis. *Obstet. Gynecol.*, **74**, 536-41.
7. Amsel, R., Totten, P. A., Spiegel, C. A., Chen, K. C. S., Eschenbach, D. and Holmes, K. K. (1983). Nonspecific vaginitis. Diagnostic criteria and microbial and epidemiologic associations. *Am. J. Med.*, **74**, 14-22.
8. Smotkin, D. (1993). Human papillomavirus infection of the vagina. *Clin. Obstet. Gynecol.*, **36**, 188-194.
9. Faro, S. (1991). *Chlamydia trachomatis*: female pelvic infection. *Am. J. Obstet. Gynecol.*, **164**, 1767-70.
10. Milsom, I., Arvidsson, L., Ekelund, P., Molander, U. and Eriksson, O. (1993). Factors influencing vaginal cytology, pH and bacterial flora in elderly women. *Acta Obstet. Gynecol. Scand.*, **72**, 286-91.
11. Halbe, H. W. (1994). *Tratado de Ginecologia.* (São Paulo: Roca).
12. Ford, L. C., Hammill, H. A., DeLange, R. J., Bruckner, D. A., Suzuki-Chavez, F., Mickus, K. L. and Lebherz, T. B. (1987). Determination of estrogen and androgen receptors in *Trichomonas vaginalis* and the effects of antihormones. *Am. J. Obstet. Gynecol.*, **156**, 1119-21.
13. Stein, I. and Cope, E. (1933). *Trichomonas vaginalis. Am. J. Obstet. Gynecol.*, **25**, 819-25.
14. James, J. A., Thomason, J. L., Gelbart, S. M., Osypowski, P., Kaiser, P. and Hanson, L. (1992). Is trichomoniasis often associated with bacterial vaginosis in pregnant adolescents? *Am. J. Obstet. Gynecol.*, **166**, 859-63.

Cytology in cervical screening for carcinoma and HPV infection: which role?

S. Masoni, R. Parducci, G. Giovannetti, C. Salvestroni, M.C. Papa, M.A. Celano, G. Guazzelli and C. De Punzio

Department of Gynecology and Obstetrics, University of Pisa, Pisa, Italy

INTRODUCTION

Since the Bethesda System was created in 1988 (1), it has drawn criticism from experts. Ambiguous terms such as "koilocytotic atypia" or "dyskaryosis" have been eliminated and an attempt has been made to correct the excessive schematism of the original Papanicolaou classification. Nevertheless many questions are left unanswered on whether to gather together CIN2 and CIN3, or CIN1 and koilocytosis and on the criteria of adequacy of the smear, especially as it concerns the presence of endocervical cells.(2)(3)

The Bethesda System has borderline aspects, not definable but by exclusion, that do not fulfil the criteria for defined benign reactive changes or Squamous Intraepithelial Lesions (SIL): these are the Atypical Squamous Cells of Undetermined Significance (ASCUS).(1)

Koss thinks that ASCUS are not frequent (4), but some often use this category in order to deceive the protocols that do not provide for colposcopy in case of persistent inflammatory atypia (2); others use it for minimal or focal lesions that otherwise could cause overdiagnosis and overtreatment in case of koilocytosis, so that terms are used such as "ASCUS that *could* represent HPV" (3) or "cellular changes *suggestive* of a specific viral infection" (5).

Even on the meaning of koilocytosis itself there are some questions, so that some Authors ask for confirmatory tests before they classify even frank koilocytosis in the SILs low grade (6), while others attach great importance to the contemporaneous finding of dyskeratosis-parakeratosis and karyorrhexis (7) and others consider koilocytosis in superficial or intermediate cells a sufficient issue (8).

Other Authors have found other borderline aspects, such as the "borderline nuclear abnormalities", which could include CIN3 and invasive carcinoma too, probably with a better prognosis compared to cases with frank nuclear abnormality. Follow-up cytology alone may be falsely reassuring in these patients.(9)

To make the problem more complicated, there are intraobserver and interobserver variability (10), and School variability too, which is related to the different approach toward the use of colposcopy, to the kind of personnel that carry out the Pap smears, to a different cost-benefit ratio.

In the United States, the Pap smear is usually carried out by paramedic personnel and even in the case of ASCUS some Authors choose to perform naked eye examination after acetic acid wash or cervicography rather than colposcopy, considered to be much too expensive(11).

In the Italian context, financial budgets often leave few space for the quality assurance, but there is a good network of colposcopists and Pap tests are often carried out under direct medical control.

These characteristics can help us to better understand colposcopic and histologic correlates of the cytologic findings of ASCUS with possible HPV presence (ASCUS-HPV), SIL low-grade (L-SIL) and SIL high-grade (H-SIL).

We have undertaken this study in order to verify the incidence and the meaning of such findings and the opportunity in these cases to perform colposcopy and possible punch biopsy.

MATERIALS AND METHODS

Among the 6512 Pap smears referred to the Laboratory of Cytology of our Department from January 1st to December 1st 1994, we selected the cases of ASCUS-HPV , L-SIL and H-SIL.

From these we went back to colposcopy and histology whenever possible. In fact, several smears come to the Laboratory from other Centers, which can make first instance colposcopies autonomously.

Colposcopic and histologic aspects of ASCUS-HPV , L-SIL and H-SIL were then compared.

RESULTS

We found an incidence rate of 4,59% for ASCUS-HPV (299 cases), 5,10% for L-SIL (332 cases), 1,20% for H-SIL (78 cases) and 0,28% for cervical carcinoma (18 cases).

Colposcopies were performed at our Department in 78/299 ASCUS-HPV, 266/332 L-SIL, 67/78 H-SIL and 17/18 carcinomas. Colposcopic results are shown in Table 1.

	ASCUS-HPV		L-SIL		H-SIL		CARCINOMA	
	N°cases	%	N°cases	%	N°cases	%	N°cases	%
NORMAL CERVIX	12	15,38	37	13,91	6	8,96	0	0,00
OTHER BENIGN PATTERN	6	7,69	22	8,27	7	10,45	2	11,76
AnTZ G0	2	2,56	4	1,50	1	1,49	0	0,00
AnTZ G1	54	69,23	177	66,54	25	37,31	0	0,00
AnTZ G2	4	5,13	26	9,77	28	41,79	1	5,88
CARCINOMA		0,00	0	0,00	0	0,00	14	82,35
TOTAL	78	100	266	100	67	100	17	100

Tab.1 - Colposcopic correlates

Most of the ASCUS-HPV and L-SIL cases are in AnTZ G1 category, while H-SIL are mostly represented in AnTZ G2 category and carcinomas are colposcopically confirmed in 82,35% of the cases.

Nevertheless, 23,07 of the ASCUS-HPV, 22,18 of the L-SIL, 19,41 of the H-SIL and 11,76 of the carcinomas show benign patterns at colposcopy.

54 of 78 ASCUS-HPV , 138 of 266 L-SIL, 51 of 67 H-SIL and 17/17 carcinomas had punch biopsy. Histologic results are shown in Table 2.

	ASCUS-HPV		L-SIL		H-SIL		CARCINOMA	
	N°cases	%	N°cases	%	N°cases	%	N°cases	%
NEGATIVE	23	42,59	40	28,99	6	11,76	0	0,00
SUGGESTIVE OF HPV	22	40,74	36	26,09	5	9,80	0	0,00
FLAT CONDYLOMA	4	7,41	36	26,09	6	11,76	0	0,00
CIN 1	4	7,41	18	13,04	6	11,76	0	0,00
CIN 2	0	0,00	6	4,35	10	19,61	0	0,00
CIN 3	1	1,85	2	1,45	18	35,29	1	5,88
CARCINOMA	0	0,00	0	0,00	0	0,00	16	94,12
TOTAL	54	100	138	100	51	100	17	100

Tab.2 - Histologic correlates

Most of ASCUS-HPV were negative for HPV (many of them showed just chronic cervicitis), but 40,74% were suggestive for HPV, 7,41% had flat condyloma, 7,41% had CIN1 and 1 case had CIN3.

Negative cases decreased as we considered L-SIL (28,99%), H-SIL (11,76%) and carcinoma (absent) but they still are the prevalent category in L-SIL.

Most of H-SIL cases, instead, had CIN3 at histology and 94,12% of carcinomas were histologically confirmed.

DISCUSSION

The Pap test has proven to be effective in the screening for cervical cancer.(12) It allows us to recognize some asymptomatic cases that a colposcopic test does not suspect, especially if the lesion affects the endocervix.

Nevertheless its role in the individualization of HPV infections has to be defined. ASCUS-HPV is a scarcely considered entity, as just 78 of 299 women with such cytological diagnosis undergo colposcopic tests. In our study, if we also consider ASCUS-HPV cases, Pap test seems to be very sensitive, but it has too many false positives (23,07% of colposcopies were negative for HPV and so were 42,59% of biopsies). If we reduce the diagnoses to L-SIL cases, we could miss many HPV and CIN positive cases (in our study we even had 1 CIN3 with ASCUS-HPV).

So we deem it necessary to take ASCUS-HPV aspects into account and to gather them in a new category, using more accurate and widely accepted criteria. In the near future, after the complete computereization of our Cytology Laboratory, we are going to follow-up ASCUS-HPV cases, in order to understand their evolution.

At this point the problem is to integrate the Pap test with viral identification techniques, which have to be just as much sensitive and as cheap, but more specific.

We have tested these techniques, but we have found them to be unfeasible for mass screening at this moment.(13)

Considering the availability and the relative low cost of colposcopy in Italy, we deem useful to perform it not only in L-SIL cases, but in ASCUS-HPV cases as well. In such a case it could be important to administer before an anti-inflammatory therapy, if phlogosis aspects join ASCUS, or an oestrogenic therapy, if the woman is in her climacteric age. In any case, we think it is very important to respect the spirit of the Bethesda System, that calls for a close collaboration between clinicians and pathologists.

REFERENCES
1)   National Cancer Institute Workshop: "The 1988 Bethesda System for reporting cervical/vaginal cytologic diagnoses".
      JAMA 262:931-934:1989
2)   Bottles K, Reiter RC, Steiner AL, Zaleski S, Bedrossian CWM, Johnson SR: "Problems encountered with the Bethesda System: the University of Iowa experience".
      Obstet.Gynecol.78:410-414:1991
3)   Broso PR e Buffetti G: "Dalla classificazione di Papanicolaou al Bethesda System"
      Minerva Ginecol. 45:557-563:1993
4)   Koss LG: "The new Bethesda System for reporting results of smears of the uterine cervix"
      J.Natl.Cancer Inst. 82:988-991:1990
5)   Vooijs GP: "Does the Bethesda System promote or endanger the quality of cervical cytology?" (lett)
      Acta Cytol. 34:455-457:1990
6)   Kuhler-Obbarius C, Milde-Langosch K, Loning T, Stegner HE: "PCR-assisted evaluation of low and high grade SIL cytology and reappraisal of the Bethesda System".
      Acta Cytol. 38:681-686:1994
7)   Tanaka H, Chua KL, Lindh E, Hjerpe A: "Patients with various types of HPV: covariation and diagnostic relevance of cytological findings in Papanicolaou smears".
      Cytopathology 4:273-283:1993
8)   Tabbara S, Saleh AM, Andersen WA, Barber SR, Taylor PT, Crum CP: "The Bethesda classification for squamous intraepithelial lesions: histologic, cytologic and viral correlates".
      Obstet.Gynecol. 79:338-346:1992
9)   Stewart CJR, Livingstone D, Mutch AF: "Borderline nuclear abnormality in cervical smears: a cytological review of 200 cases with histological correlation".
      Cytopathology 4:339-345:1993
10)   Klinkhamer PJJM, Vooijs GP, de Haan AFJ: "Intraobserver and interobserver variability in the diagnosis of epithelial abnormalities in cervical smears".
      Acta Cytol. 32:794-800:1988
11)   Slawson DC, Bennett JH, Simon LJ, Herman JM: "Should all women with cervical atypia be referred for colposcopy: a HARNET study".
      J.Fam.Pract. 38:387-392:1994
12)   Van der Graaf Y, Vooijs GP, Zielhuis GA: "Cervical screening revisited".
      Acta Cytol. 34:366-372:1990
13)   Masoni S, Parrini D, Avantaggiato A,Guazzelli G,De Punzio C, Fioretti P: "HPV typization in cervical smears by an original application of the polymerase chain reaction."
      Aggiornamenti in Scienze Ginecologiche Ostetriche, (Ed. P. Fioretti), CIC Ed., Roma 1992, Vol. I, pag. 155-157

HPV infections in male sexual partners

E. Giannone, N. Di Giulio and V. Lauro

Department of Oncologic Gynecology and Institute of Gynecology and Obstetrics, University of Perugia, Italy

SUMMARY

In many case of women with recurrent cervical-vaginal and vulvar human papilloma virus (HPV) infection has frequently demonstrated recurrent penile HPV infection of male partners. HPV might be localized anywhere on the penis, genital area or distal urethra. The AA. used a Zeiss colposcope with a magnification of 8X and 20X. Their experience has confirmed the importance of examination the male partners. The peniscope examination has been positive in 57.35% (195/340) of male partners of women with recurrent HPV genital infection, with important implications as far as the therapeutic success is concerned.

Key words: Papillomavirus - Male infection - Peniscope

INTRODUCTION

The interest towards the HPV infection has gone increasing side-by-side with the rapidly increasing incidence of condylomata accuminata observed in the last 10 years together with the discovery of the association for the first time 50 years ago on a rabbit (1).
It does esist an epidemiological evidence that the cervical cancer is transmitted through sessual ruote and it has been demonstrated the presence of HPV 16 and 18 in more than 80% of the invasive squamose carcinoma of the cervix, of the vulva and of the penis, likewise in patients with severe (CIN3) cervical intraepithelial neoplasia. We are progressively becoming aware of the fact that panting the penile skin with acetic acid in men that have had sexual intercourse with women affected by condilomata whitish areas are noticed. Biopsy has revealed that these whitish areas are affected by HPV. Many authors (2-3-4-5) have reported in their research that the male infection from women with genital infection by HPV ranges from 64-85%.

MATHERIAL AND METHODS

We made colposcopic exams to 340 men having women with HPV genital infection or cervical (CIN+HPV, flat condilomata). The colposcopic exam was made 3-5 minutes after the application of a 5% acetic acid solution. A ureteral Pap test of the balano-prepucial sulcus and the corona of the gland was made before making the colposcoping exam. An accurate anamnesis was made to all of these men, with particular attention concerning the sexuality (number of partners, their number of sexual intercorses with prostitutes, number of homosexual or heterosexual intercurses, clinical symptoms, previous veneral diseases). In some of these men, we made a biopsy on the suspected areas after a local anaesthesia.

RESULTS

Peniscoplc exam was carried out on 340 men at risk with female partners having recurrent HPV infection and/or affected by dysplasia of various grades. All of them were subjected to urine cytologic exam, to Papanicolau smear obtained from the uretral meatus and to colposcopic exam. Symptoms reported by patients, were absent in 215 out of 340 (63.23%),while 135 out of 340 (39.70%) referred the presence of papillae on the corona or on the balano-prepucial sulcus, prepuce of penis, frenulum, or on penil skin. Only 40/340(11.76%) of these papillae were florid condyloma.

Pap-smear has been positive for koilocytosis in 20/340(5.88%). This examination show low sensibility.
We frequently found white points 175/340(51.47%), flat condyloma 80/340(32.52%),florid condyloma 40/340(11.76%) and negative 45/340(13.23%). In 235/340 cases (white points and flat condyloma) executed biopsy of the lesion. Histologic diagnosis was positive for condyloma i 155 cases.

COMMENT

The increasing incidence of HPV, the risk of trasmission of viruses oncogenic for the uterine cervix need for a treatment of all male genital lesion. The male, in our study, partners of women with reccurent HPV genital infection were in total 195/340(57.35%) considering only the undoubeted cases (florid condyloma and histologic diagnosis).
Only 20/340(5.88%) had positive Pap-smear, most probably in relation with careful genital toilette and inadequate smear.
Peniscopic investigation and biopsy of lesion have a greater reliability and confirms the importance of examining the male partners of women with HPV genital infection for correct and effective treatment of the couples.

REFERENCES

1) Rous P. and Beard J.W: Exp. Med. 1935,62,523.

2) Baggish H.S.: "Treating viral venereal infections with the CO2 laser". J. Reprod. Med.27:137,1982.

3) Ferenczy A.: "Evaluation and management of male partners of condyloma patients". Colposcopy and Gynecology, Laser Sur. 2:12,1986.

4) Huovinen K., Huovinen S.: Koilocytotic ano-genital lesions in women and their male partners. European Journal of Gynaecological Oncology. 447,1987.

5) Levine R.U. et Al.: "Cervical papillomavirus infection and intraepithelial neoplasia: a study of male sexual partners." Obstet. Gynecol. Vol. 64, n.1, 16-20 1984.

HPV infection: cytocolpohystologic correlations in patients affected by condylomatosis of external genitalia

G. Piras, F. Esposito, M.P. Bagella, L. Pinna Nossai, P. Lecca, L. Manca, A. Scapinelli and P.L. Cherchi

Università degli Studi di Sassari, Clinica Ostetrica-Ginecologica, Sassari, Italy

The wide variety of cutaneous and mucous lesions HPV induced, their multifocal action and cancerous capacity (variable according to sex, location and associated cofactors) are well known.
We studied, in case of external genitalia condylomatosis, the frequency and the features of viral vaginal and cervical disease considering the high frequency of dysplasic (8.4%) and neoplastic (2.8%) lesions HPV induced (1,3,4).

MATERIALS AND METHODS

We studied 34 patients affected by genital condylomatosis arrived to our Center for Prevention and Precocious diagnosis of gynecological neoplasias.
Every patient underwent a careful general and gynecological anamnesis.
The mean age of our patients was 30 years (range 19-74) and 55% of them were less than 29 years old, the age of their first intercourse resulted between 14 and 47 years (mean age: 30.5); the number of partners resulted to be 1 in 41.1% of cases, 2-3 in 47% and >3 in 11.7%, the contraceptive method was hormonal in 61.7%, IUD in 5.8%, barrier in 2.9%, nothing (no method) in 29.4%.
44.1% of patients were used to smoking. (Tab. 1)
After a vulvar exam according to standard methods every patient underwent a colpocytologic sample and a colposcopic exam; furthermore, we made vaginal or cervical biopsy under colposcopic indication.

701

Table 1 Analysis of cases.

Mean age	30 (range 19-74)
age of first sexual intercourse	30.5 (range 14-47)
N. of partners :	
1	N. 14 (41.1%)
2-3	N. 16 (47 %)
>2	N. 4 (11.7%)
Contraception :	N. 21 (61.7%)
hormonal	N. 2 (5.8%)
barrier	N. 1 (2.9%)
nothing	N. 10 (29.4%)
Smokers	N. 21 (61%)

RESULTS

We evaluated about the viral cervicovaginal disease, the cytology, the colposcopy and the hystology, showing our results in the following table 2 .

Table 2 Results

VULVOSCOPY	COLPOSCOPY	HYSTOLOGY	CYTOLOGY
ACUMINATED CONDYLOMATA n° 6 (17.6%)	ANTZ 1 n°2 (33.3%) ANTZ 2 n°1 (16.6%)	ECV n°1 (16.6%) L.D.+ECV n°2 (33.3%)	ECV n°2(33.3%) L.D. n°1 (16.6%) D.L. + ECV n°1(16.6%)
FLOURISHING CONDYLOMATA n° 9 (26.4%)	ECV n°9 (100%) VAGINAL CONDYLOMATOSIS n°4 (44.4%)	L.D. + ECV n°2 (22.2%) M.D. + ECV n°3 (33.3%)	ECV n°1 (11.1%) L.D. + ECV n°5(55.5%) M.D. + ECV n°3(33.3%)
MICROFLOURISHING CONDYLOMATOSIS n° 8 (23.5%)	ANTZ 1 n°3(37.5%)	METAPLASIA n°1(12.5%) L.D. n°2(25%)	ECV n°2(25%) L.D. n°2(25%)
MICROPAPILLARY CONDYLOMATOSIS n° 11 (32.3%)	ANTZ 1 n°1(9%) ANTZ 2 n°3(27.2%) VIRAL COLPITIS n°1(9%)	ECV n°1 (9%) L.D. n°2 (18.1%) M.D. n°1 (9%)	L.D.+ECV n°2(18.1%) M.D. n°2(18.1%)
TOTAL 100%	61%	53%	64%

At vulvoscopic examination we observed:
condylomata acuminata: 6/34 (17.6 %)
flourishing condylomata : 9/34 (26.4 %)
microflourishing condylomatosis : 8/34 (23.5%)

micropapillary condylomatosis : 11/34 (32.3%)

By colposcopic examination, out of 6 patients with condylomata acuminata, 2 cases of ANTZ 1 (33.3%) and 1 case of ANTZ 2 (16.6 %) were diagnosed, which underwent guided biopsy. The hystologic result confirmed the presence of 2 cases (33.3%) of light dysplasia ECV associated and 1 case (16.6%) with only ECV.

Cytologic diagnosis was: 1 case (16.6%) of light dysplasia, 1 (16.6%) of light dysplasia ECV associated and 2 cases (33.3%) with only ECV.

In patients affected by vulvar flourishing condylomata colposcopic observation showed the presence of the virus in the cervix in all cases (100%), and in 4 cases (44.4%) there was an associated vaginal condylomatosis.

Hystological diagnosis confirmed in all cases (100%) the presence of ECV, with 3 cases (33.3%) of moderate dysplasia and 2 cases (22.2%) of light dysplasia.

Also cytology confirmed the presence of viral infection: 5 cases (55.5%) of light dysplasia ECV associated 3 cases (33.3%) of moderate dysplasia ECV associated and 1 case (11.1%) with only ECV.

Out of patients affected by microflourishing condylomatosis, we found 3 cases (37.5 %) of ANTZ 1.

The hystopathological response was: 2 cases (25%) of light dysplasia and 1 case (22.5%) of metaplasia.

Cytological examination showed 2 cases (25%) of light dysplasia and 2 cases (25%) of ECV infection.

Patients with micropapillar vulvitis HPV associated showed the following colposcopic patterns: 1 case (9%) of ANTZ 1, 3 cases (27.2%) of ANTZ 2 and 1 case (9%) of viral colpitis. The remaining colposcopic pictures were suggestive for HPV infection.

The performed biopsies had the following responses: 2 cases (28.1%) of light dysplasia, 1 case (9%) of moderate dysplasia and 1 case (9%) ECV associated.

Papanicolaus smears underwent the following classification: 2 (18.1%) second classes (II), 2 (18.1%) not classificable for intense phlogosis, 2 cases (18.1%) of moderate dysplasia.

DISCUSSION AND CONCLUSION

Our data showed a positivity for ECV equal to 64% of cases at cytology, 61% at colposcopy and 53% at hystology.

These results appear to be different from those obtained from Walker and coll. (7) that noticed significant colposcopic pictures in 40% of patients against 29% of cytological positivity.

However, it's necessary to underline that in those women also affected by vaginal and cervical condylomatosis the percentage of cases with cytologic and colpohystologic reports, HPV infection suggestive, appears to be higher.

Purola and Savia (5) observed similar results showing significant cytologic pictures in 33% of cases with condylomatosis limited to external genitalia and in 66% of cases with vaginal and cervical involvement.

Furthermore, cases with indicative cytology for HPV in our study appear to be less frequent in those women that presented micropapillary and microflorid condylomatosis.

On the other side, we observed the presence of colposcopic and/or cytologic diagnostic pictures or strongly suggestive for HPV infection, in 66.1% of our patient.

In our opinion the absence of colposcopic or cytologic infective signs doesn't rule out the presence of the virus inside cells, in a lot of women affected by vulvar condylomatosis.

Recently some Authors (6) noticed that in about 50% of cases, which appeared positive to the virus research into cervical vaginal epithelium, there weren't cytologic or colposcopic alterations.

Our data confirm what previously observed by Purola and Savia (5), which found 2 cases of serious dysplasia and 22 cases of light/moderate dysplasia out of a group of 192 women with "condylomata acuminata", among wich only 94 underwent biopsy.

In conclusion, we can affirm that patients affected by external genital condylomatosis present a high incidence of uterine cervical alterations HPV-correlated, and considering dysplastic and neoplastic lesions they represent a high risk group.

Therefore we remark that in patient affected by external genital condylomatosis the colposcopic and cytologic exam are advisable.

REFERENCES

1. De Palo, G.(1984). Virus e displasie della cervice uterina. Atti II Giornate di Firenze, Soc. It. Colp. e Patol. cervico-vaginale, 137.
2. Giosa, F., Negosanti, M., Camerlo, M. et al.(1988). Quadri colposcopici e colpocitologici in pazienti affette da condilomi dei genitali esterni. In Rondanelli, G., Danesino, V. "Le infezioni in ostetricia e ginecologia", pp. 645-651 (Bologna, Monduzzi Eds).
3. Mencaglia, L. et al.(1992). Testo atlante di microscopia e patologia cervicale. Milano, cap. 6-7-8.
4. Monsonego, J.(1988) Dysplasies du col utérine et papilloma virus humains. Paris, Maloine, 32-37, 48-49.
5. Purola, E., Savia, E. (1977) Cytology of gynecologic condyloma acuminatum. Acta Cytol.,21,26-31.
6. Scheneider, A., Sawava, E., Gissmann, L., Shah, K. (1987). Human papilloma viruses in women with a history of abnormal

Papanicolau smears and their male partners. Obstet.Gynecol.,69,554-562.

7. Walker, P., Colley, N., Crubb, C., Tejerina, A., Oriel, J.(1983) Abnormalities of the uterine cervix in women with vulvar warts. Br.J.Vener.Dis.,59,120-123.

Combined treatment (sytemic and topical) with α-interferon in genital HPV infections

A. Azzena, G. Cerri, V. Brunetti, J. Dal Maso, C. Vasile and F. Vasoin

Università degli Studi di Padova, Istituto di Ginecologia ed Ostetricia "G.B. Revoltella", Padova, Italy

SUMMARY

In the last decade, Human Papilloma Virus (HPV) infections with vulvar, vaginal and perineal location are representing frequent routine diagnosed pathologies in fertile patients.

The Authors of this study suggest a new therapeutical approach in the treatment of HPV lesions, using α-interpherone (α-IFN), in systemic and local administration.

Seventeen patients with an age ranged between 16 and 39 years, suffering from genital condylomas, previously diagnosed by colposcopy and cytology, were evaluated in this study.

All 17 patients were treated with α-IFN in systemic administration: 1 phial of 3.000.000 UI i.m. 2 times a week for 1 month (a total of 8 phials), associated with local jell applications of α-IFN (3 applications a day for 1 month).

The effects of the treatment were evaluated 1 month, 3 months and 6 months after the suspension of the last administration .

Nine (52.9%) cases completely remitted after 3 months, while another 3 (17.6%) demonstrated a complete recovery after 6 months.

The remaining 6 patients (35.5%) were subsequently treated with surgery (diathermocoagulation), in order to obtain a complete cure of the infection.

The side-effects of the drug (α-IFN) were poorly remarkable and, in any case didn't determine the treatment suspension; therefore, all the patients had a complete cycle of treatment.

These data demonstrate the utility and effectiveness of the combined treatment with α-IFN, in genital HPV infections, either for the complete remission as for the prevention of relapses.

Besides, we stress the low social cost (economic and human) of the treatment with α-IFN in comparison with surgery, certainly more expensive for the society and invasive for the patient.

Key words: HPV disease; α-IFN combined treatment

INTRODUCTION

Vulvar, vaginal and perineal condylomas represent the typical expression of HPV extrernal genital infection, due to mild viral types (6,11), while other more aggressive types (16,18,31,35,51) are usually associated with pre-neoplastic or frankly invasive female genital lesions (1,2,4).

Colposcopically, a condyloma is described as a white or snown-white, shining, aceto-reactive, indent borders, irregular area located inside or outside the transforamation zone (2).

Condylomas may be diagnosed by eye inspection or mostly using a magnifying glass, are located in the external genital and perineal zone and present a typical, elevated, acetorective aspect (2).

The terapeutical trends of this type of viral infection are based on systemic and local pharmacological agents as Pedofiline, 5-Fluorouracile, Trichloracetic acid, Interpherons or surgery (coagulation laser criosurgery) but all this approaches even if associated, do not eliminate relapses completely (1-5).

Relapses or lack of response after the treatment may be caused by the presence of the virus in the undamaged perilesional zone or influenced by immunological factors.

Recently, the use of pharmacological products containing α or β-interpherone became more and more important and their way of administration is multiple: endolesional, topical (cream, jell, ointment) or sistemic (intramuscle, intravenous) (1-5).

α- and β-interpherone are produced by the fibroblasts, macrophagies, epithelial cells, B and T lymphocytes and represent an immunologic response at the contact between the human organism and various bacterial, viral and tumoral antigens; in particular the antiviral action of α-IFN could be explained by the inhibition of the viral replication associated with an immunomodulating action (production of cytokines, elevation of macrophages activity, increased cytotoxic and natural-killer activity of T lymphocytes) (1,2,4,6,7).

MATERIALS AND METHODS

Seventeen fertile patients with the age ranged between 16 and 39 years (mean age 26 years), with various parity and different social categories, suffering from multiple genital condylomatas, outpatient examined underwent all investigations of the diagnosis protocol for HPV infection in order to clinically confirm the disease: Pap test, colposcopy, vulvoscopy and target biopsies.

Condylomas were located at vulvar, vaginal, perineal, cervical and anal level and their greater incidence was noted in the vulvar, vaginal, perineal area.

The exclusion criteria included patients suffering from immunologic diseases, systemic pathologies, immunological deficiency, drug abusers and pregnant women.

All patients were treated with 2 α-IFN (obtained from human normal lymphocites) in a dose of 3.000.000 UI i.m. 2 times a week for 1 month (a total of 8 administrations), associated with a topical therapy with α-IFN jell (3 applications a day for 1 month).

During the therapy. none of the patients was using drugs as cortisone, indomethacine, acetilasalicilic acid, which may interphere with the α-IFN activity and there was no need of treatment suspension because of the side effects of intherpherone (fever, astenia, musclepain, headache, nausea).

At the end of the therapy, were carried out at three and six months by colposcopy, colpocytology and vulvoscopy.

The effectiveness of the therapy was evaluated as Complete Response (CR) in the cases which underwent a complete remission of the lesions, as Partial Response (PR) when reduction in number and size of the lesions could be seen and as Null Response (NR) when no sign of remission and even progression of the disease was noted.

RESULTS

While for some patients it has been noted clinically, a positive response, 1 month after treatment, the real effectiveness of the therapy was evaluated after three months, by performing routine controls.

Nine patients presented a CR with a total disappearance of the lesions, five patients had a PR, with a clear reduction in number an size of the lesions, while in only 3 cases a NR with progression of the disease was seen.

After 6 months from the suspension of the therapy 3 out of 5 patients with PR had a CR and the 3 cases with NR presented an subsequent extension of the disease.

One case out of nine with CR relapsed, therefore all the 6 patients with remaining HPV infection underwent diathermocoagulation of the lesion, in general anesthesia (Tab.1).

Tab. 1: Clinical cases, type and site of the condylomata lesion, therapeutical response.

Cases	Age	Pathology	Site	Follow-up 3 months	Follow-up 6 months	Compl.ry treatment
1	39	C. Acumin.	vulva-vagina	C.R.	C.R.	-
2	30	C. Acumin.	vulva-vagina-portio	P.R.	C.R.	-
3	25	Micro-cond.	vulva	C.R.	C.R.	-
4	19	Micro-cond.	vulva	C.R.	C.R.	-
5	33	Micro-cond.	vulva	C.R.	C.R.	-
6	28	Micro-cond.	vulva	C.R.	C.R.	-
7	23	Micro-cond.	vulva-vagina	C.R.	C.R.	-
8	16	Micro-cond.	vulva	P.R.	C.R.	-
9	28	C. Piano	vulva-vagina-perineo	P.R.	P.R.	DTC
10	26	C. Florida	vulva-vagina-anus	P.R.	P.R.	DTC
11	25	C. Florida	vulva-vagina-portio-anus	N.R.	N.R.	DTC
12	21	C. Piano	vulva-perineo	P.R.	C.R.	-
13	23	C. Acumin.	vulva-vagina-portio	C.R.	Relapse	DTC
14	25	Micro-cond.	vulva	C.R.	C.R.	-
15	25	Micro-cond.	vulva	C.R.	C.R.	-
16	28	C. Florida	vulva-perineo-anus	N.R.	N.R.	DTC
17	32	C. Florida	vulva-vagina-portio-perineo-anus	N.R.	N.R.	DTC

C. R.= Complete Response; P. R.= Parzial Response; N. R.= None Response
DTC= Diathermocoagulation

The side effects of the drug were unremarkable; most frequently (5 cases) fever could be noted but never superior 38°C.

The best therapeutical results were seen for the acuminate condylomata and for microcondylomatas, with vulvar and vestibular location, while 4 out of 6 patients treated with coagulation presented flourishing condylomas with 1 cm superior diameter vegetation one was a diffuse plane condylomata and last 1 a relapse lesion.

CONCLUSIONS

Our experiences does confirm the validity of the medical combined local and systemic treatment with α-IFN in genital condylomats as an alternative for surgery, anyway as a presurgical therapy or even a complementary post-surgical approach in the flourishing cases.

The unremarkable, rare, side effects all mild (in no case so important in order to determine the termination of the treatment),the short-term clinical effectiveness and the optimal compliance for the patients led us to consider the pharmacological treatment with α-IFN a "therapy of choice" in the management of the genital condilomas, to be initiated in all the cases, before tempting the surgical approach.

We find important that even patients who present big lesions, usually treated by surgery undergo firstly a cycle of therapy with α-IFN, as its pharmacological action does not interest only the macroscopic lesions but also the apparently undamaged skin and the mucosa close to the lesion.

Subsequently, surgery is to be performed in order to eliminate all the unresponsive lesions completely and more than that, in all this cases, combined medical and surgical treatment increased the possibilities of a complete, definitive remission of the disease, reduced the risk of relapses, as α-IFN sterilizes the perilesional areas.

It must be not be undervalued the fact that surgical therapy for condylomas is often followed by relapses because surgery cannot "sterilize" the microscopic lesions.

In "mild" condylomas and mostly in micropapillary forms the treatment with α-IFN is potentially succesfull by eliminating subsequent surgery and not at last, when the extension of the lesion is important by avoiding unesthetical healing at the external genital level.

Moreover, medical treatment is able to avoid hospitalization and general anaesthesia wich represents either benefit for the patients as a saving in the public health budget (operating room and hospital costs) and determins the reduction of the "crowded hospital", so that a great number of women which can receive an outpatient therapy are substituted by patients with severe pathologies who need a more special surveillance.

REFERENCES

1) Pescetto G., De Cecco L., Pecorari D., Ragni N. (1989): Manuale di Ginecologia ed Ostetricia. Volume I. II Edizione. Società Editrice Universo-Roma, pag. 368-372.

2) De Palo G. (1994): Manuale di colposcopia e patologia del tratto genitale inferiore. II Edizione. Masson Editore, pag. 135.

3) Gall S.A., Constantine L. and Koukol D. (1991): Therapy of persistent human papillomavirus disease with two different interferon species. Am. J. Obstet. Gynecol., 164: 130-134.

4) Zarcone R., Cardone G., Voto I., Deconciliis B., Cardone A. (1992): Schemi terapeutici per il trattamento delle infezioni dda HPV mediante l'uso di intrferon alfa

per via topica. Nostra esperienza nelle infezioni vulvari. Minerva Ginecol., 44: 189-191.

5) Gentile G., Formelli G., Busacchi P., Pelusi G. (1994): Systemic interferon therapy for female florid genital condylomata. Clin. Exp. Obst. Gyn., 3: 198-202.

6) Baron S., Coppenhaver D.H., Dianzani F., Fleischmann W.R. jr., Hughes T.K. jr., Klimpel G.R., Niesel D.W., Stanton J. and Tyring S.K. (1992): Introdution to the interferon system. Interferon principles and medical applications. First Edition. Editors: Baron S., Coppenhaver D.H., Dianzani F., Fleischmann W.R. jr., Hughes T.K. jr., Klimpel G.R., niesel D.W., Stanton J. and Tyring S.K. The University of Texas Medical Branch at Galveston.Galveston, TX U.S.A..

7) Gewrt D., Finter N. (1992): Antiviral effects of interferons:studies in animals and at the cellular level. Interferon principles and medical applications. First Edition. Editors: Baron S., Coppenhaver D.H., Dianzani F., Fleischmann W.R. jr., Hughes T.K. jr., Klimpel G.R., niesel D.W., Stanton J. and Tyring S.K. The University of Texas Medical Branch at Galveston.Galveston, TX U.S.A.

SECTION 6

Gynecological Oncology

Sex steroid receptors, LH/hCG receptor, and oncogene expression in endometrial carcinomas

I. Konishi, M. Koshiyama, M. Mandai, T. Komatsu, S. Yamamoto, K. Nanbu, S. Fujii*, Ch. V. Rao** and T. Mori

Department of Gynecology and Obstetrics, Faculty of Medicine, Kyoto University, Sakyo-ku, Kyoto, 606, Japan, *Department of Obstetrics and Gynecology, Shinshu University School of Medicine, Matsumoto, Japan and **Department of Obstetrics and Gynecology, University of Louisville, Kentucky, USA

Endometrial carcinoma is one of the most common malignant neoplasms of the female genital tract. Development of endometrial carcinomas is strongly associated with a specific hormonal milieu such as unopposed estrogen due to polycystic ovary, perimenopause, or hormone replacement therapy. Such estrogen-related carcinomas usually show histology with endometrioid type, well to moderately differentiated adenocarcinoma, and are believed to arise through the precursor lesion, endometrial hyperplasia. On the other hand, several lines of evidence suggest that there is another type of endometrial carcinoma which develops in older postmenopausal women, and frequently exhibits non-endometrioid histology or poorly-differentiated carcinoma. However, little is known about the difference of intracellular events that occur in the tumorigenesis between the two types of endometrial carcinoma.

In women of reproductive age, growth and differentiation of normal endometrium is regulated by estrogen and progesterone of the menstrual cycle through their specific receptors, estrogen receptors (ER) and progesterone receptors (PR). In addition, luteinizing hormone (LH)/human chorionic gonadotropin (hCG) receptor has recently been demonstrated in normal endometrium. Since endometrial hyperplasias and carcinomas are defined as lesions that have escaped the regulatory mechanisms for normal growth and differentiation, expression pattern for sex steroid receptors and LH/hCG receptor may be aberrant in these lesions. Oncogenes and anti-oncogenes are essentially involved in development of human cancers. Endometrial

715

carcinomas are known to possess an alteration of Ki-*ras* oncogene or p53 anti-oncogene, as well as overexpression of growth factor receptors such as c-*erb*B-2 protein and epidermal growth factor receptor (EGFR). In this paper, we report immunohistochemical expression of ER, PR, LH/hCG receptor, p53 gene mutation and overexpression, as well as localization of c-*erb*B-2 protein and EGFR in 43 cases of endometrial carcinoma examined with reference to the two types of endometrial carcinogenesis.

Immunohistochemical expression of ER or PR was found in 30 of the 43 (70%) carcinomas, and 13 (30%) were negative for both. Positivity for ER or PR was not related with FIGO stage disease, but was significantly correlated with endometrioid histology (p<0.05) and with well differentiated state of the tumor (p<0.01). Furthermore, in stage I, well-differentiated, endometrioid-type adenocarcinoma of premenopausal patients, strong expression for ER and PR was observed in the cells of hyperplasia and carcinoma, whereas normal endometrial glands in the same patient exhibited down-regulated expression of ER and PR during the secretory phase of the menstrual cycle or upon the administration of progestins (Fig. 1). LH/hCG

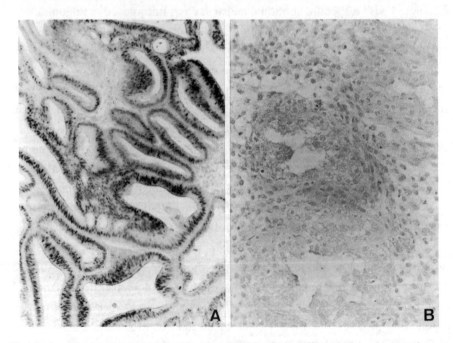

Fig. 1. Immunohistochemical expression of ER in well differentiated adenocarcinoma (A) and in the adjacent normal endometrium (B) from a premenopausal patient during the secretory phase. Carcinomatous glands exhibit strong positivity for ER, whereas normal secretory glands are ER-negative. X400.

receptor expression was found in 23 of the 35 (66%) carcinomas, and was more strong in cancer cells compared with that in normal endometrial glands.

LH/hCG receptor positivity in endometrial carcinoma was significantly correlated with younger age (p<0.05) and higher body mass index of the patient (p<0.05), and PR positivity of the tumor (p<0.01). Endometrial hyperplasias also exhibited strong immunoreactivity for LH/hCG receptor.

p53 gene mutation was identified in only one of the 7 cases analyzed by PCR-SSCP method, and immunohistochemical overexpression of p53 protein was found in 6 of the 38 (16%) cases. p53 positivity was found in carcinomas occurring in patients more than 3 years after menopause, and was significantly correlated with non-endometrioid histology (p<0.05) and with loss of both ER and PR in the tumor cells (p<0.01)(Fig. 2). In addition, both endometrial hyperplasias and carcinomas accompanied by hyperplasia were p53-negative. With regard to c-erbB-2 protein and EGFR expression, 22 of the 34 (65%) cases were c-erbB-2-positive and EGFR-negative, 8 (24%) were positive for both c-erbB-2 protein and EGFR, and 4 (12%) were negative for both. Expression of both c-erbB-2 protein and EGFR was more frequently seen in tumors of advanced stage, and was significantly correlated with poorly

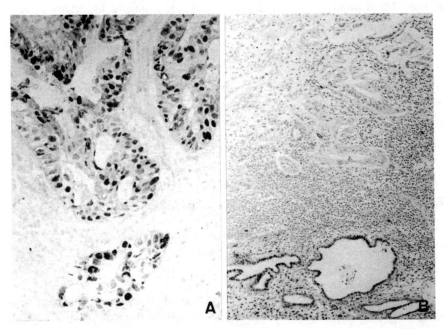

Fig. 2. Immunohistochemical overexpression of p53 protein in endometrial adenocarcinoma from a postmenopausal patient (A). The p53-positive carcinoma is present in the superficial layer of the endometrium, and is ER-negative (B). In contrast, normal endometrium below the carcinoma is ER-positive (B). A:X800, B:X200.

differentiated state (p<0.05) and with no reactivity for ER and PR (p<0.05) of cancer cells.

Endometrial carcinoma is believed to be one of the "hormone-dependent" neoplasms which may retain the responsiveness to estrogen and/or progestins. This study indicates that ER, PR and LH/hCG receptors tend to be expressed more frequently in endometrial hyperplasias and in well-differentiated carcinomas of endmetrioid-type. In addition, hyperplasias and well-differentiated adenocarcinomas in premenopausal women show strong expression of ER and PR irrespective of the menstrual cycle or progestins administration. Furthermore, these tumors exhibit stronger expression of LH/hCG receptor compared with normal endometrial gland. Consequently, estrogen-related pathway of endometrial carcinogenesis is characterized by constitutive expression of sex steroid receptors as well as overexpression of LH/hCG receptor.

p53 gene mutation is one of the most common genetic events in human cancers, and immunohistochemical overexpression of p53 protein is usually associated with p53 gene mutation. In endometrial carcinomas, however, p53 mutation and overexpression is less frequent compared with other malignant tumors. In this study, p53 overexpression is not found in hyperplasias or in well-differentiated carcinomas of pre- and perimenopausal patient, and is inversely correlated with sex steroid receptor status of the tumor. Therefore, p53 gene mutation and overexpression seems to be involved in estrogen-unrelated pathway of tumorigenesis and/or loss of hormone-dependency of endometrial carcinomas. c-*erb*B-2 protein overexpression has been reported to correlate with advanced stage disease and poor patient prognosis. This study suggests that the expression of EGFR in addition of c-*erb*B-2 protein is linked with poorly differentiated state or with progression of endometrial carcinomas. In conclusion, different intracellular events are present between the two types of estrogen-related and unrelated carcinoma of the endometrium.

References

1. Koshiyama M, Konishi, I, Wang DP, Mandai M, Komatsu T, Yamamoto S, Nanbu K, Naito MF, and Takahide Mori. (1993) Immunohistochemical analysis of p53 protein overexpression in endometrial carcinomas: inverse correlation with sex steroid receptor status. *Virchows Archiv A Pathol Anat* 423:265-271.

2. Naito M, Satake M, Sakai E, Hirano Y, Tsuchida N, Kanzaki H, Ito Y, and Mori T. (1992) Detection of p53 gene mutations in human ovarian and endometrial cancers by polymerase chain-single strand conformation polymorphism analysis. *Jpn J Cancer Res* 83:1030-1036.

3. Wang DP, Konishi I, Koshiyama M, Mandai M, Nanbu Y, Ishikawa Y, Mori T, and Fujii S. (1993) Expression of c-*erb*B-2 protein and epidermal growth factor receptor in endometrial carcinomas: correlation with clinicopathologic and sex steroid receptor status. *Cancer* 72:2628-2637.

Tumor-associated markers of stromal origin as indicators of clinical course of ovarian cancer

A. Kauppila, G. -G. Zhu, C. Tomás, U. Puistola, M. Santala, F. Stenbäck, S. Kauppila, J. Risteli and L. Risteli

Departments of Gynecology and Obstetrics, Clinical Chemistry, Medical Biochemistry and Pathology, University of Oulu, Oulu, Finland

Interstitial stroma participates in the development, growth, spread and regression of malignant tumors in many ways. In these processes the fibrillar type I and type III collagens, the most abundant soft tissue collagens in the human organism, play many important roles. First, as they are necessary for the integrity of all kind of soft tissues, the formation of collagenous network is essential for the development and growth of the neoplasms. Secondly, the host organism reacts to the presence of malignant neoplasm by fibroproliferation which involves formation of fibrotic barrier to surround the tumor and to resist its invasive spread. Thirdly, several proteolytic enzymes produced by the tumor cells or other cells activated by malignancy, may cause destructive changes in the surrounding tissues, including disruption and degradation of type I and type III collagens. Collagen turnover is thus continuously enhanced in the organism affected by a malignant tumor. In this phenomenon synthetic and degradative changes take place simultaneously.

Type I and type III procollagens are synthesized by fibroblasts and are enzymatically converted into their respective collagens in the extracellular space. The carboxyterminal propeptide of type I collagen (PICP) and the aminoterminal propeptide of type III collagen (PIIINP) are cleaved off during synthesis of respective collagens and before their assembly into the collagenous network. They are thus indicators of synthesis of type I and type III collagens, respectively **(Table 1)**. Some of the PIIINP molecules, however, remain in the mature collagen in the tissue and are cleaved off during its degradation. Therefore PIIINP has been regarded rather as an indicator of metabolism than only synthesis of type III collagen. The cross-linked carboxyterminal telopeptide of type I collagen (ICTP), on the other hand, is an indicator of degradation of a mature, type I collagen. The radioimmunoassays for PIIINP, PICP and ICTP **(Table 1)** has created interesting possibilities for the investigation of type I and type III collagen metabolism in patients suffering from malignant disease. We have therefore systematically evaluated the value of PIIINP, PICP and ICTP as tumor-associated markers in ovarian carcinoma, and to some

Table 1. Radioimmunoassays for investigating metabolism of type I and type III collagens. In parentheses, the methods available soon.

	Synthesis	Degradation
Type I collagen	PICP (PINP)	ICTP
Type III collagen	PIIINP *	(IIINTP)

* PIIINP is predominantly a marker of synthesis, although a part of it may be released into the circulation during the degradation of type III collagen.

721

extent in other gynecological malignancies as well (1). In these studies, employing biochemical, immunohistochemical and in situ hybridization methods, we have demonstrated that type I and type III collagens are abundant in large amounts in ovarian carcinoma tissues (1, 2).

In this context it is worth noticing that several other connective tissue elements are involved in the transactions between healthy and carcinomatous tissues including migrating cells of the hematopoietic system. An example of such tumor markers is the macrophage colony stimulating factor -1 (M-CSF-1), which can been measured by radioimmunoassay and has been found to be present in increased concentrations in association with ovarian, endometrial and some other soft tissue tumors (3). It may be clinically useful in the follow-up of endometrial carcinoma (4).

With the present paper, we want to summarize our results of studies on collagen metabolism in ovarian carcinoma using biochemical, immunohistochemical and in situ hybridization techniques (1,2, 5-9)

PIIINP

Type III collagen is a pure soft tissue collagen and differs thus from type I collagen which is present also in the mineralized part of the bones. It is abundant in the female genital tract and in gynecological tumors. PIIINP serves as an indicator of the metabolism of type III collagen taking place in the soft tissues.

Advanced ovarian cancer appeared to be associated with an increased serum concentration of PIIINP in about half to three quarters of our patients (1,3-6). In an early disease, the serum PIIINP level was often normal as was also the case for CA 125, the established tumor marker in ovarian cancer. It is important that the serum concentration of PIIINP followed the behaviour of the disease; steadily pathologic or increasing levels were typical of advancing disease and decreasing values were typical of regressing carcinoma. Follow-up studies also revealed that in about 75 % of patients, PIIINP and CA 125 gave similar information on the clinical course of malignancy (5). In the remaining cases, they were complementary to each other **(Fig. 1)**.

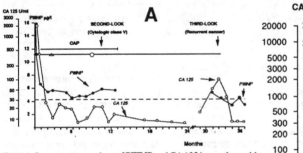

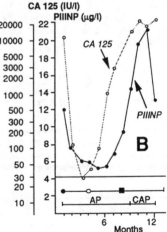

Fig. 1A. Serum concentrations of PIIINP and CA 125 in a patient with a complete response to cytotoxic chemotherapy of advanced ovarian cancer after explorative laparotomy. CA 125 concentration decreased to normal whereas PIIINP remained elevated before and during clinical remission. PIIINP measurements were stopped at the time of second-look operation, which gave no evidence of a macroscopical tumor, which, however, was found at the third-look operation about one year later.

Fig. 1B. Serum concentrations of PIIINP and CA 125 in a patient with an inoperable advanced ovarian cancer presented a short-term decrease followed by a rapid and strong increase; changes which closely correlated with the clinical course of the malignancy.

For the symbols: In the response line, the closed circle indicates the presence of a measurable tumor; the open triangle, a partial response; the open circle, a complete response; and the closed square, a clinical progression. CAP and AP indicate combinations of cyclophosphamide, adriamycin and cis-platinum, and alkeran + cis-platinum, respectively.

It is also significant that in patients with a tumor nonresponsive to cytotoxic chemotherapy the serum concentration of PIIINP indirectly correlated with survival time (6). Furthermore, in patients with complete or partial response to therapy, the persistently increased serum PIIINP level or its increase from normal to pathologic predicted always the recurrent disease. It thus complemented CA 125, which often failed in this situation. These findings stress the importance of type III collagen in the malignancy-induced reactions inside the tumor and its surroundings. It is, however, an unspecific tumor marker as increased PIIINP values have also been observed at times in patients with endometriosis, pelvic inflammatory disease and uterine fibroids (10). Hence, PIIINP resembles CA 125 in this respect. The propeptides of type I and type III collagens are eliminated via the liver. Therefore increased PIIINP values have been recorded also in association with liver diseases (2).

PICP and ICTP

Type I collagen is the most abundant type of collagen in the human body. It forms approximately 90% of the organic matrix of mineralized bone. Therefore, the metabolites cleaved off during the synthesis (PICP) or degradation (ICTP) of type I collagen are predominantly derived from the bones. Indeed, PICP and ICTP have been found to be clinically useful indicators of bone metabolism in many circumstances, e.g. rheumatoid arthritis and the formation and disappearance of bone metastases (2). Because type I collagen is the most abundant collagen also in the soft tissues including normal and malignant female genital tract tissues, we investigated the behaviour of PICP and ICTP in ovarian carcinoma.

With PICP, we observed that the changes in its serum concentration followed the pattern of changes taking place in PIIINP concentrations (7). However, PICP changes mostly took place within the reference interval and serum PICP concentration only exceeded the upper limit of the reference interval during the final progression of the disease **(Fig. 2)**. It thus does not add anything new to that available by PIIINP determinations when following clinical course of ovarian carcinoma.

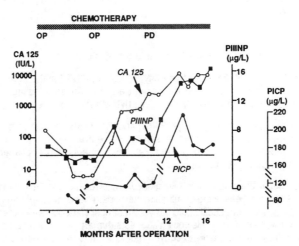

Fig. 2. Serum concentration of PIIINP (black square), PICP (black dot) and CA 125 in a patient with advanced ovarian malignancy treated with operations (OP) and cytotoxic chemotherapy. CA 125 and PIIINP predicted progression of the disease (PD) by four months. During progression, PICP also increased to a pathologic level. Solid line indicates the upper limit of reference interval for each variable.

The serum concentrations of ICTP also correlated with that of PIIINP during the follow-up of ovarian cancer patients. In many cases the individual response lines and the shapes of the concentration curves for ICTP and PIIINP were similar (8) **(Fig. 3)**. Changes in ICTP levels occur, however, often later than those in CA 125 and PIIINP levels in association with the early stage of ovarian cancer progression.

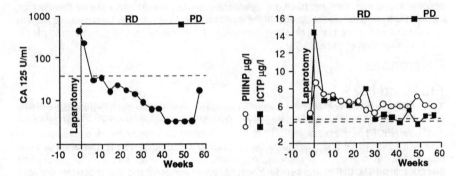

Fig. 3. Serial measurement of PIIINP, ICTP and CA 125 in a patient with advanced ovarian cancer. The disease responded to cytotoxic chemotherapy with regression (RD) followed by progression (PD). The curves of the markers resembled each other. However, PIIINP and ICTP remained pathologic all the time while CA 125 was mostly at the normal level despite the presence of malignancy.

In conclusion, our results indicate that advanced ovarian cancer also affects the metabolism of type I collagen. The strong background effect of the bone metabolism on the serum PICP and ICTP concentration limits their clinical value in monitoring the course of an advanced ovarian malignancy.

Biochemical and immunohistochemical investigations

To explore the origin of the excessive PIIINP, PICP and ICTP in the serum of patients with an advanced ovarian carcinoma we continued our studies using biochemical and immunohistochemical methods (9) and in situ hybridization techniques.

In these studies we observed that PIIINP and PICP concentrations in the ascitic fluid were manifold higher than the respective serum concentrations (9), suggesting that ovarian malignancy affects by either autocrine or paracrine mechanisms the collagen metabolism taking place within the peritoneal cavity.

The next step in our biochemical investigations was to characterize the molecular forms of the PIIINP and PICP antigens using gel filtration methods. These investigations revealed that some of PICP molecules in the ascitic fluid of ovarian cancer patients are present only in a partially processed large-sized form. This finding suggests that an overproduction of immature material exceeds the enzymatic capacity to convert molecules into free propeptides.

Immunohistochemical studies using specific antibodies for PIIINP, PICP and ICTP showed that the assembly and deposition of type I and type III collagen fibres, exhibited few changes in borderline tumors and marked irregularities in malignant tumors, particularly in poorly differentiated and anaplastic ones (9). The observations obtained in studies employing in situ hybridization techniques support the concept of severely disorded collagen metabolism in anaplastic ovarian malignancies (unpublished results).

The findings from biochemical and immunohistochemical studies confirm that ovarian carcinoma induces an intensive fibroproliferative reaction within the peritoneal space and in the tumor tissue (9). Type I and III collagens seem to be active participants in these biochemical events, and could be necessary for the further growth of the malignancy. Increased serum concentrations of PIIINP and ICTP are reflections of these phenomena and may therefore be useful in following the clinical course of the disease.

References

1. Risteli L, Risteli J, Puistola U, Tomás C, Zhu G-G, Kauppila A. Aminoterminal propeptide of type III procollagen in ovarian cancer - a review. *Acta Obstet Gynecol Scand Suppl* **71** 155, 99-103,1992

2. Risteli L, Risteli J. Biochemical markers of bone metabolism. *Ann Med* **25**, 385-93,1993

3. Kacinski BM. CSF-1 and its receptor in ovarian, endometrial and breast cancer. *Ann Med* **27**, 79-85,1995

4. Hakala A, Kacinski BM, Stanley ER, Kohorn E, Puistola U, Risteli J, Risteli L, Tomás C, Kauppila A. Macrophage colony-stimulating factor 1 (CSF-1), a clinically useful tumor marker in endometrial carcinoma. Comparison with CA 125 and the aminoterminal propeptide of type III procollagen. *Am J Obstet Gynecol*, In press

5. Kauppila A, Puistola U, Risteli J, Risteli L. Aminoterminal propeptide of type III procollagen: A new prognosis indicator in human ovarian cancer. *Cancer Res* **49**, 1885-89, 1989

6. Tomás C. The clinical usefulness of the aminoterminus of type III procollagen (PIIINP) in gynecologic malignancies. Thesis. *Acta Universitatis Ouluensis*, Series D Medica **298**. University of Oulu, Printing Center, 1994.

7. Zhu G-G, Puistola U, Risteli J, Risteli L, Kauppila A. Type I and type III procollagen metabolites and CA 125 in epithelial ovarian cancer. *Int J Oncol* **4**, 669-74, 1994

8. Santala M, Risteli L, Puistola ,U, Risteli J, Kauppila A. Elevated serum ICTP concentrations reflect poor prognosis in patients with ovarian carcinoma. *Ann Med*, **2**, :57-61,1995

9. Zhu G-G. Type I and type III collagens in ovarian neoplasia. Thesis. *Acta Universitatis Ouluensis*, Series D, Medica **317**, University of Oulu, Printing Center 1994

10. Puistola U, Risteli L, Risteli J, Kauppila A. Collagen metabolism in gynecologic patients: Changes in the concentration of the aminoterminal propeptide of type III procollagen in serum. *Am J Obstet Gynecol* **163**, 1276-81,1990

Steroid hormones and breast cancer

J.A. Pinotti and R. Hegg

Department of Obstetrics and Gynecology, São Paulo University Medical School, São Paulo, Brazil

---

This is perhaps the most controversial issue concerning the risks of estrogen therapy at present. It is well recognised that an early menarche, late menopause and many other reproductive factors are associated with an increased risk of breast carcinoma.

An increased number of menstrual ovulatory cycles (MOC) represents a risk factor, what was demonstrated in a large epidemiological study, carried out in the State University of Campinas, from 1975 to 1979 (Pinotti et al., 1984). These authors studied 174 women with breast cancer and, at least, one control for each case. The average number of menstrual cycles among women with breast cancer was 313.6 while in controls the average number was 279.7 (p < 0.00001). Breast cancer relative risk was 3.3 in women with more than 300 MOC. Therefore, it is not unreasonable to assume that "delaying the menopause" with estrogen therapy may also increase this risk.

Most of the recent epidemiological studies of breast cancer were performed in the USA and the vast majority of women were taking unopposed conjugated estrogens. Four case controlled studies (Ross et al., 1980; Brinton et al., 1981; Hoover et al., 1981; Hiatt et al., 1984) reported an

727

increase in relative risk (1.3 - 1.9) with long-term estrogen use, and three of these reported a dose-dependent association. In contrast, three other studies found no evidence to suggest that breast cancer risk was increased overall or with long term use (Kelsey et al., 1981; Kaufman et al., 1984; Wingo et al., 1987).

Many of these studies have tried to establish whether there is a particular group most at risk. A large-scale study of estrogen users from the American National Cancer Institute (Brinton et al., 1986) has demonstrated that with 5 years of use, the relative risk was 0.89 for estrogen users, whereas for 20 or more years of use the risk was 1.47.

The most recent controversy is whether progestogen addition modifies the risk of breast cancer. A prospective Swedish study suggested that the risk of breast cancer was highest among women who took combination estrogen/ progestogen therapy for extended periods (Bergkvist, 1989). A study from Denmark also found an increased risk among combination estrogen/progestogen users (Ewertz, 1988).
Breast and endometrial tissue may respond differently to the effects of progestogen. Anderson et al. (1982) studied breast tissue in perimenopausal women and found that DNA synthesis in breast epithelium does not appear to be supressed by endogenous progesterone. The Consensus Conference on Progestogens concluded that there were insufficient data on breast protection to recommend the routine prescribing of progestogens to hysterectomised women taking estrogens (Whitehead & Lobo, 1988). The problem, from the basic or biologic point of view, is as complex as the epidemiological one.

Breast tissue is subject to modifications along the menstrual cycle and according to the different lifetime periods. Even though breast tissue does not show the classical endometrial phases of proliferation and secretion, many authors could recognize cyclic morphological changes contrasting with those of the

728

endometrium: the maximal proliferative activity was observed in the second phase of the menstrual cycle, by the 21st day, suggesting a synergistic proliferative action.

Experimental studies show that estrogens stimulate the mammary gland epithelial proliferation in rodents and humans, not necessarily through a direct action, but interacting with growth factors systems and different hormones, some of them from the pituitary. Estrogens could change the function of different growth factors, acting directly in their secretion or interfering with their receptors.

Most part of the clinicians are in favor to prescribe HRT to the majority of menopausal women because of its comproved benefits. Nevertheless, we should advert them of a possible risk of breast cancer with more than 8-10 years of use; the same clinicians are divided over the advisability of prescribing HRT to women with a history of breast carcinoma. The majority counsel against its use because of the potential for stimulating growth in metastatic carcinoma cells, but most part of us seem to accept that each case should be considered individually.

ABSTRACT

We have enough evidences that hormone replacement therapy (HRT) can increase breast cancer risk when used for more than 10 years. Nevertheless results from the studies carried out did not draw a final conclusion; besides, some of their methodologies have been criticised.

Probably progestogens cannot change estrogens influence on breast cancer risk in the same way it does with the endometrium. So, women who have undergone histerectomy can use HRT without progesterone.

Other studies, larger and with longer follow-up, are needed, aiming to define in a better way the groups for which estrogens (or progestogens) can change breast cancer risk.

In the daily practice, however, we must bear in mind that the use must not exceed 8 to 10 years, and for histerectomized patients, there is no need to add progesterone.

As a precaution, for the patients who have already presented breast cancer we must avoid HRT; nevertheless, the cases should be individually analysed, considering the patient prognosis and her quality of life.

REFERENCES

BRINTON, LA; HOOVER, R; FRAUMENI, JF — Menopausal oestrogens and breast cancer risk: an expanded case-control study. Br. J. Cancer, 54: 825 – 32, 1986

BRINTON, LA; HOOVER, RN; SZKLO, M; FRAUMENI, JF — Menopausal estrogen use and risk of breast cancer. Cancer, 47: 2517 – 22, 1981

EWERTZ, M — Influence of non-contraceptive exogenous and endogenous sex hormones on breast cancer risk in Denmark. Int. J. Cancer, 42: 832 – 8, 1988

HIATT, RA; BAWOL, R; FRIEDMAN, GD; HOOVER, R — Exogenous estrogens and breast cancer after bilateral oophorectomy. Cancer, 54: 139 – 44, 1984

HOOVER, R; GLASS, A; FINKLE, WD et al — Conjugated estrogens and breast cancer risk. J. Natl. Cancer Inst., 67: 815 – 20, 1981

KAUFMAN, DW; MILLER, DR; ROSENBERG, L; HELMRICH, SP — Noncontraceptive estrogen use and the risk of breast cancer. JAMA, 252: 63 – 7, 1984

KELSEY, JL; FISCHER, DB; HOLFORD, JR et al — Exogenous estrogens and other factors in the epidemiology of breast cancer. J. Natl. Cancer Inst., 67: 327 – 33, 1981

PINOTTI, JA; HARDY, EE; FAÚNDES, A — Ciclos menstruales ovulatorios y cáncer de mama. Boletín de la Academia Nacional de Medicina de Buenos Aires, 61: 117 – 20, 1984

ROSS, RK; PAGANINI-HILL, A; GERKINS, VR — A case control study of menopausal estrogen therapy and breast cancer. JAMA, 243: 1635 – 40, 1980

WHITEHEAD, MI; LOBO, RA — Progestogen use in postmenopausal women. Consensus Conference. Lancet, ii: 1243 – 4, 1988

WINGO, PA; LAYDE, PM; LEE, NC; RUBIN, G; ORY, HW — The risk of breast cancer in postmenopausal women who have used estrogen replacement therapy. JAMA, 257: 209 – 15, 1987

Expression of bcl-2 and p53 in human breast cancer: relationships with proliferative activity and clinical findings

M. Massobrio, L. Bianchi Malandrone*, A. Demurtas*, A. Durando, O. Gaiola*, M. Geuna*, A. Ramella**, A. Ravarino**, M. Sberveglieri, B. Torchio** and G. Palestro*

Clinic of Gynecology and Obstetrics, *Department of Biomedical Sciences and Human Oncology, University of Turin and **Department of Pathology, Mauriziano Hospital, Turin, Italy

---

Background. Approximately two–third of patients with breast cancer have a disease that is apparently confined to the breast, without axillary nodal involvement. The presence of tumor in axillary lymph nodes remains the strongest predictor of recurrence (1). If axillary lymph nodes are free from disease, prognosis is improved; nevertheless almost one–third of patients with lymph node–negative tumors escape local–regional treatment control recurring in ten years. (2).The importance of identifying higher–risk patients at diagnosis is supported by the evidence of an improved relapsed–free survival after chemiotherapy or hormone therapy for specific subsets of patients with lymph node–negative breast cancer (3) .

Many new biological parameters have been studied to complement and improve the prognostic value of the conventional factors, such as tumor size, lymph node status, hormone receptor status, histological grading, cytokinetics parameters, DNA Index (DI) and S–phase fraction (SPF) . The main goal of these researches is to identify patients with a significantly higher likehood of recurrence than that of the node–negative group as a whole. In this view the not conventional features investigated have been : a) proliferation markers, i.e. Ki67 (MIB–1), cyclins, PCNA (Proliferative Cell Nuclear Antigen), b) growth factors and receptors such as erbB–2/Neu, epidermal growth factor (EGF) receptor, insulin growth factor (IGF) receptor and transforming growth factor α (TGF–α), c) invasion markers such as cathepsin D, laminin receptors, plasminogen activator, collagenase IV, angiogenetic factors, d) tumor suppressor genes p53 and rb, e) others oncogenes such as nm23, ras, c–myc, bcl–2, f) other factors such as chemoresistant protein gp170 (MDR–1) and pS2 protein (4).

In the last few years, beside cell proliferation, apoptosis (the main pathway of programmed cell death) has been increasingly recognized as a crucial event in regulating tumor growth (5).

Experimental evidence supports the role of oncogenes and tumor suppressor genes in regulating apoptotic cell death (6). The bcl–2 proto–oncogene encodes an inner mitochondrial membrane protein responsible for specific prevention of apoptosis in several cell types (7).

The p53 suppressor gene encodes for a nuclear phoshoprotein able to regulate the cell cycle and also induces the apoptotic pathway (8). The p53 gene is the most commonly altered tumor suppressor gene in human malignancies and its alteration probably represents a relatively early event in cancer progression (4). About 30% of human breast cancers have mutations in p53 gene, and in as many as 60% of tumors p53 is detectable by immunohistochemistry. The presence of mutant p53 in tumor cells is associated with poorer prognosis, but it remains uncertain whether p53 is an independent prognostic factor (9).

In this study we analyzed flow cytometric findings (DNA Index – DI and S phase fraction – SPF) in association with clinicopathological features and p53 and bcl–2 protein expression in order to investigate if oncogene expression correealtes with either cytokinetic activity and conventional clinicopathological prognostic factors.

Methods and results. In 51 breast cancer we performed on fresh/frozen tumor fragments flow cytometric evaluation of DI (ploidy) by mean of propidium iodine staining (Cycletest Plus, Becton Dickinson, San Josè, Cal). On 43 (84%) of them we also could calculate SPF, using a cut–off of 7% calculated on the basis of the median value. The expression of bcl–2 and p53 protein was detected on the same group of tumors through an immunohistochemistry method using the avidin–biotin complex (LSAB, Dako) and the monoclonal antibodies MoAb 124 (Dako, Glostrup, Denmark) and MoAb DO7 (specific for both wild type and mutant protein, Medac, Germany) respectively. For this purpose we used tissue sections obtained from the same formalin fixed and paraffin embedded tissue blocks on which breast cancer was diagnosed. The cut–off considered for bcl–2 and p53 was ≥30% and <5% stained tumor cells respectively (10, 11).

The main features of the 51 breast cancers studied are reported in Table 1, where the cases are divided on the basis of their clinicopatological characters (pT, pN and grading), cytokinetics parameters (DI and SPF) and protein bcl–2 and p53 expression. bcl–2 and p53 were inversely related (R=–0.44, p=0.001) (Table 2) as well as bcl–2 and nuclear grading (R=–0.35, p=0.01). Moreover, bcl–2 positive tumors were also significantly related to a lower proliferative activity, as detected by SPF (R=–0.38, p=0.01). By contrast, p53 expression was associated with a greater proliferation (R=0.4, p=0.007). No statistical difference was found between tumor size, lymph node status, hormone receptor status, DI and both bcl-2 and p53 protein expression. (Table 3).

Analyzing only node negative tumors (27 cases), a significant opposite relation was found between progesterone–receptor positivity and p53 expression: only 18% of p53 positive tumors were PR+, whereas 69% of p53 negative tumors were PR+ (p=0.01).

Table 1. Distribution of clinicopathological and biological features in 51 breast cancers.

	no. of cases	%
Tumor size		
pT2cm	21	41.1
pT>2cm	30	58.9
Lymph node status		
pN=0	27	52.9
pN=1	24	47.1
Nuclear grading		
G1	12	23.5
G2	21	41.2
G3	18	35.3
Hormone receptor status		
ER+	38	74.5
ER–	13	25.5
PR+	18	35.3
PR–	33	64.7
DNA index (ploidy)		
DI=1	13	25.4
DI1	38	74.6
S–phase fraction		
SPF<7	21	48.8
SPF7	22	51.2
Oncoprotein		
Bcl–2+	38	74.5
Bcl–2–	13	25.5
p53+	23	45.1
p53–	28	54.9

Table 2. Combined bcl-2 and p53 expression in 51 breast cancer cases (Pearson's correlation coefficient R=-0.44, p=0.001

Oncogenes	no of cases	%
bcl-2+/p53+	14	27
bcl-2+/p53-	24	47
bcl-2-/p53+	9	18
bcl-2-/p53-	4	8

Table 3. Correlations between bcl-2 and p53 and clinicopathological features.

bcl-2 versus	R	p	p53 versus	R	p
tumor size	-0.09	0.9	tumor size	0.12	0.4
lymph node status	-0.04	0.9	lymph node status	-0.04	0.78
grading	-0.35	0.01	grading	0.15	0.3
ER	-0.1	0.5	ER	0.15	0.27
PR	-0.14	0.3	PR	0.14	0.3
DI	-0.21	0.14	DI	-0.03	0.84
SPF	-0.38	0.01	SPF	0.40	0.007

Conclusive remarks. In this preliminary study, the analysis of bcl-2 and p53 protein expression, investigated in a series of 51 invasive breast cancers may be summarized as follow. The expression of bcl-2 was found in high percentage of breast cancers and was inversely related to proliferative activity. This result may suggest that bcl-2 expression, beside protecting the cell from apoptosis, may also be involved in processes controlling (slowing down) the cell proliferation. As a consequence of this, bcl-2 positive tumors could be genetically more stable and could have a more favourable clinical course (10, 12). This hypotesis is also supported by the higher degree of differentiation that we observed in bcl-2 positive tumors.

By contrast, p53 expression seems to be correlated to a higher proliferation of tumor cells, and, at least in node negative tumors, to the absence of PR receptors. The last finding is in keeping with previous reports (13) suggesting that mutations and subsequent accumulation of the non-functional p53 protein can enhance clonal expansion of primary tumor cells, conferring selective growth advantage to p53-immunoreactive breast cancer.

The strong inverse correlation between bcl-2 and p53 provides a further demonstration of the opposite roles played by these genes in the control of cell growth. Moreover, recently it has been proposed an inhibitory activity of mutant p53 on bcl-2 expression (14).

Silvestrini et al (10) have found a good correlation between bcl–2 and some pathological features (tumor size and oestrogen receptors) in a series of breast cancer patients. The difference between these and our results may be due to different criteria in patient selection: in the former serie only cases without lymph node involvement were considered.

In our serie the lack of correlation between p53 and tumor size, lymph node status and hormone receptor is in agreement with previous reports (13,15). However, an over–expression of p53 is thought to be an independent prognostic factor (11,15). Further studies are in course to better assess the prognostic value of bcl–2 and p53 expression and to understand the role of these genes in the control of the biological and clinical behavior of breast cancer.

References.

1) McGuire WL, Clark GM (1992):Prognostic factors and treatment decisions in axillary–node–negative breast cancer, *N Engl J Med* **326**: 1756–61.

2) Dorr FA (1993): Prognostic factors observed in current clinical trials, *Cancer* **71**: 2163–8.

3) Early Breast Cancer Trialists'Collaborative Group (1992): Systemic treatment of early breast cancer by hormonal, citotoxic, or immune therapy. 133 randomised trials involving 31.000 recurrences and 24.000 deaths among 75.000 women. *Lancet* **339**: 1–15.

4) Shapiro CL and Henderson IC eds (1994) *Hematol Oncol Clin North Am* **vol 8**, no 1.

5) Kerr JFR, Winterford CM, Harmon BV (1994): Apoptosis, *Cancer* **73**: 2013–26.

6) Osborne BA, Schwartz LM (1994): Essential genes that regulate apoptosis *Trends Cell Biol* **4**: 394–8.

7) Korsmeyer SJ (1992): Bcl-2 initiates a new category of oncogenes: regulators of cell death *Blood* **80**: :879–86.

8) Perry ME, Levine AJ (1993): Tumor–suppressor p53 and the cell cycle *Curr Opin Genetics Develop* **3**: 50–4

9) Thor AD, Moore II DH, Edgerton SM, Kawasaki ES et Al (1992): Accumulation of p53 tumor suppressor gene protein: an independent marker of prognosis in breast cancer *J Natl Cancer Inst* **84**: 845–55

10) Silvestrini R, Veneroni S Daidone MG, Benini E et Al (1994): The Bcl-2 protein : a prognostic indicator strongly related to p53 protein in lymp node–negative breast cancer patients *J Natl Cancer Inst* **86**: 499–504.

11) Silvestrini R, Benini E, Daidone MG, Veneroni S et Al (1993): p53 as an independent prognostic marker in lymph node–negative breast cancer patients *J Natl Cancer Inst* **5**: 965–70.

12) Pezzella F, Turley H, Kuzu I, Tusgekan M F et al (1993): bcl–2 protein in non–small–cell lung carcinoma *New Engl J Med* **329**: 690–4

13) Caleffi M, Teague M W, Jensen R A, Vnencak–Jones C L et al (1994): P53 gene mutations and steroid receptor status in breast cancer *Cancer* **73**: 2147–56

14) Haldar S, Negrini M, Monne M, Sabbioni S et al (1994): Down–regulation of bcl–2 by p53 in breast cancer cells *Cancer Res* **54**: 2095–7

15) Friedrichs K, Gluba S, Eidtmann H, Jonat W (1993): Overexpression of p53 and prognosis in breast cancer *Cancer* **72**: 3641–7.

Endocrine management of breast cancer

H.P.G. Schneider

Munster, Germany

Hormonal therapy for breast cancer began more than a hundred years ago with the observation that bilateral oophorectomy caused tumour regression in selected premenopausal patients. In the first half of this century, besides extending ablation of ovarian function to photon irradiation, surgical adrenalectomy and hypophysectomy were introduced, and hormonal additive therapies such as the use of androgens, estrogens, progestins, and glucocorticoids were established. Clearly defined objective regression rates for advanced breast cancer with all types of endocrine therapy at this point did not exceed 35 %.

The demonstration that adjuvant systemic therapy (i. e. systemic therapy given at the time of primary local treatment in the absence of demonstrated metastases) can prolong the disease-free interval and improve overall survival has been a major advance in the management of breast cancer. The rationale was to control or eliminate micrometastases before the onset of tumour recurrence.

The antiestrogen Tamoxifen was chosen for the majority of studies since the mid-1970s. Since the first report of a successful treatment in patients with metastatic breast cancer, the number of treated women worldwide has reached over three million. Objective response rates (CR and PR following UICC) in unselected patients is 34 %. An additional 19 % experience no change, the mean duration of remission being 9 to 12 months.

The non-steroidal antiestrogen Tamoxifen has been used successfully to treat both pre- and postmenopausal women with all stages of the disease. It is used both as a palliative treatment for women with advanced disease, and as an adjuvant treatment following surgery for node negative or node positive disease. If the patients are regrouped for analysis based on the estrogen and progesterone receptor (ER and PR) status of their primary tumour, patients with ER + /PR + disease have a 70 % - 80 % likelihood of responding favourably to Tamoxifen. In an overview analysis of 30,000 patients from 40 trials of adjuvant Tamoxifen, a significant increase was found in both disease-free and overall survival. When patients were separated by nodal status, statistically significant increases were observed in disease-free and overall survival for both node positive and node negative patients. Women over 50 appear to benefit most from Tamoxifen treatment, experiencing highly significant increases in disease-free and overall survival regardless of nodal status. Women under 50 years of age treated with Tamoxifen experience a trend towards increased disease-free and overall survival compared to control patients, yet not of statistical significance. Tamoxifen can be used for treatment of breast cancer of any stage with some success. However, since Tamoxifen primarily acts as a cytostatic and not cytotoxic agent, most patients ultimately experience disease recurrence or progression during or after therapy.

Newer antiestrogens include Trioxifene, Toremifene and Droloxifene (3-OH-Tamoxifen). Randomized, prospective studies are still under way to prove their clinical superiority or not.

Progestins exert direct antiproliferative effects in human breast cancer cell lines. They may also exert direct antiestrogenic action by increasing the oxidative activity of 17ß-hydroxy-steroid-dehydrogenase, thereby facilitating the conversion of estradiol to estrone, an estrogen of lower potency. This effect appears to be mediated through interaction with the progesterone receptor. Progestins may exert additional antiestrogenic effects due to their suppression of ER levels. In addition, progestins besides binding to progesterone receptors also recognize androgen and glucocorticoid receptors in human breast cancer, thus spreading their direct anti-tumour action. As they also cause estrogen deprivation indirectly through suppression of pituitary ACTH secretion, resulting in reduced production of adrenal androgen precursors, both low- and high-dose regimens have been studied. High doses of MPA and MA apparently produce similar clinical effects to Tamoxifen, whereas conventional low doses seem to be less effective. Most side effects include hypertension, hyperglycemia, edema, congestive heart failure, diarrhea, and hypercalcemia, mostly because of the glucocorticoid-like activity of high-dose progestins.

Aromatase inhibition in premenopausal women leads to interruption of estrogen biosynthesis; the reflex rise in FSH, however, stimulates production of new aromatase enzyme, and the LH increment results in enhanced ovarian steroidogenesis in the thecal compartment and specifically higher amounts of the aromatase substrate androstenedione. These two effects tend to counteract the inhibitory action of aromatase-blocking drugs on the ovary.

In postmenopausal women, extraglandular aromatase is present predominantly in fat, liver, muscle, and hair follicles. Aminoglutethimide was initially recognized to be an inhibitor of cytochrome P-450-mediated steroid hydroxilations and particularly of those involving the cholesterol side-chain cleavage enzyme. Clinical use of Aminoglutethimide for breast cancer thus attempted to produce a "medical adrenalectomy". A dose of 1,000 mg Aminoglutethimide daily produced 95 to 98 % inhibition of aromatase in postmenopausal women with breast cancer. The regimen of Aminoglutethimide plus hydrocortisone inhibited plasma and urinary estradiol to levels comparable to those observed after surgical adrenalectomy. A combination of clinical responses to Aminoglutethimide plus glucocorticoid in women with breast cancer reveals results similar to those expected with other forms of endocrine therapy. Overall, one-third of women experience either complete or partial tumour regression whereas 54 % with ER positive tumours responded with objective regressions. Responses persist for a mean of 13 months, and patients survive for an average of 20 months. Side effects include drug rash, fever and lethargy.

The development of improved aromatase inhibitors includes steroidal derivatives such as 4-Hydroxyandrostenedione and non-steroidal compounds such as Pyridoglutethimide; in addition, Imidazole drugs have been introduced as they exert potent effects on a number of cytochrome P-450-mediated steroid hydroxilation steps. These include Ketoconazole, CGS 16949 A, and R 76713.

Preliminary clinical data with 4-Hydroxystenedione demonstrated a 33 % objective regression rate of breast cancer in postmenopausal women previously treated with multiple endocrine therapies. Optimal daily doses of 250 to 500 mg/day of Aminoglutethimide appear to be most effective as second-line hormone therapy. Wide-range clinical experience with the newer aromatase inhibitors is still lacking.

As comparative trials of aromatase inhibitors and Tamoxifen with surgical adrenalectomy and hypophysectomy demonstrated similar response rates to each of these therapies, other medical approaches are investigated. As they do not require hospitalization and major surgery, they have largely supplanted ablative treatment.

GnRH analog therapy has been suggested to exert a direct anti-tumour action in addition to the indirect effects mediated by pituitary suppression. Various studies with Leuprolide, Zoladex, and its depot form Goserelin in summary revealed a 41 % objective response rate in unselected patients and 51 % in women with ER positive tumours. Although there are no data from randomized trials, the results of therapy with GnRH analogues are similar to those expected from oophorectomy.

Emerging new endocrine treatments involve RU-486 (Mifeprestone) and bromocryptine/somatostatine analog therapy. RU-486 with its antiprogestational and antiglucocorticoidal effects has been used in recent pilot clinical trials as a second- or third-line therapy in women with advanced breast cancer. RU-486 administration has been found to increase circulating levels of ACTH, cortisol, androstenedione, and estradiol. The potential adverse effect on tumour growth of high circulating levels of estradiol could be offset by concomitant Tamoxifen administration. The role, if any, of antiprogestin therapy needs to be defined by larger clinical trials in less heavily pretreated patients.

It may be possible with the combined administration of dopaminergic drugs and the newly developed somatostatin analogues to inhibit both PRL and GH secretion and thus completely block lactogenic activity with the ultimate goal of inducing breast cancer regression. Preliminary pilot experience has not yet proven the therapeutic potential of this form of treatment in metastatic breast cancer.

There appears to be little clinical advantage to combining various forms of hormonal therapy. One hypothesis proposes to utilize the endocrine dependency of human breast cancer to hormonally modified tumour cell kinetics as a mean of increasing the efficacy of cytotoxic chemotherapy. The strategy involves an arrest of hormonal-sensitive cells in the G_0 state through estrogen deprivation and a sequential phase of physiological estrogen repletion to induce synchronized cell replication. Chemotherapy is then given at the time of peak DNA synthesis when chemosensitivity is presumably at its best. The published randomized clinical trials indicate benefit from estrogen priming is modest and restricted to previously untreated patients.

In conclusion, when breast cancer is first detected, there are 7 % distant metastases; at the time of original surgery, 50 % of patients are found to be node negative, yet in one-third cancer will return. Tumour changes linked to poor prognosis concern ER, PR status, angiogenesis, as well as erb B_2 gene and NM 23 gene. A better understanding of the mechanisms of endocrine tumour dependence on a basic level is required in order to further improve treatment strategies.

Surgical management of breast cancer

F.R. Pérez-López

Department of Obstetrics and Gynecology, Hospital Clínico and University of Zaragoza Faculty of Medicine, Zaragoza, Spain

1. INTRODUCTION

Although in the second century AD Galen depicted cancer as a systemic disease, diverse findings obtained during the 19th century led Halsted to formulate the basis for breast cancer radical surgery that has been systematically used for almost a century. The radical surgical procedures were submitted to several technical modifications with only minimal reduction of local relapses and without improvement in the mortality rate.

The management of breast cancer has undergone remarkable changes over the last two decades. Meticulous conservative surgery with the use of relatively innocuous breast radiation eliminates the need for breast radical surgery. The changes produced in breast cancer surgical management have been the consequence of prospective studies showing similar final results in terms of survival and disease-free interval for either radical surgery and less agressive procedures when used appropiately in women with tumors of less than 3 cm (1-3). The breast-conserving approach has been also used in patients with larger tumors (4-6). However, in reality, conservative surgery is being used much less extensively than expected. Nattinger *et al.* (7) indicate that only 10-20 % of American women are treated with conservative surgery. Regional variations were also reported among the nine regions in the United States covered by the Surveillance, Epidemiology, and End Results (SEER) program of the National Cancer Institute (8). Iscoe *et al.* (9) report that in the Canadian province of Ontario breast-conserving therapy is performed in 31 % of breast cancer patients. Fear of recurrence has raised a controversy between those favouring mastectomy and those advocating a less radical operation.

The psychological morbidity of radical surgery has been recognised for many years, although anxiety and depression are also frequent after conservative surgery for breast cancer. Psychological morbidity may be related to the lack of information, fear of cancer and its ancestral association with death, and loss of self-confidence. It seems that body image and patient satisfaction may improve by conservative surgery as compared to ablative surgery, but psychological morbidity is the same in both groups.

Polychemotherapy and hormonal therapy after local treatment of breast cancer can reduce the annual risk of recurrence by some 25% and mortality by around 17% (10). However, the best drug combination and the optimal program of systemic treatment remains to be determined because at the present time similar results are reported in terms of disease free interval and survival with different approaches. Furthermore, many published results are only descriptive of empiric combinations with substantial costs, with few advantages over previous treatments and with doubtful benefit to individual patients. Future investigation of systemic treatment should be based on randomized studies with careful evaluation that includes quality of life and cost-benefit analysis in addition to the traditional disease free interval and survival.

During the last 20 years we have performed different surgical techniques for the treatment of breast cancer. Until the early 80's the Halsted procedure was used for non-metastatic breast cancer. Therefore, we have shifted toward performing a less mutilating procedure: axillar lymphadenectomy together with either mastectomy as suggested by Madden (11, 12) or wide excision of the primary tumor with grossly normal margins. Postoperative radiotherapy is included as standard treatment when breast-preserving approaches are used.

Elderly patients should receive similar surgical management to any other woman, although axillar surgery should be avoided unless grossly involved. Exclusive medical treatment (without surgery) of elderly patients with breast cancer has a high local morbidity with the need to perform secondary salvage surgery in those women with a worse general condition than at the initial time of diagnosis.

2. EARLY BREAST CANCER

For suspicious palpable breast tumors we perform a peroperatory excision biopsy with wide free margins; if the pathological study indicates invasive breast cancer, definitive surgical treatment is performed in the same step. Cytological examination of the aspiration of cysts or solid lesions and core biopsy for histological examinations have the disadvantage of not always sampling the target tissue, thus leading to false-negative results. Since these invasive techniques may also induces multiple and unpredictible biological changes, we prefer to perform a pathologic diagnosis, sampling for steroid receptors and definitive surgical treatment in one step.

The limitations of mammography to define specific findings, in order to differentiate benign and very early malignant lesions, and the risk to get a false cytological or drill biopsy led us to use wide excision of mammographic suspicious lesions. In non-palpable suspicious lesions stereoataxic-guided biopsy is performed and the pathologic study is delayed to have a secure diagnosis. We perform hook-wire needle biopsies inserted aseptically into the breast by the radiologist. An incision is made overlying the questionable area and a tunnel created through aiming at this area. During biopsy it is important to preserve the pectoralis major muscle and its fascia in order to prevent possible tumor cell implantation, specially in the two-step procedures. To identify the area removed and the mammographic finding that precipitated the decision for biopsy, specimen radiography is mandatory.

The assessment of axillary lymph node status is associated with a significant incidence of error both in false-positive and false-negative clinical impresions as compared to pathologic diagnosis. The therapeutic role of axillary surgery in breast cancer has been challenged, although the presence of axillar lymph node metastasis is still the best prognostic marker. Axillar surgery allows staging and thus a rational decision regarding systemic therapy may be made. Level I and II dissection provides sufficient information in most patients and if these nodes are not invaded the probability of tumor invasion for higher nodes is less than 1 % (13, 14). Dissection of the internal mammary lymph nodes is unnecessary since these are rarely invaded if the axillary nodes are negative (15).

The incidence of multicentric breast cancer ranges from 9-75 %, including nonpalpable early stages (16, 17), and the incidence of occult micrometastatic disease can reach 30 % in stages I or II (18). Therefore, the choice of surgical procedures is not always an easy decision in individual patients. Furthermore, the prognostic factors currently used are not good endpoints for the risk of later metastatic disease (19, 20).

Conservative surgery

The cosmetic results of conservative surgery are related to both surgery and radiation. A proper selection of the surgical conservative procedure minimizes the first factor, whilst the degree of breast induration, telangiectasia and scar retraction are related to the dose and metod of irradiation.

Non-metastatic invasive malignant breast tumors may be treated with either quadrantectomy or wide excision with grossly normal margins and lymphadenectomy. The main characteristic of the quadrantectomy is the radial direction of the resection including the tumor and the whole ductal tree of the gland. Lumpectomy with wide normal margins is a less extensive operation and gives better cosmetic results than quadrantectomy.

The best skin incision is usually curvilinear, placed over the tumor following the Langer's lines. In peripheral tumors the circumareolar technique should not be performed given that the margins are difficult to distinguish and hinder a meticulous hemostasia. Furthermore, the tunnel through the tumor is removed may raise problems regards planning the boost dose of radiotherapy. The radial incision may be useful to perform a quadrantectomy and for the wide excision of tumors from the lower mammary half. Preservation of the subcutaneous fat and the avoidance of the skin flaps is important in maintaining the normal breast contour.

To obtain an adequate pathologic evaluation the tumor should be removed as a single piece of tissue. Gross inspection of the specimen in the operating room will allow the identification of positive close margins facilitating immediate re-excision. However, careful histological evaluation of the margins of resection is important and re-excision or mastectomy may be mandatory if tumor removal was inadequate. Since re-excision produces a poor cosmetic result in some cases, it is better to perform an initial wide enough biopsy-excision.

Meticulous hemostasis after tumor excision is important to prevent a large hematoma that may hinder the differential diagnosis with local recurrence, although a small hematoma or seroma may lead to better cosmetic results. It is also convenient to mark the cavity outline with vascular clips in order to facilitate the subsequent radiotherapy. The incision should be sutured in two layers: the subcutaneous cellular tissue with absorbable suture of size 2-0 and skin with non-absorbable monofilament 5-0 or silk 3-0.

The axillar dissection is best performed by a different skin incision, although for tumors from the upper lateral quadrant it may be possible to perform tumor excision and lymphadenectomy through the same skin incision. We perform a complete dissection of all the fat and lymphatic tissue in the triangle bordered by the axillary vein superiorly, the latissimus dorsi laterally, and the serratus anterior medially. Identification of the axillar vasculoneural trunk, and the thoracodorsal and long thoracic nerves avoids injury to these structures during dissection. The number of axillar nodes obtained with this procedure ranges from 10 to 20.

Early bilateral synchronous breast cancer can be managed by conservative surgery. Contraindications to breast conserving-surgery includes multicentric tumors, diffuse microcalcifications, extensive intraductal component in patients with infiltrating ductal carcinoma, breast cancer detected in the first or second trimester of pregnancy, pre-existing collagen vascular disease, and prior therapeutic irradiation to the breast region. Relative contraindications include history of collagen vascular disease, presence of a large tumor in a small breast and central lesions. In women with large or pendulous breasts poor cosmetics results are achieved.

So far there is no consensus about the optimal negative margin for tumor excision. The presence of microscopic tumor at the margins is associated with a significant increase in the number of local relapses (21-24). Re-excision should be performed in patients with unknown margins and in those with extensive amounts of microscopic tumor at margins of excision due to the risk of a significant tumor burden. Less clear is the need to re-excise when minor microscopic exists at the margin of resection. However, in patients with microscopically positive margins an increase in radiation from 60 Gy to 65 Gy or an increase in boost doses from 10 Gy to 20 Gy permits the control without any further surgery (25-28).

Early-stage breast cancer with an extensive intraductal component may be associated with a high risk of local recurrence in the treated breast, although this possibility is still open to some question (29). In such patients wider resections or boost irradiation may ameliorate local control. In patients with infiltrating lobular carcinoma with discontinuous foci, close margins may be considered for re-excision. It appears that infiltrating lobular carcinoma does not have a worse local recurrence rate compared with infiltrating ductal carcinoma when each is treated with breast-conserving therapy (30, 31).

Re-excision is associated with the sacrifice of large amounts of breast. It should be disregarded if the primary tumor was big with wide and extensive infiltrated margins and, therefore, a mastectomy would be preferable in these cases since conserving surgery will not allow good cosmesis.

Modified radical mastectomy

Mastectomy associated with lymphadenectomy may be performed when tumor/mammary size does not guarantee a good cosmetic result, when there is a risk for multicenter lesions, and in women that prefer the radical procedures. It should be emphasized that despite the increasing trend toward conservative surgery, many women still want a mastectomy for breast cancer treatment.

Most patients with breast cancer may be subjected to the Madden modified radical mastectomy which is less mutilating than the Halsted operation. The pectoral muscles are preserved with better functional results and a secondary breast reconstruction is allowed, and level I-II lymph node dissection is enough for staging purposes since lymphadenectomy is not curative. The entire breast, axilla and arm are prepared in a sterile manner. At a minimum, a 4-cm skin margin an elliptical incision is outlined around the biopsy site and the nipple-areolar complex (Stewart incision). This allows a oblique scar with good cosmetic result that facilitates later breast reconstruction. Thin skin flaps are dissected to the outer limit of the breast in all directions. The breast is dissected from the major pectoral and left laterally until axillar dissection is completed. Dissection of the apex of the axilla may be accomplished with gentle retraction of both the pectoralis major and minor muscles. All the fat and lymph nodes are dissected from the top to bottom taking care to avoid injuring the neurovascular structures that course to the arm and the thoracodorsal nerve and vessels. After the removal, en masse, of the mammary gland and the axillar content, two suction drains are placed and the skin closed.

Contraindications to modified radical mastectomy include: extended inflammatory cancer, supraclavicular lymph node metastasis, chest wall fixation of the primary tumor, ipsilateral arm edema, satellite lesions beyond skin incision, distant metastasis and anesthetic contraindications.

Breast reconstruction after mastectomy may eliminate or at least palliate the psychosocial morbidity due to mastectomy. Breast reconstruction is controversial with regard to the indications for the procedure, the type of technique, and the appropiate time. Since immediate reconstruction may compromise adjuvant treatment, may interfere with the the detection of locoregional recurrences, and also increase the risk of these recurrences, we prefer delayed breast reconstruction. Although all women are affected psychologically by mastectomy, the majority of Spanish women aged over 60 years are not willing to undergo secondary surgical reconstruction.

Timing of surgery

There is evidence that breast tumor manipulation and invasive procedures increase the cancer cell dissemination. Attention has been focused on the timing of surgical treatment and the effect of the menstrual cycle on the survival outcome. A number of retrospective studies have been reported with apparently conflicting results (32-36).

Gnant *et al.* (35) found that the last menstrual period does not provide any prognostic information for breast cancer surgery outcome. In the Danish Breast Cancer Cooperative Study (36) the 5 and 10 years survival were not influenced by the time of surgery in relation to the last menstrual period.

Other recent publications indicate that in premenopausal women high circulating progesterone levels may reduce cell cancer dissemination and may improve prognosis and survival (37-39). The mechanisms by which progesterone exerts a *"protective"* effect is unknown and independent of the tumor steroid receptors. This effect on survival may be related to changes in proteolytic activity; surgery activates a physiological inflammatory response associated with increased vascular permeability.

These conflicting results justify a future prospective study with strict criteria in which the cycle phase at the time of surgery is biochemically determined in order to evaluate the effect of the endocrine milieu on survival outcome.

Surgical complications

The surgical procedures described have relatively few complications. Wound infection is infrequent, although it may be increased when re-excision is done and therefore the use of prophylactic antibiotics may be convenient. Skin necrosis may be related to thin skin flap dissection and to incomplete flap dissection with high suture tension.

Seroma is probably the most common postoperative problem and related to obesity, bulky lymph nodes, poor hemostasia, and the two-step procedure. The drains should be maintained in place with a high prevalence of wound infection. Pressure dressings are not effective in reducing seromas and may cause skin necrosis.

Keidan *et al.* (40) reported a 6 % of delayed breast abscess after breast conserving surgery and radiotherapy that may be related to fat necrosis in the area of tumor excision.

Early postoperative lymphedema is usually associated with wound infection. The later development of lymphedema is a complication of axillar dissection and is more frequent following radiotherapy. Low grade infection will aggravate and preventive measures includes avoidance of blood sampling and injections into the ipsilateral extremity to breast surgery. Massage of the arm with an anti-inflammatory and heparinoid may partially improve circulatory alterations and prevent further complications.

Disabling pain is related to surgical nerve injury, although general tightness of the chest wall is frequently reported during the first days after surgery. The administration of analgesics and vitamin B complexes usually improve the parastesic symptoms and alleviate pain.

Adjuvant radiotherapy after conservative surgery

Locoregional control remains a therapeutic concern because the treated breast has a cumulative risk of 2 % per year of disease recurrence after conservative therapy, and the risk increases if conservation surgery is not followed by radiation therapy (1, 41, 42). Systemic treatment should be initiated a few days after surgery whilst radiotherapy should be initiated when breast wound healing is adequate. It appears that a delay up of up to 8 weeks in the interval between the breast surgery and the start or radiotherapy is not associated with an increased risk of recurrence (43).

A number of factors related to radiotherapy have been associated with the cosmetic results after conservative surgery: the use of whole breast doses exceeding 50 Gy, fraction sizes exceeding 2Gy/day, imprecise matching of the tangential fields and the anterior field to treat the axillary or supraclavicular region or both, and the use of a large volume boost or boost dose of greater of 18 Gy (44).

The dose of radiotherapy may influence the risk of locoregional recurrence. Apparently, 75 Gy gives a lower local failure rate than when 50 to 65 Gy are given (24). Patients with large and pendulous breasts should use a special breast holding mask, depending on the individual mammary size, in order to improve dose homogeneity and cosmetic outcome.

Radiotherapy for breast cancer contributes little to the already high risk of a second malignancy or a recurrence (45, 46).

3. CARCINOMA *IN SITU*

Breast carcinoma *in situ* may be either ductal or lobular according to the histologic characteristics and patterns of growth (47-49). Prior to the wide use of mammography, ductal carcinoma *in situ* (DCIS) accounted for only a small fraction of all breast cancers. The palpable DCIS is a rare form of presentation as compared to the high proportion of microcalcifications and calcifications associated with earlier steps of this type of cancer (50, 51). If DCIS is suspected from mammography, a hook-wire localization is done and a wide excision performed to include all the area and to guarantee free margins.

Although the natural history of DCIS remains unclear it seems that not all DCIS advance to invasion (49, 52). The histologic features of DCIS are important to know the risk of progression to invasive carcinoma. Five patterns of DCIS can be considered: comedo, cribiform, papillary, micropapillary and solid. The comedo type is agressive, with a high rate of multicentricity and of invasion, whilst the micropapillary forms very often affect multiple breast quadrants. The pathologic features predicting for local recurrence are the presence of comedo carcinoma, necrosis, high nuclear grade, and nipple discharge. Tumor size (> 25 mm) is a separate risk factor for multicentricity (53). Axillar invasion is very rare in DCIS (54, 55).

Simple mastectomy is the safest therapeutic option for DCIS and with nearly 100% long-term survival (54, 56). As not all patients with DCIS will progress to invasive cancer, other possibilities have been explored, although the clinical selection for less agressive surgical procedures is not easy. DCIS can also be treated with subcutaneous mastectomy and either cosmetic prosthesis or plastic reconstructive surgery, and breast preserving surgery associated with radiotherapy. The incidence of local recurrence after conservative surgery without radiation is up to 25 % (57).

Breast preservation surgery with radiotherapy may be considered in non-invasive ductal carcinoma if the lesion is smaller than 25 mm, with free microscopical surgical margins, without previous personal or family history of breast cancer, and if the patient fully understands the risks and accepts a strict follow-up (57, 58). For the patient with intraductal carcinoma on initial breast biopsy, there is a risk of an occult microinvasive carcinoma in the remainder of the breast. Histologically negative margins do not guarantee the absence of other lesions and residual DCIS may still be present in the breast. Although axillar invasion is very rare, lymphadenectomy is well tolerated and the histological confirmation of negative nodes may lend emotional support to the patient.

The management of DCIS with microinvasion is a controversial subject. In a small series it seems that modified radical mastectomy or wide excision with or without lymphadenectomy are legitimate options (59, 60). The subcutaneous mastectomy with prosthesis placement may be considered in some women. Since some failures were reported with this procedure, we include 6 months of chemotherapy ir order to improve the results.

Lobular carcinoma *in situ* (LCIS) refers to a lesion characterized by a solid proliferation of small cells in breast lobules, with small, uniform, round-to-oval nuclei and variably distinct cell borders. Its frequency is about 15-20 % of all non-invasive breast cancer and with a high risk of affecting several mammary quadrants, a low presence of invasive lesions, and a high prevalence in premenopausal women (61-63). Invasive cancer will develop in 20-35 % of women with LCIS, although in many women this occurred after 15 years, sometimes in the contralateral breast, with the most common type being infiltrating ductal (52, 54, 64, 65). Therefore, LCIS may be considered a premalignant lesion or as a marker for subsequent cancer. The surgical options are wide excision and long term follow-up and uni- or bilateral subcutaneous mastectomy with prosthesis implantation or breast reconstruction. Since the LCIS may affect both mammary glands, bilateral surgical treatment should be considered. The value of preventive treatment with tamoxifen remains to be determined (66).

4. ADVANCED BREAST CANCER

The surgical management of locally advanced breast cancer is controversial subject and individualized indications should be used. Inflammatory breast cancer has a high mortality rate and surgery is best accomplished after 3-6 cycles of neo-adjuvant chemotherapy, and therefore consolidation chemotherapy should follow, associated or not to radiotherapy.

Neglected advanced breast cancer usually has a slower clinical evolution than inflammatory breast cancer and surgery ameliorates the local cosmetic situation and reduces bulky tumors. The objective of surgery is to reduce tumor burden, to ameliorate the aesthetic local condition and to *"clean"* the thoracic area. Preoperative polychemotherapy may reduce tumor size and skin infiltration. In some patients radiotherapy may be administered preoperatively to the breast in question and regional lymph nodes to reduce the tumor mass. This program is agressive with morbidity that includes wound infections, necrosis, delayed healing, upper extremity lymphedema and seromas (67).

In some locally advanced breast tumors the Halsted radical mastectomy may be the procedure of choice when there are large and bulky tumors involving the pectoralis major muscle, or fascia or if there is grossly involved interpectoral nodes affecting the posterior fascia of the muscle. The dissection technique for radical mastectomy is quite similar to that for modified radical mastectomy, with regard to incision placement and flap dissection, although the breast and pectoralis major fascia are not removed from the muscle and the dissection is carried out laterally until pectoralis minor muscle is encountered. Axillary dissection is easier than in the Madden procedure because muscles have been removed. The beneficial effects of postoperative adjuvant radiotherapy should be considered to obtain locoregional control. Systemic treatment may be used instead of or together with radiotherapy for patients who have other sites of metastases.

The locoregional treatment of metastatic breast cancer can only be considered in order to ameliorate the local cosmetic conditions and to reduce tumoral mass in order to obtain a better response with systemic therapy.

5. SALVAGE SURGERY

Local and regional recurrence after conservative management of breast cancer occurs in up to 22 % of the cases (68, 69). Evident distant metastases are concomitant in only 5 % of patients at the time of local relapse (70). Although a number of factors predict an increased risk of local relapse after breast-preserving surgery, none so obviously compromises survival that breast conservation is contraindicated (71). The prognosis for breast recurrence after conservative surgery is better than that for chest wall or nodal recurrences after mastectomy. The size of local recurrence and number of positive axillary lymph nodes at the time of salvage surgery influence the prognosis (72).

Most recurrences occur during the first 2 years after the primary treatment, are found by the patient herself or during medical physical examination, and are located within the breast or near the axilla. Mammography plays an important role, complementary to physical examination, in the detection of locoregional relapse following breast-conserving therapy. The early diagnosis of locoregional relapse is dependent on exhaustive 3- to 6- month follow-ups. The changes induced by radiation therapy may hinder a recurrence, especially in young women.

Local and regional recurrence may follow the initial treatment of invasive cancer or DCIS with breast-conserving surgery and definitive breast irradiation. When the initial lesion was a DCIS at the time of recurrence the lesion may be invasive ductal or intraductal carcinoma and, exceptionally, Paget's disease (73).

Salvage mammary surgery is indicated in women with recurrent or a new cancer after conservative surgery and radiotherapy. Locoregional recurrences are managed with wide mastectomy and axillar dissection of lymph nodes if necessary. Wedge excision may be an adequate alternative to mastectomy when there is an isolated recurrence, 2 cm or less, mobile and with low growth (74). Since these patients have already received irradiation and chemotherapy, wound healing is significantly impaired. In some cases surgical ablation results in a large soft-tissue defect that may be covered by a myocuatenous flap with increased operative morbidity. The local treatment should be support by systemic therapy.

Locoregional recurrence may also appear in 5-30 % patients treated by Halsted radical or modified radical mastectomy (75, 76). The incidence is primarily influenced by the number of initially positive axillary lymph nodes. At the time of locoregional recurrence one third of the patients have already developed obvious distant metastases (77). Surgical excision may be useful in local relapse after the Madden operation to eliminate tumor mass that would facilitate radiotherapy and/or systemic therapy. The best results are obtained if a complete resection of all gross disease can be accomplished and with at least 45 Gy irradiation administered to comprehensive fields. Systemic treatment may reduce local disease progression and prevent subsequent distant metastases.

The excision of solitary metastases may be considered to reduce bulk tumors. In metachronous bilateral breast cancer the Madden modified radical procedures may be considered.

6. CONCLUSIONS

The gynecologist holds a unique position as a primary care physician whom women consult about breast diseases or hormone therapy. Therefore, gynecologists must actively search for early breast carcinomas. The wide use of mammography for the screening of asymptomatic women and for the evaluation of specific symptoms of breast diseases has ameliorated the early detection of breast carcinoma. More and more women are advised to undergo breast biopsy based on radiologic findings. Thus, the diagnosis of malignancy is often made on the basis of these nonpalpable findings by applying stereotaxic techniques in order to localize and excise small lesions.

It appears that breast cancer is a systemic disease at the time of diagnosis in almost all cases. The Halstedian principles supporting radical surgical procedures have been challenged and at the present time a more conservative surgical approach predominates. Breast conservative surgery is the preferred surgical treatment for most, if not all, patients with stage I and II breast cancer. However, many menopausal women believe that mastectomy offers a better prognosis than conservative surgery.

The value of surgery in advanced breast cancer is to reduce bulky mammary tumors and to "*clean*" the thoracic area. The ominous prognosis is determined by the high amount of tumor cells in metastatic disease. Salvage surgery may be useful in local relapse and may be accompanied by radiotherapy and sytemic supportive treatment.

Although adjuvant cytotoxic and hormone therapy have been widely employed, the mortality rates due to breast cancer have not significantly decreased during the past years. With some exceptions, the strategy of killing the last cancer cell has not been successful (78, 79). At the present time, early diagnosis and treatment are the most important factors to reduce the mortality rate due to breast cancer and gynecologists should play a major role in accomplishing these objectives.

REFERENCES

1. Fisher, B., Redmond, C., Poisson, R. *et al.* (1989). Eight year results of a randomized clinical trial comparing total mastectomy and lumpectomy with or without irradiation in the treatment of breast cancer. *N. Engl. J. Med.*, **320**, 822-8
2. Kurtz, J.M., Amalric, R., Brandone, H., Ayme, Y. and Spitalier, J.M. (1991). How important is adequate radiotherapy for the long term results of breast conserving treatment? *Radiother. Oncol.*, **20**, 84-90

3. Veronesi, U., Luini, A., Del Vecchio, M. *et al.* (1993). Radiotherapy after breast-preserving surgery in women with localized cancer of the breast. *N. Engl. J. Med.*, 328, 1587-91

4. Bonadonna, G., Veronesi, U., Brambilla, C. *et al.* (1990). Primary chemotherapy to avoid mastectomy in tumors with three centimeters or more. *J. Natl. Cancer Inst.*, 82, 1539-45

5. Khanna, M.M., Mark, R.J., Silverstein, M.J., Juillard, G., Lewinsky, B. and Giulano, A.E. (1992). Breast conservation management of breast tumors 4 cm or larger. *Arch. Surg.*, 127, 1038-43

6. Calais, G., Berger, C., Descamps, P. *et al.* (1994). Conservative treatment feasibility with induction chemotherapy, surgery, and radiotherapy for patients with breast carcinoma larger than 3 cm. *Cancer*, 74, 1283-8

7. Nattinger, A.B., Gottlieb, M.S., Veum, J., Yahnke, D. and Goodwin, J.S. (1992). Geographic variation in the use of breast-conserving treatment for breast cancer. *N. Engl. J. Med.*, 326, 1102-7

8. Samet, J.M., Hunt, W.C. and Farrow, D.C. (1994). Determinants of receiving breast-conserving surgery. The Surveillance, Epidemiology, and End Results program, 1983-1986. *Cancer*, 73, 2344-51

9. Iscoe, N.A., Naylor, C.D., Williams, J.I. *et al.* (1994). Temporal trends in breast cancer surgery in Ontario: can one randomized trial make a difference? *Can. Med. Assoc. J.*, 150, 1109-15

10. Early Breast Cancer Trialists' Collaborative Group (1992). Systemic treatment of early breast cancer by hormonal, cytotoxic or immune therapy. *Lancet*, 339, 1-15, 71-85

11. Madden, J.L. (1965). Modified radical mastectomy. *Surg. Gynecol. Obstet.*, 121, 1221-30

12. Madden, J.L., Kandalaft, S. and Bourque, R.A. (1970). Mastectomía radical modificada. *Prensa Med. Argentina*, 57, 1421-3

13. Pigott, J., Nichols, R., Maddox, W.A. and Balch, C.M. (1984). Metastases of the upper levels of the axillary nodes in carcinoma of the breast and its implications for nodal sampling. *Surg. Gynecol. Obstet.*, 158, 255-9

14. Veronesi, U., Rilke, F., Luini, A. *et al.* (1987). Distribution of axillary node metastases by level of invasion. *Cancer*, 59, 682-7

15. Saunders, C.M. and Baum, M. (1994). Management of early breast cancer. *Oncol. Practice*, 3, 4-8

16. Schwartz, G.F., Patchesky, A.S., Feig, S.A. *et al.* (1980). Multicentricity of nonpalpable breast cancer. *Cancer*, 45, 2913-6

17. Holland, R., Solke, H.J.V., Mravunac, M. *et al.* (1985). Histologic multifocality of Tis, T1-2 breast carcinomas. *Cancer*, 56, 979-90

18. Pantel, K., Schlimok, G., Braum, S. and Riethmüller, G. (1994). Characterisation of micrometastatic tumor cells in bone marrow. In: Fox, R. (ed.). *The Lancet Conference: The challenge of breast cancer*, p 18. (London: The Lancet)

19. Boyd, J. (1994). Molecular medicine quietly comes of age. New opportunities in the treatment of patients with breast cancer. *Cancer*, 74, 2215-7

20. Harada, Y., Katagiri, T., Ito, I. *et al.* (1994). Genetic studies of 457 breast cancer. Clinicopathologic parameters compared with genetic alterations. *Cancer*, 74, 2281-6

21. Van Dongen, J.A., Bartelink, H., Fentiman, I.S. *et al.* (1992). Factors influencing local relapse and survival and results of salvage treatment after breast conserving therapy in operable breast cancer: EORTC trial 10801, breast conservation compared with mastectomy in TNM stage I and II breast cancer. *Eur. J. Cancer*, 28A, 801-5

22. Anscher, M.S., Jones, P. and Prosnitz, L.R. (1993). Local failure and margin status in early stage breast carcinoma treated with conservation surgery and radiation therapy. *Ann. Surg.*, 218, 22-8

23. Borger, J., Kemperman, H., Hart, A. *et al.* (1994). Risks factors in breast-conservation therapy. *J. Clin. Oncol.*, 12, 653-60

24. Harris, J.R. and Gelman, R. (1994). What have we learned about risk factors for local recurrence after breast-conserving surgery and irradiation? *J. Clin. Oncol.*, 12, 647-9

25. Solin, L.J., Fowle, B.L., Schultz, D.J. and Goodman, R.L. (1991). The significance of the pathology margins of the tumor excision on the outcome of patients treated with definitive irradiation for early stage breast cancer. *Int. J. Rad. Oncol. Biol. Phys.*, 21, 279-87

26. Schmidt-Ullrich, R.A., Wazer, D.E., DiPetrillo, T. *et al.* (1993). Breast conservation therapy for

early stage breast carcinoma with outstanding local control rates: A case for aggressive therapy to the tumor bearing quadrant. *Int. J. Rad. Oncol. Biol. Phys.*, 27, 545-52

27. Schnitt, S.J., Abner, A., Gelman, R. *et al.* (1994). The relationship between microscopic margins of resection and the risk of local recurrence in patients with breast cancer treated with breast-conserving surgery and radiation therapy. *Cancer*, 74, 1746-51

28. Spivack, B., Khanna, M.M., Tafra, L., Jullard, G. and Giuliano, A.E. (1994). Margin status and local recurrence after breast-conserving surgery. *Arch. Surg.*, 129, 956-7

29. Krishnan, L., Jewel, W.R., Krishnan, E.C., Cherian, R. and Lin, F. (1992). Breast cancer with extensive intraductal component: treatment with immediate interstitial boost irradiation. *Radiology*, 183, 273-6

30. Osteen, R.T. (1994). Selection of patients for breast conserving treatment. *Cancer*, 74, 366-71

31. White, J.R., Gustafson, G.S., Wimbish, K. *et al.* (1994). Conservative surgery and radiation therapy for infiltrating lobular carcinoma of the breast. The role of preoperative mammograms in guiding treatment. *Cancer*, 74, 640-7

32. Hrushesky, W.J.M., Bluming, A.Z., Gruber, S.A. and Sothern, R.B. (1981). Menstrual influence on surgical cure of breast cancer. *Lancet*, ii, 949-52

33. Goldhirsch, A., Gelber, R., Forbes, J. *et al.* (1991). Timing breast cancer surgery. *Lancet*, 338, 691-2

34. Rageth, J.C., Wyss, P., Unger, C. and Hochuli, E. (1991). Timing of breast cancer surgery within the menstrual cycle: influence of lymph-node involvement, receptor status, postoperative metastatic spread and local recurrence. *Ann. Oncol.*, 2, 269-72

35. Gnant, M.F.X., Seifert, M., Jakesz, R., Adler, A., Mittboeck, M. and Sevelda, P. (1992). Breast cancer and timing of surgery during menstrual cycle: A 5-year analysis of 385 pre-menopausal women. *Int. J. Cancer*, 52, 707-12

36. Kronan, N., Hojgaard, K.W., Andersen, K.W. *et al.* (1994). Timing of surgery in relation to menstrual cycle does not predict the prognosis in primary breast cancer. *Eur. J. Surg. Oncol.*, 20, 430-5

37. Badwe, R.A., Wang, D.Y., Gregory, W.M. *et al.* (1994). Serum progesterone at the time of surgery and survival in women with premenopausal operable breast cancer. *Eur. J. Cancer*, 30A, 445-8

38. Saad, Z., Vincent, M., Bramwell, V. *et al.* (1994). Timing of surgery influences survival in receptor-negative as well as receptor-positive breast cancer. *Eur. J. Cancer*, 30A, 1348-52

39. Veronesi, U., Luini, A., Mariani, L. *et al.* (1994). Effect of menstrual phase on surgical treatment of breast cancer. *Lancet*, 343, 1545-7

40. Keidan, R.D., Hoffman, J.P., Weese, J.L. *et al.* (1990). Delayed breast abscess after lumpectomy and radiation therapy. *Am. Surg.*, 54, 440-4

41. Kurtz, L., Amalric, R., Delouche, G., Pierquin, B., Roth, J. and Spitalier, J. (1987). The second ten years: long term risks of breast conservation in early breast cancer. *Int. J. Radiat. Oncol. Biol. Phys.*, 13, 1327-32.

42. Liljegren, G., Holmberg, L. and Adami, H.O. (1994). Sector resection with or without postoperative radiotherapy for stage I breast cancer: five-year results of a randomized trial. Uppsala-Orebro Breast Cancer Study Group. *J. Natl. Cancer Inst.*, 86, 717-22

43. Nixon, A.J., Recht, A., Neuberg, D. *et al.* (1994). The relation between the surgery-radiotherapy interval and treatment outcome in patients treated with breast-conserving surgery and radiation therapy without systemic therapy. *Int. J. Radiat. Oncol. Biol. Phys.*, 3, 17-21

44. de la Rochefordière, A., Abner, A.L., Silver, B., Vicini, F., Recht, A. and Harris, J.R. (1992). Are cosmetic results following conservative surgery and radiation therapy for early breast cancer dependent on technique? *Int. J. Radiat. Oncol. Biol. Phys.*, 23, 925-31

45. Boice, J.D., Harvey, E.B., Blettner, A., Stoval, M. and Flannery, J.T. (1992). Cancer in the contralateral breast after radiotherapy for breast cancer. *N. Engl. J. Med.*, 326, 781-5

46. Zucali, R., Merson, M., Placucci, M., Di Palma, S. and Veronesi, U. (1994). Soft tisse sarcoma of the breast after conservative surgery and irradiation for early mammary cancer. *Radiother. Oncol.*, 30 L, 271-3

47. Broders, A.C. (1932). Carcinoma in-situ contrasted with benign penetrating epithelium. *JAMA*, 99, 1670-4

48. Foote, F.W. and Stewart, F.W. (1941). Lobular carcinoma in-situ: A rare form of mammary

cancer. *Am. J. Pathol.*, 17, 491-6

49. Bellamy, C.O.C., McDonald, C., Salter, D.M., Chetty, U. and Anderson, T.J. (1993). Noninvasive ductal carcinoma of the breast: The relevance of histologic categorization. *Hum. Pathol.*, 24, 16-23

50. Gump, F.E., Jicha, D.L. and Ozello, L. (1987). Ductal carcinoma in-situ (DCIS): A revised concept. *Surgery*, 102, 790-5

51. Dershaw, D.D., Abramson, A. and Kinne, D.W. (1989). Ductal carcinoma in-situ. Mammographic findings and clinical implications. *Radiology*, 170, 411-5

52. Rosen, P.P., Braun, D.W. and Kinne D.W. (1980). The clinical significance of preinvasive breast carcinoma. *Cancer*, 46, 919-25

53. Lagios, M.D., Westdahl, P.R., Margonic, F.R. and Rose, M.R. (1982). Duct carcinoma in-situ. Relationship of noninvasive disease to the frequency of occult invasion, multicentricity, lymph node metastases and short term treamtent failures. *Cancer*, 50, 1309-14

54. Kinne, D.W., Petrek, J.A., Osborne, M.P. *et al.* (1989). Breast carcinoma in-situ. *Arch. Surg.*, 124, 33-6

55. Silverstein, M.J., Gierson, E.D., Colburn, W.J., Rosser, R.J., Waisman, J.R. and Gamagami, P. (1991). Axillary lynphadenectomy for intraductal carcinoma of the breast. *Surg. Gynecol. Obst.*, 172, 211-4

56. Frykberg, E.R. and Bland, K.I. (1994). Overview of the biology and managment of ductal carcinoma in situ of the breast. *Cancer*, 74, 350-61

57. Lagios, M.D. (1990). Duct carcinoma in situ: pathology and treatment. *Surg. Clin. North Am.*, 70, 618-24

58. Solin, L.J., Yeh, I.T., Kurtz, J. *et al.* (1993). Ductal carcinoma in situ (intraductal carcinoma) of the breast treated with breast-conserving surgery and definitive irradiation. Correlation of pathologic parameters with outcome of treatment. *Cancer*, 71, 2532-42

59. Rosner, D., Lane, W.W. and Penetrante, R. (1991). Ductal carcinoma in situ with microinvasion: A curable entity using surgery alone without need for adjuvant therapy. *Cancer*, 67, 1498-503

60. Silverstein, M.J., Gierson, E.D., Waisman, J.R., Senofsly, G.M., Colburn, W.J. and Gamegani, P. (1994). Axillary lymph node dissection for T1a breast carcinoma. Is it indicated? *Cancer*, 73, 664-7

61. Haagensen, C.D., Lane, R., Lattes, R. *et al.* (1978). Lobular neoplasia (so-called lobular carcinoma in situ) of the breast. *Cancer*, 42, 737-69

62. Tinnemans, G.M., Wobbes, T., Holland, R. *et al.* (1987). Mamographic and histopathological correlation of nonpalpable lesions of the breast and the reliability of frozen section diagnosis. *Surg. Gynecol. Obstet.*, 165, 523-9

63. Holland, R., Hendricks, J.H.C.L., Verbeek, A.L.M. *et al.* (1990). Extent, distribution and mammographic/histological correlation of breast ductal carcinoma in situ. *Lancet*, 335, 519-22

64. Rosen, P.P., Lieberman, P.H., Braun, D.W. *et al.* (1978). Lobular carcinoma in situ of the breast. *Am. J. Surg. Pathol.*, 2, 225-51

65. Gump, F.E. (1993). Lobular carcinoma in situ (LCIS): pathology and treatment. *J. Cell Biochem. Suppl.*, 17G, 53-8

66. Van Dongen, J.A., Fentiman, I.S., Harris, J.R. *et al.* (1989). In-situ breast cancer; report of the EORTC consensus meeting. *Lancet*, ii, 25-7

67. Sauter, E.R., Eisenberg, B.L., Hoffman, J.P. *et al.* (1993). Postmastectomy morbidity after combination preoperative irradiation and chemotherapy for locally advanced breast cancer. *World J. Surg.*, 17, 237-41

68. Rutgers, E.J.T., van Slooten, E.A. and Kluck H.M. (1989). Follow-up after treatment of primary breast cancer. *Br. J. Surg.*, 76, 187-90

69. Osborne, M.P. and Simmons, R.M. (1994). Salvage surgery for recurrence after breast conservation. *World J. Surg.*, 18, 93-7

70. Stotter, A., McNeese, M., Ames, F., Oswald, M. and Ellerbroek, N. (1989). Predicting the rate and extent of locoregional failure after breast conservation therapy for early breast cancer. *Cancer*, 64, 2217-25

71. Osteen, R. (1994). Risk factors and management of local recurrence following breast conservation surgery. *World J. Surg.*, 18, 76-80

72. Cajucom, C.C., Tsangaris, T.N., Nemoto, T., Driscoll, D., Penetrante, R.B. and Holyoke, E.D. (1993). Results of salvage mastectomy for local recurrence after breast-conserving surgery without radiation therapy. *Cancer*, 71, 1774-9

73. Solin, L.J., Fourquet, A., McCormick, B. *et al.* (1994). Salvage treatment for local recurrence following breast-conserving surgery and definitive irradiation for ductal carcinoma in situ (intraductal carcinoma) of the breast. *Int. J. Radiat. Oncol. Biol. Phys.*, 30, 3-9

74. Kurtz, J.M., Amalric, R., Brandone, H., Ayme, Y. and Spitalier, J.M. (1988). Results of wide excision for mammary recurrence after breast-conserving therapy. *Cancer*, 61, 1969-72

75. Crowe, J.P. Jr., Gordon, N.H., Antunez, A.R. *et al.* (1991). Local-regional breast cancer recurrence following mastectomy. *Arch. Surg.*, 126, 429-32

76. Demicheli, R., Terenziani, M., Valagussa, P., Moliterni, A., Zambetti, M. and Bonadonna, G. (1994). Local recurrences following mastectomy: Support for the concept of tumor dormancy. *J. Natl. Cancer Inst.*, 86, 45-8

77. Borner, M., Bacchi, M., Goldhirsch, A. *et al.* (1994). First isolated locoregional recurrence following mastectomy for breast cancer: results of a radiation Swiss Group for Clinical Cancer Research. *J. Clin. Oncol.*, 12, 2071-7

78. Clavel, M. and Catimel, G. (1993). Breast cancer: chemotherapy in the treatment of the advanced disease. *Eur. J. Cancer*, 29A, 598-604

79. Schipper, H., Wang, T.L. and Goh, C.R. (1994). Revising the cancer paradigm: must we kill to cure? In: Fox, R. (ed.). *The Lancet Conference: The challenge of breast cancer*, p 58. (London: The Lancet)

Hormonotherapy for advanced or recurrent breast cancer

P. Sismondi and F. Genta

Cattedra di Ginecologia Oncologica, Istituto di Ginecologia e Ostetricia, Università di Torino, Turin, Italy

INTRODUCTION

In past decades the hope of curing breast cancer by chemotherapy overshadowed hormonal therapy (HT) which, over a century after Beatson (1896), proved unable to cure. Afterwards HT wone bach its role, not only thanks to new drugs. The criteria of selection (age, menopause, receptors, prolonged disease-free survival, site of metastasis) are not changed and in selected subgroups we might obtain more than the usual 30%, gained overall by HT. If we get over the idea of a single drug effectiveness, we meet the real problem, that is to outline a treatment strategy for patients bearing a not rapidly growing breast cancer.

REVIEW

All drugs, if singly administered, did show a proven effectiveness to obtain the stabilization (SD) or the partial remission (PR) of the disease and, in few cases, the complete remission (CR) too. Sequential or concomitant administrations did never obtain better results.

Since no treatment in metastatic breast cancer (MBC) resulted till now in a better chance of survival, but cross-over studies showed further responders to HT, we have now to think in terms of quality of life and of extending time to progression. Analysing only comparative studies among single drugs we will be able to prove the real clinical impact of HT.

Tamoxifen (TAM) has the same effectiveness of progestins on objective remissions (OR) (Tables 1-2), but these have more side effects, leading to 10-15% of discontinuations. Higher doses of medroxyprogesterone acetate (MPA) obtained better results, but they were charged by higher and higher side effects.

New anti-estrogens did not show impressive OR (1-5) so far.

Table 1. Comparative studies on TAM (40mg) vs MPA (900-2000mg) in ABC

Authors (ref)	Cases	TAM OR (%)	MPA OR (%)
Mattson 1980 (6)	58	15/32 (47)	14/26 (54)
Pannuti 1982 (7)	53	7/26 (27)	10/27 (37)
Robustelli 1982 (8)	54	5/26 (19)	8/28 (28)
Silva 1985 (9)	265	40/133 (30)	53/132 (40)
Fosser 1985 (10)	274	27/99 (27)	63/175 (36)
Van Veelen 1986 (11)	129	24/68 (35)	27/61 (44)
Garcia-Giralt 1987 (12)	103	28/51 (55)	23/52 (44)
Varini 1989 (13)	116	19/63 (30)	28/53 (53)
Marchetti 1990 (14)	101	20/50 (40)	21/51 (41)
Muss 1991 (15)	171	13/86 (15)	45/85 (53)
Castiglione 1993 (16)	119	19/64 (30)	27/55 (50)
TOTAL	1443	217/698 (31)	319/745 (43)

Table 2. Comparative studies on TAM (40mg) vs MA (160mg) in ABC

Authors (ref)	Cases	TAM OR (%)	MA OR (%)
Ingle 1982 (17)	55	7/27 (26)	5/28 (16)
Morgan 1985 (18)	94	17/48 (36)	14/46 (31)
Ettinger 1986 (19)	190	42/99 (42)	32/91 (35)
Muss 1988 (20)	125	20/64 (31)	16/61 (26)
Paterson 1990 (21)	156	27/79 (34)	26/77 (34)
Gill 1993 (22)	184	32/92 (35)	27/92 (29)
TOTAL	804	145/409 (35)	120/395 (30)

Old (Table 3) and new (27) aromatase inhibitors (AI) showed similar results in OR and in comparison to tamoxifen or progestins (Tables 4-5). Tam-responders have shown higher OR percentages to AI, resulting in longer time to progression and survival.

Table 3. Comparative studies on TAM (20mg) vs AG (500-1000 mg) in ABC

Authors (ref)	Cases	TAM OR (%)	AG OR (%)
Smith 1981 (23)	117	18/60 (30)	17/57 (30)
Lipton 1982 (24)	75	15/39 (38)	13/36 (36)
Alonso-Munoz 1988 (25)	65	18/34 (53)	15/31 (48)
Gale 1994 (26)	216	29/108 (27)	49/108 (45)
TOTAL	473	80/241 (33)	94/232 (41)

Table 4. Comparative studies on AG (500) vs MPA (1000) in ABC

Authors (ref)	Cases	AG OR (%)	MPA OR (%)
Canney 1988 (28)	218	29/106 (27)	35/112 (31)
Garcia-Giralt 1988 (29)	245	46/127 (36)	39/118 (33)
TOTAL	463	75/233 (32)	74/230 (32)

Table 5. Comparative studies on AG (500) vs MA (160) in ABC

Authors (ref)	Cases	AG OR (%)	MA OR (%)
Lundgren 1989 (30)	150	26/76 (34)	23/74 (31)
Congdon 1991 (31)	140	13/69 (18)	8/71 (11)
TOTAL	290	39/145 (27)	31/145 (21)

In premenopausal patients ovarian suppression by LHRH analogues (Table 6) or ovariectomy vs Tamoxifen (Table 7) showed similar results.

Table 6. Studies on LHRH An in ABC in premenopause

Authors (ref)	Cases	OR (%)
Klijn 1984 (32)	22	9 (41)
Harvey 1985 (33)	25	11 (44)
Williams 1986 (34)	45	14 (31)
Santen 1986 (35)	25	11 (44)
Walker 1989 (36)	16	5 (38)
Anderson 1989 (37)	13	5 (38)
Milsted 1990 (38)	228	83 (36)
Dixon 1990 (39)	75	25 (33)
Dowsett 1990 (40)	12	5 (42)
Bianco 1990 (41)	53	16 (30)
Brambilla 1991 (42)	22	7 (32)
Kaufmann 1991 (43)	118	53 (45)
Blamey 1991 (44)	153	43 (28)
Bajetta 1994 (45)	38	17 (45)
TOTAL	845	300 (35)

Table 7. Comparative studies on Ovariectomy vs TAM in ABC

Authors (ref)	Cases	OVX OR (%)	TAM OR (%)
Buchanan 1986 (46)	107	11/53 (21)	13/54 (24)
Ingle 1986 (47)	53	10/27 (37)	7/26 (27)
TOTAL	160	21/80 (26)	20/80 (25)

Another important question is: does HT improve the results of chemotherapy and vice versa? Tables 8-13 show that it is definitely so, both in premenopausal and in postmenopausal patients.

Table 8. Comparative studies on Chemotherapy (CMF-like or polichemo including ADR) vs Chemotherapy + Tam in MBC

Authors (ref)	Chemoth.	Cases	% Ch OR	% Ch+Tam OR
Boccardo 1985 (48)	ADR	68	42	75
CALBG 1985 (49)	ADR	474	55	64
ANZBCTG 1986 (50)	ADR	226	45	41
Perry 1987 (51)	ADR	101	62	70
TOTAL	ADR	869	53	60
Cocconi 1983 (52)	CMF	133	51	74
Krook 1985 (53)	CMF	122	66	60
Mouridsen1985 (54)	CMF	220	49	75
Viladiu 1985 (55)	CMF	98	46	71
TOTAL	CMF	573	53	71
TOTAL ADR+CMF		1442	53	64

Table 9. Comparative studies on OVX vs OVX + Chemotherapy in ABC in premenopausal patients

Authors (ref)	Cases	OVX OR (%)	Ch+OVX OR (%)
Ahmann 1977 (56)	52	7/26 (27)	10/26 (38)
Falkson 1979 (57)	148	7/38 (18)	75/110 (68)
Cavalli 1983 (58)	109	12/54 (22)	25/55 (46)
TOTAL	309	26/118 (22)	110/191 (58)

Table 10. Comparative studies on Chemotherapy vs Chemotherapy + OVX in ABC in premenopausal patients

Authors (ref)	Cases	Ch OR (%)	Ch+OVX OR (%)
Brunner 1977 (59)	42	10/23 (43)	14/19 (74)
Falkson 1987 (60)	81	29/38 (76)	36/43 (84)
TOTAL	123	39/61 (64)	50/62 (81)

Table 11. Comparative studies on Tam vs Tam + Chemotherapy in ABC in postmenopausal patients

Authors (ref)	Cases	Tam OR (%)	Ch+Tam OR (%)
Bezwoda 1982 (61)	50	15/24 (63)	17/26 (65)
Cavalli 1983 (58)	297	25/145 (17)	61/152 (40)
ANZBCTG 1986 (50)	226	25/113 (22)	58/113 (51)
TOTAL	573	65/282 (23)	136/291 (47)

Table 12. Comparative studies on Chemotherapy vs Chemotherapy + Tam in ABC in postmenopausal patients

Authors (ref)	Cases	Ch OR(%)	Ch+Tam OR (%)
Cocconi 1983 (52)	133	36/71 (51)	46/62 (74)
Viladiu 1985 (55)	67	15/33 (45)	24/34 (71)
Mouridsen 1985 (54)	220	51/105 (49)	86/115 (75)
ANZBCTG 1986 (50)	226	51/113 (45)	58/113 (51)
TOTAL	646	153/322 (48)	214/324 (66)

Table 13. Comparative studies on Chemotherapy vs Chemotherapy + MPA in ABC in postmenopausal patients

Authors (ref)	Cases	Ch OR (%)	Ch+MPA OR (%)
Robustelli 1984 (FAC) (62)	80	22/40 (55)	30/40 (75)
Robustelli 1984 (VAC) (62)	224	50/107 (47)	66/117 (56)
Viladiu 1985 (55)	64	15/33 (45)	21/31 (68)
TOTAL	368	87/180 (48)	117/188 (62)

Reviewing cross-over studies (Table 14), we can state that: a) aminoglutethimide or MPA after tamoxifen are more effective than vice versa; b) aminoglutethimide is effective after MPA in postmenopause; c) Tam is effective after ovarian blockage by LHRH agonists; d) megestrole acetate (63) and aromatase inhibitors (64), after poli-HT, resulted in high percentages of SD in previously responders.

Table 14. Results of cross-over studies: % of OR to second line treatments

Resistence to	MPA	MA	Tam	AG
Tam	34	15		36
MPA			22	27
MA			15	16
AG			19	
LHRHAn			29	0

CONCLUSIONS

Pooling all data (Figures 1-2), we can deduce a treatment strategy which considers biology of breast cancer, age and symptoms of patients and previous therapy.

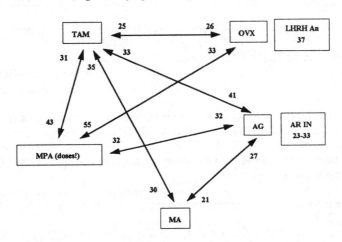

Figure 1. Objective remissions reported by the comparative studies among HT.

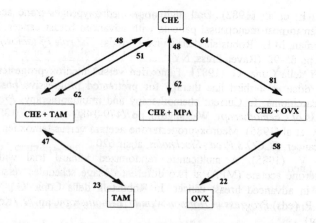

Figure 2. Objective remissions reported by the studies comparing hormono- and chemotherapies given sequentially or in combination.

Patients affected by fast progressive disease, with visceral metastases and ER-negative breast cancer, are firstly candidates to chemotherapy and afterwards to HT.

Patients affected by ER-positive advanced or recurrent breast cancer, after a long disease-free interval, are firstly candidates to HT. If pain, anorexia or slimming are the main symptoms, progestins will be firstly chosen, followed by AI. Otherwise we could use LHRH agonists in premenopause and AI in postmenopause, since Tamoxifen has nearly always been pre-used as adjuvant setting. In all cases the chemotherapy and the remaining HT will represent a second line choice.

REFERENCES

1. Nomura, Y. et al. (1993). Clinical evaluation of NK 622 (toremifene citrate) in advanced or recurrent breast cancer. A comparative study by a double blind method with tamoxifen. *Gan To Kagaku Ryoho* 20(2), 247-258

2. Coopman, P. et al. (1994). Anti-proliferative and anti-estrogenic effects of ICI 164,384 and ICI 182,780 in 4-OH-tamoxifen-resistant human breast-cancer cells. *Int.J.Cancer* 56(2), 295-300

3. Buzdar, A.U. et al. (1994). Phase I trial of droloxifene in patients with metastatic breast cancer. *Cancer Chemother.Pharmacol.* 33(4), 313-316

4. Marschner, N. et al. (1994). Droloxifene for postmenopausal female patients with metastatic breast cancer. Double-blind randomized phase II study. *Onkologie* 17(suppl), 32-39

5. Pyrhonen, S. et al. (1994). High dose toremifene in advanced breast cancer resistant to or relapsed during tamoxifen treatment. *Breast Cancer Res.Treat.* 29(3), 223-228

6. Mattsson, W. (1980). A phase III trial of treatment with tamoxifen versus treatment with high-dose medroxyprogesterone acetate in advanced postmenopausal breast cancer. In Iacobelli, S., Di Marco, A. (eds) *Role of Medroxyprogesterone Acetate in Endocrine Related Tumors*, pp.65-71. (Raven Press, NY)

7. Pannuti, F. et al. (1982). Oral high dose medroxyprogesterone acetate versus tamoxifen in post menopausal patients with advanced breast cancer. In Iacobelli, S., Lippman, M.E., Robustelli della Cuna, G. (eds) *The role of tamoxifen in breast cancer*, pp.85-92. (Raven Press, NY)

8. Robustelli della Cuna, G. (1982). Tamoxifen versus medroxyprogesterone acetate loading dose as a third line therapy for pretreated progressive postmenopausal breast carcinoma. In Current chemotherapy and immunotherapy. *Proc. 12th Int. Congress of Chemotherapy*. Washington, pp.1479-1480

9. Silva, A. et al (1985). Medroxyprogesterone acetate versus tamoxifen in advanced breast cancer. *ECCO 3 Proc., Stockholm*, abstr.620

10. Fosser, V. (1985). A multicentre randomized clinical trial with medroxyprogesterone acetate (MPA) at two different dosage schedules versus tamoxifen (TMX) in advanced breast cancer. In Robustelli della Cuna, G., Nagel, G.A., Lanius, P. (eds) *Progress in Hormono- and Chemotherapy*, pp.79. (Kehrer Verlag, Freiburg)

11. Van Veelen, H. et al. (1986). Oral high-dose medroxyprogesterone acetate versus tamoxifen. *Cancer* 58, 7-13

12. Garcia Giralt, E. et al. (1987). Breast cancer first line hormonotherapy: a multicentric randomized trial comparing TAM with MPA and their sequential administration. *ASCO Proc.* 6, 61

13. Varini, M. et al. (1989). High response to high dose medroxyprogesterone acetate does not improve overall survival of postmenopausal patients with metastatic breast cancer. *ASCO Proc.* 8, 46

14. Marchetti, P. et al. (1990). Sequential hormonal treatment (TAM/MPA) of advanced breast cancer. *J.Cancer Res.Clin.Oncol.* 116, 395

15. Muss, H. et al. (1991). Tamoxifen versus high-dose oral medroxyprogesterone acetate as first line endocrine therapy for metastatic breast cancer: a randomized trial of the Piedmont oncology association. *ASCO Proc.* 10, 41

16. Castiglione Gertsch, M. et al. (1993). Primary endocrine therapy for advanced breast cancer: to start with tamoxifen or with medroxyprogesterone acetate? *ASCO Proc.* 12, 188

17. Ingle, J.N. et al. (1982). Randomized clinical trial of megestrol acetate versus tamoxifen in paramenopausal or castrated women with advanced breast cancer. *Am.J.Clin.Oncol.* 2, 155-158

18. Morgan, L.R. (1985). Megestrol acetate vs tamoxifen in advanced breast cancer in postmenopausal patients. *Sem.Oncol.* 12(suppl.1), 43-47

19. Ettinger, D.S. et al. (1986). Megestrol acetate vs tamoxifen in advanced breast cancer: correlation of hormone receptors and response. *Sem.Oncol.* 13(suppl.4), 914

20. Muss, H.B. et al. (1988). Megestrol acetate versus tamoxifen in advanced breast cancer: 5-year analysis. *J.Clin.Oncol.* 6, 1098-1106

21. Paterson, A.H.G. et al. (1990). Comparison of antiestrogen and progestogen therapy for initial treatment and consequence of their combination for second-line treatment of recurrent breast cancer. *Sem.Oncol.* 17(suppl.9), 52-62

22. Gill, P.G. et al. (1993). Randomized comparison of the effects of tamoxifen, megestrol acetate, or tamoxifen plus megestrol acetate on treatment response and survival in patients with metastatic breast cancer. *Ann.Oncol.* 4(9), 741-744

23. Smith, I.E. et al. (1981). Tamoxifen versus aminoglutethimide in advanced breast carcinoma: a randomized cross-over trial. *Br.Med.J.* 283, 1432-1434

24. Lipton, A. et al. (1982). A randomized trial of aminoglutethimide versus tamoxifen in metastatic breast cancer. *Cancer* 50, 2265-2268

25. Alonso Munoz, M.C. et al. (1988). Randomized trial of tamoxifen versus aminoglutethimide and versus combined tamoxifen and aminoglutethimide in advanced post-menopausal breast cancer. *Oncology* 45, 350-353

26. Gale, K.E. et al. (1994). Hormonal treatment for metastatic breast cancer: an Eastern Cooperative Oncology Group phase III trial comparing aminoglutethimide to tamoxifen. *Cancer* 73(2), 354-361

27. Pérez Carrión, R. et al. (1994). Comparison of the selective aromatase inhibitor formestane with tamoxifen as first-line hormonal therapy in postmenopausal women with advanced breast cancer. *Ann.Oncol.* 5(suppl.7), 19-24

28. Canney, P.A. et al. (1988). Randomized trial comparing aminoglutethimide with high-dose medroxyprogesterone acetate for advanced breast carcinoma. *J.Natl.Cancer Inst.* 80, 1147-1151

29. Garcia Giralt, E. et al. (1988). Second line hormonotherapy in breast cancer: a multicentric randomized trial comparing MPA with AG in patients who have become resistant to tamoxifen. *ASCO Proc.* 7, 113

30. Lundgren, S. et al. (1989). Megestrol acetate versus aminoglutethimide for metastatic breast cancer. *Breast Cancer Res.Treat.* 14, 201-206

31. Congdon, J. et al. (1991). Megestrol acetate and aminoglutethimide/hydrocortisone in sequence or in combination as second line endocrine therapy of estrogen receptor positive metastatic breast cancer. *ASCO Proc.* 10, 45

32. Klijn, J.G.M. et al. (1984). Antitumor and endocrine effects of cronic LHRH agonist treatment (buserelin) with or without tamoxifen in premenopausal metastatic breast cancer. *Breast Cancer Res.Treat.* 4, 209-220

33. Harvey, H.A. et al. (1985). Medical castration produced by the GnRH analogue leuprolide to treat metastatic breast cancer. *J.Clin.Oncol.* 3, 1068-1072

34. Williams, M.R. et al. (1986). The use of an LH-RH agonist (ICI 118630, Zoladex) in advanced premenopausal breast cancer. *Br.J.Cancer* 53, 629-636

35. Santen, R.J. et al. (1986). Gonadotropin releasing hormone (GnRH) analogs for the treatment of breast and prostatic carcinoma. *Breast cancer Res.Treat.* 7, 129-145

36. Walker, K.J. et al. (1989). Endocrine effects of combination antioestrogen and LH-RH agonist therapy in premenopausal patients with advanced breast cancer. *Eur.J.Cancer Clin.Oncol.* 25, 651-654

37. Anderson, E.D.C. et al. (1989). Response to endocrine manipulation and oestrogen receptor concentration in large operable primary breast cancer. *Br.J.Cancer* 60, 223-226

38. Milsted, R.A.V. et al. (1990). A review of the International Experience with the LHRH agonist Zoladex in the treatment of advanced breast cancer in pre- and perimenopausal women. In Glodhirsch, A. (eds) *ESO Monograph Series* pp.59-65

39. Dixon, A.R. et al. (1990). Combined goserelin (zoladex) and tamoxifen in premenopausal advanced breast cancer. *Breast Cancer Res.Treat.* 16, 193-6

40. Dowsett, M. et al. (1990). A dose-comparative endocrine-clinical study of leuprorelin in premenopausal breast cancer patients. *Br.J.Cancer* 62, 834-837

41. Bianco, A.R. et al. (1990). GnRH analogue goserelin (zoladex) in the treatment of pre- and perimenopausal women with metastatic breast cancer: results of a multicentric study. *Eur.J.Cancer* 26, 176

42. Brambilla, C. et al. (1991). Medical castration with zoladex: a conservative approach to premenopausal breast cancer. *Tumori* 77, 145-150

43. Kaufmann, M. et al. (1991). The depot GnRH analogue Goserelin in the treatment of premenopausal patients with metastatic breast cancer: a 5-year experience and further endocrine therapies. *Onkologie* 14(1), 22-30

44. Blamey, R.W. et al. (1991). Randomized trial comparing zoladex with nolvadex plus zoladex in pre-menopausal advanced breast cancer. *5th Breast Cancer Working Conference Leuven*, A77

45. Bajetta, E. et al. (1994). Goserelin in premenopausal advanced breast cancer: clinical and endocrine evaluation of responsive patients. *Oncol.Switz.* 51(3), 262-269

46. Buchanan, R.B. et al. (1986). A randomized comparison of tamoxifen with surgical oophorectomy in premenopausal patients with with advanced breast cancer. *J.Clin.Oncol.* 4, 1326-1330

47. Ingle J.N. et al. (1986). Randomized trial of bilateral oophorectomy versus tamoxifen in premenopausal women with metastatic breast cancer. *J.Clin.Oncol.* 4, 178-185

48. Boccardo, F. et al. (1985). Chemotherapy with or without tamoxifen in post-menopausal patients with late breast cancer. A randomized study. *J.Steroid Biochem.* 23(6B), 1123-1127

49. Perry, M.C. et al. (1985). Chemotherapy with cyclophosphamide, adriamycin and 5-fluorouracil compared to chemotherapy plus hormonal therapy with tamoxifen in the treatment of advanced breast cancer. *J.Steroid Biochem.* 23(6B), 1135-1140

50. The Australian and New Zealand Breast Cancer Trials Group, Clinical Oncological Society of Australia (1986). A randomized trial in postmenopausal patients with advanced breast cancer comparing endocrine and cytotoxic therapy given sequentially or in combination. *J.Clin.Oncol.* 4, 186-193

51. Perry, M.C. et al. (1987). Chemohormonal therapy in advanced carcinoma of the breast: Cancer and Leukemia Group B protocol 8081. *J.Clin.Oncol.* 5, 1534-1545

52. Cocconi, G. et al. (1983). Chemotherapy versus combination of chemotherapy and endocrine therapy in advanced breast cancer. A prospective randomized study. *Cancer* 51, 581-588

53. Krook, J.E. et al. (1985). Randomized clinical trial of cyclophosphamide, 5-FU and prednisone with or without tamoxifen in postmenopausal women with advanced breast cancer. *Cancer Treat.Rep.* 69(4), 355-361

54. Mouridsen, H.T. et al. (1985). Combined cytotoxic and endocrine therapy in postmenopausal patients with advanced breast cancer. A randomized study of CMF vs CMF plus tamoxifen. *Eur.J.Cancer Clin.Oncol.* 21, 291-299

55. Viladiu, P. et al. (1985). Chemotherapy versus chemotherapy plus hormonotherapy in postmenopausal advanced breast cancer patients. A randomized trial. *Cancer* 56, 2745-2750

56. Ahmann, D.L. et al. (1977). An evaluation of early or delayed adjuvant chemotherapy in premenopausal patients with advanced breast cancer undergoing oophorectomy. *N.Engl.J.Med.* 297, 356-360

57. Falkson, G. et al. (1979). Improved remission rates and remission duration in young women with metastatic breast cancer following combined oophorectomy and chemotherapy. A study by Cancer and Leukemia Group B. *Cancer* 43, 2215-2222

58. Cavalli, F. et al. (1983). Concurrent or sequential use of cytotoxic chemotherapy and hormone treatment in advanced breast cancer: report of the Swiss Group for Clinical Cancer Research. *Br.Med.J.* 286, 5-8

59. Brunner, K.W. et al. (1977). Combined chemo- and hormonal therapy in advanced breast cancer. *Cancer* 39, 2923-2933

60. Falkson, G. et al. (1987). Treatment of metastatic breast cancer in premenopausal women using CAF with or without oophorectomy: an Eastern Cooperative Oncology Group Study. *J.Clin.Oncol.* 5, 881-889

61. Bezwoda, W.R. et al. (1982). Treatment of metastatic breast cancer in estrogen receptor positive patients. A randomized trial comparing tamoxifen alone versus tamoxifen plus CMF. *Cancer* 50, 2747-2750

62. Robustelli della Cuna, G. et al. (1984). Medroxyprogesterone acetate in combination with chemotherapy for advanced breast cancer: updated results and criticisms. In Pellegrini, A. et al. (eds) *Role of Medroxyprogesterone acetate in endocrine-related tumors*, pp.91-104. (Raven Press, NY)

63. Brufmann, G. et al. (1994). Megestrol acetate in advanced breast carcinoma after failure to tamoxifen and/or aminoglutethimide. *Oncology Switz.* 51(3), 258-261

64. Dowsett, M. et al. (1994). The clinical and endocrine effects of the oral aromatase inhibitor vorozole in human breast cancer. *ASCO Proc.* 13, 85

GnRH-agonists for treatment of benign and malignant breast disease

A.E. Schindler

Department of Gynecology and Gynecological Oncology, University of Essen, Essen, Germany

GnRH-agonists have found broad clinical application in gynecology for benign and malignant condition. Among the benign lesions are: endometriosis, myoma, PCO-syndrom, fertility problems and benign breast disease; among the malignant conditions are: ovarian cancer, endometrium cancer and breast cancer.

The mechanisms of action are the following:

1. Constant and profound suppression of the endogeneous ovarian estrogen secretion and thereby decrease of estrogen receptors.

2. Possible direct action at the cellular level with proliferation inhibition and tumor growth inhibition.

3. Decrease of ovarian androgen secretion with decrease of extraglandular estrogen production.

4. Decrease of prolactin secretion.

So far, three possibilities for the use of GnRH-agonists in breast treatment are to be considered:

1. Benign breast disease

2. Malignant breast disease

3. Prevention

BENIGN BREAST DISEASE

In benign breast disease, mastalgia and fibrocystic disease have been studied. In cyclic mastalgia an effect of up to 90% was found (1). In fibrocystic disease complete response was observed in 53% (2).

Further improvement could be reached by combination with tamoxifen in estrogen-receptor positive cases and with cyproterone acetate in progesterone positive cases (2).

MALIGNANT BREAST DISEASE

In patients with breast cancer the following basic conditions have to be considered:

1. Premenopausal

a. adjuvant

b. metastatic recurrence

2. Postmenopausal

Furthermore, single agent or combination therapies can be applied. Most studies have been published regarding metastatic breast cancer recurrence in premonepausal women. A summary of these data is shown in table 1.

Table 1: Studies on GnRH-agonists for the treatment of premenopausal women with recurrent metastatic breast cancer

GnRH-Agonist	Number of patients	Response (CR + PR)		Median time to progression in weeks	Reference
		N	%		
Goserelin	75	25	33,0	./.	3
Goserelin	61	16	32,0	17	4
Goserelin	22	7	32,0	64	5
Goserelin	118	53	44,9	59	6
Goserelin	228	83	36,4	44	7

It should be pointed out that response was also seen in estrogen-receptor negative cases. In case of progression of the disease, a combination with tamoxifen in addition to GnRH-agonist treatment revealed complete and partial response in nearly 30% and in addition no change was found in 32% (6). Also the addition of aminoglutethimid showed a response (6). GnRH-agonists in depot-form are to be preferred compared with nasasl application.

In postmenopausal women with metastatic breast cancer GnRH-agonists have also been tried and found that there is a decrease of FSH and LH reducing also ovarian androgen secretion and a decrease in peripheral aromatization of androgens to estrogens. The response rate appears to be around 10% (8).

BREAST CANCER PREVENTION

A further aspect of GnRH-agonist therapy is prevention of breast cancer. It was suggested that a 10 year treatment of a premenopausal women with GnRH-agonists to suppress endogeneus ovarian estradiol secretion and to substitute as add-back with 0,625 mg conjugated estrogens and 10 mg MPA for 12 days every 4 months. Under such regiment a bone density decrease of 1.9% per year was found (9). In order to prevent this, a small dose of androgens was suggested.

The goals to be accomplished are:

1. Live time risk reduction of up to 50% to develop breast cancer and in addition contraception is provided.

REFERENCES

1. Hamed, H., Chaudary, M.A., Caleffi, M., Fentiman, I.S. (1990). LHRH analogue for treatment of recurrent and refractory mastalgia. J. Royal Coll. Surg. Engl. 72, 222-4.

2. Monsenego, J., Estable, M.D., De Sanit Floren, G., Amouroux, J., Kouyoumdjan, J.-C., Haour, F., Breau, J.-L., Israel, L., Comaru-Schally, A.M., Schally, A.V. (1991). Fibrocystic disease of the breast in premenopausal women: Histohormonal correlation and response to luteinizing hormone releasing hormone analogue treatment. Amer. J. Obstet. Gynecol. 164, 1181-4

3. Dixon, A.R., Robertoson, J.F.R., Jackson, L., Nicholson, R.I., Walker, K.J. Blamey, R.W. (1990). Goserelin (Zoladex) in premenopausal advanced breast cancer: duration of response and survival. Cancer 62, 868-70.

4. Bianco, A.R., Roso, R., Galabresi, F., Fiorentino, M., Lopez, M., Sismondi, P.G., Lenti, R., Fosser, V., De Placido, S., Perrone, F., Pronzato, P., Carlini, P., Loranasiero, A., Veltri, W., Zola, P., Farinacci, M., Gulisani, M., Artioli, R. (1991) LH-RH analogue Zoladex in the treatment of pre- and perimenopausal women with metastatic breast cancer. Eur. J. Gynecol. Oncol., 12, 429-37

5. Brambila, C., Escobedo, A., Artioli, R., Lechuga, M.J., Motta, M., Bonadonna,G. (1991) Medical castration with Zoladex: A conservativ approach to premenopausal breast cancer. Tumori 77, 145-50.

6. Robertson, J.F.R., Walker, K.J., Nicholson, R.I., Blamey, R.W. (1989) Comined endocrine effect of LHRH-agonist (Zoladex) and Tamoxifen (Nolvadex) therapy in premenopausal women with breast cancer. *Brit. J. Surg.* 75, 1262-65.

7. Blamey, R.W., Jonat, W., Kaufmann, M., Bianco, A.R., Namer, M. (1992) Goserelin Depot in the treatment of premenopausal advanced breast cancer. *Eur. J. Cancer* 28a, 810-4

8. Saphner, T., Troxel, A. B., Tormey, D.C., Neuberg, D., Robert, N.J., Pandya, K.J., Edmonson, J.H., Rosenbluth, R.J., Abeloff, M.D. (1993) Phase II Study of Goserelin for patients with postmenopausal mestatic breast cancer. *J. Clin. Oncol.* 11, 1529-35.

9. Pike, M., Ross, R.K., Lobo, R.A., Key, T.J., Potts, M., Henderson, B.E. (1989) LHRH agonists and the prevention of breast and ovarian cancer. *Brit. J. Cancer* 60, 142-8

Mammary and metabolic changes induced by tamoxifen

F.R. Pérez-López, I. Morollón, J. Hergueta and R. Pérez Sanz

*Department of Obstetrics and Gynecology, Hospital Clínico and University of
Zaragoza Faculty of Medicine, Zaragoza, Spain*

INTRODUCTION

Tamoxifen (TAM) is a triphenylethylene antiestrogen widely employed as first
line endocrine therapy for breast cancer in postmenopausal women with
positive estrogen receptor proteins. TAM efficacy is equivalent to oophorectomy
for breast cancer treatment. This drug is also useful in the treatment of
melanoma, adenocarcinoma of the pancreas, some brain tumors and in hepatic
carcinoma. Although TAM blocks estrogen binding to the nuclear estrogen
receptor, it also participates in cell replication through the release or activation
of autocrine growth factors, induces changes in angiogenesis, protects
membranes against oxidative damage, and induces immunologic changes (1-6).
These effects may explain the low but consistent response frequency reported
in breast cancer patients when steroid receptors are absent.

In recent years the importance of TAM has been stressed to reduce the
incidence of a new malignant tumor in the remaining mammary gland from
breast cancer patients (7, 8). Furthermore, TAM is also useful for the treatment
of mastalgia and fibrocystic disease of the breast (9, 10) and it may be feasible
for the chemoprevention of breast cancer (8). Women under TAM may express
side effects in target cells. These effects may be advantageous as is the case on
bone metabolism, the antiatherosclerotic and cardioprotective benefcts; or
negative like the genital neoplastic changes (11-16).

TAMOXIFEN IN BENIGN BREAST DISEASES

Mastalgia, of varying duration and intenstity throughout the menstrual cycle, is a frecuent disturbance which has been related to non-demonstrated supposed hormonal changes, alterations in mammary vascularization and psychological dysfunctions. The administration of TAM notably improves these disturbances, with similar or better effectiveness than other treatments. However, it should be pointed out that in some women the administration of a placebo improves the symptomatology.

Controversy exists as to the existence of fibrocystic disease of the breast (FDB) and its limits (17, 18). However, a large amount of women experience exaggerated breast tenderness, pain, swelling, increased fibrous components, and radiologic evidence of high density. This clinical situation has been considered an *"exaggerated response"* to the normal endocrine and paracrine regulatory mechanisms, although steroid and pituitary hormones are within the normal range (19). Dietetic factors, microvascular alterations and psychological abnormalities have also considered. FDB is usually a benign and progressive process which starts at the age of 20-30 years with a lobular or diffuse increase in glandular tissue. A proportion of these patients develop duct ectasia, fibrosis and small cysts. Although large cysts may appear at all stages of FDB, they are a relatively late phenomenon.

TAM treatment induces a significant reduction in breast pain, swelling and nodular or fibrous areas in FDB. Clinical objective improvement and mammographic changes are obtained after 6 months of treatment (10, 20). During treatment the most frequent complaints are spotting, headache and nervousness. The clinical improvement obtained with TAM persists after treatment, althouth some women have a tendency to relapse. The reinstauring of treament with this antiestrogen continues to be effective in successive therapeutical administrations.

Gorodeski *et al.* (21) reported that a single dose of TAM resulted in activation and up regulation of endometrial estrogen receptor and progesterone receptor concentrations. In women with FDB, TAM treatment induced a significant reduction in endometrial estrogen receptors and a significant increase in circulating estradiol without significant changes in either other plasma steroids or endometrial progesterone receptors (22).

TAM is not effective as treatment for mammary fibroadenoma, although the tumor remains stable during treatment. In fact, the mammary fibroadenoma does not usually respond to other hormonal treatments either, and surgical removal should be considered when the presence of the tumor creats anxiety, is painful or suddenly in increases in size.

TAMOXIFEN IN BREAST CANCER

Postmenopausal women with breast cancer are usually administerd TAM over a period of several years, althouth there is no concensus regarding the most convenient duration of this treatment. There is a significant increase of the risk of developing a second breast tumor in patients with breast cancer. Administration of TAM not only treats primary breast cancer, but also in addition reduces the risk of developing a mammary malignancy in the contralateral breast (7, 8). However, TAM can also act by stimulating the mammary tumors growth in certain cell populations (23, 24). The mammary changes induced in patients are scarcely visible in mammographs.

The administration of TAM in young women with breast cancer induces significant hormonal changes and induces menstrual disturbances including amenorrhea, although the woman continues to ovulate and is at risk of becoming pregnant (25). On the other hand, in postmenopausic women, TAM produces few changes in steroid hormones and circulating gonadotropines (table 1). However, the hormonal and metabolic situation may differ in women who develop a genital pathology. Furthermore, the effects on target organs could be much greater than those effects detected in the circulating hormones.

In the Scottish trial on adjuvant TAM, patients who received the drug for a 5-year period experienced a reduction of fatal myocardial infarction of more than 50 % compared to placebo treated women (12) whilst there are conflicting

Table 1 Mean ± SEM plasma hormones in postmenopausal women with breast cancer without hormone therapy as compared to women treated with TAM for 25.7±2.3 months. * p<0.05; ** p<0.01

	Control group (n=16)	Under TAM (n=15)
Years since menopause	17.7±2.0	18.6±3.5
Weight (kg)	69.7±2.5	71.7±5.5
LH (ml.U./ml)	14.8 ± 2.3	9.9 ± 1.5 *
FSH (ml.U./ml)	57.7 ± 7.4	35.9 ± 5.0 **
Prolactin (ng/ml	11.3 ± 1.8	8.2 ± 1.7
Estradiol (pg/ml)	23.3 ± 2.3	39.5 ± 10.3
DHEA-S (ng/ml)	634.9 ± 108.0	670.6 ± 93.9
Androstendione (ng/ml)	1.8 ± 0.4	2.1 ± 0.3
Cortisol (μg/dl)	16.8 ± 2.9	23.7 ± 2.3 *

results about thromboembolic complications (26-28). The factors involved in coronary illnesses are extremely diverse, including metabolic alterations and changes in coagulation, hypertension, tobacco addiction and life style. The cardioprotective benefits of TAM could be related to modifications of the lipid metabolism (13). However, in a group of women with breast cancer treated with TAM, the levels were not significantly different to the values of women who received no form of hormone therapy (table 2). The cardioprotective benefits of TAM could also intervene protecting cardiac membranes against the damage caused by lipid peroxidation, reducing plasma homocysteine, or by other unknown mechanisms (5, 29).

Steroid receptors have been detected in bone tissue. The effects of TAM on bones are contradictory (11, 30, 31). In women who received TAM , the levels of circulating osteocalcin were found to be lower than in women who had not received hormone therapy (table 3), suggesting a favourable effect on the formation of bone tissue. However, it remains to be demonstrated whether these changes are accompanied by a reduction in the number of bone fractures.

Table 2 Mean ± SEM plasma lipids and lipoproteins in women with breast cancer without hormone therapy as compared to women treated with TAM for 24.4±2.0 months

	Control group (n=13)	Under TAM (n=13)
Years since menopause	16.6±1.9	16.6±3.8
Weight (kg)	69.1±6.7	67.7±2.7
Total cholesterol (mg/dl)	192.8±6.7	207.4±8.1
HDL-cholesterol (mg/dl)	53.2±4.6	56.2±2.4
LDL-cholesterol (mg/dl)	117.3±5.5	123.9±7.3
Triglicerydes (mg/dl)	112.7±16.3	133.9±15.8

Long term TAM treatment is associated to several risks that cannot be avoided. Women under TAM treatment have a remarkably high prevalence of pathological genital changes including endometrial cancer (14-16). In most postmenopausal women under TAM the endometrium remains atrophic but epithelial metaplasia, endometrial hyperplasia, polyps, ovarian cysts and endometrial cancers have been reported.

Table 3 Mean ± SEM plasma osteocalcin, calcitonin, parathyroid hormone (PTH), calcium, inorganic phosphorus, and alkaline phosphatase in women with breast cancer without hormone therapy as compared to women treated with TAM for 25.8±2.3 months. *p<0.01

	Control group (n=15)	Under TAM (n=14)
Years since menopause	16.7±2.2	15.9±3.4
Weight (kg)	69.5±5.8	69.1±2.7
Osteocalcin (ng/ml)	7.5±0.9	4.1±0.2 *
Calcitonin (pg/ml)	7.3±0.9	8.0±0.7
Intact PTH (pg/ml)	47.9±3.9	49.9±4.7
Calcium (mg/dl)	9.2±0.1	9.0±0.4
Inorganic P (mg/dl)	3.7±0.1	3.8±0.4
Alkaline phosphatase (U/l)	79.9±10.2	63.0±6.7

The genital lesions associated to treatment with TAM usually show very little symptomology and should, therefore, be located sistematically forming part of the clinical follow-up of women with cancer. It seems that the risk of endometrial cancer is related to the duration of drug intake. However, endometrial tumors that arise after TAM treatment for breast cancer are not consistent with the types generally linked to exogenous estrogen intake (32, 33).

Although new pure antiestrogens are currently under study, it seems that the special characteristics of TAM and its different mechanisms of action and the side effects deserve future research. Some estrogenic actions of TAM may cause delayed gynecologic side effects that must be carefully monitored.

REFERENCES

1. Pollock, M., Costantino, J. and Polychronakos, C. (1990). Effect of tamoxifen on serum insulin-like growth factor 1 levels in stage 1 breast cancer patients. *J. Natl. Cancer Inst.*, **82**, 1693-7

2. Butta, A., MacLennan, K., Flanders, C. *et al.* (1992). Induction of transforming growth factor-ß 1 in human breast cancer in vivo following tamoxifen treatment. *Cancer Res.*, **52**, 4261-4

3. Gagliardi, A. and Collins, D.C. (1993). Inhibition of angiogenesis by antiestrogens. *Cancer Res.*, **53**, 533-5

4. Noguchi, S., Motomura, K., Inaji, H., Imaoka, S. and Koyama, H. (1993). Down-regulation of transforming growth factor α by tamoxifen in human breast cancer. *Cancer*, **72**, 131-6

5. Wiseman, H. (1994). Tamoxifen: new membrane-mediated mechanisms of action and therapeutic advances. *Trends Pharmacol. Sci.*, **15**, 83-9

6. Berry, J., Green, B.J. and Matheson, D.S. (1987). Modulation of natural killer cell activity by tamoxifen in stage I post-menopause breast cancer. *Eur. J. Cancer Clin. Oncol.*, **23**, 517-20

7. Fisher, B., Costantino, J., Redmond, C. *et al.* (1989). A randomized clinical trial evaluating tamoxifen in the treatment of patients with node-negative breast cancer who have estrogen-receptor-positive tumors. *N. Engl. J. Med.*, **320**, 479-84

8. Gray, R. (1993). Tamoxifen: how boldly to go where no women have gone before.

J. Natl. Cancer Inst., **85**, 1358-60

9. Fentiman, I.S., Caleffi, M., Hamed, H. and Chaudary, M.A. (1988). Dosage and duration of tamoxifen treatment for mastalgia: a randomised trial. *Br. J. Surg.*, **75**, 845-8

10. Pérez-López, F.R. (1992). Effects of tamoxifen in women with fibrocystic disease of the breast. In. Genazzani, A.R., Genazzani, A.D. and D'Ambrogio, G. (eds.). *Recent developments in gynecological endocrinology*, pp. 509-16. (Carnforth: The Parthenon Publishing Group)

11. Kristensen, B., Ejlertsen B., Dalgaard, P. *et al.* (1994). Tamoxifen and bone metabolism in postmenopausal low-risk breast cancer patients: A randomized study. *J. Clin. Oncol.*, **12**, 992-7

12. McDonald, C.C. and Stewart, H.J. (1991). Fatal myocardial infarction in the Scottish adjuvant tamoxifen trial. *Br. Med. J.*, **303**, 435-7

13. Thangaraju, M., Kumar, K., Gandhirajan, R. and Sachdanandam, P. (1994). Effect of tamoxifen on plasma lipids and lipoproteins in postmenopausal women with breast cancer. *Cancer*, **73**, 659-63

14. Seoud, M.A.F., Johnson, J. and Weed Jr, J.C. (1993). Gynecologic tumors in tamoxifen-treated women with breast cancer. *Obstet. Gynecol.*, **82**, 165-9

15. Fisher, B., Costantino, J.P., Redmond, C.K. *et al.* (1994). Endometrial cancer in tamoxifen-treated breast cancer patients: findings from the National Surgical Adjuvant Breast and Bowel Project (NSABP) B-14. *J. Natl. Cancer Inst.*, **86**, 527-37

16. Van Leewen, F.E., Benraadt, J., Coeberg, J.W.W. *et al.* (1994). Risk of endometrial cancer after tamoxifen treatment of breast cancer. *Lancet*, **343**, 448-52

17. Hutter, R.V.P. (1985). Goodbye to "fibrocystic disease". *N. Engl. J. Med.*, **312**, 179-81

18. Cancer Committee of the College of American Pathologists (1986). Consensus meeting: Is "fibrocystic disease" of the breast precancerous? *Arch. Pathol. Lab. Med.*, **110**, 171-3

19. Pérez-López, F.R., Hergueta, J., Blasco, C. and Juste, G. (1992). Plasma pituitary and steroid hormones and endometrial steroid receptors in women with fibrocystic disease of the breast. *Neuroendocrinology Lett.*, **14**, 113-7

20. Pérez-López, F.R. (1994). Treatment of fibrocystic disease of the breast with tamoxifen. *Int. J. Obstet. Gynecol.*, **46 (Suppl.1)**, 106

21. Gorodeski, G.I., Beery, R., Lunenfeld, B. and Geier, A. (1992). Tamoxifen increase plasma estrogen-binding equivalents and has an estradiol agonistic effect on

histologically normal premenopausal and postmenopausal endometrium. *Fertil. Steril.*, **57**, 320-7

22. Pérez-López, F.R. and Blasco Comenge, M.C. (1993). Effects of tamoxifen on endometrial estrogen and progesterone receptor concentrations in women with fibrocystic disease of the breast. *Gynecol. Endocrinol.*, **7**, 185-9

23. Horwitz, K.B. (1993). Can hormone "resistant" breast cancer cells be inappropriately stimulated by tamoxifen? *Ann. N. Y. Acad. Sci.*, **684**, 63-74

24. Maenpaa, J., Wiebe, V., Koester, S. *et al.* (1993). Tamoxifen stimulates in vivo growth of drug-resistant estrogen receptor-negative breast cancer. *Cancer Chem. Pharmacol.*, **32**, 396-8

25. Jordan, V.C., Fritz, N.F., Langan-Fahey, S., Thompson, M. and Tormey, D.C. (1991). Alteration of endocrine parameters in premenopausal women with breast cancer during long-term adjuvant therapy with tamoxifen as the single agent. *J. Natl. Cancer Inst.*, **83**, 1488-91

26. Taylor, S.F. IV, Kalish, L.A., Olson, J.E. *et al.* (1985). Adjuvant CMFP versus CMFP plus tamoxifen versus observation alone in postmenopausal, node positive breast cancer patients: Three year results of an Eastern Cooperative Oncology Group study. *J. Clin. Oncol.*, **3**, 144-54

27. Rutqvist, L.E. and Mattsson, A. (1993). Cardiac and thromboembolic morbidity among postmenopausal women with early-stage breast cancer in a randomized trial of adjuvant tamoxifen. The Stockholm Breast Cancer Study Group. *J. Natl. Cancer Inst.*, **85**, 1398-406

28. Rivkin, S.E., Green, S., Metch, B. *et al.* (1994). Adjuvant CMFVP versus tamoxifen versus concurrent CMFVP and tamoxifen for postmenopausal, node-positive, and estrogen receptor-positive breast cancer patients: A Southwest Oncology Group Study. *J. Clin. Oncol.*, **12**, 2078-85

29. Anker, G., Lonning, P.E., Ueland, P.M., Refsun, H. and Lien, E.A. (1995). Plasma levels of the atherogenic amino acid homocysteine in postmenopausal women with breast cancer treated with tamoxifen. *Int. J. Cancer*, **60**, 365-8

30. Gotfredsen, A., Christiansen, C. and Palshof, T. (1984). The effect of tamoxifen on bone mineral content in premenopausal women with breast cancer. *Cancer*, **53**, 853-7

31. Fentiman, I.S., Caleffi, M., Rodin, A. *et al.* (1989). Bone mineral content of women receiving tamoxifen for mastalgia. *Br. J. Cancer*, **60**, 262-4

32. Magriples, U., Naftolin, F., Schwartz, P.E. and Cargangiu, M.L. (1993). High grade

endometrial carcinoma in tamoxifen-treated breast cancer patients. *J. Clin. Oncol.*, **11**, 485-90

33. Barakat, R.R., Wong, G., Curtin, J.P., Vlamis, V. and Hoskins, W.J. (1994). Tamoxifen use in breast cancer patients who subsequently develop corpus cancer is not associated with a higher incidence of adverse histologic features. *Gynecol. Oncol.*, **55**, 164-8

Breast cancer and breast implants: can a chronic granulomatous inflammation provoked by a breast implant with rough-spongious surface produce acquired immunity against tumors? – the role of IFN-γ and TNF secreting epithelioid cells

I. Lyras, P. Rapti*, T. Nassif, G. Cotta-Pereira and I. Pitanguy

Department of Plastic Surgery, IPGMCC, PC University, Rio de Janeiro, Brazil and *Department of Endocrinology, "Lito" Maternity Hospital, Athens, Greece

INTRODUCTION

A great deal of recent scientific progress in the fight against cancer has been achieved in the direction of immunoprotection and immunotherapy. Nowadays, induction of prospective immunity to tumors can actually be accomplished by active immunization procedures.

Recent experiments demonstrate that in some cases of disease, intense inflammatory infiltrates accumulate around cytokine-secreting tumors[1]. (Eosinophils and macrophages dominate IFN-γ secreting tumors and massive lymphocyte infiltrates, surround IL-2 producing tumors). This way, depending on the type of infiltrate cells recruited around a tumor or a granuloma by diferent cytokines, diferent effector as well as accessory cell functions lead to the the optimal activation of T cells. Local production of cytokines and lymphokines may augment specific T cell responses to tumor antigens.

Until 1991, silicone gel-filled breast implants, (used since 1960 for breast augmentation and breast reconstruction) were considered safe, biocompatible medical devices. For the past 4 years their use has been restricted because of the great public and scientific concern related to the complications they provoke, although recent reports demonstrate that breast cancer is rarer and of better prognosis in women that carry breast implants.[2,3,4]

The present study is based mainly on the importance of surface morphology of the implants and how it affects the healing process on the site of their inclusion.

The results of the present study have offered us good reasons for further investigations in colaboration with other centers. Currently, we are investigating the variations of interferon, tumor necrosis factor and other lymphokine blood levels in women with breast prostheses before and after the implantation of these devices for both aesthetic and reconstructive reasons. Another experimental study, currently underway in our

787

laboratory examines the effects of the presence of specially designed and patented by Dr. I. Lyras, medical implants in animals suffering from provoked or diagnosed cancer.

MATERIAL AND METHODS

Fourty-eight, adult Wistar rats weighting about 270 grams at the time of implantation were used for this experimental study. One smooth, one textured and one spongious (polyurethane covered) surface silicone 2 ml mini implants, were placed subcutaneously through three lateral 2 cm long incisions into the back of each animal.

All animals were obtained from the same supplier, were conditioned for a period of four weeks before use and were maintained with a standard laboratory chow and water ad libitum. 400 days after implantation we examined the tissue reaction - implant complex.

Light, polarization and electron microscopy was performed on the material (capsules and liver) harvested from the animals. We used H-E, Gomori and Picrosirius staining techniques and gold impregnation for scanning electron microscopy (Jeol 100 Cx eletron microscope). Immunohistochemistry is underway.

RESULTS

Four hundred days after inclusion, the following situations were documented:

1) Smooth surface implants

Completely balanced reaction. All fibroblasts had become myofibroblasts. Almost no residual inflammatory cells were observed inside the capsule which was dense, thick, compact and practically avascular. Complete insolation of the implant from the host organism through fibrotic repair (type I collagen fibres) of the connective tissue (Synovial Metaplasia) was acomplished. Very few lymphocytes and eosinophils were present inside the capsule. No inflamatory exudate was observed.

2) Textured surface implants

Fibroblasts formed a strange type of capsule. They hang on multiple vascular axons the way "birthday party flags" hang on cords, being always vertical to the surface of the implant in a perfect organization. Among them much exudate, some type III collagen fibrilles, some lymphocytes and eosinophils and a variable number of epitelioid cells in contact with the silicone were observed. Angiogenesis was moderate.

3) Polyurethane foam covered implants

The entire foam was filled with adipocytes, occupying the place of the present initially but totally absent in this phase fibroblasts. Multinucleated giant cells were covering completely the particles of polyurethane, and a great number of epitelioid cells were found in contact with internal membrane of the implants. Some lymphocytes and eosinophils were actively present inside a discrete quantity of inflammatory exudate. Angiogenesis was very intense. No collagen was observed.

788

4) Infection

Three cases of tissue necrosis with infection occured 30 days after implantation. The causative pathogen was enterobacter. The implants involved were carrying a rough surface (two foams and one textured).

5) Liver

No pathology related to the presence of polyurehane or silicone was observed in the liver. Some macrophages and lymphocytes were observed inside small vassels of the liver parenchyma.

6) Carcinogenesis

No carcinogenesis was observed to any of the animals.

7) Degradation of biomaterials

Some degradation of the rough surfaces was observed without altering the characteristics of the implants.

DISCUSSION

The qualitative nature of the inflammatory response to a surgical procedure may vary with the kind of injury produced and the presence of foreign bodies at the site of the injury. In most noncontaminated surgical wounds, the acute inflammatory reaction subsides and recognizable repair commences in three to five days. When the wound contains foreign material this reaction becomes chronic. As a general principle the body reacts to any insoluble foreign material either by extruding it if it can be moved or by walling it off by a granulomatous-type reaction. The intensity and the extent of the reaction vary widely, depending on both the physical and chemical nature of the foreign body[6]. Repair of the reacting tissue is accomplished both by regeneration of parenchymal cells and replacement by connective tissue which in time produces fibrosis and scaring when the foreign body has a smooth surface. There are four components to this process:

• Formation of new blood vessels (angiogenesis)

• Migration and proliferation of fibroblasts

• Deposition of extracellular matrix

• Maturation and reorganization of the fibrous tissue, also known as remodeling.

Migration of fibroblasts and their subsequent proliferation are mediated by growth factors such as PDGF, PGF, EGF, FGF, VPF, VEGF, somatomedins and TGF-β. TGF-β is particularly critical in favouring fibrous tissue deposition. It induces fibroblast migration and proliferation as well as increased collagen synthesis and decreased collagen degradation of excess cellular matrix biometalloproteinases. TGF-β is thus thought to play an important role in chronic inflammatory fibrosis.

Formation of a fibrous capsule around an implant is markedly aided if very fine lines are etched on the surface of this implant[5]. On absolutely smooth surfaces, fibroblasts move bidirectionally and when they come in contact they soon acquire active contractive properties, with the formation of a fibrous capsule.

The reaction of the host organism against foreign bodies with rough surface is dramatically diferent to the one against foreign bodies with smooth surface, practically leading to a chronic granulomatous inflamation. This type of reaction is characterized by <u>granulomas</u> -small collections of modified macrophages.[1]

Macrophages are central figures in chronic inflammation because of the great number of biologically active products they can secrete. They are derived from peripheral blood monocytes that have been induced to emigrate across the endothelium by chemotactic agents. The latter include C5a, fibrinopeptides, cytokines (MCP-1), platelet-derived growth factor (PDGF), and collagen and fibronectin fragments. Macrophages can be activated to secrete numerous facrors, including neutral proteases, chemotactic factors, arachidonic acid metabolites, reactive oxygen species, complement components, coagulation factors, growth factors, cytokines (such as IL-1 and TNF), and other factors (e.g. PAF and a-interferon).[6] Macrophage activation in inflammation is triggered by lymphokines (γ-interferon) produced by immune activated T cells, or by nonimmune factors (e.g. endotoxin).[7,8,9,10] The secretory products of macrophages induce the changes characteristic of chronic inflammation, tissue destruction (proteases and oxygen-derived free radicals), neovascularization, fibroblast proliferation (growth factors), connective tissue accumulation (cytokines and growth factors), and remodeling (collagenases). Macrophages when modified acquire abundant pink cytoplasm and are called epithelioid cells. Epithelioid cells may coalese to form multinucleate giant cells. Lymphocytes, plasma cells, neutrophils, and central necrosis may also be present in a granuloma.

There are two types of granulomas:

1. Foreign body granulomas, incited by relatively inert foreign bodies as in the case of our textured surface implants.

2. Immune granulomas, formed by immune T cell-mediated reactions to poorly degradable antigens. Lymphokines, principally γ-interferon from activated T cells, cause transformation of macrophages to epithelioid cells and multinucleate giant cells as in the case of our polyurethane foam covered implants.[1]

Granulomas are characteristic of certain diseases caused by particular infectious agents (e.g., tuberculosis), mineral dusts (e.g. silicosis), or other unknown conditions (e.g. sarcoidosis).[10]

Formation of granulomas around foreign bodies is also influenced by:

• Lymphocytes modilized by antibody and cell-mediated immune reactions. Lymphocytes have a unique reciprocal relationship to macrophages in chronic inflamation. They can be activated by contact with the implant. Activated lymphocytes produce lymphokines, and these (particularly γ-interferon) are major stimulators of monocytes and macrophages.

• Plasma cells. They produce antibodies dierected against foreign antigen.

• Eosinophils. Their granules contain (toxic) major basic protein (MBP).

• Intracellular adhesion molecule (ICAM) and major histocompatibility complex (MCH). Very important defence mecanisms against tumors.

Some authors have recently noticed a slight degrease of the expected incidence rates of primary or second primary breast cancer[2,3,4] in women that have undergone breast augmentation and breast reconstruction with breast implants. These observations are somehow important and one could suggest that there must be a biological reason involved in this situation.

The fact that around implants, specially the ones with rough-slongious type of surface (as in polyurethane foams), phagocygosis will not subside even after one year, makes chronic inflamation continue and acquire the characteristics of a granulomatous disease like tubercusis or sarcoidosis.[6]

One could observe a strange similarity in this type of cellular and hymoral disorder of the cell-mediated immune response to diferent antigens. Tuberculosis is a good example of a disease in which protective cell-mediated immunity after some time will lead to antigenic stimulation and T cell and macrophage activation with formation of granulomas. Reaction to sarcoidosis is also very much alike in most cases.

On the other side, this type of immune reaction could also lead to a delayed type of hypersensitivity which could cause tissue injury, or under certain conditions, (preexisting undiagnosed tumors) to immune or genetic accidents of tumor growth stimulation or tumor escape, evasion or "genetic instability" instead of a much desired tumor suppression, repression and regression. Tolerogens are believed to play an important role in preventing these accidents[1]. The fact that medical implants are sterile devices, certainly is important because this way the antigenic stimulus is not recognised by the host organism, neither as an extra or intracellular bacteria, nor as a virus or a parasite. This leads to a situation where an implant behaves as a nonspecific, (polyclonal) antigen, leading to a general increase of both the humoral and the cellular types of immune response. The regulation of this immune reaction to the foreign body (breast implant) seems to be self-limited since no clinical sign of disease was noticed to any of the animals examined. Reports on patients are still inconclusive. Further large scale research on the subject is required.

In any way, it has already been accepted that although immunization against tumors would likely be used in patients with already established tumors, general "vaccinations" against tumor antigens could conceivably be performed profilactically in populations at high risc for certain cancers.[1]

CONCLUSION

A different model of active immunization against tumors is presented. By a specially designed high quality biocompatible medical implant (with rough-spongious surface morphology) placed somewhere inside the body, we can provoke a permanent low grade granulomatous chronic inflammation and this way a nonspecific stimulation of the immune system of patients. The mecanism of this stimulation involves a markedly increased humoral response, lymphocyte memory enhancement and continuous antigenic activity and is based on the rationale that an implant containing granuloma behaves and should be considered as a cytokine and lymphokine-secreting tumor. Interferon-γ (IFN-γ), tumor necrosis factor (TNF) and interleukin (IL)-secreting lymphocytes and epithelioid cells are key factors of this process. We propose that this method of preventive nonspecific stimulation of the immune system should be seriously considered as a useful approach for achieving acquired immune defence against cancer.

REFERENCES

1) Abbas, A.K. Lichtman, A.H, Rober, J.S. (1994) Immunity to tumors. In: *cellular and molecular Immunology, W.B. Saunders (Edt) Second Edition: 357-375.*

2) Dreapen, D.M, Brody, G.S. (1992) Augmentation Mammoplasty and Breast Cancer: A 5-year update of the Los Angeles study. *Plast Reconstr. Surg. 89:660.*

3) Petit, J.Y., Lê, M.G., Mouriesse, H., Rietjens M., Gill, P. Contesso, G. Lehmann, A. (1994). Can Breast reconstruction with Gel-Filled Silicone Implants Increase the risk of death and second Primary Cancer in Patients treated by mastectomy for Breast cancer. *Plast Reconstr. Surg. 94. 1-115-125.*

4) Birdsell, D.C., Jenkins, H., Berkel, H. (1993). Breast Cancer Diagnosis and Survival in women with and without Breast implants. *Plast Reconstr. Surg. 92; 5:795-800.*

5) Raso, D.S., Crymes, L.W. Metcalf, J.S. (1994). Histological assessement of Fifty Capsules from smooth and textured augmentation and reconstruction mammoplasty prostheses with emphasis on the role of Sinovial Metaplasia. *Mod. Pathol. 7; 3:310-316.*

6) Peacock, E.E. Jr., Van Winkel, W. Jr. (1976). *Wound repair. W.B. Saunders Company, Second edition, 1-145.*

7) Fiers, W., Bouckaert, P., Guisez, Y. et al. (1986). Recombinant interferon-gamma and its synergism with tumor necrosis factor in the human and mouse systems. *In: Schellekens, H., Stewart, W.E. (Eds), The Biology of the interferon System. p. 241, Elsevier Amsterdam.*

8) Marequet, R.L., Ijzermans, J.N.M., Bruin, R.W. Fetal (1987). Antitumor activity of recombinant mouse tumor necrosis factor (TNF) on colon Cancer in rats is promoted by recombinant rat interferon-gamma: toxicity is reduced by indomethacin. *Int. J. Cancer, 40-550.*

9) Hosang, M. (1988). Recombinant interferon-γ inhibits the mitogenic effect of platelet-derived Growth Factor at a level distal to the Growth Factor receptor. *J. Cell. Phys. 134:396-404.*

10) Kindler, V. et al. (1989). The inducing role of tumor necrosis factor in the development of Bacterial granulomas during BCG infection. *Cell 56:731-740.*

Needle localization of clinically occult breast lesions

G. Ragonesi, L. Nuzzo, A. Decko, E. Alba, M. Fenocchio, L. Corvetto and S. Maffei

Department of Gynecology and Obstetrics, Cattedra B, Turin, Italy

Mammography as screening, can detect early lesions before they are clinically palpable. Non palpable cancers are shown as a mass with or withouth calcifications or as clustered calcifications only. Accurate surgical excision can be most difficult since there are no gross manifestations at surgery to localize the site of calcification. In our experience percutaneous needle localization is reliable and easy to perform, permiting high accurancy in mapping procedures. Fixing the wire in the tissue reduces the possibility of the localizer changing position with breast motion and facilitates operative procedures.

INTRODUCTION

Breast lesions detected by mammography may not be evident on physical examination because of small size, deep location within the breast or confinement to the ducts.

Most of these lesions remain non-individuable even when physical examination is performed with knowledge of the mammographic findings. With the increasing number of mammograms performed for screening purposes, the identification of non palpable lesions is increasing in frequency (3).

For example the incidence of calcifications present in breast cancer as determined by clinical mammography varies from series to series, Levitan 29% - Egan 45% - Zuckerman 63% (6).

In patients with clustered tiny microcalcifications, however, the incidence of cancer, especially intraductal and lobular carcinoma in situ is increased (1).

793

In a patient with suspicious clustered microcalcifications therefore, there is a significant possibility that

a) a carcinoma is present

b) an early non invasive breast cancer without metasteses may be found.

Exact localization and excision of these microcalcifications is imperative.

In spite of state of the art equipment and technique a certain number of pre-clinical tumors will be radiologically interpreted as borderline or benign lesions (5).

Biopsy of these lesions is a logical consequence in order to arrive at a sure diagnosis.

Using mammograms and biopsy together, and examination of the literature reveals benign lesion / malignant tumor ratio of 3:1. This ratio may thus be considered as a standard of good quality (7).

The method employed for the localization of the lesion must allow for both adeguate resection of the lesion and limited cosmetic damage, while at the same time offering minimals possibilities for diagnostic error. In addition the biopsy should not complicate an eventual therapeutic procedure, should it be required.

METHOD

If we depict the breast as a three dimensional graph with the nipple as the origin, then the position of any lesion within the breast can be defined by the means of three coordinates.

The x coordinate (horizontal) descibes the medial or lateral distance from the nipple.

The distance above or below the nipple determines the y coordinate (vertical).

These two coordinates are measured from the craniocaudal and lateral mammograms respectively and together are transcribed as a single point on the patients skin.

Through this point the needle is inserted along the axis towards the chest wall.

The depth of lesions (z coordinate) from the nipple can be determined from either the lateral or craniocaudal mammogram.

To secure its placement the needle is inserted to its full extent, even if it extends beyond the z coordinate.

The point of insertion is marked on the patient's skin with a ballpoint pen and the area is then cleansed with alcohol.

In our experience we used Omer Mammalok Plus Breast Needle Wire Localizer, working together with the radiologists of our department.

The Omer Breast Needle consists of a two part stabilizer, 20 gauche needle and unique "J" wire.

Having selected the correct Homer Mammalok needle length according to the lesion depth, we retract the "J" curve into the needle. After prepping and draping, we insert the needle into the breast to the desired depth.

By pushing on the stabilizer, the wire advances into the breast until the stabilizer butts against the hub. This ensures formation of the "J" curve in the parenchyma.

Insertion of the marker precisely into the suspicious area is not necessary: mammography is repeated at once with the marker in position so that surgeon and radiologist can together determine the relation of the guide wire to the suspected lesion and plan the biopsy approach.

In our experience with fourteen patients the localizing procedure required less than 20 minutes and facilitated small, rapid and accurate biopsy, while always including the lesion within the biopsy specimen, upon x-ray control.

Anestesia time is shortened and breast disfigurement minimized.

Specimen radiographs are necessary to verify the removal of suspicious area. In the operating room, with the patient under general anesthesia a circumareolar incision is outlined, with its center in line with the needle.

The lesion along with a small amount of surrounding breast tissue is excised. The quantity of excised tissue never exceeded 25 grams. If the lesion described by mammography contains calcifications specimen radiography must be performed to ensure that they are contained in the biopsy specimen.

While the patient is still on the operating room table, the surgeon is informed by the radiologist of the x-ray results of the specimen.

If the calcifications are not all visible on specimen x-ray, he is advised to excise additional tissue, which is also radiographed.

DISCUSSION

A number techniques have been developed to aid in the biopsy of nonpalpable lesions.

Non invasive methods include simple extrapolation of areas on the mammogram to the actual breast and skin markers.

These methods are often unsatisfactory, particulary in pendulous breasts. The injection of dye and contrast media into the breast has been used successfully but the dispersion of these media, particulary within ducts, makes this procedure less precise than the needle method.

This tecnique differs from other needle localization methods in that only a single needle is used, the thin wire marker rather than the needle is left in the tissue and this marker is anchored in place by its hooked tip: the self-retaining feature is important to avoid displacement of the marker during subsequent mammograghy and preparation for surgery.

Nonpalpable cancers found in this manner appear to have a lower rate of axillary-lynphnode involvement and a lower case fatality rate than palpable breast cancers.

REFERENCES

1. Frank HA, Hall FM, Steer ML. (1976). Preoperative localization of nonpalpable breast lesions demonstrated by mammography. N Engl J Med 295:259-260.

2. Homer MJ. (1979). Percutaneous localization of breast lesions. J Can Assoc Radiol 30:238-241

3. Feig SA. (1983). Localization of clinically occult breast lesions. Radiol Clin North Am 21: 155-172.

4. Kopans DB, Swann CA. (1989). Preoperative imaging-guided needle placement and localization of clinically occult breast lesions. Am J Roentgenol 152: 1-9.

5. Homer MJ. (1983). Transsection of the localization hook wire during breast biopsy. Am J Roentgenol 141: 929-930.

6. Helvie MA, Ikeda DM, Adler DD. (1991). Localization and needle aspiration of breast lesions: complications in 370 cases. Am J Roentgenol 157:711-714.

7. Berger SM., Curcio BM. (1966).Mammographic localization of unsuspected breast cancer. Am J Roentgenol 96: 1046-1052.

8. Patton RB, Poznanski AK. Pathologic examination of specimens containing nonpalpable breast discovered by radiography. Am J Clin Pathol 46: 330-334;1966.

9. Curcio BM. (1970)Techinque for radiographic localization of nonpalpable breast tumors Radiol Technol 42: 155-160.

10. Stevens JM. (1971). Mammographically directed biopsy of nonpalpable breast lesions Arch Surg 102: 292-295.

Intra-operative ultrasound in non-palpable mammary lesions

A. Di Giorgio, L. Cersosimo, P. Arnone and A. Canavese

I Institute of Clinical Surgery, University of Rome "La Sapienza", Italy

INTRODUCTION

An increasing number of small nonpalpable breast lesions can now be detected for which is suitable (2, 4, 11, 12).
Excision is undoubtedly the most reliable method of biopsy in order to assure a correct diagnosis. Surgical excision entails significant disadvantages, especially in the localizing of the lesions, which require extremely accurate marking techniques and an immediate analysis of results by means of radiologic or histologic control of the specimens (5, 6, 1, 8, 7). The excision of such lesions can be quite difficult and laborious to perform and may result in the unnecessary removal of a large portion of the surrounding breast tissue (3).
On the basis of this premise, we have developed a simple and accurate excisional biopsy technique for nonpalpable nodes using an intraoperative sonographic technique in which the sterilized transducer of an ultrasound scanner is inserted directly into the breast through the surgical wound.

MATERIALS AND METHODS

An sterilizable high-resolution ultrasound scanner is used to obtain an accurate intraoperative localization of the lesion to be removed.
The transducer is sterilized with formaldehyde or Cydex.
The operation is performed with the aid of local anesthesia.
A periareolar incision is made 20-30 mm along the curve in the quadrant where the lesion has been localized.
A blunt dissection of the subcutaneous connective tissue from the glandular parenchyma is performed, thereby creating a pocket where the transducer may be inserted (Fig.: 1). The scanner aids in determining the depth of the lesion and selectively guides the surgeon towards the target zone. To facilitate imaging, the blunt dissected zone has been filled with a physiologically sterile solution which replaces the gel normally used on the skin.
Once the site of the lesion in the glandular parenchyma has been localized, it is pulled forward with the help of Kocher forceps and very small retractors (Fig.: 2). This helps in delineating the zone of incision and aids in determining the depth needed to reach the lesion. It also aids in determining what modality of exeresis is to be used: enucleation of the lesion (in the case of fibroadenoma) or exeresis of a portion of the parenchyma (in the case of lesion whose borders are not

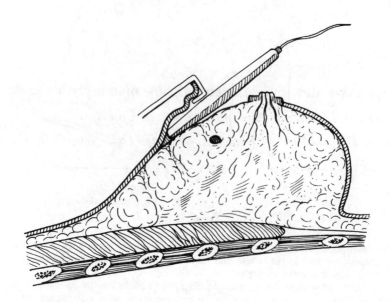

FIG. 1

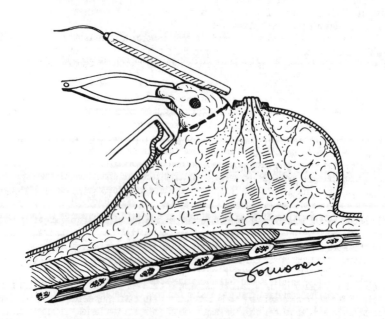

FIG. 2

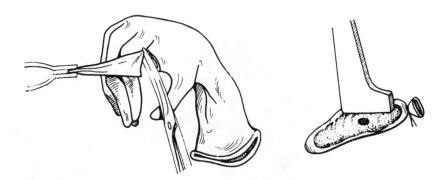

FIG. 3

well defined, such as neoplasm and fibrocystic mastopathies). When the specimen has been removed, a
further intraoperative check is run to make sure that exeresis has been complete and that no other
structures previously undetected are present.
Before being sent to pathologist for an immediate histologic examination, the specimen is scanned
with the ultrasound scanner in order to compare the post-operative images with the pre and intraoperative ultrasonograms. This will confirm whether or not the operation has been performed successfully. To facilitate this, the specimen may be placed in a finger of surgical glove filled with
physiological solution (Fig.: 3).
When the correct execution of the method has been confirmed, the mammary parenchyma, the subcutaneous tissue and the skin incision are then closed.

PATIENTS AND RESULTS

In this study conducted by the Special Service of Surgical Technology at the I Institute of Clinical Surgery of the University of Rome "La Sapienza" in 1993, 27 patients with nonpalpable breast
lesions underwent ultrasound-guided excisional biopsy (Table 1). The average age was 40.4, median
40 (range 17-68; S.D. 14.16). In 12 of the 27 patients, the lesion was found in the right breast
with localization in the upper outer quadrant (UOQ) in 58.3% of cases; in 15 patients with lesions
of the left breast, the UOQ was involved in 73.3% of cases.The pre-operative ultrasonographic findings showed a nodular hypoechogenic image in 17 patients (63.0%) and a hypoechogenic image with
hyperechogenic areas in 9 cases (33.3%). In one case found to be histologically neoplastic, the
mammographic screening revealed a suspicious neoplastic-like abnormality of 6mm while the ultrasonographic findings revealed only the presence of an architectural distortion of the parenchyma,
slightly hyperechogenic. The size of the lesion when measured with the scanner varied from a maximum of 16 mm to a minimum of 5 mm (average= 10.9 mm; median = 11 mm; S.D.= 2.97).The size of specimen removed varied from a maximum of 30 mm to a minimum of 6 mm with an average of 17.2 mm (median=
16 mm; S.D.= 5.6). (Fig.: 4). The total number of lesions encountered in 27 biopsies was 29, with a
maximum diameter of 16 mm and minimum of 2 mm (Fig.: 5) (average= 8.9 mm; median= 8 mm; S.D.=3.52).
Histologic examination of the specimen diagnosed 2 invasive ductal carcinomas (6.9%), 8 fibroadenomas (27.6%), 18 fibrocystic masthopathies with apocrine metaplasia (62.1%) and 1 case of atypical
ductal hyperplasia (3.4%). An ultrasound intraoperative scanning after the excision and immediate
post-operative examination confirmed that the lesion had been completely removed in all cases. The
re were no complications worthy of note except for three cases of subcutaneous seroma.
Later scarring proved to be cosmetically acceptable and in the follow-up six months later, findings
revealed nothing worthy of note.

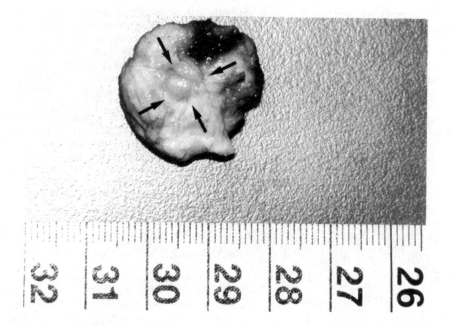

FIG. 4

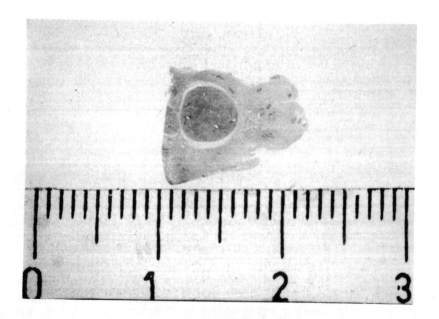

FIG. 5

DISCUSSION

The technique discussed here is original and in the literature only one author, Schwartz (10, 9) has reported using a similar technique in his description of a study concerning the biopsy of non-palpable breast nodules. However, Schwartz's methodology is not described in detail and the ultrasound transducer itself is not sterilized but inserted in a sterilized sheath filled with gel. In our case, instead, the transducer is sterilized and used directly and with greater manegeability thanks to the use of the physiological solution with which the wound and blunt dissected area are filled. The solution creates a liquid interface between the tissue and the transducer which is necessary in order to obtain a high resolution image.

The technique we are proposing here can be used exclusively in those cases in which the lesion can be localized by an ultrasound scanner. It is not applicable in cases of parenchymal abnormalities which can be identified only throuh mammographic screening. However, thanks to the availability of high resolution scanners on the market, the number of lesions which may be detected by radiographic means but which are undetectable through ultrasonography has been reduced. Clinical practice has shown that in many instances ultrasonography is able to detect abnormalities of pathological significance in the mammary parenchyma which were not revealed by mammographic screening. At the present state it may be sustained that only in the case of microcalcifications has mammography been shown to be superior to ultrasonography in the identification of pathological areas (13).

In this regard, however, our experience has shown that even though ultrasonography does not aid in identifying microcalcifications, it is useful in evaluating abnormalities in the tissue where the microcalcification is found.

The method we are proposing has the following advantages:

- it is extremely accurate in identifying the site of the abnormality. Since the skin and subcutaneous connective tissue no longer pose a barrier to the scanner, a high resolution image is obtained;
- it allows for greater precision in removing the mass as the surgeon is constantly guided by the scanner;
- the accuracy of the biopsy may checked immediately by examining the removed specimen with the scanner;
- the exeresis of a limited section of the breast parenchyma may be performed without the useless and sometimes harmful sacrifice of healthy breast tissue;
- when the transducer is inserted in the wound, it allows the surgeon to examine the state of the mammary gland immediately after the specimen has been removed;
- it is able to detect other lesions which were not previously apparent.

The procedure described above was used in 27 cases of patients with nonpalpable breast lesions. All patients underwent a mammographic screening as well as an ultrasonographic examination. In 24 patients, the radiological findings corresponded to the ultrasonographic findings, thus they were able to undergo the procedure described above. In three cases, the ultrasound scanner revealed abnormalities which did not show up in the mammographic findings.

The validity of this technique was clearly evident after the results were analysed. In all cases the abnormal area was removed with extreme accuracy. The analysis of the dimension of the lesion measured with the scanner showed an average of 10.9 mm and a median value of 11 mm. As we can see from these values, it was possible to perform biopsies of extremely small dimensions in that the average diameter of the biopsies was equal to 17.2 mm, with a median of 16 mm while the histologic dimensions of the lesions were found to be equal to 8.9 mm as an average value and 8 mm as a median value. Thus we have shown that through this procedure the exeresis of a limited area of the tissue may be performed. We have also shown that ultrasonography is reliable in the identifying of pathological or suspicious areas since the dimensions of the lesions measured with the scanner correspond significantly to the dimensions of the lesions when measured histologically.

In some cases, the lesions removed were found to be larger than 10 mm in diameter. These were also nonpalpable, both due to the large dimensions of the breast and (in 2 cases) to intracanalicular fibroadenomas whose consistency was similar to normal breast tissue and therefore nonpalpable.

In most cases these lesions were found to be benign fibroadenomas. In 2 cases carcinomas were found, one of 6 mm and one of 8 mm. In both cases the biopsy allowed for a complete removal of the tumor and in the histologic examination following the mastectomy, no residual tumor was found in the parenchyma.

All cases were performed in an out-patient setting with local anesthesia and patients were able to return to normal activities just a few hours after the operation. In all patients the operation was performed through a periareolar incision and in no case was draining necessary. Only in 3 cases was the appearance of serous secretion from the wound noted and this phenomenon regressed after proper medication. An excellent cosmetic effect was obtained.

The procedure we have proposed here merits further confirmation over a prolonged period of study and experimentation. To this end, the use of very small and more easily manageable transducers with more angles of aperture and higher resolution power would be of great benefit.

REFERENCES

1) Choucair, R.J., Holcomb, M.B., Mathews, R., Hughes, T.G.: Biopsy of nonpalpable breast lesions. The American Journal of Surgery, 1988, 156: 453-456.

2) Frank, H. A., Hall, F.M., Steer, M. L.. Preoperative localization of nonpalpable breast lesions demonstrated by mammography.
New Engl. J. Med, 1976, 295: 259-60.

3) Jacobsen, U., Karesen, R., Skaane, P., and Others. Out-patient surgical for nonpalpable breast lesions. Technique, results and consequences.
Acta Chir Scand., 1989, 155: 313-316.

4) Kopans, D.B., De Luca. S.: A modified needle-hookwire technique to simplify preoperative localization of occult breast lesions.
Radiology, 1980, 134: 781.

5) Lefor, A.T., Numann, P.J., Levinsohn. E. M.: Needle localization of occult breast lesions. The American Journal of Surgery, 1984, 148: 270-274.

6) Mahoney, L.: Intraoperative localization of occult breast tumours. The Canadian Journal of Surgery, 1985, 28:329-331.

7) Meyer, J. E., Kopans, D. B. Preoperative roentgenographically guided percutaneous localization of occult breast lesions, three year experience with 180 patients and description of a method.
Arch. Surg.,1982, 117: 65-68.

8) Papatestas, A. E., Hermann, D., Hermann, G., and Others. Surgery for nonpalpable brest lesions.
Arch. Surg.,1990, 125:399-402.

9) Schawartz, G. F., Goldberg, B. B., Rifkin, M. D. and D'Orazio, S. E.: Ultrasonography: an alternative to x-ray-guided needle localization of nonpalpable breast masses.
Surgery, 1988, 104: 870-873.

10) Schwartz, G. F., Goldberg, B. B., Rifkin, M. D. , D'Orazio, S. E.: Ultrasonographic localization of nonpalpable breast masses.
Ultrasound Med. Biol., 1988, 14 suppl.: 23-25,

11) Silverstone, Wyshak, G.: nonpalpable breast lesions: recommendations for biopsy based on suspicion of carcinoma at mammography.
Radiology, 1988, 167:353-358.

12) Symmonds, R. E., Jr, Roberts, J. W.: Management of nonpalpable breast abnormalities.
Ann. Surg., 1987, 520-528.

13) Weber, W. N., Sickles, E. A., Callen, P. W., Filly, R. A.: Nonpalpable breast lesion localization: limited efficacy of sonography.
Radiology, 1985, 155: 783-784.

A follicular cyst complicating tamoxifen therapy in a premenopausal breast cancer woman: a case report

L. Leo, A. Re, M. Tessarolo, R. Bellino, G. Gordini*, A. Venuti, M. Rosso**, T. Wierdis and A. Lanza

Department B of Gynecology and Obstetrics Institute, University of Torino, *Department of Pathology and **Department of Clinical Chemistry, S. Anna Hospital, Torino, Italy

INTRODUCTION

Tamoxifen citrate (TAM) is commonly employed as adjuvant therapy after primary surgery for invasive breast cancer for its favourable effect on the disease-free and overall survival with few side effects. In fact the patients who should quit taking TAM because of its side effects are only 2-4% (1). In addition, it is one of the drugs most commonly used to induce ovulation in infertile women.

This report describes a premenopausal woman who developed unilateral ovarian follicular cyst with adnexal torsion after receiving adjuvant tamoxifen therapy for 4-month. She had an increase in the blood estradiol concentration, while luteinizing hormone (LH) and follicle-stimulating hormone (FSH) corresponded to those normally observed immediately before ovulation. There may be a direct effect of TAM on ovary, without altered gonadotropins level, causing an increase on E2 secretion and block of the oestrogen receptors of the hypothalamic- pituitary axis (2).

The purpose of our observation is to report the clinical course of this patient with emphasis on her steroid blood profile.

CASE REPORT

A 49-year-old premenopausal woman with 2 pregnancies and deliveries underwent a modified radical mastectomy and axillary lymphadenectomy for a left lower inner quadrant infiltrating lobular breast carcinoma, stage I, with negative lymphnodes (0/24). Estrogen and progesterone receptors were positive.

803

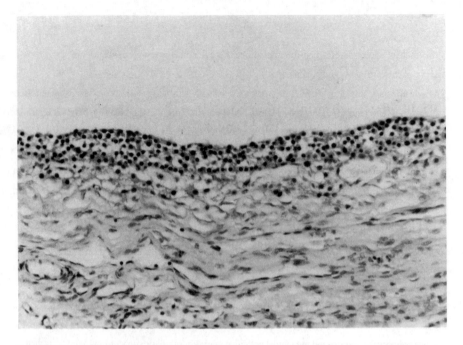

Figure 1   Follicular cyst with evident superficial layer of follicular cells

She started a low dose Tamoxifen citrate treatment, 10 mg three times a day, as adjuvant therapy on the 14th postoperative day.

After four months the patient developed severe intermittent lower abdominal pain. Her status on admission did not show atypical uterine bleeding and the uterus was normal in size while a tender left ovarian mass was palpable. Her abdomen was soft, painfull at palpation, more in the left than in the right side, accompanied by nausea without vomiting or diarrhea. The patient had a temperature of 37°C. Vaginal sonography confirmed the presence of a large left ovarian cyst approximately 6 cm x 3.5cm while the right ovary and uterus were normal.

Laboratory values revealed serum estradiol level (E2) of 785 pg/ml , progesterone of 2,19 ng/ml, CA125 of 8,6 IU/l and testosterone of 0,61 ng/ml while LH and FSH corresponded to those normally observed immediately before ovulation. Ten days before E2 was 783 pg/ml .

She underwent laparotomy which revealed two left ovarian cysts with a blue-black left salpinx. A bilateral salpingo-oophorectomy and pelvic washing were performed.

By day 10th after surgery E2 decreased markedly until stabilizing on 10 pg/ml, while the gonadotropins increased.

Pathological findings revealed two follicular cysts in the left ovary (4x4cm and 2x2,9cm) with a granulosa cells inner layer and an outer luteinized teca interna layer. The cysts contained pale yellow serum. An associated corpus luteum was also found. (Fig.1).

The patient has continued taking tamoxifen at the same dosage since surgery with no further complication.

DISCUSSION

Tamoxifen is one of several non-steroidal triphenylethylene derivates all of which are non-steroidal and are partial estrogen agonist/antagonist (3).

The side effects of this drug are few and women who should quit taking TAM because of its side effects are only 2-4%; the most frequent adverse reaction are hot flushes, nausea, vomiting, vaginal bleeding, and skin rushes. However, they are not well described in premenopausal women.

TAM is structurally similar to clomiphene and equivalent to this for induction of ovulation (4).

If it is easy to find ovarian enlargement in patients treated with TAM as ovulation inducer because of an increase in secretion of the pituitary gonadotrophs, in the present premenopausal patient TAM did not increase FSH and LH secretion, but caused a marked increase of E2 level and the development of a large ovarian follicular cyst.

Some authors have observed that FSH and LH remain unchanged during of TAM treatment in premenopausal patients, while in some cases serum estradiol levels might elevate to as high as 2500 pg/ml (5,6,7). Chronic high level of serum E2 normally decreases FSH and LH incretion.

These observations suggest that TAM may act directly on the ovaries to increase steroidogenesis with an excessive proliferation of the granulosa cells that causes abnormal elevation of E2 level so the balance between its agonist and antagonist activities maintain pituitary gonadotropin incretions at near normal levels.

An explaination of this could be related with an increased production of the growth-factor TGF-β, an important mediator of TAM action, in ovarian cells; it might strengthen FSH action on aromatase of granulosa cells with a metabolic impulse, without interfering on the proliferation of the granulosa cells, resulting in a follicular liquid formation (8,9,10).

This hormonal status does not appear to interfer with the antiproliferative action of TAM on breast cancer, nevertheless it is not clear why only few patients on TAM could develop ovarian cyst (11).

These findings confirm that tamoxifen has mild estrogenic activity, but its carcinogenic potential on the genital tract is low and the beneficial effects as an adjuvant therapy for breast cancer outweigh its theoretical risks.

Shulman et al. observed in two premenopausal patients that serum estrogen decreased to postmenopausal concentrations and ovarian cysts completely resolved during and following simultaneous treatment with TAM and gonadotropin-releasing hormone agonist (12).

The patients treated with TAM might costitute a new "risk" group so we must prevent this iatrogenic side effect with regular clinical examinations, blood analysis, and with a correct instrumental surveillance of the genital tract of patients taking TAM for adjuvant therapy and for chemo-prevention of breast cancer (13).

Acknowledgment: the authors thank Pharmacia / Farmitalia Carlo Erba

REFERENCES

1. Leo, L.,Lanza, A.,Re, A.,Tessarolo, M.,Bellino, R.,Lauricella, A.,Wierdis, T. (1994). Leiomyomas in patients receiving Tamoxifen. *Clin. Exp. Obst. Gyn.*,**2**,94-98

2. Sunderland, M.C., Osborne, C.K.(1991). Tamoxifen in premenopausal patients with metastatic breast cancer: a review. *J.Clin.Oncol.*,**9**,1283-1297

3. Sunderland, R.L., Jordan, V.C.(1981). Non-steirodal antioestrogens. Sydney,Academic Press

4. Cole, M.B.,Jones, C.T.A.,Todd, I.D.H. (1985). A new anti-oestrogenic agent in the late breast cancer: an early clinical approach of ICI 1464 74. *Brit.J.Cancer*,**25**,237-238

5. Ravdin, P.M.,Fritz, N.F.,Tormey, D.C.,Jordan, V.C.(1988). Endocrine status of premenopausal node positive breast cancer patient following adjuvant chemotherapy and long term tamoxifen. *Cancer Res.*, **48**,1026-1029

6. Jordan, V.C.,Fritz, N.F., Langan-Fashey, S.,Thompson, M.,Tormey, D.C.(1991). Alteration of endocrine parameters in premenopausal women with breast cancer during long term adjuvant tamoxifen therapy. *J.Natl.Cancer Inst.*,**83**,1488-1491

7. Manni, A., Pearson, O.H.(1980). Antiestrogen-induced remission in premenopausal women with stage IV breast cancer:effects on ovarian function.*Cancer Treat.Rep.*,**64**,779-785

8. Re, A.,Wierdis, T.,Tessarolo, M.,Leo, L.,Bellino, R.,Lauricella, A.,Lanza, A.(1994). Two cases of ovarian cysts in postmenopausal patient under antiestrogen treatment.*Clin. Exp. Obst. Gyn.*,**4**,221-224

9. Terada, S.,Uchide, K.,Suzuki, N.,Akasofu, K.(1993). A follicular cyst during tamoxifen therapy in premenopausal breast cancer woman. *Gynecol. Obstet. Invest.*,**35**,62-64

10.Neven, P., Shepherd, J.H. Lowe, D.G. (1993). Tamoxifen and gynaecologist. *Brit. J. Obstet. Gynaec.*,**100**,893-897

11.Wolf, D.M., Jordan, C.V. (1992). Gynecologic complications associated with long-term adjuvant tamoxifen therapy for breast cancer. *Gynec.Oncol.*, **45**,118-128

12.Shulman, A., Cohen, I., Altaras, M.M., Maymon, R., Ben-Nun, I., Tepper, R., Beyth, Y. (1994). Ovarian cyst formation in two pre-menopausal patients treated with tamoxifen for breast cancer. *Hum. Reprod.*, **9(8)**, 1427-9

13.Lanza, A., Alba, E., Re, A., Tessarolo, M., Leo, L., Bellino, R., Lauricella, A., Wierdis T. (1994). Endometrial carinoma in breast cancer patients treated with tamoxifen. *Eur.J.Gynaec.Oncol.*, **6**, 455-9

Oncogenes and ovarian cancer

M. Marzola, F. Morali*, G. Balconi*, M.G. Cantù, S. Rota and C. Mangioni

Ospedale S. Gerardo, Monza, University of Milan and *Istituto di Ricerche Farmacologiche M. Negri, Milan, Italy

Recent advances in cancer research have led to a greater understanding of the involvement of specific genes in the development and progression of cancer. Molecular studies have largerly focused on oncogenes and tumor suppressor genes. Proto-oncogenes (the normal genes relates to oncogenes) encode for proteins that play positive effector roles in cell growth, while tumor suppressor genes encode for proteins that exert inhibitory effects on cell growth. Mutations of proto-oncogenes increase their normal functions and enhance cellular proliferations. These mutations result in a dominant phenotype. Because mutations or allelic loss of tumor suppressor genes abrogate their normal inhibitory effects, the net result is also an enhanced cellular proliferation. Mutations or loss of tumor suppressor genes result in a recessive phenotype. To date, more than 50 oncogenes and tumor suppressor genes have been identified and, for some tumors (colorectal cancer, thyroid cancer), a molecular model of the multistep process of cancer development and progression has been proposed. However relatively little is known on the oncogenes involved in ovarian cancer. Several investigators have reported a high frequency of loss of heterozigosity on chromosomes 3p, 6, 11p and 17q and p, suggesting the presence of tumor suppressor genes important in ovarian tumorigenesis on these chromosomes. As regards genes HER-2/Neu (erb B-2), c-myc oncogenes and p53 tumor suppressor gene have been investigated in this neoplasm. HER-2/Neu oncogene, related to the EGF receptor, has a not well established role in the cell growth regulation. HER-2/Nen protein, p 185, is reported to be overexpressed in approximately 20-30% of advanced ovarian cancer, due to gene amplification or overexpression. The c-myc oncogene encodes for a protein that binds to regulatory elements in DNA. Growing cells exhibit increased amount of nuclear c-myc protein. Amplification of

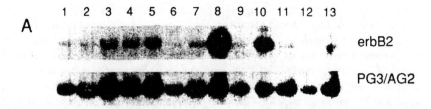

A

Lane 8 clearly indicates the amplification of ERB B-2 of the positive
case.
DNA from the SK Br 3 cell line was loaded in lane 10 as positive
control.
The other lanes correspond to DNA from other tumor biopsies or from
normal lymphocytes (lane 1, 7, 11) showing a similar intensity
corresponding to one copy of the ERB B-2 gene.

this gene has been observed in 33% of ovarian carcinomas. The p53
tumor suppressor gene is located on the short arm of chromosome 17 and
plays an inhibitory role on cell proliferation. Loss of p53 activity
can result from two events, allelic deletion or point ¬mutation
resulting in a non-functional protein that accumulate and can be
detected by unimmunostaining tecniques in 50-70% of advanced ovarian
carcinomas. Because p53 protein is found in high percentage only in
advanced stages probably it is involved in the late steps of cancer
progression. Recently several studies investigated the effects of
oncogenes and tumor suppressor genes on prognosis but results are
conflicting. The aim of our study was to investigate the frequency of
amplification and overexpression of erb B-2 and c-myc in highly
purified ovarian cancer cells deriving from surgical samples and to
analyze the relationship between these events and prognosis. Ovarian
cancer cells were freed from stroma by a previously assessed tecnique
based on enzymatic digestion and filtrations, in order to avoid bias
of the analysis due to the presence of other cell populations. DNA was
analysed by the Southern blot tecnique in 75 samples from 62 patients
who underwent first look laparotomy for ovarian cancer (50 primary
tumors, 2 of which were borderline, 20 metastases and 5 ascitic
fluids). The SK Br 3 cell line was used as a positive control for the
amplification and overexpression of erb B-2. Amplification of
Her-2/Neu was found only in one case (Fig. 1). Histological sections
of 65 samples were tested using the immunoperoxidase tecnique to
define the overexpression of p185. Staining was positive in 12 cases
(18.5%). No correlation was found between p185 positivity and
pathological and clinical features or theraputic outcome: the analysis
of 51 cases evaluable for the response to chemotherapy, assessed by a
second look laparotomy, revealed p185 positivity in 25% of the
patients with a complete response, in 13% of those with a partial
response and in 28% of non responders. On the same filters (from 75

specimens) on which erb B-2 amplification was tested, we analysed also m—myc amplification. Amplification was found in 20 specimens from 14 patients. From these 20 positive cases, 12 were also evaluable for mRNA. Overexpression of c-myc was also seen in 3 further cases in which DNA was not amplified. At present our project is to assess the specific role of p53 by analysing in a retrospective study, a large number of ovarian cancer paraffin embedded specimens aiming at defining its prognostic significance and the involvement in the progression of advanced ovarian carcinoma.

REFERENCES

1) Phillips N, Ziegler M et al. Allelic loss on chromosome 17 in human ovarian cancer. Int. J. Cancer 1993, 54: 85-91.

2) Slamon DJ, Godolphin W, Jones LA et al. Studies of the HER-2/Nen proto—oncogene in human breast and ovarian cancer. Science 1989, 244: 707-712.

3) Morali F, Cattabeni M et al. Overexpression of p185 is not related to erb B-2 amplification in ovarian cancer. Ann. of Oncol. 1993, 4: 775+779.

4) Hartman LC, Podratz KC et al. Prognostic significance of p53 immunostaining in epithelial ovarian cancer. J. Clin. Oncol. 1994, 12: 64-69.

5) Borsari S, Viale G et al. p53 accumulation in ovarian carcinomas and its prognostic implications. Hum. Pathol. 1993, 24: 1175-1178.

Cytokines in ovarian cancer

A. Gadducci, M. Ferdeghini, O. Gagetti, C. Prontera*, A. Bonuccelli,
V. Facchini, R. Bianchi* and A.R. Genazzani*

Department of Gynecology and Obstetrics and **Institute of Nuclear Medicine,
University of Pisa, Italy

Cytokines are low molecular weight peptide cell regulatory
factors able to display several biological activities. As
far as ovarian cancer is concerned, constitutive production of some cytokines, such as Interleukin-6 (IL-6),
Macrophage-Colony Stimulating Factor (M-CSF) and Tumor
Necrosis Factor (TNF) by human ovarian cancer cell lines
or tissues has been demonstrated (1-4). Conversely, normal
ovarian surface epithelium does not express mRNA or protein for IL-6, M-CSF, or TNF (4). Dysregulated cytokine
production could occur during the transformation from
normal to malignant epithelium. Cytokines and cytokine
receptors are also released by tumor-infiltrating macrophages and lymphocytes. Whereas an abnormal endogenous
production of some cytokines may lead to an autocrine or
paracrine stimulation of tumor cells (4), others cytokines
can directly or indirectly inhibit neoplastic growth and
their recombinant forms can be used in cancer therapy (5).
While the biological role of cytokines in the pathogenesis of ovarian cancer is still controversial, the serum
assay of some cytokines or cytokine receptors may offer
useful information for the management of patients with
this tumor.
Elevated serum IL-6 levels have been detected in patients
with different malignancies including gynecological cancers (1,6-8). Berek et al. (1) found that the mean ($\pm$SD)
serum IL-6 concentrations were higher in 36 ovarian cancer
patients than in 12 controls (0.24 ± 0.04 vs 0.12 ± 0.03 U/ml,
p< 0.05). The mean values were related to the extent of
disease at the time of laparotomy. Serum IL-6 levels were
elevated (> 0.20 U/ml) in 18% of 22 ovarian cancer patients with serum CA125 <35 U/ml and in 86% of 14 patients
with serum CA125 >35 U/ml. Patients whose IL-6 levels at
the time of laparotomy were elevated survived a mean of
12.5 months compared with 27.2 months for those patients

with normal levels (p< 0.001). Moreover, serial IL-6 levels correlated with the clinical course of disease.

Scambia et al. (6) confirmed that ovarian cancer patients with low serum IL-6 values had a better median survival than those with elevated values. These Authors also found that patients unresponsive to chemotherapy had higher IL-6 levels when compared to responsive patients. Conversely, Plante et al. (7) reported that serum and ascites IL-6 levels did not correlate with survival, tumor stage, grade, residual disease after debulking surgery, and serum CA125 levels.

We measured the serum levels of soluble receptor for IL-6 (sIL-6R) in 59 patients with ovarian cancer and in 50 patients with benign ovarian masses, and found no difference in antigen values between the two groups (mean value $+SD = 29.2+12.4$ vs $31.4+10.2$ ng/ml, p= NS) (9). Moreover, in ovarian cancer patients no difference in sIL-6R levels was detected according to FIGO stage. Among patients with advanced tumor, preoperative serum sIL-6R levels were similar in the 17 patients who died of disease or were alive with clinically detectable disease and in the 7 patients who were alive without clinically detectable disease after 2 years from first surgery $(28.3+13.3$ vs $31.7+13.9$ ng/ml, p= NS) (10). The serum sIL-6R assay seems to have no value for the management of ovarian cancer patients.

M-CSF is a chemoattractant for monocytes which in turn can release several cytokines. Xu et al. (2) found that the mean $(+SD)$ serum M-CSF levels were 2.6-fold higher in 69 patients with clinically evident ovarian cancer than in 80 controls $(3.02+1.72$ vs $1.15+0.65$ ng/ml). Elevated M-CSF levels (> 2.5 ng/ml) were detected in 56% of 25 patients with clinically evident ovarian cancer and serum CA125 <35 U/ml, and in 31% of 29 patients with persistent disease at second-look and serum CA125 <35 U/ml.

We measured M-CSF levels in blood samples drawn from ovarian cancer patients at different times from first surgery. The mean $(+SD)$ M-CSF values were higher in the 76 samples from patients with clinical evidence of disease than in the 73 samples from patients without clinical evidence of disease $(2.8+2.1$ vs $1.8+1.9$ ng/ml, p= 0.002). The mean M-CSF levels before second-look laparotomy were similar in the 17 patients who had persistent disease and in the 9 patients who achieved the pathological complete response $(1.5+0.8$ vs $1.4+1.2$ ng/ml, p= NS).

Naylor et al. (3) detected expression of the gene for TNF in 71% of 63 biopsies from ovarian cancer. Differently from other tumors such as colorectal and breast cancer in which TNF was localized in infiltrating macrophages, in ovarian cancer TNF expression was confined predominantly to the neoplastic epithelial cells. Ovarian carcinomatous tissues were also found to contain receptors for TNF (TNF-R). Both TNF and soluble TNF-R (55 and 75 kDa sTNF-R) have been detected in serum and ascites of ovarian cancer patients (3,11).

Grosen et al. (11) noted that the serum levels of 55 and 75 kDa sTNF-R were significantly higher in 79 patients with ovarian, endometrial and cervical cancer compared to 16 controls. Moreover, these authors reported that among ovarian cancer patients the levels of both receptors were significantly higher in patients with active disease than in those without clinical evidence of active disease.

We recently assessed the preoperative serum levels of TNF, sTNF-R, and soluble CD14 (sCD14, monocyte-derived glyco-protein) in 66 patients with ovarian cancer and 59 patients with benign ovarian masses as controls (data in press). The mean ($\pm$SD) values of these antigens were significantly higher in the former patients (TNF= 12.8$\pm$10.3 vs 7.6$\pm$5.6 pg/ml, p= 0.001; 55 kDa sTNF-R= 3.6$\pm$ 1.8 vs 2.0$\pm$0.6 ng/ml, p< 0.0001; 75 kDa sTNF-R= 16.4$\pm$12.3 vs 11.5$\pm$11.0 ng/ml, p= 0.022; sCD14= 5.7$\pm$1.8 vs 3.7$\pm$1.3 ug/ml, p< 0.0001). Preoperative TNF levels did not correlate with FIGO stage, histologic grade, and residual disease after first surgery. 55 kDa sTNF-R levels were higher in stage III-IV than in stage I disease (p< 0.0001). Among patients with advanced malignancy, preoperative 55 kDa sTNF-R concentrations correlated with stage (IV vs III, p= 0.008) but not with histologic grade or residual disease after first surgery. 75 kDa sTNF-R levels were similar in stage III-IV and in stage I disease. Among patients with advanced malignancy, preoperative 75 kDa sTNF-R levels correlated with FIGO stage (IV vs III, p=0.01) but not with histologic grade or tumor residuum. sCD14 concentrations were higher in stage III-IV than in stage I disease (p=0.005). Among patients with advanced malignancy, sCD14 levels correlated with none of the common prognostic variables. We examined in more detail 24 patients with stage III-IV ovarian cancer, who had received six cycles of chemotherapy with cisplatin- or carboplatin-based regimens. After two years from first surgery, 17 patients had died of disease or were alive with clinical evidence of disease (group A), while the other 7 patients were alive without clinical evidence of disease (group B). Preoperative serum levels of 55 and 75 kDa sTNF-R were higher in group A than in group B (p= 0.03 and p<0.0001, respectively). Conversely, TNF and sCD14 levels were similar in the two groups. TNF, 55 and 75 kDa sTNF-R, and sCD14 levels were also measured in several blood samples drawn from these 24 patients at different times from first surgery. 55 and 75 kDa sTNF-R levels were higher in the samples collected from patients with clinical evidence of disease than in those from patients without clinical evidence of disease (p= 0.004 and p= 0.029, respectively). Conversely, TNF and sCD14 levels were not significantly different in the two groups. According to the present data, the measurement of serum TNF and sCD14 seems to be of no clinical value for the management of patients with ovarian cancer. Conversely, the assay of serum 55 and 75kDa sTNF-R might have a potential clinical relevance for both prognostic purposes and assessment of disease status. As suggested by Grosen et al. (11), the soluble receptors for TNF might have an immunoregulatory role either on TNF or other cytokines and immune cells, or they might exert a protective effect against the tumor-destructive activity of TNF.

Interleukin-2 (IL-2) is a cytokine produced by T-helper lymphocytes, which promotes the growth of T-lymphocytes by interaction with a specific cell surface receptor. Activated T-lymphocytes release in the blood a soluble form of IL-2 receptor (sIL-2R). Elevated serum sIL-2R levels have been detected in patients with different malignancies (12).

We measured the preoperative serum sIL-2 levels in 47 patients with ovarian cancer and 113 patients with benign ovarian disease undergoing laparotomy (13). The mean ($\pm$SD) values of serum sIL-2R were higher in the former patients (227+219 vs 37+50 U/ml, p< 0.0001), and correlated with FIGO stage ($\overline{\text{III}}$-IV vs I-II, p= 0.048). Among patients with advanced malignancy, preoperative sIL-2R levels were higher in patients who developed progressive disease than in those who were progression-free (p= 0.02) after a median follow-up time of 18 months. Serial CA 125 levels correlated better than sIL-2R levels with the clinical course of disease. Therefore serum sIL-2R assay seems to be of limited value in monitoring patients with ovarian cancer. Our data showed that increased serum preoperative sIL-2R levels had a poor prognostic significance for patients with advanced ovarian cancer. Since sIL-2R is able to bind IL-2, elevated levels of this receptor could contribute to the bad prognosis by blocking IL-2-mediated cytotoxic activities of lymphocytes.

Multivariate analysis on a larger number of patients is needed to assess the prognostic relevance of serum sTNF-R and sIL-2R in ovarian cancer.

REFERENCES

1) Berek JS, Chung C, Kaldi K et al. Am. J. Obstet. Gynecol. 164, 1038, 1991.

2) Xu FJ, Ramakrishnan S, Daly L et al. Am. J. Obstet. Gynecol. 165, 1356, 1991.

3) Naylor MS, Stamp GWH, Foulkes WD et al. J. Clin. Invest. 91, 2194, 1993.

4) Malik S, Balkwill F. Br. J. Cancer 64, 617, 1991.

5) Fioretti P, Gadducci A. In: "Frontiers in Gynecologic and Obstetric Investigation" (Genazzani AR et al Eds), The Parthenon Publishing Group, Carnforth, New York 1993, p. 287.

6) Scambia G, Testa U, Benedetti Panici P. et al. Anticancer Res. 13, 1754, 1993 (Abstr. 105).

7) Plante M, Rubin SC, Wong GY et al. Cancer 73, 1882, 1994.

8) Ferdeghini M, Gadducci A, Prontera C et al. Anticancer Res. 14, 735, 1994.

9) Ferdeghini M, Gadducci A, Prontera C et al. In: "XXIInd Meeting ISOBM '94", Groningen, September 18-22, 1994, p. 196, abstr. O 12.3.

10) Gadducci A, Ferdeghini M, Prontera C et al. In: "XXIInd Meeting ISOBM '94", Groningen, September 18-22, 1994, p.203, abstr. P 12.5.

11) Grosen EA, Granger GA, Gatanaga M et al. Gynecol. Oncol. 50, 68, 1993.

12) Lissoni P, Barni S, Rovelli F et al. Eur. J. Cancer 26, 33, 1990.

13) Gadducci A, Ferdeghini M, Malagnino G et al. Gynecol. Oncol. 52, 386, 1994.

Serum CA 125 assay in the management of ovarian cancer

A. Gadducci, M. Ferdeghini*, C. Castellani, C. Annicchiarico*, A. Perutelli, V. Facchini, R. Bianchi* and A.R. Genazzani

Department of Gynecology and Obstetrics and *Institute of Nuclear Medicine, University of Pisa, Italy

CA 125 is an antigenic determinant on a high-molecular weight glycoprotein defined by a murine monoclonal antibody obtained against a serous ovarian carcinoma cell line (1). CA 125 has been found in tissue sections and serum samples from patients with epithelial ovarian cancer of all histologic types. However mucinous tumors espress the antigen less frequently than serous tumors.

As for discriminating a benign from a malignant ovarian mass, the literature reported that serum CA 125 assay had a sensitivity of 78%-100% and a specificity of 60-94% using the value of 35 U/ml as cut-off, and, respectively, a sensitivity of 50-93% and a specificity of 80-99% using 65 U/ml as cut-off (2-4). The combined evaluation of other tumor-associated antigens could be of clinical usefulness (3). In our experience the association of serum CA 125 (cut-off=65 U/ml) and CA 19.9 (cut-off= 40 U/ml) had a significantly higher sensitivity (93.2% vs 81.1%, p= 0.03) and a similar specificity (78.9% vs 86.0%, p= NS) when compared to serum CA 125 assay alone in the differential diagnosis of ovarian masses in patients older than 50 years (5).

Serum CA 125 assay can increase the diagnostic accuracy of clinical examination and ultrasound in the preoperative assessment of ovarian masses, expecially in postmenopausal women (6). Moreover, in our experience the combined evaluation of abdominal ultrasound, CA 125, CA 19-9 or TAG-72 had a significantly higher sensitivity and a not significantly different specificity when compared to ultrasound alone in postmenopausal women (7).

An International multicentric study (8) on 228 patients showed that the individual accuracy of pelvic examination, transvaginal ultrasound, and serum CA 125 assay (cut-off = 35 U/ml) in discriminating a benign from a malignant pelvic mass was quite the same (76%, 74%, and 77%, respec-

817

tively). However it is worth noting that no cancer was found in patients in whom all three methods were negative. An Italian multicentric study (9) on 290 patients undergoing surgery for a postmenopausal pelvic mass revealed that the diagnostic accuracy of serum CA 125 (cut-off = 65 U/ml) was 83%, of abdominal ultrasound was 81%, and of serum CA 125 plus ultrasound was 94%. Therefore the association of ultrasound plus serum CA 125 might support the clinical judgement and identify a significant percentage of those women who are most likely to benefit from prompt intervention.

Among patients with histologically proven ovarian cancer, changes in CA 125 levels have been found to correlate with the clinical course of disease in about 90% of instances (1,10). Elevated CA 125 levels at the time of second-look surgery are quite always predictive of persistent disease, while normal antigen concentrations can be associated with both positive and negative second-look findings. CA 125 levels raise before the clinical detection of recurrence in about 70-94% of cases, with a median lead time of 3-4 months (10-12). In our experience, serum CA 125 correlated with disease course better than serum CA19-9, TAG-72, CA 15-3, and tumor-associated trypsin inhibitor (TATI) (10). Moreover, serum CA 125 usually raised earlier or in a higher percentage of cases than the other antigens before the diagnosis of neoplastic progression by noninvasive techniques. Therefore in patients with positive CA 125 assay at diagnosis, the combined evaluation of these other antigens did not give information better than that of CA 125 assay alone. Conversely, the determination of the other antigens could be of great clinical usefulness in patients with negative CA 125 assay.

Recently some authors investigated the relationship among the decline of CA 125 levels during early chemotherapy, second-look findings and survival of ovarian cancer patients. Several parameters of evaluation of serum CA 125 assay during treatment have been suggested. Patients with serum CA 125 <35 U/ml three months after the start of chemotherapy have a good chance to achieve a pathological complete response, while persistent disease after the end of treatment is quite always detected in patients with serum three-month CA 125 >35 U/ml (10,13). Sevelda et al. (14) found that serum CA 125 three months after surgery was an independent prognostic variable for survival in 132 patients with stage I-IV ovarian cancer. Fayers et al. (15) observed that the absolute value of serum CA 125 before the third cycle of chemotherapy was the single most important factor for predicting progression at 12 months in a series of 248 patients with stage I-IV ovarian cancer.

The dynamics of serum CA 125 half-life are complex: patients with residual neoplastic cells continue to secrete CA 125 after surgery, and laparotomy alone can increase antigen levels even when no cancer is present (16,17). The decline of serum CA 125 in effectively

treated ovarian cancer patients follows the exponential
regression model described by Buller's equation (18).
Van der Burg et al. (19) calculated serum CA 125 half-life
in 37 patients with stage I-IV ovarian cancer, and detected that patients with a half-life $\geq$ 20 days had a 3.2
times as high progression rate (p = 0.01) and a significantly shorter median time to progression (11 months vs
43 months) when compared to patients with a half-life <20
days. Several other papers confirmed the prognostic relevance of serum CA125 half-life (20-22). In a series of 51
women with stage I-IV ovarian cancer, Rosman et al. (22)
found that stage, residual disease, minimum CA 125 value,
and CA 125 half-life individually were predictive of
persistent disease or recurrence within 3 years of diagnosis with sensitivities of 97%, 70%, 34%, and 49%, respectively, and specificities of 33%, 83%, 100%, and 83%,
respectively. A patient with $\leq$1 cm residual disease, a
CA 125 half-life < 12 days, and the minimum level of
CA 125 < 35 U/ml had a chance of 100%, 93% and 85% of
remaining disease-free during the first year, the
first 2 years, and the first 3 years after diagnosis,
respectively.
An Italian multicentric study has recently assessed the
prognostic relevance of serum CA 125 half-life during
early chemotherapy in 225 advanced ovarian cancer patients
treated with platinum-based chemotherapy at the
Departments of Gynecology and Obstetrics of the University
of Pisa, Torino, Monza , Brescia and Padova (Gadducci et
al. Gynecol. Oncol. in press) . In agreement with the
literature, this study found that serum CA 125 half-life
(cut-off= 25 days) was an independent prognostic variable
for the chance of achieving a pathological complete response and survival.
An EORTC phase III trial comparing a combination of taxol-
platinum versus a combination of cyclophosphamide-platinum
in advanced ovarian cancer patients is currently ongoing.
An important aspect of the trial will be the prospective
confirmation that CA 125 half-life during chemotherapy is
a strong predictor of survival, whether the patient has or
has not received taxol in her front-line regimen.

REFERENCES

1) Jacobs I, Bast RC Jr. Hum. Reprod. 4, 1-12, 1989.

2) Malkasian GD jr, Knapp RC, Lavin PT, et al. Am. J.
Obstet. Gynecol. 159, 341-346, 1988.

3) Soper JT, Hunter VJ, Daly L, et al. Obstet. Gynecol.
75, 249-254, 1990.

4) Di-Xia C, Schwartz PE, Xinguo L, Zhan Y. Obstet. Gynecol. 72, 23-27, 1988.

5) Gadducci A, Ferdeghini M, Prontera C, et al. Gynecol. Oncol. 44, 147-154, 1992.

6) Finkler NJ, Benacerraf B, Lavin PT et al. Obstet. Gynecol. 72, 659-664, 1988.

7) Gadducci A, Capriello P, Ferdeghini M et al. Cancer J. 4, 249-253, 1991.

8) Schutter EMJ, Kenemans P, Sohn C, et al. Cancer 74, 1398-1406, 1994.

9) Maggino T, Gadducci A, D' Addario V et al. Gynecol. Oncol. 54, 117-123, 1994.

10) Fioretti P, Gadducci A, Ferdeghini M et al. Gynecol. Oncol. 44, 155-169, 1992.

11) Niloff JM, Knapp RC, Lavin PT et al. Am. J. Obstet. Gynecol. 155, 56-60, 1986.

12) Schilthuis MS, Aalders JG, Bouma J et al. Br. J. Obstet. Gynaecol. 94, 202-207, 1987.

13) Lavin PT, Knapp RC, Malkasian G, et al. Obstet. Gynecol. 69, 223-227, 1987.

14) Sevelda P, Schemper M, Spona J. Am. J. Obstet. Gynecol. 161, 1213-1216, 1989.

15) Fayers PM, Rustin G, Wood R, et al. Int. J. Gynecol. Cancer 3, 285-292, 1993.

16) Brand E, Lidor Y. Obstet. Gynecol. 81, 29-32, 1993.

17) Van der Zee AGJ, Duk JM, Aalders JG, et al. Br. J. Obstet. Gynaecol. 97, 934-938, 1990.

18) Buller RE, Berman ML, Bloss JD, et al. Am. J. Obstet. Gynecol. 165, 360-367, 1990.

19) van der Burg MEL, Lammes FB, van Putten WLJ, Stoter G. Gynecol. Oncol. 30, 307-312, 1988.

20) Hogberg T, Kagedal B. Acta Obstet. Gynecol. Scand. 69, 423-429, 1990.

21) Willemse PH, Aalders JG, de Bruyn HW, et al. Eur. J. Cancer 27, 993-995, 1991.

22) Rosman M, Hayden CL, Thiel RP, et al. Cancer 74, 1323-1328, 1994.

Immunoscintigraphy in ovarian cancer

M. Ferdeghini, A. Gadducci*, G. Boni, F. Matteucci, C.R. Bellina, M. Grosso, B. Prato*, V. Facchini*, A.R. Genazzani* and R. Bianchi

Institute of Nuclear Medicine and *Department of Gynecology and Obstetrics, University of Pisa, Italy

Serum CA125 assay using monoclonal antibodies represents an useful biochemical tool for differentiating malignant from benign ovarian masses and for monitoring the disease course in patients with ovarian cancer (1,2). Conversely, the clinical usefulness of the in vivo administration of radiolabeled monoclonal antibodies for tumor imaging is still under evaluation.

Several radioisotope-labeled monoclonal antibodies have been tested for radioimmunodetection of ovarian cancer, such as HMFG1, OC125, B72.3, and MOv18 (3,4). The suitability of a radioisotope depends on its half-life (T1/2) and on the mode and physical properties of its decay (3,5). Most studies have employed isotopes of iodine (131-I, 123-I), Indium-111 (111-In) and Technetium-99m (99mTc). 131-I and 123-I have T1/2 of 8 days and 13 hours, respectively, and a gamma emission energy of 364 and 159 KeV, respectively. Iodine isotopes can be directly linked to monoclonal antibodies. 131-I is not optimal for imaging, because of its physical properties and its beta emission which can cause local tissue destruction. 123-I has an appropriate gamma energy but its short T1/2 makes it very difficult to employ in clinical practice. When iodine-labeled monoclonal antibodies are used, the thyroid gland must be blocked with iodine. 111-In has T1/2 of 67 hours and is characterized by two peaks of gamma emission energy (173 and 247 KeV, respectively). However 111-In is aspecifically uptaken by liver, spleen, and kidneys. This isotope can be attached to monoclonal antibodies by an indirect technique using a chelating group. 99mTc is a good radioisotope for imaging because of its physical properties (gamma energy emission = 140 Kev, T1/2 = 6 hours). Labeling techniques with this isotope consist of either direct labeling of endogenous sulphydryl groups on monoclonal antibodies or indirect labeling by conjugation of a pre-

formed 99mTc-chelate (6).
The amount of injected monoclonal antibodies which actually binds to tumor tissues depends on several pharmacological and biological factors, but in any case it is very low
($\leq$ 0.005% per gram/tissue) (7). In order to increase tumor
uptake of monoclonal antibodies, some authors are investigating methods for increasing tumor blood flow and
vascular permeability (8). These methods are based on
either physical procedures, such as hyperthermia, or
drugs, such as alpha-adrenergic agonists and beta-adrener-
gic antagonists.
Immunoscintigraphy is a safe procedure (9). Only few anap-
hylactic-type reactions have been reported in the literature. However the development of human anti-mouse antibodies can occur in 25%-68% of the patients and can increase
after multiple administrations. Human anti-mouse antibodies can cause false-positive CA125 values in routine
serum radioimmunometric assays (10), and moreover they can
alter the clearance and biodistribution of monoclonal
antibodies upon readministration and affect the quality
of the image (11). The administration of lower monoclonal
antibody doses, as well as the use of monoclonal antibody
fragments or mouse-human chimeric monoclonal antibodies or
further humanized monoclonal antibodies or totally human
monoclonal antibodies might reduce the production of human
anti-mouse antibodies (8,9).
Papers published on immunoscintigraphy in ovarian cancer
generally include few patients (12-22). The smallest
lesions detected by this method range from 1.5 to 2 cm.
The overall sensitivity of immunoscintigraphy in the
detection of recurrences is about 60-80% (13,17). In the
series of Landoni et al. (23), who employed 131-I labeled
OC125, the association of immunoscintigraphy and CT scan
revealed a greater number of recurrences than each technique alone. However, immunoscintigraphy seems to be of
limited value in detecting subclinical residual disease in
patients with normal CA125 levels after first-line chemotherapy (24). Crippa et al. (16) reported that the sensitivity of immunoscintigraphy performed with 131-I labeled
OC125 was 50% in a group of 13 patients undergoing second-
look surgery.
Our preliminary experience on radioimmunodetection of
ovarian cancer includes 23 patients who underwent immunoscintigraphy before second-look laparotomy (n.6) or
before surgery performed for suspected recurrent disease
(n.17). At that time, serum CA 125 levels were greater
than 35 U/ml in 1 of the former 6 patients and in 14 of
the latter 17 patients. At diagnosis, all patients had
FIGO stage III-IV disease. Histologically, 16 carcinomas
were serous, 3 undifferentiated, 2 endometriod and 2
mucinous.
Different radiolabeled monoclonal antibodies were used:
111-In OC125 (111 MBq) that recognizes CA 125 antigen
(6 patients), 131-I MOv18 (111-185 MBq) (6 patients) and
99mTc MOv18 (555-740 MBq) (11 patients). MOv18 is a G1 K

isotype immunoglobulin recognizing a 38 kD glycoprotein (a folate binding protein) expressed on the cell membrane of about 90% of non mucinous ovarian carcinomas (4).

After intravenous administration of the radiolabeled monoclonal antibodies, immunoscintigraphy was performed using wide field gamma-cameras (General Electric Starcam 3000/XC and XRT). Whole body and regional abdomen and pelvis planar images were acquired at 6-20 hours (99mTc MOv18), 48-72-96 hours (111-In OC125), and up to 120 hours (131-I MOv18). Moreover, single photon emission computed tomography (SPECT) images (64 images/360, 64x64 matrix, total time = 30-60 minutes) of the abdomen and pelvis were obtained at 6-20 hours (99mTc MOV18) and 48-72 hours (111-In OC125). Images were reviewed and interpreted by two nuclear medicine physicians. Planar and SPECT (transaxial, coronal, and sagittal) images obtained at different times were compared to detect persistent uptake areas corresponding to tumor lesions. Furthermore, in doubtful cases, a scintigraphic landmarking of organs with aspecific distribution of the radiopharmaceutical (bone, kidneys, bladder, and liver) and the estimate of temporal variation of the target-background uptake ratio were sometimes used.

Immunoscintigraphy and CT scan data were compared with surgical findings.

The surgical exploration detected histologically proven tumor in pelvis in 2 patients, in abdomen in 4 patients, and both in pelvis and abdomen in 14 patients.

The table shows the diagnostic reliability of the two methods in the detection of persistent or recurrent ovarian cancer.

DIAGNOSTIC RELIABILITY OF IMMUNOSCINTIGRAPHY (IS) AND CT SCAN IN THE DETECTION OF PERSISTENT OR RECURRENT OVARIAN CANCER

- PELVIC LESIONS	IS	CT	IS or CT
SENSITIVITY	10/16 (63%)	11/16 (69%)	13/16 (81%)
SPECIFICITY	7/7	7/7	7/7
DIAGNOSTIC ACCURACY	17/23 (74%)	18/23 (78%)	20/23(87%)
- ABDOMINAL LESIONS	IS	CT	IS or CT
SENSITIVITY	8/18 (44%)	10/18(56%)	13/18 (72%)
SPECIFICITY	5/5	5/5	5/5
DIAGNOSTIC ACCURACY	13/23 (57%)	15/23 (65%)	18/23(78%)

The diagnostic accuracy of immunoscintigraphy was better for pelvic than for abdominal lesions. This was partly due to an aspecific hepato-splenic uptake of In111-labeled monoclonal antibodies.
According to our preliminary experience, immunoscintigraphy seems to be less sensitive than CT scan for the detection of persistent or recurrent ovarian cancer. However, the association of the two techniques has a greater diagnostic reliability than CT alone for both pelvic and abdominal disease.

REFERENCES

1) Gadducci A, Ferdeghini M, Prontera C, et al. Gynecol. Oncol. 44, 147, 1992.

2) Fioretti P, Gadducci A, Ferdeghini M, et al. Gynecol. Oncol. 44, 155, 1992.

3) Rubin SC. Cancer 71, 1602, 1993.

4) Coney LR, Tomassetti A, Carayannopoulos L, et al. Cancer Res. 51, 6125, 1991.

5) Larson SM, Cheung NK, Leibel SA, et al. In: "Biologic therapy of cancer" (De Vita VTJ et al. Eds), Philadelphia: JB Lippincott 1991, p. 496.

6) Reilly RM. Nucl. Med. Commun. 14, 347, 1993.

7) Larson SM, Carrasquillo JA, Reynolds JC. Cancer Invest. 2, 353, 1984.

8) McKearn TJ. Cancer 71, 4302, 1993.

9) Delaloye AB, Delaloye B. Cancer 73 (3 Suppl), 900, 1994.

10) Muto MG, Lepisto EM, Van den Abbeele AD, et al. Am. J. Obstet. Gynecol. 161, 1206, 1989.

11) Reynolds JC, DelVecchio S, Sakahara H, et al. Nucl. Med. Biol. 16, 121, 1989.

12) Patensky N, Philipp K, Sevelda P, et al. Gynecol. Obstet. Invest. 24, 211, 1987.

13) Chatal JF, Fumoleau P, Saccavini JC, et al. J. Nucl. Med. 8, 1807, 1987

14) Fotiou S, Skarlos D, Tserkezoglou A, et al. Eur. J. Gynaecol. Oncol. 9, 304, 1988.

15) Brokelmann J, Bockisch A, Vogel J, et al. Arch. Gynecol. Obstet. 244, 193, 1989.

16) Crippa F, Presti M, Marini A, et al. Int. J. Biol. Markers 5, 103-108, 1990.

17) Peltier P, Wiharto k, Dutin JP, et al. Eur. J. Nucl. Med. 19, 1006, 1992.

18) Neal CE, Baker MR, Hilgers RD, et al. Clin. Nucl. Med. 18, 472, 1993.

19) Krag DN, Ford P, Smith L, et al. Arch. Surg. 128, 819, 1993.

20) Chung JK, Kang SB, Lee HP, et al. J. Nucl. Med. 34, 1651, 1993.

21) Perkins AC, Symonds IM, Pimm MV, et al. Nucl. Med. Commun. 14, 578, 1993.

22) Surwit EA, Childers JM, Krag DN, et al. Gynecol. Oncol. 48, 283, 1993.

23) Landoni F, Arosio M, D'Amico P, et al. In: "Up-dating on tumor markers in tissues and in biological fluids" (Ballesta AM et al. Eds), Ed. Minerva Medica, Torino 1993, p.507.

24) Hempling RE, Piver MS, Baker TR, et al. Am. J. Clin. Oncol. 17, 331, 1994.

Laparoscopic treatment of serous and mucinous ovarian cystoadenomas

D. Cirillo, A. Tolino, G. Passannanti, E. Sole, A. Petrone, V. Graziano, P. Ferrara and C. Nappi

Faculty of Medicine and Surgery, Obstetrics and Gynecology, University of Naples "Federico II", Naples, Italy

Introduction

Serous and mucinous ovarian cystadenomas from the histogenetic point of view are classified as ovarian tumors formed from the coelomatic or mullerian epithelium, and by definition are benign epithelial ovarian tumors. However, rather frequently does it happen that the histological examination of these masses reveals abnormalities which are considered malignant, even if with only a low or very low potential which characterizes them as borderline forms (6).

In our study we meant to stress the limits of endoscopic surgery in the treatment of serous and mucinous ovarian cystomas. However we did not mean to offer a solution to the problem which is being examined in this work.

Materials and methods

In the five years between 1990 and 1994 we treated 29 patients with serous ovarian cystadenoma and 6 patients with mucinous ovarian cystadenoma by laparoscopic route. All the women had undergone ovariostatic therapy for 3 to 6 months before surgery.

Before the laparoscopic surgery the patients underwent a preoperative diagnostic management which included: personal anamnesis, accurate clinical examination, accurate echographic examination, abdominal and pelvic x-rays and an NMR and/or a CT-scan in the uncertain cases, plasma assays of tumor markers (Ca125, A-FP, CEA, Ca19-9) (7).

The combination of the morphological, instrumental and clinical data for the diagnosis in all cases indicated the presence of benign ovarian cysts. We did not observe any sign or symptom of malignancy, which would have made us choose traditional surgery for the treatment of the patient. In no case we had high levels of the assayed tumor markers in the plasma.

In addition to all that, the age of our patients ranged between 23 and 36 years, an age when the index of malignancy of ovarian cysts is just 4.5 per 100.000 cases (9). In all patients, before proceeding with the enucleation of the cysts, we performed an accurate laparoscopic examination of the pelvis and paid particular attention to the peritoneal, omental, mesenteric surfaces, etc., which supported the data obtained from the preoperative management, as it did not reveal any suspected lesion.

Nevertheless it must be considered that so far no diagnostic instrument is able to completely exclude the malignancy of an ovarian cyst before operating on it, and this in spite of the improvement of the diagnostic potentials of the tools we have available today.

For this reason in all cases we tried to treat the ovarian tumefactions according to Semm's technique (2), i.e. we tried to enucleate the whole cyst without breaking its wall. Upon finding the cleavage planes between the cystic wall and the cortical wall of the ovary, we removed the mass and placed it into a plastic bag. Where it was possible we aspired the content of the cyst so as to decrease its size and thus facilitate its extraction out of the abdominal cavity by means of a 12 mm trocar.

As a matter of fact this technique was feasible only in 13 patients. In the other 22 we still tried to enucleate the intact cysts, but these accidentally broke and in some cases produced abundant fluid discharge .

Since we were aware of the risks we faced, we requested the presence in the operating theatre of an anatomical pathologist to perform an extemporaneous examination of the endocystic fluid, of the bioptic fragments, of the cystic capsules, of the peritoneal washing, and of the cystic content, especially in the cases when the cyst accidentally broke and there was a spillage in the peritoneum.

In all cases the results the extemporaneous histological and cytological examinations were not of malignancy.

On the margins of the ovarian wound we applied a Roeder's double snare and produced a definitive hemostasis by coagulating the bleeding points by means of a monopolar electrocoagulator. At the end of every surgery we performed peritoneal washings with abundant, warm lactated Ringer's solution. All the patients were then administered an oestroprogestative therapy (Minulet – Triminulet) for 6 to 12 months to place the ovary at rest.

These patients were also followed for a period of 6 to 12 months. Their follow-up consisted of a clinical examination and a vaginal echography every 3 months.

Results

Besides the extemporaneous examination in the operating theater we also had a definitive histological examination of the cystic capsules performed. Twenty nine patients had a serous cystadenoma and six patients had a mucinous cystadenoma .

Although the final histological test did not give any result of cystadenocarcinoma, we were however rather negatively struck by the result from a test performed on the cystic wall of a serous cystoma, which revealed the presence of proliferative activity of the epithelial cells with nuclear abnormalities, but without infiltrative or destructive growth. This is considered a borderline (1) condition, i.e. potentially malignant, although very slightly so. As concerns the postoperative course, only in 1 case the hospitalization lasted about 7 days. This was the case of a patient who had a mucinous ovarian cystoma of 10 cm, which accidentally broke during the operative maneuvers and caused the extravasation of the endocystic fluid. This patient presented hyperthermia from peritoneal reaction, which was treated and cured with the common antibiotic and anti-inflammatory therapies.

The hospitalization of the other patients was never longer than 48 hours, with an average of 36 hours, and the period of convalescence ranged between 10 to 15 days, and the patients resumed their normal working activities without any problem.

The postoperative follow-up did not reveal any long-term complication for the patients or recidive ovarian masses.

The patient with the borderline serous cystoma was and still is being closely controlled. Every 2-3 months the patient undergoes an echography and a plasma assay of ovarian tumor markers. In agreement with the patient, who is young and without children, we did not perform a radical surgery. Her control investigations are still negative after about 3 years from surgery.

Discussion

The combined use of morphological (vaginal echography), clinical (objective examination) and lately also fluxometry (echographic color doppler) data brought about an improvement in the diagnostic potential for the recognition of malignant forms. A careful endoscopic examination before surgery on the mass can improve the diagnosis even more. If we were faced with a mass with even a single suspected sign of malignancy we would immediately choose a traditional surgery.

There is however a condition which, in spite of an accurate preoperative management, is not recognized at all, and this is the borderline ovarian cysts.

Borderline serous ovarian cystadenomas are the most frequent among all borderline epithelial ovarian tumors, as they account for 47% to 67% of these tumors; while the incidence of the mucinous ones is between 20 and 48% (4).

It must be also considered that the survival rate at 10 years of patients with the serous histotype in its borderline form is between 70% and 75%. The survival rate with borderline mucinous tumors ranges between 68% and 96%. Although the survival rate is rather high, these data nevertheless indicate the possibility of an unfavourable diagnosis at 10 years from the finding of the tumor (5).

It is however also true that the diagnosis depends on a whole series of parameters of great prognostic significance which could improve the survival rate. This however does not eliminate the concern caused by the finding of malignant cells in a mass, although it was enucleated, which is still such that we cannot maintain that the neoplastic process was completely removed.

Among all the considerations above there is also that we believe that handling masses containing atypical cells by endoscopic route could favour intraoperative spillages, and this could worsen the prognosis for the patient.

There is by now general agreement in the world literature on the fact that an ovarian carcinoma in stage Ia, whose cystic capsule is accidentally broken during the maneuvers, can at the most change its stage into Ic, and that this provoked and not spontaneous modification does not at all affect the quo ad vitam prognosis of the patients (3 - 8 - 10).

In spite of the support of the literature data we however wondered whether we would have still treated the patient by laparoscopic route, could we have diagnosed her case with certainty before surgery.

Unfortunately there is no diagnostic means to recognize such an event before surgery. This surely does not change our opinion on the validity of endoscopic surgery for the treatment of ovarian cysts in young patients.

However, we always suggest the presence of an anatomical pathologist in the operating theater so as to have the first cytological and histological data on the peritoneal washing fluid and on the bioptic fragments of the accidentally broken cystic capsules already during the surgery.

BIBLIOGRAPHY

1) Yoonessi M., Crickard K., Celik C., Yoonessi S.: "Borderline epithelial tumors of the ovary: ovarian intraepithelial neoplasia." Obstet. Gynecol. Survey 43 pag. 435-444

2) Mecke H., Lehmann-Willenbrock E., Ibrahim M., Semm K.: "Pelviscopic treatment of ovarian cysts in premenopausal women." Gynecol Obstet. Invest. 1992. 34 pag. 36-42

3) Sevelda P., Dittrich C., Salzer H.: Prognostic value of the rupture of the capsule in stage I epithelian ovarian carcinoma." Gynecol. Oncol. 1989; 35: 321-322

4) Rossiello R.: "Tumori epiteliali borderline: aspetti anatomopatologici e correlazioni cliniche." Atti del Congresso: "L'ovaio: fisiopatologia benigna e maligna." Napoli 24 - 26 Febbraio 1994

5) Robbins S.L., Cotran R.S., Kumar V.: " Apparato genitale femminile: l'ovaio." in "Pathologic basis of disease" Ed. Italiana Piccin 1987

6) Pescetto G., De cecco L., Pecorari D., Ragni N.: "Tumori ovarici" in " Manuale di Ginecologia" Ed. S.E.U. Roma 1990

7) Vasilev S., Schlaerth J., Campean J., Morrow P.: "Serum Ca-125 levels in preoperative evaluation of pelvic masses." Obstet Gynecol. 1988. 71: 751-756

8) Annual Report on the Rsults of Treatment in Gynecological Cancer. Stockholm, Radiummhemmet, Vol. 20. 1986

9) Nezhat C., Winer W.K., Nezhat F.: "Laparoscopic removal of dermoid cysts." Obstet. Gynecol. 1989. Feb. 73(2): 278-80

10) Finn C.D., Luesley D.M., Buxton E.J., et al.: "Stage I epithelial ovarian cancer overtreated both surgically and systematically? Results of a five-year cancer registry review." Br. J. Obstet. Gynecol. 1992, 99: 54-8

Laparoscopic treatment of dermoid cysts

D. Cirillo, A. Tolino, A. Petrone, G. Passannanti, S. Ronsini, E. Sole, P. Ferrara and C. Nappi

Faculty of Medicine and Surgery, Obstetrics and Gynecology, University of Naples "Federico II", Naples, Italy

Introduction

The dermoid cyst or benign cystic teratoma is the benign ovarian neoplasia of greatest clinical interest among all teratoid tumors. It accounts for 15% of all primary gonadial tumors in women (1 - 2 - 3).
Presently, thanks to the progresses in techniques and instruments, it is possible to treat almost all ovarian cysts by laparoscopic route. In the case of dermoid cysts in young patients the limits of surgical laparoscopy are mainly related to the possible spillage of endocystic matter in the abdominal cavity. In the case this happens and causes a chemical peritonitis, the well-known advantages of laparoscopy over traditional laparotomy are nullified. In this work the authors stress the importance of an accurate preoperative laparoscopic evaluation such as to help the surgeon choose the most suitable surgical (laparoscopic or laparotomic) technique which implies the least risks for the patient.

Materials and Methods

In the six years from 1989 to 1994 we examined 18 patients with ovarian dermoid cysts, which we diagnosed by means of vaginal ultrasonography . Out of the patients aged between 18 and 37 years 7 were nulliparas and 11 pluriparas. They complained pain in the adnexal seat with or without alterations of their menstrual cycles. Moreover 2 out of the 18 patients had a positive anamnesis of previous endometriosis.
The preoperative management consisted of the echographic color doppler vaginal examination and of the assay of tumor markers (Ca 125, Ca 19.9, CEA, alpha-

833

fetoprotein). In 2 cases with large dermoid cysts with uncertain echographic pictures we performed also an abdominal-pelvic CT-scan which revealed the cysts to be completely benign in both patients . All the patients were first examined by us after they had been using oestroprogestatives for at least three months, which in no case had modified the cystic echostructures.

Out of our 18 patients 16 underwent surgical laparoscopy in general anesthesia according with the following technique : in 9 cases with small cysts these were enucleated intact. We made an incision of about 3-5 cm by means of an electrosurgical knife on the cortex of the ovary. Once revealed the capsule, the cysts have been removed from the cortex by means of clamps and scissors. We reached the pedicle, cut it and electrocoagulated it. By this method we tried to enucleate the cysts without breaking their walls, so as to prevent a possible peritoneal spillage. Larger cysts were removed from the peritoneal cavity either through a colpotomic incision which was then sutured, or by means of a trocar of 22 or 11 mm.

In 5 other cases the cysts were first emptied by means of a 16 mm aspirator introduced through a 22 or 11 mm trocar. In one case 2 dermoid cysts were enucleated from the same ovary, placed in the space of Retzius and aspired, and then taken outside through a 16 mm trocar. In one last case one cyst measuring 10 x 9 cm accidentally broke during the maneuver for its detachment from the cortex, and caused an abundant spillage of endocystic matter (dense fluid full of hairs and small solid formations), in spite of the previous aspiration.

As concerns the residual ovarian breach. in 2 cases with bleeding points we electrocoagulated them and left the ovarian breach open. In 10 cases where the ovarian breaches appeared to have too large borders and did not bleed too much we used Roeder's double snares. Eventually, in 4 cases where scarce ovarian tissue was left and the margins bled quite a bit, we sutured the ovarian breach . In all treated cases, during our surgeries we always have an anatomical pathologist with us in the operating theater, to make an extemporaneous histological and cytological examination.

To all patients we suggested an oestroprogestative therapy (Triminulet, Wyeth) for a period of six months and a laparoscopic second look, which was performed after 7 to 12 months, so as to exclude the formation of postoperative pelvic adhesions.

Eventually for 2 out of our 18 patients we chose the traditional laparotomic surgery in consideration of the remarkable sizes of the cysts (11x12 cm and 13x11.5 cm) and of the contemporary presence of pelvic adhesion syndrome. We believe these conditions make laparoscopic surgery not suitable because of the high risk of short-term (chemical peritonitis) and long-term (adhesion syndrome) complications.

In all treated patients the histological examination confirmed the benign diagnosis. Out of the 16 patients operated in laparoscopy only 8 (5 nullipara and 3 pluriparas) underwent the laparoscopic second look .
In 6 out of these patients we did not observe the formation of significant adhesions. In one patient (pluripara with bilateral ovarian cysts) we observed thin periovarian and peritubal adhesions which were easily removed.

The patient who had the accidental rupture of the cyst, in spite of our attempt to aspire its matter and the abundant and scrupulous washing of the peritoneal cavity with lactated Ringer's solution, developed a chemical peritonitis with consequent hyperthermia and an hospitalization of 10 days. She was administered the normal antibiotic and anti-inflammatory therapies. Moreover at the laparoscopic second look 9 months later we observed an adhesion syndrome with both thin and velar adhesions and thick and vascularized ones.

Discussion and Conclusion

The limits of surgical laparoscopy in case of dermoid cysts in young patients are mainly related to the possible spillage of the endocystic matter in the abdominal cavity (4, 5, 6). Such an event, like the one we reported, can nullify the desired advantages of laparoscopic surgery: i.e. little invasion with reduced formation of adhesions and complications for the future fertility of the patient, fast healing with short hospitalization, and a great compliance from the patient. From what we said so far it is evident the importance of a careful preoperative laparoscopic evaluation in patients with dermoid cysts. Even if today, thanks to the progresses in the technique, in modern instruments, and to the experience gained, it is possible to treat almost all ovarian cysts, we believe that not always all that is possible is also useful.

BIBLIOGRAPHY

1) Scaccia A., Di Girolamo P., Voghera P.
   Dermoid cysts of the ovary
   Min. Chir. 1990, 45 (13-14): 993-5

2) King M.E. et al.
   Immature teratoma of the ovary grade 3, with karyotype analysis. Int. J. Gynecol. Pathol. 1990, 9 (2): 178-84

3) Spaun E., Rix P.
   Benign cystic monodermal teratoma of neurogenic type.
   Int. J. Gynecol. Pathol., 1990, 9 (3): 283-90

4) Nezhat C., et al.
   Laparoscopic removal of dermoid cysts.
   Obstet e Gynecol., 29 Feb., 73 (2): 278-80

5) Cirillo D., Tolino A., et al.
Valutazioni sul trattamento delle cisti dermoidi
dell'ovaio: chirurgia endoscopica e laparotomica a
confronto."Attualità in tema di terapia in Ginecologia
Oncologica" Copanello, Ott. 1992, pag. 101-7

6) Cirillo D., et al.
Endoscopic treatment of ovarian cysts: endosuture
techniques and complications.
Current investigation in Gynecology and Obstetrics
The Partenon Publishing Group, page 321-31
Madonna di Campiglio, Feb. 1993

Laparoscopic treatment of ovarian cysts

G.L. Bracco, M.E. Coccia, E. Scatena and G. Scarselli

Department of Obstetrics and Gynecology II, University of Florence, Italy

INTRODUCTION

During the last few years operative laparoscopy has had a remarkable diffusion and we can consider it an indispensable component of modern gynecological surgery particularly in the treatment of ovarian cyst

The surgical treatment followed by the histopathological examination is the appropriate treatment to obtain an early diagnosis of the ovarian cancer. The traditional treatment of ovarian cysts is the laparotomy but this is characterized by an elevated morbility and it often showes the benign nature of the ovarian cyst (1).

The main problem regarding the laparoscopic approach to the ovarian cyst is the risk of treating an ovarian cancer and the worsening of the prognosis due to the spillage at the time of surgery. Some authors have reported that the rupture of the capsule in stage I ephitelial ovarian cancer during the operation has an adverse influence on survival prognosis, while others in retrospective studies have showed any influence on the prognosis (2,3). However the majority of ovarian cysts are benign and eligible for endoscopic treatment.

The appropriate selection of the patient for laparoscopic ovarian surgery necessitates the availability of information on the characteristics of the cyst which can be obtained by ultrasound examination. One of the most important advance in gynecological ultrasound diagnosis has been the introduction of transvaginal sonography which gives a good image of the pelvic organs due to close distance of the ultrasound transducer to these organs. More recently by the application of color doppler on echography it has been possible to have information about the state of neovascolarization of the ovarian cyst wall (4,5).

Actually a laparoscopic ultrasound imaging (L.U.I.) has been introduced. Laparoscopic ultrasound imaging transducer is designed for easy insertion through the trocar and it is applyable to a normal ultrasound equipment.

Using the operative laparoscopy we perform the enucleation and the remotion of the cyst (women in fertile age), the ovariectomy or adnexectomy (women in post-menopause) with the advantages of this type of surgery: minor post-operative pain, minor formation of adhesion, minimum of hospitalization (24-48 hours), rapid return to the normal activity (7-10 days).

MATERIALS AND METHODS

120 patients (age range between 16-64 years) who had adnexal cysts were treated by operative laparoscopy. All the patients underwent to our protocol that was strictly observed and consisted in appropiate preoperative evaluation, careful patient selection considering patient's age, laboratory tests, dosage of CA 125 , CA 19-9, CEA, TPA, aFP, beta-hCG, transabdominal and transvaginal ultrasound examination.

96 patients were under 40 years of age (Group A: media 27 ± 5 years) and 24 were over 40 years (Group B: media 54 ± 7 years). 18 patients were in post-menopause.

In Group A the patients were treated after three months of observation or therapy with GnRH agonists or oral estroprogestinic. In Group B the women in fertile age and with diameter's cyst <50 mm were treated as the Group A; the patients in post-menopause or with a cyst >50 mm in diameter were immediately treated by laparoscopy.

The dimension of the cyst in the Group A was mm 42 ± 17 (media 47mm; range 12-82mm). The dimension of the cyst in the Group B was mm 51 ± 13 (media 52mm; range 36-93mm).

Using the instrumentation of Karl Storz (West-Germany) we performed in patients in fertile age the enucleation of the cyst after cystoscopy with 5 mm laparoscope. The ovary was not sutured and in cases of cysts very large we have approached the ovary's borders with bipolar electrocoagulation or using glue of fibrine (Tissucol). Patients in post-menopause were treated with ovariectomy or adnexectomy (with simultaneous histologic evaluation).

Diagnosis of the cysts was confirmed during laparoscopy and we performed aspiration of the peritoneal fluid sample, careful examination of the cystic ovary, complete inspection of the pelvic peritoneum, controlateral ovary and omentum.

More recently we have introduced during laparoscopy a laparoscopic ultrasound probe for an intraoperative ultrasonic examination. The transducer (UST-5521, Aloka , Japan) is a 7.5 MHz linear array designed for easy insertion through a 10 mm trocar and it is applicable to our SSD 620 (Aloka, Japan) ultrasound equipment.

When the cyst appeared to be macroscopically benign and the laparoscopic ultrasound imaging showed benign features, cyst puncture, aspiration using an aspirating needle or the 5 mm suvrapubic trocar, was performed taking care to minimize spillage. The cyst was then opened using laparoscopic scissors and examined to look for papillary structures inside. In post-menopausal patients and in cases of dermoid cysts we used endoscopic bags to avoid the "spillage".

Patients were controlled with ultrasound after 3,6 and 12 months.

RESULTS

After laparoscopic diagnosis 120 patients were treated by operative laparoscopy. Only one patient was converted to laparotomy for a major bleeding into the ovary.

The transvaginal sonography (TVS) showed a very good concordance with definitive pathologic diagnosis and with macroscopic examination.

32 cases of endometriosis were classified as Stage III (30 cases) and Stage IV (4 cases) of the AFSR Classification. In 30 patients the enucleation of endometrioma was completely done, while in 4 cases, medically pre-treated with GnRH agonists, was impossible.

All cases presented benign feature at laparoscopy.

In one case at LUI examination we found an iperechogenic structure inside the endometrioma cyst undiagnosed at TVS. When the cyst was opened this structure appeared black stone like haemosiderin. LUI application was particularly usefull especially in one case where the cyst was very small and deep in the ovary. The laparoscopic ultrasound probe showed the correct point where perform a small incision on the ovary and every step was followed on the ultrasound monitor. The disappearance of the iperechogenic structure on the screen showed that the cystectomy was completed.

The histopathological examination diagnosed:

34 endometrial cysts, 27 serous cysts, 22 cystic teratomas, 15 paraovarian cysts, 11 serous cystoadenomas and 11 mucinous cystoadenomas.

There were not post-operative complications.

In Group B, on the base of the benign ultrasound features and the dosage of CA 125 <35U/mL, was diagnosed any malignant tumor at the histology. The correlation between echographic and histopathologic diagnosis in Group A showed the concordance of 100% in endometrial cysts, 82% in cystic teratomas and 75% in paraovarian cysts.

The time of the laparoscopic operation was 70±37 minutes (media 60min, range 30-180 min) in Group A and 64±18 (media 46min, range 25-90min) in Group B. The time of hospitalization was 2,1±1,1 days (media 3 days, range 1-6 days). We effected clinical and ultrasound controls at 3,6 and 12 months (follow-up'range: 3-40 months).

DISCUSSION

In our experience operative laparoscopy represents a valid alternative in the treatment of benign adnexal masses. We have obtained 100% in sensibility and negative predictivity in the diagnosis of malignant tumors at ultrasonography and laparoscopy.

Surely it is very important the selection of the patients based on a multimodal approach in which transvaginal ultrasound, dosage of CA 125, clinical examination and anamnesis represent a fundamental diagnostic time to avoid the treatment of malignant masses. It is very important to evaluate the ovarian cyst with a careful ultrasound study and the dosage of tumoral markers.

The echographic criteria of benignity are: unilaterality, uniloculariety, absence of septa >3mm and intracystic vegetations, pure borders (6-7). If such criteria, evaluated by a transvaginal probe, are respected and the dosage of CA 125 is <35 U/mL (8), the probability of a benign formation is very high.

During laparoscopy we can obtain information observing the cyst and the peritoneal cavity. Actually we can use endoscopic bags to remove the cyst or the whole ovary without spillage performing immediately the histological examination. In this way it is possible to reduce the risk of treating by laparoscopy an ovarian cancer.

Regards the laparoscopic treatment of ovarian cysts in women over 40 years of age under appropriate criteria of selection, were not described in literature cases of malignant tumors (9-11).

Some authors noted that using specific ultrasonographic criteria the negative predictivity is 96% (6) and in post-menopause 95-100% (12,13). When an ovarian mass is sonographically defined as unilocular and anechogenic cyst, the positive predictivity is between 90% and 95% (6,14). Some authors proposed the association of clinical examination, CA125 dosage and transvaginal ultrasound as 100% in specificity (8,15).

Regards the problem of the suture of the ovary after the enucleation of the cyst, we never performed this suture and the following ultrasound controls revealed a normal ovarian morphology. We consider the ovarian suture unnecessary: it does not influence the formation of adhesions or the pregnancy rate

In the comparison between transvaginal ultrasound and histological diagnosis we obtained a very good concordance : 100% in endometrial cysts, 82 % in cystic teratomas, 75% in paraovarian cysts.

In two cases (25%) of paraovarian cysts the ultrasound diagnosis was as ovarian cysts but the two patients were in menopause and the evaluation of the atrophic ovary is surely more difficult and somtimes impossible.

In conclusion we consider the laparoscopic treatment of the ovarian masses useful and safe even in post-menopausal patients under appropriate conditions: benign sonographic aspect, CA 125 <35 U/mL, benign laparoscopic feature.

REFERENCES

1 Creasman, W.T., Soper, J.T. (1986). The undiagnosed adnexal mass after the menopause. *Clin Ostet Gynecol* ,29:,446.
2. Webb, M.J., Decker D.G., Mussey, E.,et al (1973). Factors influencing survival in stage I ovarian cancer. *Am.J.Obstet.Gynecol.*, 116,222-8.
3. Dembo, A.J., Davy, M., Stenwig, A.E.,et al (1990). Prognostic factors in patients with stage I epithelial ovarian cancer. *Obstet. Gynecol.*,75, 263-72.
4 Leibman, A.J., Kruse, B., Mc Sweeney, M.B. (1988). Transvaginal sonography: comparison with transabdominal sonography in the diagnosis of pelvic masses. *Am.J.of Roentgenology*,151,89-92.
5 Kurjak, A., Zulad,I., Alfirevic, Z.(1991). Evaluation of adnexal masses with transvaginal colour ultrasound. *Journal of Ultrasound in Medicine.*,10,295-97.

6. Herrmann, U.J., Locher, G.W., Goldhirsch, A (1987). Sonographic patterns of malignancy: Prediction of malignancy. *Obstet Gynecol* , **69**, 777-81.

7. Grandberg, S., Nostrom, A., Wikland, A (1990). Tumors in the pelvis as imaged by vaginal sonography. *Gynecologic Oncology* , **37**, 224.

8   Finkler, N.J., Benacererraf, B., Lavin, P.T., Wojciechowski, C., Knapp, R.C. (1988). Comparison of serum CA125, clinical impression and ultrasound in the preoperation evaluation of ovarian masses. *Obstet Gynecol.*, **72**, 659-64.

9.   Levine, R.L.(1990). Pelviscopic surgery in women over forty. *J Repr Med* , **35,** 597-600.

10. Parker, W., Berek, J.(1990). Management of selected cystic adnexal masses in postmenopausal women by operative laparoscopy: A pilot study. *Am J Obstet Gynecol* .,**163,** 1574.

11. Mann, W.J., Reich, H.(1992). *J Repr Med* , **37**:,254-56.

12 Rulin, M.C., Preston, A.L.(1987) Adnexal masses in postmenopausal women. *Obstet Gynecol* **70,**578.

13. Goldstein, S.R., Subramanyam, B., Snyder, J.R. et al.(1989) The postmenopausal cystic adnexal mass: the potential role of ultrasound in conservative management. *Obstet Gynecol* **73**, 8-10.

14 Meire, H.B., Farrant, P., Gutha, T. (1978). Distinction of benign from malignant ovarian cysts by ultrasound. *Br J of Obstet Gynecol,* **85,**893.

15. Jacobs, I., Stabile, I., Bridges, J. et al.(1988) Multimodal approach to screening for ovarian cancer. *Lancet* **1,** 268.

Usefulness of presurgical staging in the prognostic evaluation of endometrial cancer

P.L. Cherchi, F. Sbernardori, G. Ruiu, F. Esposito, G.B. Franco, M.P. Bagella and A. Ambrosini

Università degli Studi di Sassari, Clinica Ostetrica-Ginecologica, Sassari, Italy

---

The surgical staging introduced by FIGO in the World Congress of 1988 has modified the terapeutic approach in the endometrial carcinoma, especially with the introduction of systematic pelvic and para-aortic lymphadenectomy.

Presurgical staging was also introduced to correct the diagnostic error caused by surgical staging, that did not allow a correct prognostic evaluation with an understaging up to 50%.

However in about 2/3 of the cases, apparently confined to the uterine body, hysterectomy alone appears as an adequate surgical treatment, without any need of limphadenectomy, that sometimes is difficoltous to be performed, because of the severe obesity, poor general condition, etc.

The clinical staging, with the last generation imaging techniques, can detect low risk cases that will undergo only to hysterectomy.

Many Authors have studied this problematic, suggesting a selective approach in the surgical staging and it has been proposed to personalize the treatment with an intraoperative evaluation of lymphonodal status and of myometrial invasion.

Burke in 1990 (2) proposed a staging based on clinical and instrumental assessments, and dividing low risk cases (endometrioid carcinoma, G1 grading, superficial myometrial invasion, serum Ca 125 < 35 U/ml) and high risk cases (clear cell or adenosquamous or serous papillary carcinoma, G2 or G3, deep myometrial invasion, high Ca 125 serum levels, etc.). The treatment of low risk cases was based on hysterectomy alone, followed by an intraoperative evaluation of grading, myometrial invasion, peritoneal washing and cervical invasion; in case of severe patterns, these patients underwent to the same treatments of high risk cases: para-aortic and pelvic limphadenectomy, peritoneal and diaphragmatic biopsies. Using this approach the Authors performed hysterectomy in 60-70% and a more intensive treatment in 30-40% of the cases.

Shim et al. (8) found a good diagnostic reliability using uterine frozen sections soon after hysterectomy, whereas Doering et al. (4) proposed a simple macroscopic intrasurgical evaluation.

The aim of our study was to assess if presurgical staging can detect high risk cases, that will undergo to a more aggressive treatment, and at the same time to observe if there are important differences between clinical and surgical staging.

MATERIALS AND METHODS

From 1991 to 1994 we studied 50 patients, affected by endometrial carcinoma apparently confined to the uterine body, aged between 46 and 83 years (median 64 years), 8 were in pre-menopause and 42 in post-menopause. We performed the following examinations for presurgical staging:

-clinical examination;
-hysteroscopy, for cervical extension, tumoral size;
-hystotype and hystological grading;
-trans-vaginal ultrasonography (TVU), for myometrial invasion assessment;
-pelvic and upper abdominal ultrasonography for liver, pelvic and limphonodal assessments;
-abdomen-pelvis C.T. for limphnodal status;
-presurgical serum levels of Ca125.

Considering the previous assessments, we gave a score for different risks (score 1-3 by risk level) according to following parameters: hystological grading and hystotype, myometrial invasion, histology of non invaded endometrium, cervical involvement, lymphonodal status, serum Ca125, and, before the surgical operation, we found three groups: low risk (score 9-12), medium risk (13-17) and high risk (18-23) patients (tab. 1).

Table 1   Parameters considered of risk score

RISK SCORE	1	2	3
GRADING	G1	G2	G3
HYSTOTYPE	Endometrioid	clear cell squamous	papilliferous
MYOM. INVASION	no invasion	< 50%	> 50%
NODAL STATUS	N-	Single N+	N+ >3
SIZE OF TUMOR NON INVADED	focal	<2 cm	>2 cm
ENDOMETRIUM	hyperplasic	normal	atrophicum
CERVICAL INV.	no invasion	focal	deep
EXTRAUTERINE DIS.	negative	adnexal	pelvic
SERUM CA 125	<35 U/ml	35-50 U/ml	>50 U/ml

After the presurgical staging, the high-risk patients underwent to minimal surgery (abdominal hysterectomy alone), to pelvic limphadenectomy (medium risk-pts) and para-aortic limphadenectomy (high risk-pts). The surgical approach was also influenced by intraoperative evaluation of myometrial and cervical invasion, or by intra-abdominal assessment (presence of adenophaty, extrauterine invasion). We had 10 low risk (20%), 17 medium risk (34%) and 23 high risk cases (46%).

We performed abdominal hysterectomy in the 10 low risk patients, abdominal hysterectomy + L.A. in 26 patients (52%), abdominal hysterectomy + pelvic and para-aortic L.A. in 14 patients (28%). In the pelvic L.A. group the limphnodal positivity was 7.6% (2/26) and in the para-aortic L.A. group was 21,4% (3-14) (tab. 2).

Table 2   Surgical treatment

	N. CASES	%	N+	%
HYSTERECTOMY ALONE	10	20.0	- -	- -
PELVIC L.A.	26	52.0	2	7.6
PELVIC AND PARA-AORTIC L.A.	14	28.0	3	21.4
TOTAL	50	100.0	5	12.5

RESULTS AND DISCUSSION

Using   risk group score   and FIGO 1988 staging, we diagnosed in the 10 low risk cases 7 IA and 3 IB, with a good corrispondence. In the 17 medium risk cases we found 2 IA and 15 IB without any limphnodal positivity in the patient who underwent to lymphadenectomy. In the 23 high risk cases we found 16 IC, 2 IIIA (focal unilateral adnexal invasion) and 5 IIIC (N+ that were not presurgically detected in 2 cases for the presence of micrometastasis, and for a limphnodal invasion <3 nodes).

The presurgical myometrial invasion assessment by T.V.U. and C.T. detected 18 cases without invasion, 21 with superficial invasion (<50%) and 11 with deep (>50%) myometrial invasion.

The comparison between clinical and surgical staging showed a good correlation in 40/50 of cases (80%), with a   poor diagnostic error: 5 IIIC (N+ previously not detected by T.V.U. and C.T.), 2 IIIA (focal adnexal invasion) and 3 IB in which surgical diagnosis did not manage to detect myometrial invasion (tab.3).

Table 3   Presurgical staging vs FIGO stage

RISK SCORE	N.	FIGO STAGE (1988)				
		I A	IB	IC	IIIA	IIIC
LOW	10	7	3	--	--	--
MILD	17	2	15	--	--	--
HIGH	23	--	--	16	2	5
TOTAL	50	9	18	16	2	5

In our study the diagnostic error was 14%, 7 cases in which clinical staging was I but postsurgical staging was III.

Anyway, in endometrial carcinoma limphnodal status assessment is very difficultous, because nor with RMN neither with C.T. it is possible to detected the presence of limphnodal metastasis less than 1,5-2 cm of diameter.

Comparing the histologic results with macro-intraoperative evaluation of myometrial invasion we found a concordance of 55% for M0, 91,3% for superficial myometrial invasion and of 72,2% for deep myometrial invasion. The overall correlation was 78% (tab.4).

Table 4   Intraoperative evaluation of myometrial invasion vs hystology

MYOMETRIAL INVASION	N.	MO	<50%	>50%	%
MO	9	5	4	--	55.5
<50%	23	--	21	2	91.3
>50%	18	--	5	13	72.2
TOTAL	50	5	30	15	78.0

Also the histological grading showed a difference between the presurgical bioptical patterns and the definitive diagnosis: we had 4 of 15 presurgical G1 cases who became G2, of the 25 G2 cases we had 2 cases who became G1 and 2 G3, and of the 10 G3 cases 1 became G2. This indicate that the presurgical histologic grading has a reliability of 80% (tab. 6).

Table 5   Histologic grading

GRADING	PRE	POST	POST
G1	15	G1 11	13
		G2 4	
		G3 --	
G2	25	G1 2	26
		G2 21	
		G3 2	
G3	10	G1 --	11
		G2 1	
		G3 9	

The correlation between clinical and intraoperative evaluation of myometrial invasion and histologic findings showed better results (table 6) for the intraoperative evaluation than for diagnostic imaging, with respectively 78% and 67,4%, especially in the absence of myometrial invasion and in the deep myometrial invasion (in the superficial myometrial invasion both the techniques showed 91,3% reliability).

Table 6 Preoperative and intraoperative evaluation of myometrial invasion vs histology

MYOMETRIAL INVASION (HYSTOLOGY)	N.	CORRELATION	
		PREOPERATIVE %	INTRAOPERATIVE%
MO	9	50.0	55.5
<50%	23	91.3	91.3
>50%	18	61.1	72.2
TOTAL	50	67.4	78.0

CONCLUSION

In conclusion our study showed a good correlation between clinical and surgical staging concernig the detection of risk cases, for specific surgical indication we correctly evaluated 40/50 cases. We had an understaging of 14% (7/50) with a little percentage compared to the figures we found in literature (the understaging, with the old FIGO classification was up to 50%), even if we have to admit that because this is a prospectic study selected patients had a very accurated presurgical staging.

Many difficulties still exist for the limphnodal evaluation, because the actual imaging can not identify micrometastasis and nodes larger less than 2 cm. There is a good reliability for the myometrial invasion evaluation, especially for the superficial invasion; this assessment could be improved with recently introduced gadolinium MNR. The macro-intraoperative evaluation is anyway very useful to modulate the surgical approach, and to avoid an undertreatment, that in the past was the most frequent cause of long term failures for this neoplasia.

REFERENCES

1. Anderson, B. (1992). Diagnosis understaging in endometrial carcinoma. Clin Obst.Gyn.,25,75.
2. Burke, T.W.(1990). Selective approach to surgical staging. Cancer Bull.,42,80.

3. Cowles, T.A., Magrina, J.F., Masterson, B.J. et al. (1985). Comparison of clinical and surgical staging in patients with endometrial carcinoma. Obst.Gynecol.,66,3.

4. Doering, D.L., Barnahill, D.R., Weiser, E.B., et al (1989). Intraoperative evaluation of depth of myometrial invasion in stage I endometrial adenocarcinoma. Obst.Gynecol.,74,930.

5. Girardi, F., Petru, E., Haas ,J., et al.(1993). Pelvic lymphadenectomy in the surgical treatment of endometrial cancer. Gynecol.Oncol.,49,177.

6. Larson, D.M., Johnson, K., Olson, K.(1992). Pelvic and paraaortic lymphadenectomy for surgical staging of endometrial cancer: morbidity and mortality. Obstet.Gynecol.,79,998.

7. Mangioni ,C., De Palo ,G., Marubini, E.(1993). Surgical pathologic staging in apparent stage I endometrial carcinoma. Int. J. Gynecol. Cancer, 3, 373.

8. Shim,J., Rose, P., Reale, F., et al.(1992). Accuracy of frozen sections diagnosis at surgery in clinical stage I and II endometrial carcinoma. Am.J.Obst.Gynecol.,166,1335.

SHBG level changes after high-dose danazol in postmenopausal women with endometrial cancer

A. Rigano, G. Baviera, E. Sturlese, M. Rigano and C. Pullè

Department of Gynecology, University of Messina, Italy

INTRODUCTION

Several studies (1,2,3,4,5,6,7,8.9,10,11) have pointed out a marked decrease of the serum SHBG levels, as side effect, among others, of the danazol therapy. All these studies, but one, refer to normally cycling women affected by benign breast disease or by endometriosis, and women were given danazol, at last for 6 months, at different doses, that is mg./ die 200, 400, 600, 800, . From these studies, it is worthy to note that, after danazol therapy, the decrease appears to be dose related, beeing greater with higher doses,and : a) SHBG serum levels decrease virtually immediately, after 24 hours, and reach statistical significance within 48 hours (5); b) the maximum decrease is achieved after about 4 weeks (2,7); c) the SHBG half-life is approximately 15 days (5). So, after this progressive fall, SHBG serum concentration become stable at a new steady-state.

In postmenopausal women (5) the SHBG levels appeared to be about 15 % less than in premenopausal women but, the estimated metabolic half-life was the same - about 15 days - with only somewath a wider range; the decrease, after 1 month, at whatever dose, was about 12% more than in premenopausal women. This study, as a part of the bigger one concerning premenopausal subjects, reports the effect of a midlle-dose of danazol, so, the aim of our study is to investigate the behaviour of SHBG serum levels in postmenopausal women, after 4 weeks of very high danazol therapy, g. 1,2 / die x 28, looking for correlations with several parameters.

This protocol, among others, has been selected for other purpose, namely for enhancing PR in endometrial cancer. After several attempts, the best response on PR increase was achieved with this high dose for 21-28 days, as some of us have reported in previous papers (12,13,13). Then, it appears to us very interesting to study, in this group of postmenopausal women, also the SHBG behaviour, on the basis of the above mentioned papers, because our dose was different, very high - 1/3 more higher than the previous higher ones, but the lenght of treatment - 4 weeks - was just that one with wich the maximal SHBG serum levels decrease has been seen by others.

MATERIAL AND METHODS

MATERIAL: 16 postmenopausal women affected by endometrial cancer were treated, before surgery, with danazol - g.1,2 / die (mg. 400 x 3) x 4 weeks.
SUBJECT'S CHARACTERISTICS
 - age   mean 66,43 ± SE 8,62 years (range 57-78)
 - years form menopausa: n = 15 : mean 16,83 ± 6,7 , plus one within 1 year
 - BMI : n = 5 < 24,9; n = 8 < 29,9; n = 2 < 39,9; n = 1 >40
 - BS : n = 5 =/< 1,6; n = 7 < 1,8; n = 3 < 1,9; n = 1 > 2,1
 - all but one multipara
ENDOMETRIAL CANCER
 - stage : n = 9 stage 1a-b; n = 7 stage 2a
 - grading : G 1-2
 - receptor's status : 14/16 ER "+"
                                 9/16 PR "+"
METHODS : blood samples were drawn at 8 a.m. before treatment and the day after the end of therapy. The samples were centrifuged and serum was stored at -20 C° until analysis for SHBG, total testosterone and total estradiol. SHBG   was measured by IRMA; total testosterone and estradiol were measured by RIA with commercial kits. Chromatography on celite column (14) was performed before tT RIA for avoiding danazol cross-reactivity. Free E2 and free T have been calculated as free index (FEI and FTI) according to Wilne and Utley (15). All values are espressed as mean ± SE. Significance of differences was tested by unpaired t-test.

RESULTS

Basal and after danazol therapy values (mean ± SE) are summarized below.

	basal values	after danazol
SHBG nmol/l	43,78 ± 2,91	8,24 ± 0,78
total T nmol/l	1,49 ± 0,34	0,916 ± 0,323
total E2 nmol/l	40,4 ± 6,02	25,51 ± 9,85
FEI	0,93 ± 0,132	2,87 ± 1,15FTI
FTI	0,033 ± 0,012	0,068 ± 0,031

After 4 weeks g.1,2/die danazol therapy, SHBG markedly decreases of 81,20 %, from nmol/l 43,78 to 8,24 (difference of highly statistic significance : p < 0,01) (fig.1). Total T and total E2 also decrease both by about 36 % , but the difference between basal values and after danazol therapy has no statistic significance. Free T and free E2 have a strong increase after danazol therapy, as shown by FEI by over 200% and FTI by over 100%, differences of high statistic significance (P < 0,01).

DISCUSSION

In postmenopausal women, g.1,2 / die danazol therapy for 28 days caused a strong decrease of SHBG serum levels of over 81 %. Our data are agreed with previuous above quoted

SHBG before and after danazol

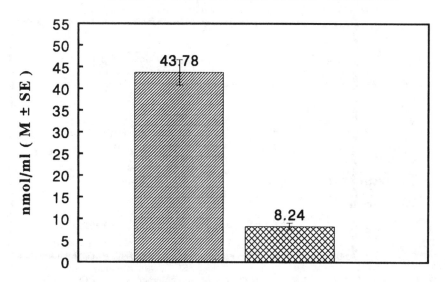

fig. 1 - SHBG serum levels before an after 4 weecks danazol therapy -
g.1,2 / die x 28 .- Decrease (M ± SD) by 81,2% ± 5,09 (p < 0,01)

Author's ones, but it is worthy to stress that this decrease is of the same degree as in premenopausal women, treated with a lower dose - mg.800/ die -, in wich the maximum decrease was achieved after 4 weeks therapy (2,7).

Previous data support the suggestion that danazol - at wathever dose - causes a marked decrease in the serum SHBG levels, but the degree of suppression appear to be more pronounced with higher dose, namely mg.800/ die. Our data point out that also a more high dose, g.1,2/die by us used, has the same effect than mg. 800/die; over this dose there is no enhancement of the SHBG decrease.

Our data point out basal levels in postmenopausal women are less than in premenopausal ones as reported by Al. (5), moreover there is a constant decrease with increased age (fig.2).

It is interesting to note that after danazol therapy, the SHBG decrease is of the same magnitude at wathever age and then wathever was the basal value. Namely we have a less fall of SHBG level after danazol therapy by about 5% in women aged over 65, with BMI >30 and with years past menopause >15, but, of course, this difference has no significance at all.

After therapy, within 4 weeks, agreed with quoted Authors, SHBG levels remain constant at a new steady stade at about 20% of basal values.

The mechanism of this effect is not completely understood. An increased metabolic rate exceeding the rate of synthesis as cause of the decrease seems unlikely. Also changes in estradiol and testosterone levels cannot be significant factors, since also these hormones

Age and SHBG

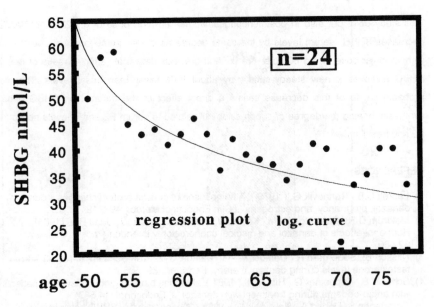

$$Y - 98,174 - ,854 * X; R (E2) - ,523$$

fig.2 - Correlation between SHBG and age in postmenopausal women.
Individual SHBG concentration are plotted against age. The 24 values have
been collected among the 16 patients in this study and a group of 8 healthy
volunteers (4 women 50-55 old at least 4 years past the menopausa, 2
women 65-68 years old and 2 over 75). The regression plot point out a
slow but constant SHBG decrease with increasing age.

were found to decrease and the difference between pre- and post- menopausal
concentrations has no statistic significance.

We are agreed with hypothesis (5) that the two most obvious possible mechanism are: a)
indirect inhibition synthesis by testosterone as result of incresed level of fT; b) direct
inhibition of epatic synthesis.

Previous studies (8, 17) have shown that danazol binds to SHBG with high affinity and
displaces T, increasing the free T values. Also our data, according to several Authors (2, 3,
6, 8), show a strong increase of fT as revealed by rise of the free index over 100%. But, the
high levels of fT don't appear sufficent to account the SHBG decrease (5) also because
there is a more higher increase of free E2, for balancing T effects.

Since the levels of albumin and other plasma proteins were unaffected by danazol therapy
(8), the most probable cause of SHBG decrease (5) is a direct specific inhibitory effect of
the drug on the epatic synthesis.

CONCLUSION.

This study point out also in postmenopausal women an high dose of g.1,2/die of danazol decreases SHBG serum levels by the same degree as in the premenopausal ones treated with a lower dose of mg 800/die. We confirm previous data that after 4 weeks of therapy SHBG achieves a new steady-state , by about 80% lower than basal levels. The most probable cause of this decrease seems a direct effect of the danazol on SHBG hepatic synthesis, beeing the degree of suppression not related to serum E2 and T levels nor to free E2 and free T index.

REFERENCES

1) Laurell C.B., Rannevik G. (1979). A comparison of plasma protein changes induced by danazol, pregnancy, and estrogens. J.Clin.Endocrinol.Metab., 49, 719.
2) Meldrum D.R., Pardridge W.M., Karow W.G., Rivier J., Vale W., Judd H.L. (1983). Hormonal effects of danazol and medical oophorectomy in endometriosis. Obst.Gyn., 62,480.
3) Nilsson B., Sodergard R., Damber M..-G., Damber J.-E., von Schoultz B. (1983). Free testosterone levels during danazol therapy. Fert.Ster., 39, 505.
4) Schwart S., Tappeiner G., Hinter H. (1981). Hormone binding globulin levels in patients with angio-oedema during treatment with danazol. J. Endocrinol. 14,563.
5) Gershagen S. Doberl A., Rannevik G. (1984). Changes in the SHBG concentration during danazol treatment. Acta Obst.Gyn.Scand. Suppl. 123, 117.
6) Evers J.L.H., Menheere P.P.C.A. (1986). The effects of danazol and gestrinone on serum androgen levels. XII World Congr.Fert.Ster., Singapore 26-31/10.
7) Bevan J.R., Dowsett M., Jeffcoate S.L. (1984). Endocrine effects of danazol in the treatment of endometriosis. Brit.J.Obst.Gyn., 91, 160.
8) Damber M.G., Damber J.E., Nilsson B., von Schoultz B., Sodergard B. (1984). Danazol displacement of testosterone and influence on free testosterone levels. Acta Obst.Gyn. Scand. suppl.123, 115.
9) Forbes K.L., Dowsett M., Rose G.L., Mudge J.E., Jeffcoate S.L. (1986) : Dose related effects danazol on sex hormone-binding globulin and free and total androgens levels. *Clin.Endocrin. 25,suppl.5,597-605.*
10) Telimaa S., Apter D., Reinila M., Ronnberg L., Kauppila A. (1990). Placebo-controlled comparison of hormonal and biochemical effects of danazol and high-dose medroxypro-gesterone acetate. Europ.J.Obst.Gyn.Reprod.Biol., 36, 97.
11) Mancini A., Fiumara C., Conte G. et Al. (1992): Plasma SHBG and IGF-1 concentrations in pre and post-menopausal women with benign breast disease. in Genazzani A.R. et Al. (Eds) *"Recent developments in Gynecological Endocrinology" pp. 517-22 - Casterton Hall UK, Parthenon Publishing Group.*
12) Rigano A., Panama S., Sturlese E., Gallippi G., Romeo F., Iuele R., Pullè C. (1992). Receptor status in endometrial cancer after danazol therapy alone and plus a-interferon an immunohistochemical study. in Genazzani A.R. et Al. (eds) *Recent developments in Gynecological Endocrinology,* pp. 454-460. (Casterton Hall, UK: Parthenon Publishing Group).
13) Rigano A., Pullè C. (1992). hormonal therapy on endometrial cancer - Current pro-blems and future development. in Genazzani A.R. et Al. (eds) *Recent development in Gynecological Endocrinology,* pp. 469-474. (Casterton Hall, UK: Parthenon Publishing Group).
14) Rigano A.,Pullè C., Panama S., Sturlese E., Gallippi G., Romeo F., Iuele R. (1993). Effects of middle-term therapy with a2-b interferon, danazol and MPA as single drug and in sequential mode on receptor status of endometrial cancer. in Genazzani A.R. et Al. (eds) *Current Investigations in Gynecology and Obstetrics,* pp 421-426 (Casterton Hall, UK: Parthenon Publishing Group).

15) Brenner P.F., Guerrero R., Cekan Z., Diczfalusy E. (1973): Radioimmunoassay method for six steroids in human plasma. *Steroids, 22,775.*

16) Wilne J.J., Utley D.J. (1987): Total testosterone free-androgen index, calculated free testosterone, and free testosterone by analog RIA compared in hirsute women and in otherwise normal women with altered sex-hormone binding globulin. *Clinical Chemistry 33, 1372-75.*

17) Nilsson B.,Sodegard R., Damber M-G., von Schoultz B. (1982). Danazol and gestagen displacement of testosterone and influence on sex-hormone-binding globulin capacity. *Fert. Ster., 38,48.*

Ploidy in endometrial carcinoma

M. Melpignano, M. Brusati, C. Merisio, L. Sansebastiano, M. Fontanesi,
A. Merialdi and E. Vadora*

*Department of Obstetrics and Gynecology and *Department of Pathology,
University of Parma, Italy*

INTRODUCTION

Endometrial carcinoma is the most common gynecological malignancy in Italy, where about 5,000 new cases are annually registered (1).

About 1,700 women eventually die of this tumor, not only for advanced stage of the disease, but also because of an unpredictable adverse evolution in a fraction of low stage and grade cases (1,2).

In recent years, a lot of research has been carried out in the attempt to identify the tumors at high risk of recurrence, where a more aggressive therapeutic approach may be used.

Many biologic factors have been investigated in the attempt to predict the tumoral behaviour. At present ,the DNA content is one of the most studied factors, and many reports support its potential role in predicting the clinical outcome in endometrial carcinoma.

The aims of this study are as follows: (1) to investigate the relationship between ploidy and other pathologic parameters, and (2) to analyse the impact of these factors on the clinical outcome of the disease.

MATERIALS AND METHODS

One hundred-one consecutive cases of endometrial carcinoma, observed in the Department of Obstetrics and Gynecology, University of Parma, between January 1989 and April 1994, were studied. Patients'age ranged from 40 to 89 years, with a median of 64 years.

All patients underwent primary surgery, that consisted in a total abdominal hysterectomy with bilateral salpingo-oophorectomy and staging laparotomy in 92 cases, while the remaining 9 patients were submitted to a vaginal hysterectomy.

In order to measure the ploidy, a suspension of tumor cells was obtained using the mincing tecnique. Every sample was then treated with RNAse and Propidium Iodide (PI) solution. The DNA analysis was performed with a flow cytometer FACSCAN (Becton-Dickinson), equipped with an Argon laser. The emission maxima light of fluorescent nuclei stained by PI was detected at 639 nm. As DNA diploid standard, human lymphocytes were used. The histograms were based on a measurement of about 30,000 cells. Every pattern different from diploid was categorized as aneuploid.

Follow-up data were available for all the 101 patients: the median of follow-up was of 35 months (ranged 6 to 73 months).

Statistical analysis.

The chi square test and, when appropriate, the Fisher's exact test were employed for the analysis of the relationship between ploidy and pathological parameters. The curves were computed by the Lifetest Procedure SAS (Kaplan-Meier method) and statistically analyzed using the Log-rank and the Wilcoxon's rank test.

These analyses were performed by statistical software of the SAS System.

RESULTS

Twenty-two (21.7%) out of 101 tumors showed an aneuploid and 79 (78.2%) a diploid pattern.

All cases were evaluable for surgical stage, depth of myometrial invasion, grading and histotype: the aneuploidy frequency according to these parameters is shown in table I.

Tab.1 Ploidy according to pathological parameters

Pathological parameters		DNA Index		p
		diploid (%)	aneuploid (%)	
Stage	I-II	66 (79.5)	17 (20.4)	0.71
	III-IV	13 (72.2)	5 (27.7)	
Myom invasion	<1/2	47 (74.6)	16 (25.4)	0.37
	>1/2	32 (84.2)	6 (15.8)	
	G1	13 (86.6)	2 (13.3)	
Grading	G2	49 (77.7)	14 (22.2)	0.64
	G3	17 (73.9)	6 (26.0)	
Hystotipe endometrioid		79 (79.7)	20 (20.2)	0.06
unfavourable		0	2 (100)	

Regarding FIGO stage, aneuploidy was found in 17 out of 83 early cancers (stage I-II) (20.4%) and in 5 out of 18 advanced cancers (stage III-IV) (27.7%).

When the tumor involved the inner half of myometrium the incidence of aneupoloidy was 25.4% (16/63) and 15.8% (6/38) when the outer half was involved.

Aneuploidy recurred in 13.3% (2/15) of well-differentiated tumors, 22.2% (14/63) of moderately differentiated and in 26% (6/23) of poorly differentiated.

However, these differences never reached the statistical significance.

The two cases with unfavourable histotype were both aneuploid.

Concerning follow-up data, there were 12 recurrences and 9 of them died. The recurrence rate was 22.7% (5/22) for the aneuploid and 8.8% (7/79) for the diploid cancers. Among the twelve patients who had a recurrence, 4 (33%) had a stage I disease, two of them were aneuploid and two diploid tumors.

The statistical analysis demonstrated that the disease free survival rate was significantly related with stage,grade and ploidy (Fig.1,2,3), while the depth of myometrial invasion failed to show any prognostic value. If we consider only the stage I tumors the disease free survival rate was not related to grade and the depth of myometrial invasion but only to ploidy (Fig.4).

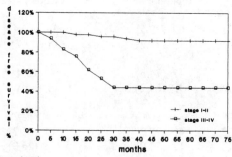

Fig.1 estimated curve according to
stage: all stages

Wilcoxon (p<0.01)
Log-rank (p<0.01)

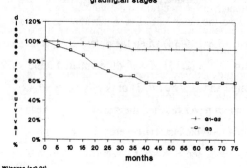

Fig.2 estimated curve according to
grading:all stages

Wilcoxon (p<0.01)
Log-rank (p<0.01)

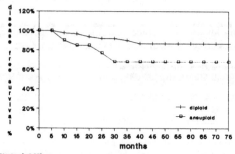

Fig.3 estimated curve according to
ploidy: all stages

Wilcoxon (p<0.05)
Log-rank (p<0.05)

Fig.4 estimated curve according to ploidy: stage I

Wilcoxon (p<0.05)
Log-rank (p<0.05)

DISCUSSION

Recently, many authors have investigated the prognostic value of ploidy in gynecological malignancies, often in a retrospective way.

With regards to endometrial cancer, it has been shown that approximately one-third is aneuploid (3), ranging from 11% (4) to 44% (5).

In our series the aneuploidy prevalence was 22%, comparable to the results of other studies, and the DNA content was not related to surgical stage, grade nor myometrial invasion.

The results discrepancy can be partially explained with the DNA heterogeneity within the same tumor as well as the contamination of the specimens from non-neoplastic tissues. In fact the histologic evaluation of endometrial carcinomas often identifies areas with different degrees of differentiation (6) and the ploidy analysis sometimes shows a diploid and aneuploid pattern in the same tumoral lesion (7). Regarding the ploidy prognostic value, many studies (8-11) found the aneuploidy an independent prognostic indicator of adverse clinical outcome. Mainly, some authors have stressed the presence of aneuploidy in early stage endometrial cancer which have recurred (12-17).

In our analysis the surgical stage, the grading and the ploidy were significantly related to disease free survival rate, while the depth of myometrial invasion failed to show any prognostic value. Recurrences and deaths were significantly related only to tumoral ploidy if we consider only the stage I cancers.

Although these results could be affected by the small number of adverse events occurred in our study, probably due to a too short follow-up period, it is remarkable that the surgical stage is the best predictor of survival.

Regarding ploidy, new data are necessary to assess its prognostic role.

At present, in our opinion it is still too hazardous to tailor the endometrial carcinoma treatment according to ploidy as previously proposed by some authors (14,18).

This work was supported in part of by funds from the Ministero della Pubblica Istruzione

REFERENCES

1. Zanelli R, Crosignani P, eds. Cancer in Italy. Incidence data from cancer registries 1983-87. Torino: Silvestrelli e Cappelletto, 1992
2. Boronow R.C. (1976). Endometrial cancer: not a benign disease. *Obstet. Gynecol.*, **47**, 630-5.
3. Burghardt E, editor Surgical Gynecologic Oncology Thieme Medical Publishers, 1993
4. Oud PS, Reubsaet-Veldhuizen JAM, Beck HLM(1986).DNA and nuclear protein measurement in columnar epithelial cells of human endometrium. *Cytometry*, 7, 325-30.
5. Quillamor RM, Furlong JW, Hoschner JA, Wynn RM. (1986). Relative prognostic significance of DNA flow cytometry and histologic grading in endometrial carcinoma. *Gynecol. Obstet. Invest.* , **26**, 332-7.
6. Mortel R, Zaino RJ, Satyaswaroop PG. (1984).Heterogeneity and progesterone receptor distribution in endometrial adenocarcinoma. *Cancer* , **53**, 113-6.
7. Ikeda M, Watanabe Y, Nanjoh T, Noda K.(1993). Evaluation of DNA ploidy in endometrial cancer. *Gynecol. Oncol.*, **50**, 25-9.
8. Britton LC, Wilson TO, Gaffey TA, Lieber MM, Wieand HS, Prodratz KC. (1989). Flow cytometric DNA analysis of stage I endometrial carcinoma. *Gynecol. Oncol.*, **34**, 317-22.
9. Britton LC, Wilson TO, Gaffey TA, Cha SS, Wieand HS, Prodratz KC. (1990). DNA ploidy in endometrial carcinoma: major objective prognostic factor. *Mayo Clin.Proc.*, **65**, 643-50.
10. Symonds DA. (1990). Prognostic value of pathologic features and DNA analysis in endometrial carcinoma. *Gynecol. Oncol.*, **39**, 272-6.
11. Iversen OE, Utaaker E, Skaarland E. (1988). DNA ploidy and steroid receptors as predictorsof disease course in patients with endometrial carcinoma. *Acta Obstet. Gynecol. Scand.* , **67**, 531-7.
12. Lindahl B, Alm P, Ferno M. (1989). Prognostic value of steroid receptor concentration and flow-cytometric DNA measurement in stage I-II endometrial carcinoma. *Acta Oncol.*, **28**, 595-9.
13. Lurain JR, Rice BL, Rademaker AV, Poggensee L, Schink J, Miller D. (1991). Prognostic factors associated with recurrence in clinical stage I adenocarcinoma of the endometrium. *Obstet. Gynecol.* , **78**, 63-9.

14. Melchiorri C, Chieco P, Lisignoli G, Marabini A, Orlandi C. (1993). Ploidy disturbances as an early indicator of intrinsic malignancy in endometrial carcinoma *Cancer* , **72**, 165-72.
15. Rosenberg P, Wingren S, Simonsen E, Stal O, Risberg B, Nordenskjold B. (1989). Flow citometric measurements of DNA index and S-phase on paraffin-embedded early stage endometrial cancer: an important prognostic indicator. *Gynecol. Oncol.*, **35**, 50-4.
16. van der Putten HWHM, Baak JPA, Koenders TJM, Kurver PHJ, Stolk HG, Stolte LAM. (1986). Prognostic value of quantitative pathologic features and DNA content in individual patients with stage I endometrial adenocarcinoma. *Cancer* , **63**, 1378-87.
17. Newbury R, Schuerch C, Goodspeed N, Fanning J, Glidewell O, Evans M. (1990). DNA content as a prognostic factor in endometrial carcinoma. *Obstet. Gynecol.*, **76**, 251-7.
18. Susini T, Rapi S, Savino L, Boddi V, Berti P, Massi G.(1994). Prognostic value of flow cytometric deoxyribonucleic acid index in endometrial carcinoma: comparison with other clinical-pathologic parameters. *Am .J. Obstet. Gynecol.*, **170**, 527-34.

Hormonal pattern after high-dose danazol therapy in postmenopausal women with endometrial cancer

A. Rigano, G. Baviera, E. Sturlese, M. Rigano and C. Pullè

Department of Gynecology, University of Messina, Italy

INTRODUCTION

It is common knowledge that danazol has an antigonadotropic and antiestrogen effect in premenopausal women, but there are conflicting reports concerning the serum hormonal pattern during or after danazol therapy. These variables results appear to be due to several factors: different dose regimens, different lenght of therapy, different phase of the menstrual cycles when therapy started, consequently data hardly can be compared.

For instance, concerning the gonadotropins, some Authors point out no changes in serum level (1,2,3,4,5,6,), others have observed the decrease of both gonadotropins (7,8) or LH decrease and FSH increase (9) or FSH unchanged and LH increase (10), or also increase of both FSH and LH (11). Moreover LH release pulses appear significantly changed (1, 2, 9,11,12).

Related to female steroid hormones, E2 clearly decreases (2,3,4,5,8,11, 12, 13, 14, 15, 16, 17) or doesn't change or has little decrease (6,12); Pg basal levels appear low and don't surge in the luteal phase (2,4,5,7,12). Data concerning androgens serum levels show DHEAS little increase (18, 19) or no change (4) while DHEA and A4 are low (10, 18, 19, 20); total T serum levels have been found low (10,19, 20,) or, on the contrary, high (18,21), but increased T levels could be unreliable because danazol cross-reactivity in RIA witout prealable chromatographic extration (18, 22, 23).

Studies of the effects of danazol on serum level of some hormones in postmenopausal women (24,25,26) have shown a constant decrease of both gonadotropins and no changes in E2 (25) or PRL (24) but no studies have been done on other hormones.

So the aim of this study is to investigate the behaviour of gonadotrophic hormones - FSH, LH, - ovarian ones - E2, fE2, 17OH-Pg, Pg - and androgens - T, fT, D4 A, DHEAS - after a short term danazol therapy, at very high dose, g.1,2 / die x 28, in postmenopausal women..

This protocol, among others, has been selected for other purpose, namely for enhancing PR in endometrial cancer. After several attempts, the best response on PR increase was achieved with this high dose for 21-28 days, as some of us have reported in previous papers (27,28,29). Then, investigations on the hormonal effect of danazol therapy, at higher dose than previous ones, in postmenopausal women appears to us very interesting, related to the new employements of this drug in some gynaecological disease. Moreover, in this study, the absence of cyclic feedback control of gonadotropins secretion, can contribute to a better knowledge of the so-called antigonadotropic action of danazol.

MATERIAL and METHODS

MATERIAL : 16 postmenopausal women affected by endometrial cancer were treated, before surgey, with danazol - g.1,2 / die (mg 400 x 3) x 4 weeks.

SUBJECT'S CHARACTERISTICS
- age mean 66,43 ± SD 8,62 years (range 57-78)
- years from menopausa : n = 15 : mean 16,83 ± SD 6,7 plus one within 1 year
- BMI: n = 5 < 24,9; n = 8 <29,9; n = 2 < 39,9; n = 1 > 40
- BS : n = 5 =/< 1,6; n = 7 < 1,8; n = 3 < 1,9; n = 1 > 2,1
- all but one multipara

ENDOMETRIAL CANCER
- stage : n = 9 stage 1 a-b ; n = 7 stage 2 a
- grading : G 1-2
- receptor's status : 14 / 16 ER "+"
                       9 / 16 PR "+"

METHODS : 3 blood samples, at 8 at 8,20 and at 8,40 a.m., were dawn before treatment and the day after the end of therapy. The samples were centriuged and serum was stored at -20 C° until analysis. LH and FSH were measured by IRMA ; tE2, Pg, 17-OH-Pg, tT, DHEAS, A-4 by RIA, all commercial kits ; free E2 and free T have been calculated as free index (FEI and FTI) (30). Chromatography on celite microcolumn (31) was performed before tT RIA for avoiding danazol cross-rectivity. Serum values of each patient are the average of the 3 drawings. All values are expressed as mean ± SE. Significance of differences among mean basal values and after therapy was tested by unpaired t-test for all hormones.

RESULTS

Basal and after danazol therapy values (mean ± SE) are summarized below.

	basal values	after danazol
LH (n=11) : U.I./l	51,3 ±6,32	44,7 ±5,25
FSH (n=11) U.I./l	76,4 ±10,5	61,37 ±10,039
tE2 (n=12) nmol/l	40,4 ±6,02	25,5 ±9,86
Pg (n=13) nmol/l	0,47 ±0,083	0,56 ±0,231
17OH-Pg (n=13) ng/ml	0,79 ±0,23	1,04 ±0,667
tT (n=12) nmol/l	1,45 ±0,34	0,92 ±0,32
DHEAS (n=11) ng/ml	829,08 ±163,98	850,77 ±180,61
A-4 (n=13) ng/ml	2,595 ±0,27	2,228 ±0,309
FEI (n=12)	0,93 ±0,13	2,87 ±1,15
FTI (n=12)	0,033 ±0,012	0,069 ±0,031

After 4 weeks g. 1,2 / die danazol therapy, the mean gonadotropin's levels are decreased LH by 13% and FSH by 19% (fig. 1), but FSH values result from a vider range; ovarian hormones have variable changes: t E2 decreases by 36% while Pg increases by 20% and 17-OH Pg by 32%. Also androgens have variable answer to danazol: tT clearly decreases by 36% , while DHEAS and A-4

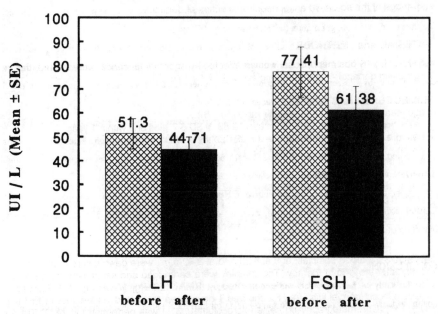

LH and FSH before and after danazol

fig.1 - Changes on serum levels of gonadotropic hormones - LH and FSH -
after danazol therapy, g.1,2 / die x 28.
LH decreases by 13% and FSH by 19%. Differences have no statistical
significance by unpaired t-test (LH: P= 0,432 - FSH: P= 0,314)

practically doesn't change. The differences of the mean serum values of each hormon between before and after danazol therapy, tested by unpair t-test, don't have statistical significance.

Free E2 and free T, calculated as free index,   have instead a strong increase after danazol therapy, as shown by FEI over 200% and FTI by over 100 %, differences of high statistical significance (P< 0,05).

DISCUSSION

In postmenopausal women, g.1,2 / die danazol therapy for 28 days caused changes in hormonal pattern. First, there it is a moderate decrease of gonadotropic hormones in all subjects, slightly greater for FSH. Since danazol has be found to reduce the gonadotropins pulse frequency (1,7,9,10) and to reduce the response to GnRH test (7, 24, 26), the decrease of FSH and LH, in absence of steroidal feedbak control in postmenopausal women, means that danazol has a specific antigonadotropic effect, acting directly   at hypophiseal level slowing down secretion and , maybe also synthesis, of the gonadotropins.

Second, danazol decreases mean values of E2 by 36%. Since in postmenopausal women ovarian estrogen synthesis is about quite absent, the fall of E2 serum levels is due to the increased clearance rate (32,33) and to the decrease of the peripheral conversion ratio of E1 to E2 (35). Some Authors (10,19) point out danazol causes a block of sulphatase activity, wich diminishes the conversion ratio of E1S to E1 and consequently E1 serum levels are low also in postmenopausal women (34), and, moreover, also some block of 17-beta steroid dehydrogenase (6) with reduced conversion of E1 to E2 (35). So, the E2 decrease is likely due to a sum of several factors. Our data are not completely agreed with the above quoted study (25), in wich E2 doesn't change, but it is very likely that with the higher dose of danazol we have used, we have got different effects than with 800 mg/ die.

Third, danazol decreases mean values of T and our data are agreed with those in premenopausal women. It is very likely that this fall is due at least to two factors: a lesser ovarian synthesis, either by direct effect or by a lesser stimulative action owing to a decreased LH serum levels, and to an increased metabolic clearance rate, caused by displacement of T from SHBG.

Fourth, we have found danazol increase free sex steroids serum levels: the estimated index as FTI for testosterone is increased by 100% and as FEI for E2 by over 200%. These high values are the results of a marked fall of SHBG by about 80% of basal values, as we have shown in previous paper (36), and, moreover, of the ability of danazol to displace sex steroids from SHBG.

Finally, other androgens of adrenal source, DHEAS and A-4, practically don't change, pointing out danazol doesn't impair adrenal function, even if danzol has be found (10, 37) to cause a slight inhibition of adrenal steroidogenesis.

CONCLUSION

In this study we have provided evidence that danazol therapy, at very high dose - g.1,2/die x 21-28, in postmenopausal women has about the same effects on hormonal pattern than in premenopausal women treated with a lesser dose, 600-800 mg/ die. It is worthy to note the constant decrease of mean serum level of FSH, LH, E2 and T. even if the difference among basal values and after therapy have no statistical significance.

REFERENCES

1) Dmowski W.P., Headley S., Dodwanska E. (1983). Effects of danazol on pulsatile gonado-tropin pattern and serum levels in normally cycling women. *Fert.Ster.,39,49.*
2) Telimaa S., Apter D., Reinila M., Ronnberg L., Kauppila A. (1991). Placebo-controlled comparison of hormonal and biochemical effect of danazol and high-dose medroxyproge-sterone acetate. *Eur.J.Obst.Gyn.Reprod.Biol. (NL), 36,97.*
3) Mauris P., Dowsett M., Rose G., Edmonds D.K., Rothwell C., Robertson W.R. (1990). The effect of danazol and LHRH agonist analogue goserelin (zoladex) on the biological activity of luteinizing hormone in women with endometriosis. *Clin.Endocrin.(England), 33,539.*
4) Chimbira T.H., Anderson A.B.M., Cope E., Turnbull A.C. (1980). Effect of danazol on se-rum gonatrophins and steroid hormone concentration in women with menorrhagia. *Brit.J. Obst.Gyn., 87,330.*
5) Kokko E., Janne O., Kauppila A., Ronnberg L., Vihko R. (1982). Danazol has progestin-like actions on the human endometrium. *Acta Endocrin. 99, 588.*
6) Barbieri R.L., Ryan K.J. (1980). Danazol: endocrine pharmacology and therapeutic appli-cations. *Am.J.Obst.Gyn., 141, 453.*

7) Leyendecker G., Wildt L., Braun P.(1985). The effect of danazol on pulsatile release, basal LH and FSH serum levels, biphasic feedback of oestradiol and GnRh induced gonatotropin release. in Baum M et Al. (eds) " *Benign Breast Disease*" - Royal Med.International Congress and Symp. , series No 76, pp 83-84.

8) Rannevik G., Thorell J.I. (1984). The influence of danazol on pituitary function and on the ovarian follicular hormone secretion in premenopausal women. *Acta Obst.Gyn.Scand., suppl..123, 89.*

9) Mauris P., Dowsett M., Edmonds D.K., Sullivan D. (1991). The effect of danazol *Fert.Ster., 55, 890.*

10) Steingold K.A., Lu J.K.H., Judd H.L., Meldrum D.R. (1986). Danazol inhibits steroidogenesis by human ovary in vivo. *Fert.Ster. 45,649.*

11) Bevan J.R., Dowsett M., Jeffcoate S.L.. (1984). Endocrine effect of danazol in the treatment of endometriosis. *Brit.J.Obst.Gyn., 91,160.*

12) Hickok L.R., Burry K.A., Cohen N.L., Moore D.E., Dahl K.d., Soules M.R. (1991). Medical treatment of endometriosis: a comparison of the suppressive effects of danazol and nafarelin on reproductive hormones. *Fert.Ster.,56, 622.*

13) Adamyan L.V., Fanchenko N.D., Alexeyeva Y.N., Novikov Y.A., Jahan I. (1993). Hormonal and immunologic methods in the diagnosis and treatment of patients with benign ovarian tumors and endometriotic cysts. *Int.J.Fert., 38,92.*

14) Rock J.A., Truglia J.A., Caplan R.J. (1993). Zoladex (goserelin acetate implant) in the treatment of endometriosis: a randomized comparison with danazol. The zoladex endometriosis study group. *Obst.Gyn., 82,198.*

15) Wood G.P., Wu C., Flickinger G.L., Mickail G. (1975). Hormonal changes associated with danazol therapy. *Obst.Gyn, 45,302.*

16) Floyd W.S. (1980). Danazol: endocrine and endometrial effects. *Int.J.Fert.,25,75.*

17) Meldrum D.R., Partdridge W.M., Karow W.G., Rivier J., Vale W., Judd H.L. (1983). Hormonal effects of danazol and medical oophorectomy in endometriosis. *Obst.Gyn., 62,480.*

18) Murakami K., Nakagawa T., Yamashiro G., Araki K., Akasofu K. (1993). Levels of androgens and danazol metabolites in serum during danazol therapy. *Fert.Ster., 60,179.*

19) Carlstrom K., Doberl A., Gershagen S., Rannevik G.(1984). Periferal levels of dehydroepiandrosterone sulfate, dehydroepiandrosterone, androstenedione, and testosterone following different doses of danazol. *Acta Obst.Gyn.Scand., suppl.123.*

20) Rannevik K.G.: Hormonal effects of danazol. (1987). in Wood C. ed. " *Benign breast disease*", London: Roy.Soc.Med.Serv., pg.93-99.

21) Evers J.L.H., Menheere P.P.C.A. (1986): The effects of danazol and gestrinone on serum androgen levels. *12° World Congress Fert.Ster.,* Singapore 26-31/10.

22) Nilsson B., Sodergard R., Damber M., Damber J., von Schoultz B. (1983). Free testosterone levels during danazol therapy. *Fert.Ster., 39,505.*

23) Schindler A.E.: Danazol for benign breast disease. (1988). *I° Intern.CongressSoc.Gyn. Endocrin.,* Crans Montana (CH), !0-14/3/1988.

24) Franchimont P., Cramilion C.(1977). The effect of danazol on anterior pituitary function. *Fert. Ster.28,714.*

25) Doberl A., Jeppsson S., Rannevik G. (1984). Effect of danazol on serum concentrations of pituitary gonadotropins in postmenopausal women. *Acta Obst.Gyn.Scand. suppl.123, 95, 1984.*

26) Cagnacci A., Melis GB., Paoletti AM., Soldani R., Fioretti P. (1991). Thermoregulatory effects of low dose of danazol in postmenopausal women: interaction with the effect of naloxone. *Life Science, 48, 1051.*

27) Rigano A., Panama S., Sturlese E. et Al.: (1992). Receptor status in endometrial cancer after danazol therapy alone and plus a-interferon.: an immunohistochemical study. in Genazzani A R. et Al. (eds). *Recent developmentin Gynaecological Endocrinology,* pp. 454-60 - (Casterton Hall, UK: Parthenon Publishing Group).

28) Rigano A., Pullè C. (1992). Hormonal therapy on endometrial cancer - Current problems and future development. in Genazzani A.R. et Al. (eds) *Recent development in Gynaecological Endocrinology,* pp 469-74 - (Casterton Hall, UK: Parthenon Publishing Group).

29) Rigano A., Pullè C. et Al. (1993). Effects of middle-term therapy with a2-b interferon, danazol and MPA as single drug and in sequential mode on receptor status of endometrial cancer. in Genazzani A:R. et Al. (eds) *Current investigations in Gynecology and Obstetrics* pp. 421-26 (Casterton hall, UK : Parthenon Publishing Group).

30) Wilne J.J., Utley D.J. (1987). Total testosterone free-androgen index, calculated free testosterone and free testosterone by analog RIA compared in hirsute women and in otherwise normal women with altered sex-hormone binding globulin. *Clinical Chem.33,1372.*

31) Brenner P.F., Guerrero R., Cekan Z., Dicfalusy E. (1973). Radioimmunoassay method for
six steroids in human plasma. *Steroids, 22,775.*

32) Mc Ginley R., Casey J.H. (1979). Analysis of progesterone in unextracted serum: A
method using danazol - a blocker of steroid binding to proteins. Steroids,33,127.

33) Schwarz S., Hinter H., Tappeiner G. (1979). Endocrinological study in 4 patients with
hereditary angioneurotic edema before and during danazol therapy: Effects on sex
hormone binding globulin. Acta Endocrin. 91, 114.

34) James V.H., Ree M.J., Purohit A. (1992). Inhibition of oestrogen synthesis in postmenopausal women with breast cancer. J.Steroid.Biochem.Mol.Biol., 43,149.

35) Nguyen B.L., Ferme I., Chetrite G., Pasqualini J.R. (1993). Action of danazol on the
conversion of estrone sulfate to estradiol and on the sulfatase activity in the MCF-7,
T-47D and MDA-MB-231 human mammary cancer cells. J.Steroid Biochem.Mol.Biol.,
46,17.

36) Rigano A., Baviera G., Sturlese E., Rigano M., Pullè C. (1995). SHBG level changes after
danazol high-dose in postmenopausal women with endometrial cancer. In press.

37) Stillman R.J., Fencl M.D., Schiff I., Barbieri R.L., Tulchinsky D. (1980). Inhibition of adrenal steroidogenesis by danazol in vivo. Fert.Ster., 33,401.

Changes of hormone serum levels in endometrial adenocarcinoma after progestin therapy

A. Re, R. Bellino, M. Rosso*, M. Tessarolo, L. Leo, A. Lauricella, A. Venuti, T. Wierdis, G. Visca and A. Lanza

Department B of Gynecology and Obstetrics Institute, University of Turin and
*Department of Clinical Chemistry, S. Anna Hospital, Turin, Italy

INTRODUCTION

Endometrial cancer is the most frequent neoplasia of the genital tract. From the data of Piedmont Register of Tumors, not yet published and courteously given us, in Turin there were 302 endometrial cancer from 1985 to 1987 with a 5-year survival crude rate of 66.6%. In our previous studies (1,2) we showed that some hormones (Estradiol, Progesterone, FSH, LH) had statistically significative differences between a group of women with endometrial tumor and a control group.

In this study we report the results obtained from women with adenocarcinoma of endometrium and from a control group in whom Androgens and SHBG, not valued in our previous works, have been checked.

MATERIAL and METHODS

We studied 28 post-menopausal women with endometrial cancer and 27 post-menopausal women as a control group. In table 1 we report the clinical features of the two groups. All the patients had ovaries and did not take substitutive hormonal therapy or glycocorticoides. The patients with endometrial adenocarcinoma were selected among 189 women with the same cancer and treated in Department B of the Institute of Obstetrics and Gynecology, University of Turin, from January 1977 to December 1994.

The surgical treatment of all the patients with cancer of the endometrium was total abdominal hysterectomy, bilateral salpingo-oophorectomy, partial vaginectomy and bioptic selective paraaortic and pelvic lymphadenectomy. Before surgery the patients were treated with MPA (1 g per os) for 30

Table 1   Clinical characteristics of patients with endometrial adenocarcinoma and controls

	Patients (No28)	Controls (No27)	Patients vs Controls (p)
Age	64.4 ± 11.2	62.5 ±10.4	N.S.
BMI (Kg\m²)	29.63 ± 3.84	23.82± 2.41	N.S.
Age at menopause	51.4 ± 2.6	50.6 ± 1.2	N.S.
Years since menpause	12.8 ± 1.2	15.0 ± 2.3	N.S.
Age at menarche (yrs)	11.4 ± 3.1	12.6 ± 1.8	N.S.
No of pregnancies	2 (0 - 3)	2 (0 - 5)	N.S.
Weight (Kg)	64.2 ± 1.7	66.6 ± 1.9	N.S.
Height (cm)	156 ± 1.7	158 ± 1.5	N.S.

days. Twenty patients were stage I (G1), two stage IIA, three stage IIB (G2), and three stage IIIA (G3) according to FIGO. Tumor was well differentiated in 18 cases, moderately differentiated in 6, and scarcely differentiated in 4.

The 27 women of the control group underwent D & C for dysfunctional methrorragia.

Blood samples were taken in patients with cancer before and after progestin therapy while in the control group only before C and D.

Body mass index (BMI) was used as a measure of obesity and expressed in Kg of weight divided by body surface in m².

Cortisol, Estradiol, Progesterone, Prolactin, Dehydroepiandrosterone sulfate, Testosterone, Androstenedione, 17α-hydroxyprogesterone, and FSH have been determined by radioimmunoassay while SHBG by an immunoradiometric technique.

Our laboratory values of all these hormones are showed in table 2.

Student's, Fisher's, and Mantel's tests have been used in statistical analysis of data and we have considered significative a p value ≤ 0.05.

RESULTS

Patients and controls were similar in clinical and anthropometric features (tab.1). We found a difference in BMI in the two populations, even though not statistically significative, while no difference was showed in adipose tissue distribution (gynoid or android type). In table 2 all hormones are described. Cortisol, progesterone, and prolactin have similar values both in patients before and after MPA and in controls. 17β estradiol and DHEAS values are significantly higher in patients before progestin therapy than in control group, where as androstenedione, testosterone, and 17α hydroxyprogesterone are higher in patients than in controls even though not significantly. The decrease of SHBG in patients with endometrial tumor and its inverse relationship with BMI are statistically significative, while the decrease of FSH in patients before treatment is not.

Table 2 Serum hormone levels in patients with endometrial carcinoma (before and after progestin therapy) and controls

Serum hormone mean levels	Values	I Controls	II Patients before progestins therapy	I vs II P	III Patients after progestins therapy	II vs III P
Cortisol (nmol/l)	165.6-607.2	325 ±52	340 ±41	N.S.	195 ±39	0.001
E₂ (pmol/l)	91.75-146.8	38 ± 20	48 ±24	0.01	36.5± 7.8	N.S.
Pg (nmol/l)	0.477-1.43	1.1± 0.6	1.4± 0.8	N.S.	1.3± 0.4	N.S.
Prolactin (µg/l)	1.4-10	5 ± 1.4	5 ± 2.1	N.S.	5 ±1.4	N.S.
Testosterone(nmol/l)	0.69-3.47	1 ± 0.5	1.3± 0.9	N.S.	0.7±0.2	0.01
DHEA-S (nmol/l)	0.76-10.5	5.1± 2.3	8.5± 2.1	0.01	4.1±1.2	0.01
A₄ (nmol/l)	0.34-10.7	3.1± 1.1	3.9± 1.2	N.S.	1.9±1.8	0.01
17OH-Pg (nmol/l)	0.303-1.81	1.1± 0.1	1.6± 0.9	N.S.	1.2±0.8	N.S.
SHBG (nmol/l)	20-100	64.2±15.6	48.5±12.1	0.01	31.4± 5.2	0.001
FSH (U/l)	18-125	47.4± 4.8	34.8± 8.2	N.S.	13.5±4	0.001

E₂ = estradiol 17β; DHEA - S = dehydroepiandrosterone sulfate; A₄ = 4 - androstene - 3,17 - dione; 17OHPg = 17α - hydroxyprogesterone

After the 30-day progestin therapy cortisol, testosterone, DHEA-S, androstenedione, SHBG, and FSH significantly decrease while the other hormonal parameters do not show any significant variation.

Eighteen patients continued with MPA therapy for six months after surgery; in 70% of these cases 17β estradiol showed a decrease. Probably this represents the percentage of patients who belong to group I (according to WHO classification) hormone responsive adenocarcinoma.

DISCUSSION

Some Authors (9,10,11,12) have described the increase of E_2 value in patients with endometrial adenocarcinoma, while Others (13,14,15)have thought it to be only due to weight gain.

Our results show a significative increase of E_2 in patients with cancer as to control group, not evidenced in previous study (1).

Regarding to androgens metabolism, the different behaviours of SHBG level, which decreases in patients with cancer, and that of androgens which increases compared to those of the controls, confirm an inhibitory effect of androgens on SHBG production (16).

In patients with adenocarcinoma there is a trend toward a male-type hepatic metabolism of steroids and SHBG (12).

The significant inverse relationship between SHBG and BMI is possibly due to a hepatic inhibition of SHBG production that depends on hyperinsulinemia of obese women.

Obesity is probably the most important factor in SHBG regulation (12,17).

The effect of progestin therapy (MPA 1g daily per os for 30 days) can be explained as:

(a) a decrease of gonadotropins and basal cortisol, whose rhythm is unchanged (6);

(b) a decrease in total E_2 that is significative after a 6-months treatment (2);

(c) a decrease of testosterone, DHEA-S, and androstenedione.

MPA therapy works on three levels (18):

1. it blocks ovarian secretion by inhibiting pituitary production of gonadotropins (2);

2. it increses the metabolic clearance of androgens reducing their trasformation into estrogens (19,20);

3. it decreases the level of intracellular estradiol by its action on estradiol metabolism (2,5) that leads to physiologic cell life.

The decrease of SHBG is probably due to an inhibitory effect on hepatic globulin synthesis.

FSH reduction is important as prognostic factor. We studied the relationship between number of mitoses and FSH level with two different type of regression. With monofactorial regression (9) both differences in the number of mitoses and FSH levels were significantly associated with the frequency of relapses. With multifactorial regression the influence of FSH levels and number of mitoses showed that FSH reduction was the decisive factor in relapse prevention (21).

872

Treatment with MPA greatly interferes on hormonal asset and peripherical metabolism of estrogens in endometrial neoplastic cell (3,4,5), data that confirm and enhance what previously was evidenced, that is a decrease of gonadotropins (2) and of basal cortisol with a normal circadian rhythm (6,7,8).

Acknowledgment: the authors thank Pharmacia / Farmitalia Carlo Erba

REFERENCES

1. Agrimonti, F., Lanza, A., Fornaro, D. (1982). Valutazioni ormonali in donne portatrici di adenocarcinoma dell'endometrio e in donne normali di controllo. *Giorn. It. Oncol.*, **2**, 255

2. Renzetti, M. E., Lanza, A., Fedele, M. (1982). Parametri ormonali di donne con adenocarcinoma dell' endometrio in corso di terapia con medrossiprogesterone acetato e ad alte dosi. *Giorn. It. Oncol.*, **2**, 282

3. Pannuti, F., Giovannini, M., Fruet, F., Rubino, I., Pieromaldi, S., Vecchi, F., Zanichelli, L. (1980). Effects of hig dose oral Medroxyprogesterone acetate (MPA) on plasma levels of T3, T4, TSH, LH, FSH, PRL, 17 β estradiol, testosterone and aldosterone. *IRCS Med. Sci.*, **8**, 764

4. Sala, G., Castegnaro, E., Lenaz, G.R., Martoni, A., Piana, E., Pannuti, F. (1978). Hormone interference in metastatic breast cancer patients treated with Medroxyprogesterone acetate at massive doses: preliminary results. *IRCS Med. Sci.*, **6**, 129

5. Tseng, L., Gurpide, E. (1975). Induction of human endometrial estradiol dehydrogenase by progestins. *Endocrinolog* ,**97**, 825

6. Agrimonti, F., Frairia, R., Fornaro, D., Lanza, A., D'addato, F., Angeli, A. (1983). Circadian profile of plasma cortisol in patients with endometrial carcinoma before and during long term treatment with high-dose medroxyprogesterone acetate. *Chronobiologia*, **10**, 107

7. Lanza, A., Fedele, M., D'addato, F., Re, A., Olivero, F., Agrimonti, F., Gordini, G., Arisio, R. (1985). Effetti ormonali e istologici della terapia pre-operatoria con medrossiprogesterone acetato (MPA) : criteri di ammissione all'ormonoterapia in pazienti affette da adenocarcinoma dell' endometrio. *Giorn. It. Oncol.* **5**, 115

8. Lanza, A., Agrimonti, F., D'addato, F., Olivero, F., Fedele, M., Re, A. (1985). Reattività ipotalamo-ipofisario in donne affette da adenocarcinoma dell' endometrio prima e dopo trattamento con medrossiprogesterone acetato ad alte dosi per via orale. *Giorn.It. Oncol.* **5**, 159

9. Benjamin, F., Deutisch, S. (1976). Plasma levels of fractionated estrogens and pituitary hormones in endometrial carcinoma. *Am. J. Obstet. Ginecol.*, **126**, 638-647

10. Petterson, B., Bergstrom, R., Joansson, E. (1986). Serum estrogens and androgens in women with endometrial cancer. *Ginecol. Oncol.* **25**, 223-233

11. Nyholm, H.C.J., Nielsen, A.L., Lyndrup, J., Dreisler, A., Haug, E. (1993). Plasm oestrogens in postmenopausal women with endometrial cancer. *Br. J. Obstet. Gynecol.*, **100**, 1115-19

12. Möllerström, G., Carlstrom, K., Lagrelius, A., Einhorn, N. (1993). Is there an Altered Steroid Profile in Patients with Endometrial Carcinoma ? *Cancer*, **72**, 173-81

13. MacDonald, P.C., et al. (1978). Effect of obesity on conversion of plasma androstenedione to oestrone in postmenopausal women with and without endometrial cancer. *Am. J. Obstet. Gynecol.*, **130**, 448 - 455

14. Nisker, J. A., et al. (1980). Serum sex hormone binding globulin capacity and the percentage of free estradiol in postmenopausal women with and without endometrial carcinoma. *Am. J. Obstet. Gynecol.*, **138**, 637-642

15. Judd, H., et al. (1980). Serum androgens and estrrogens in postmenopausal women with and without endometrial cancer. *Am. J. Obstet. Gynecol.*, **136**, 859-871.

16. Maggino, T., Pirrone, F., Velluti, F., Bucciante, G. (1993). The role of the endocrine factors and obesity in hormone dependent gynecological neoplasias. *Eur. J. Gynaecol. Oncol.*, XIV, 2, 119

17. Von Schoultz, B., Carlstrom, K. (1989). On the regulation of sex-hormone-binding globulin: a challenge of an old dogma and outlines of an alternative mechanism. *J. Steroid. Biochem.* **32**, 327-34

18. Gurpide, E., (1976). *Cancer*, **38** (suppl.), 504.

19. Gordon, G.G., Altman, K., Southren, A. L., Olivo, J. (1971). Human hepatic testosterone A-ring reductase activity. Effect of medroxyprogesterone acetate. *J. Clin. Endocrinol. Metab.*, **32**, 457.

20. Lanza, A., Fedele, M., Di Gregorio, A., Gagna, G. (1980). trattamento con medrossiprogesterone acetato di un caso di ipersurrenalismo con adenocarcinoma dell'endometrio. *Min. Gin.*, **32**, 259.

21. Lanza , A., D'Addato, F., Re, A., Zardo, L., Vigezzi, P. A., Raspollini, M., Caldarola, B., Rocca, G., Proserpio, D., Ferraris, G.(1988). Hormonal and surgical treatment of endometrial adenocarcinoma: actuarial survival. *Eur J. Gynaecol. Oncol.* **9**, 209.

Cervical cancer treated at stage I and II: evolution and surveillance

N. Surico and G. Ferraris

University of Turin, Faculty of Medicine of Novara, Department of Medical Sciences, Clinic of Obstetrics and Gynaecology, Turin, Italy

A clinical staging of cervical cancer shows itself to be exact, by alone, largely only in pre-invasive and pre-clinical stages (STAGE 0 and STAGE IA) or in the advanced stages (STAGE III and STAGE IV).

In all the other cases, a staging made on the basis of clinical elements only, results often inexact or, even, wrong.

In fact, we are exposed to a great risk of making an under- or upper-staging thru diagnostic examinations, either clinical or imaging.

We can have a real outline of the situation at clinical stages IB and II   (re-staging and risk factors) only thru a surgical control and some related exames. The predictor risks of recidivation, as reported in litterature, are:

- lymphonodal metastasis
- cancer diameter > or = to 4 cm.
- cervical meshwork deep invasion
- capillary-like spaces invasion
- adverse histotype: adenocarcinoma and adenosquamous carcinoma
- very little differenciated carcinoma
- more advanced stages: vagina and/or parametrium invasion
- cancer diffusion to uterine corpus
- woman aged less than 35

These risk factors condition the cancer evolution, and consequently, an eventual comparision of recidivations, prospect of life and, at last, survival. All this will cause some differences in follow-up and in any eventual adjuvant complemental therapies. A recidivation entity risk conditions the frequency of clinical controls and the use of imaging. The result we obtained with surgery can be stabilized with any eventual complemental therapies: at the same time we'll be able to prolongue, at least, the survival and the disease free interval.

LYMPHONODAL METASTASIS

The main prognostic factor in women operated by cervical carcinoma at stages IB and II is the presence of lymphonodal metastasis, that can condition the comparision of eventual recidivation, and also affect on survival. Some factors, however, condition the cancer evolution itself. They are:
- Micrometastasis lymphonodal invasion
- Macrometastasis lymphonodal invasion with or without capsula   invasion
- Number of invaded lymphonodes
- Mono- or bilateral invasion
- Anatomical level of the invaded lymphonodes

Lymphonodal localizations are so divided:

Ist level: obturator fossa and external ileal vessels lymphonodes
IInd level : common ileal vessels and pre-sacral lymphonodes
IIIrd level: para-aortical lymphonodes

Recidivation frequency progressively increase so as the survival reduction.
In 10% of cases of our casistic we found "skip metastasis", metastasis with skip of lymphonodal stations and levels.
We have best prognosis and less severe conditions in case of:
  - micrometastasis
  - one and alone lymphonodal monolateral invasion
  - low level of invaded lymphonodes
We'll have worst prognosis in case of:
  - lymphonodal macrometastasis
  - overcoming of lymphonodal capsula
  - elevated number of involved lymphonodes
  - bilateral invasion
  - high level of involved lymphonodes
In case of surgical diagnosis of lymphonodal metastasis, transcutaneous radiant treatment doesn't improve the survival and it doesn't extend the disease free interval. In some cases with worst prognosis we can combine polichemotherapy to radiotherapy. We also don't have significant data about the results of this therapeutic association, because of the scantiness of cases.
We derive a diagnosis of disease reprise at lymphonodal level from:

  - clinical general and pelvic evaluation
  - ultrasonography
  - computed tomography
  - magnetic resonance imaging
  - tumoral markers use
  - diagnostic laparoscopy
  - explorative laparotomy

A clinical evaluation results significative only when we have:
  - bulky tumefactions
  - severe functional alterations
These elements will be also integrated by any elements deriving from more deep investigations. The imaging (ultrasonography, computed tomography, magnetic resonance) is limited by the resolution power and so, with these limits too, is, perhaps, more useful for diagnosis of extra-abdominal than abdominal recidivation.
Also tumoral markers are useful only when a recidivation is extended. More useful for diagnosis is laparoscopy, expecially associated to bioptic specimen, even if we obtain the best diagnostic-prognostic result, regarding disease, with explorative rilaparotomy.

TUMORAL EXTENSION: >4 cm.

In these cases, even if tumoral stage is IB, we have a higher frequency of lymphonodal metastasis and, so, of recidivation of the disease itself.
Actually, we use neo-adjuvant pre-surgery polichemotherapy (instead of pre- and post-surgery radiotherapy), which can considerably reduce the neoplastic tissue until its vanishing. We also cannot say if this treatment can better the survival.

DEEP CERVICAL STROMA INVASION UNTIL EXTERNAL THIRD; CAPILLARY LIKE SPACES INVASION EXTENSION TO PARAMETRIUM and/or VAGINA

The informations coming from surgery and successive hystological exames give us more precise data if related to the pre-surgery evaluations; even if we considered them one by one, they all are adverse prognostic elements, expecially if they are related to themselves: in fact, they are index of a greater risk of disease recurrence and of a survival reduction.

The invasion of the cervical stroma external third makes worse prognosis and it reduces patients survival percentage to 5 years (see Table 1).

Capillary like spaces invasion is a very unfavourable condition (see Table 2), but also the invasion of the vagina is a very unfavourable prognostic element (see Table 3). Parametrium neoplastic invasion is a heavy prognostic factor (see Table 4).

If we evaluate the survival comparing the associations of different elements, we can see that we observed the worst prognosis for survival in case of vaginal and cervical stroma external third invasion. We always prescribed a post-surgery transdermal radiant treatment when these risk factors (cervical stroma external third, capillary like spaces, parametrium and vagina invasion) are present, even without lymphonodal metastasis.

We recently began an adiuvant polichemotherapy trial versus radiotherapy with other Italian Institutes.

UNFAVOURABLE HYSTOTYPE

Actually, Adenocarcinoma became more frequent than Squamous Carcinoma, and it strikes women more younger than in the past: it also is a very aggressive clinical form.

We recently used a pre-surgery adiuvant polichemotherapy, expecially in the treatment of exophytical form and in more advanced cases: our aim was to make operable some severe cases. We can't also judge our results, but we're not satisfied.

POOR DIFFERENTIATED CARCINOMA

In 1989 we showed that there was a correlation between cell differentiation loss and deep cervical stroma invasion ($p=0,02$) and between cell differentiation loss and invasion along cervical canal ($p=0,002$). There are many points of view about the evaluation of metastasis increase and about prognosis and so we can't give our final opinion.

UTERINE CORPUS TUMORAL EXTENSION

For a long time, FIGO classification did not considerate the tumoral extension to the uterine corpus. In our experience, this factor involves a lymphonodal invasion risk of about 30%; there is a correlation between uterine corpus invasion and presacral lymphonodes invasion ($p<0,05$); a presacral lymphonodes invasion is a very severe prognostic element.

AGE LOWER THAN 35 YEARS

The age of patients doesn't play an important role about the frequency of risk factors appearence and disease reprise; in young woman we observed a more elevated frequency of largest tumors already at the first diagnostic impact. We however showed this fact even if we are not able to explain it.

SUMMARY

The Authors show that only surgery can give a sufficiently exact stadiation and a reliable prognostic evaluation.

Prognostic risk factors about cervicocarcinoma treated at stages I and II are:

a) lymphonodal metastasis b) tumoral diameter c) cervical stroma invasion d) capillary like spaces invasion e) hystotype f) no-differenciated carcinoma g) more advanced stages (vagina and/or parametrium invasion) h) uterine corpus tumoral invasion i) patient age

These risk factors are evaluated one to one and they're compared about their mutual differences.

TAB. 1

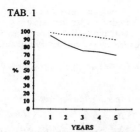

Survival related to cervical stroma external 3rd invasion:
continuous line: external 3rd NEGATIVE
broken line: external 3rd POSITIVE

TAB.2

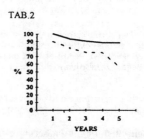

Survival related to capillary like spaces invasion:
continuous line: capillary like spaces NEGATIVE
broken line: capillary like spaces POSITIVE

TAB.3

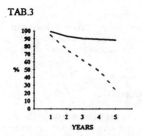

Survival related to vaginal invasion:
continuous line: vagina NEGATIVE
broken line: vagina POSITIVE

TAB.4

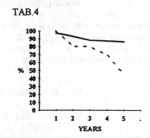

Survival related to parametrium invasion:
continuous line: parametrium NEGATIVE
broken line: parametrium POSITIVE

TAB.5

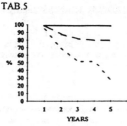

Cervicocarcinoma survival:
continuous line: vagina NEGATIVE, capillary like spaces NEGATIVE
cervical stroma external 3rd NEGATIVE
broken line: vagina NEGATIVE, capillary like spaces NEGATIVE
cervical stroma external 3rd POSITIVE
dotted line: vagina POSITIVE, cervical stroma external 3rd POSITIVE

REFERENCES

Ayhan a, Tuncer ZS, Kucukali t, Tuna T, Enunlu t
"Correlation between pathological risk factors and pelvic limph node metastases in stage I squamous carcinoma of the cervix: amultivariate analysis of 194 cases"
J Surg Onc, 48(3), 2077-209,1991

Alvarez RD, Potter ME, Soong SJ, Gayj FL, Hatch KD, Partridge EE, Shingleton HM
" Rationale for using pathologic tumor dimensions and nodal status to subclassify surgically treated stage IB cervical cancer patients"
Gynecol Oncol, 43(2), 108-112, 1991

Burke TW
" Factors affecting recurrence and survival in stage I carcinoma of the uterine cervix"
Oncology, 6(2), 111-116, 1992

Ferraris G, Andriani A, Leonardis A, Wierdis T
"L'isterectomia radicale secondo Wertheim con linfoadenectomia"
Ed. Minerva Medica, 1977

Ferraris G, Lanza A, Wierdis T, D'Addato F, Surico N, Re A, Olivero F
" Surgical staging in uterine cancer"
Proceeding of Inter Meeting of Gyn Oncology, Venice-Lido, April 1985, p. 276-284

Ferraris G, Lanza A, Re A, Raspollini M, Proserpio D, Bellino R
"The significance of the limph node status at pelvic, common iliac and paraortic levels"
Clin Obstet Gynecol, Bailliers, 2, 913, 1988

Heaps JM, Berek JS
"Surgical staging of cervical cancer"
Clin Obstet Gynaecol, 33(4), 852-862, 1990

Lanza A, Re A, D'Addato F, Morino M, Wierdis T, Caldarola B, Ferraris G
"Limph nodal metastase and the clinical stage of cervix carcinoma"
Eur J Gynaecol Oncol 8, 61-67, 1987

Malfitano JH, Keys H
"Aggressive multimodality treatment for cervical cancer with paraortic limph node metastases"
Gynaecol Oncol, 42(1), 44-47, 1991

Moore DH, Dotters DJ, Fowler WC
"Computed tomography: does it really improve the treatment of cervical carcinoma?"
Am J Obstet Gynaecol, 167(3), 768, 1992

Sironi S, Zanello A, Rodighiero MG, Vanzulli A, Taccagni GL, Belloni C, Del Maschio A
"Il carcinoma invasivo della cervice uterina (stadio IB-IIB) Confronto TC-RM nella valutazione del parametrio"
Radiol Med, 81 (5), 671-677, 1991

Smiley LM, Burke TW, Silva EG, Morris M, Gershenson DM, Warton JT
Prognostic factors in stage IB squamous cervical cancer patients with low risk of recurrence"
Obstet Gynaecol, 77(2), 271-275, 1991

Radical hysterectomy and pelvic lymphadenectomy for cervical cancer IB: a review of 72 cases

V. Vavalà, A. Monaco, M. Garizio and A. Scribanti

Ospedale Degli Infermi, Div. Ostetrico-Ginecologica, Biella, Italy

The Wertheim-Meigs radical hysterectomy is considered the most suitable operation for initial stage of cervical car_ cinoma.(1) After the experiences of Freund(2),Clark(3)and Reis(4),W ertheim in 1912 reported a series of 500 consecu_ tive cases of radical hysterectomy that included removal of the uterus with adjacent supporting tissues medial to the ureters and metastatic lynph nodes.(5) Currently this tecni_ que is classified as a type II of Piver-Rutledge.(6) In 1944 Meigs reported his radical hysterectomy technique(7) which included supporting tissues lateral to the ureters and pel_ vic lymphoadenectomy(not always practised by Wertheim): type III of Piver.

OUR METHODOLOGY

From january 1985 to december 1993,a total of 72 patients with stage IB cervical cancers underwent radical hysterecto_ my and pelvic lymphadenectomy. The pre-operative staging has provided: clinic examination(vaginal and rectal),histologi_ cal investigation,radiological investigation(CT and-or MR), cistoscopy. The abdomen is opened through a lower median incision that extends to the left at approximately five cm. above the umbilicus. We explore the liver,the right and the left para-colic gutter,the omentum,the stomac and the blad_ der. If during the operation the pre-operative staging is confirmed,we practise the Wertheim hysterectomy and pelvic lymphadenectomy. If we observe an under staging pre-operati_ ve of the cancer,we practise a larger radicality(Piver III) with particular attention at the prevention of morbility that this choice involved.

OUR DATA

From january 1985 to december 1993 a total of 72 patients
with stage IB cervical cancer underwent Wertheim radical
hysterectomy: clinic stage was confirmed in 93% of cases.
(tab.1)

```
I---------I----------I----------I----------I
I IB small I IB bulky I  IIA   I  OVER   I
     35         32         2        3
I---------I----------I----------I----------I
```

tab.1: pathologic stage of 72 patients with clinical stage
       IB.

Tumor grade,according to literature,showed statistical si_
gnificance for the prognosis.(8-9) The table 2 show our data
about tumor grade.

```
100 I
    I
    I                    G2 70%
    I                    I-----I
% 50 I                   I     I
    I                    I     I
    I                    I     I
    I       GI 16%       I     I       G3 14%
    I       I-----I      I     I       I-----I
  0 I-----I-----I-----I-----I-----I-----I-----I-----
```

        tab.2: tumor grade

Clinical stage of cervical cancer is important prognostic
factor.(1-11) In 1990 Bianchi(10) affirmed that the cell ty_
pes,with the condition of the lymph nodes,can show three
prognostic classes of patients with different five-yr survi_
val rate: R3 positive 56%,R2 negative nodes but unfavourable
cell types 83%,R1 negative nodes and favourable cell types
97.6% . Adenosquamous cell carcinoma is less frequent,but
often does nodal metastasis,like literature show(11-12-18)
although there's not according between the authors about
prognostic value of cell types(13-14-15-16). In our cases
cell types are these:(tab.3)

```
                    I
                    I       * 85%
                    I       I----I
squamous  *         I       I    I
adenoca.  +         I       I    I
adenosq.  ^         I       I    I
                    I       I    I
                 %  I       I    I
                    I       I    I
                    I       I    I    + 9%
                    I       I    I    I----I
                    I----I----I----I----I----I----I-----
                                            ^ 6%
```

        tab.3: cell types

Pelvic and paraortic nodal metastasis in cervical cancer is reported in all studies with different incidences.(17-18) In table 4 the AA.show the incidence of pelvic nodal meta_ stasis in the stage IB:

```
                              I------I
                              I IB   I
      I------------------------I------I
      I  Pelvic nodes +        I  15% I
      I------------------------I------I
```

    tab.4:lymph node metastasis

We practise postoperative irradiation to selected patients who have high-risk factors in the surgical speciment,such as poor histologic fiondings,tumor in the margins resection,po_ sitive pelvic lymph nodes and a primary lesion measures more than 4 cm. in size. Recurrence rate increase if there are nodal metastasis: IB 6.2 versus 36.7%.(19) The literature report a recurrence rate of 32.1% in stage IB with pelvic nodal metastasis.(11) In our cases, at the stage IB with no_ dal metastasis, we have registred three recurrences that ra_ present the 36.6%.(tab.5)

```
                  I--------------I
                  Istage IB lymp.I
                                +
      I---------------I--------------I
      I % recurrence  I    36.6      I
      I---------------I--------------I
```

    tab.5: recurrence rates

The survival rate five-yr. is showed in table 6.

```
I--------I---------------I
I        Isurvival 5-ys  I
I--------I---------------I
I nodes +I    65.3%      I
I--------I---------------I
I nodes -I    90%        I
I--------I---------------I
```

tab.6:Effects of pelvic nodal metastasis on survival.

CONCLUSIONS

Our data showed that cervical cancer strikes in 36% young women from 31 to 50 years old. This is very important to put in practice some surgical tricks making accettable future sexual activity of these women. On these patients we consi_ der interesting "the vaginal prolongation" maked by some au_ thors in young women.(11) Since about one year we dont make visceral peritoneum suture. Survival rate confirm the signi_ ficant prognostic indicators: clinical stage-grading,cell type,nodal metastasis. (22-23-24) Recently, important pro_ gnostic significance is ascribed to the flussocitometry, ploydia valuation and DNA index.(Trope 1994) S.C.C. assumed an important role in relapses control and in valuation of result to neoadjuvant chemotherapy.(Scambia 1994) Radiation therapy adjuvant data are debated and,actualy,an adjuvant chemotherapy is suggested in advanced and recurrent cervical cancer.(25) At this purpose,conforting results are reported with 244.S use(Cis-platinum analogous),with Ifosfamide and Dibromodulcitol.(26) Since about one year we make,in advan_ ced stages,neo-adjuvant chemotherapy with very promising results.(27-28-29)

REFERENCES

1.Morrow CP.Tumors of Cervix. Synopsis of gyn.onc.3rd ed.n. y.:wiley-sons 1987 127-130
2.Freund AW zu meiner methode der totalen uterus-extripation zentralbl gynacol 1878.
3.Clark VG. a more radical method of performing hysterectomy for cancer of uterus:1895
4.Reis E. modern treatment of carcinoma of the uterus. Chicago med.res.1895.
5.Wertheim E. the extended abdominal operation for carcinoma uteri(besed on 500 operative cases)am.j.obst1912/66169/232
6.Piver,Rutledge,Smith:five classes of extended hysterectomy for women with cervical cancer.obst.gyn.1974 44:265.
7.Meigs J. carcinoma of the cervix:the wertheim operation. surg.gyn.-obst.1944.78:195.
8.Hopkins M.P. et Al. :Stage IB squamous cell cancer of the cervix:clinic-pathologic features related to survival. Am. J.Obst.Gyn.1991 164 1520-9.
9.Underwood PB. et Al.: radical hysterectomy:a critical re_ view of 22 years experience.Am.J.Obst.gyn.1979 134:889.
10.Bianchi U.et al.:Primary radical hysterectomy in stage IB cervical cancer:possible role adjuvant of the radiotherapy Eur.J.Gyn.Onc. Vol.12 N 3-4.
11.Averette H.E.:radical hysterectomy for invasive cervical cancer. Cancer1993 1422-1437.
12.Jones W.:Cancer febb.1993,1451.
13.Gallup DG.et al.:Poor prognosis in patients with adeno_ squamous cell carcinoma of the cervix. Obst.gyn.1985/65 416-22.
14.Saigo P.E. et al.:Prognostic factors in adenocarcinoma of the uterine cervix. Cancer 1986,57:1584.
15.Klein W.et al.:Prognosis of adenocarcinoma of the cervix uteri:a comparative study. Gyn.Onc.1989;35:145.
16.Kilgore LC.:adenocarcinoma of the uterine cervix.Clin.Ob. Gyn.1990.33:863-71.
17.Delgado G.et al.:prospective surgical-pathological study

of disease free interval in patients with IB squamous cell carcinoma of the cervix:a gyn. onc. gruop study:gyn. onc. 1990.38:353-7.

18.Terada K.Y.: Gyn. Onc. 31 :389-395 nov. 1988

19.NG HT GYN. ONC. 26.355.

20.Ayanh A.: radical histerectomy with linfoadenectomy for treatment of
early stage cervical cancer clinical experience of 278 cases.j
surgical oncol.1991;47:175-7.

21.Simmonds RD morbidity and complications of radical hysterectomy with
pelvic lymphonodo.am.j.obst.gyn. 1966;94:663-78.

22.Park RC et al:treatment of stage IB carcinoma of the cervis.obst.
gyn.1973; 41:117-22

23.Morley GW et al:radical pelvic surgery versus radiation therapy for
stage IB carcinoma of the cervix (exclusive microinvasion) Am.journ.
obst.gynec. 1976;126: 785-98.

24.Lerner HM et al.: radical surgery for the treatment of early carcinoma (IB) review of 15 yeras experience. Obst.Gynec. 1980 56: 413-
418.

25.KinneyW.K. et al: Value of adjuvant whole-pelvis after Werteim
hysterectomy for early-stage squamous carcinoma of the cervix with
pelvic nodal metastasis:a matched-control study-Gin.Oncology 1989;
34:258.

26.Park R.C. et al.: Chemotherapy in advanced and recurrent cervical
cancer. Cancer 1993;71,1446.

27.Mancuso S.: XIII Corso Agg. Fisiop.Riprod. Umana Genn.1990

28.Massi et Al: Rivista di Ost. e Gin. Aprile 93

29.Di Re et al.:Progetto finalizzato C.N.R.: carcinoma della cervice
localmente avanzato; chemioterapia neo adiuvante seguita da chirurgia radicale versus radioterapia esclusiva.
Febbraio 1992

HPV and cervical intraepithelial neoplasia

G. Piras, M.P. Bagella, F. Esposito, L. Pinna Nossai, P. Lecca, M. Putzolu, A. Scapinelli and P.L. Cherchi

Università degli Studi di Sassari, Clinica Ostetrica-Ginecologica, Sassari, Italy

Since the last century, many epidemiological studies had demonstrated the closely related correlation between cervical carcinoma and sexual activity, with particular reference to the promiscuity, to the precocity of the sexual intercourses and to the sexually transmitted diseases (11).

The important role played by certain types of Papilloma virus in the neoplastic lesions of uterine cervix is generally accepted.

Our study has been conducted with the purpose of evaluating the association between HPV and cervical carcinoma in the patients come to clinical observation at the Center for the Prevention and Precocious Diagnosis of lower female genital tract neoplasias, of the Gynaecologic and Obstetric Institute of University of Sassari.

MATERIALS AND METHODS

During the period from january 1992 to september 1993, at the Center for the Prevention and Precocious Diagnosis of the female genital tumours, 2972 colposcopic examinations have been performed and, during the exam, 847 mirate biopsies have been done. A colposcopic report has been compiled for every patient, in which a familar, personal and gynaecological anamnesis has been included.

Before colposcopy, a Pap test was performed, which was examined at our Institute, while biopsies were sent for examination to the Institute of Pathological Anatomy of the same University.

In the cases resulted positive for HPV, where CIN 3 was also associated, we examined the cyto-colpo-hystological correlation, the relation between the patient's age, coitarche, the number of partners declared, parity and cigarette smoke.

Out of 2972 colposcopic exams, we diagnosed 10 cases (O.3 %) of CIN 3, which were successively submitted to cervical conization. From the examined data, we found that the patient's mean age was 37, the youngest was 25 and the oldest 70.

The first intercourse occurred at about 17 (with a range from 15 to 19 years of age). 70% of patients declared one partner, 10% 2 partners, 20% more than 2. 30% of the patients didn't have any pregnancy; 70% is represented by pluriparae (20% had more than 2 pregnancies). 60% of patients were smokers (Tab. 1).

Table 1   Features of the patients positive for CIN 3 HPV associated

Mean Age	37 (range 25-70)
Age of first sexual intercourse	17 (range 15-19)
N. of partners: 1 2 >2	(70%) (10%) (20%)
Parity : nulliparae pluriparae	30% 70%
Smokers	60%

RESULTS

In the 10 cases of CIN 3 that we have examined, the cytological diagnosis was of serious dysplasia in 8 cases (80%), 6 of which presented a moderate dysplasia, 1 case ECV associated (10%). The colposcopic exams showed only 1 case (10%) of ANTZ G1 (white thin epithelium), 8 cases (80%) of ANTZ G2 and 1 case (10%) of leucoplakia. The hystological exam, which was performed over mirate cervical biopsies, diagnosed 8 cases (80%) of serious dysplasia-K in situ, of which one was ECV associated, while in 2 cases there was a light-moderate dysplasia.

All bioptical samples underwent immunohystochemical research for HPV, always with negative results (Tab. 2).

Tab. 2: Results of the different used tecniques.

RESEARCH	N° OF CASES	OUTCOME
hystology	9(90%) 1 (10%)	CIN 3 CIN 3 + E.C.V.
cytology	1 (10%) 1 (10%) 8 (80%)	E.C.V. light dysplasia+ E.C.V. serious dysplasia
colposcopy	1 (10%) 8 (80%) 1 (10%)	ANTZ G1 ANTZ G2 leucoplakia
immunohystochemistry	10(100%)	negative

DISCUSSION AND CONCLUSION

The analysis of our results allows to make some observations. According to literature, our study has demonstrated that HPV infections CIN 3 associated are more frequent in the pluriparae than in the nulliparae.

Regarding the cigarette smoke, a positive correlation exists with CIN 3 (smoke acts as cofactor, promoting the integration of viral genoma in the cells of cervical epithelium) (5,10,13).

We believe that the data about sexual promiscuity are not always accurate, while we have found that the premature coitarche is an important factor.

The cyto-colpo-hystologic data were agreeing with CIN 3 in 90 % of cases. In one case (10%) there was a cytological response of light dysplasia ECV associated and of ANTZ G1 at colposcopy.

The hystology did not result to be an adequate technique for the diagnoses of the HPV infections (with a sensivity limited to 10 % of cases), contrary to the cytology, which in our study resulted positive in 80 % of cases (according to the data of the National Institute of Tumours, the sensivity of cytology is 88 %).

We believe that probably the mirate biopsies are not always able to show the typical reports of this infection, contrary to the cytology, with a larger possibility of identification.

Moreover, the typical Koilocitic cell, also repeatable in the experimental HPV infection, marking the cytohystological diagnosis of genital condyloma, is variously present in the CIN lesions and occasionaly present in the invasive carcinoma (8).

The colposcopic pictures of HPV are often indistinguishable from the ones typical of CIN: the flourishing cervical condylomata are less frequent; we can more often see the "flat condyloma" which can show the vascular pattern of the "mosaic" or "punctuation" and so on.

Immunohystochemistry is an easy technique, but it presents a with scarse accuracy (50 %); it resulted negative in all of our cases.

The recente massive introduction of molecular hybridization techniques has allowed to identify the presence of HPV with high specificity and sensitivity(8). It would be desirable, for a better diagnostic certainty and for the successive follow-up (expecially in the cases resulted positive for the viral types at high risk for carcinoma), the routinary use of "in situ" hybridization.

REFERENCES

1. Bergeron, C. (1989). Conduite a teneir devant une infection a HPV pendant la grossesse. J. Ginecol.Obstet.Biol.Reprod.,18,895.

2. Boselli, F., Garuti,G., Gennazzani A.R. (1991). Infezione da HPV e neoplasia cervicale. Oncol. Ginecol., 10, 223-230.
3. Campion, M.J., McCance, D.J., Cuzick, J., Singer, A.(1986). Progressive potential of mild cervical atypia: prospective, cytological, colposcopic and virological study. Lancet, 2,237.
4. Colgan, T.J., Percy, M.E., Suri, M., Shier, R.M., Andrews, D.F., Lickrish, G.M.(1989). Human papillomavirus infection of morphologically normal cervical epithelium adjacent to squamous dysplasia and invasive carcinoma. Hum. Pathol., 20,316.
5. Crum, C.P., Burckett, B.J.(1989). Papillomavirus and vulvovaginal neoplasia. J. Reprod. Med., 34,566.
6. Ferenczy, A., Winkler, B. (1987). Cervical intraepithelial neoplasia and condyloma.In Kurman ed. Blaustein's Pathology of the female Genital tract, 177.
7. Kreider, J.W., Howett, M.K., Wolfe, S.A.,Bartlett, G.L., Zaino, R.J., Sedlacek, T.U., Mortel, R. (1985). Morphological trasformation in vivo of human uterine cervix with papillomavirus from condylomata acuminata. Nature, 317,639.
8. Nuovo, G.J., Friedman, D., Richart, R.M.(1990). In situ hybridization analysis of human papillomavirus DNA segregation patterns in lesions of the female genital tract. Gynecol. Oncol., 36,256.
9. Rapp, F., Jeckins, F.J.(1981). Genital cancer and viruses. Gynecol. Oncol., 12, 325.
10. Syrjanen, K.J. et al.(1988). Factors associated with progression of cervical human papillomavirus (HPV) infections into carcinoma in situ during a long term prospective follow-up. Br.J.Obstet.Gynecol.,95,1096-1102.
11. Syrjanen, K.J.(1989). Epidemiology of HPV infections and their associations with genital squamous cell cancer. APMIS, 97,957-970.
12. Zur Hausen, H.(1987). Papillomaviruses in human cancer. Cancer res., 49, 4677-4681.
13.Winkekstein, W.J.(1977). Smoking and cancer of the uterine cervix: hypothesis. Am.J. Epidemiol.,106,257.

Aggressive angiomyxoma of the vagina: case report and review of the literature

A. Azzena, R. Salmaso*, F. Vasoin, G. Cerri, M. Gardiman and T. Zen

Università degli Studi di Padova, Istituto di Ginecologia ed Ostetricia "G.B. Revoltella" and *Istituto di Anatomia Patologica, Padova, Italy

SUMMARY

Aggressive angiomyxoma of the vagina is a rare neoplasia of the soft tissue histologically characterized by low cellularity and scarce mitosis, with fusiform or stellate cells, collagene fibrils and numerous vessels in the mixoid stroma. In 1983 Stepper and Rosai published a study on 13 cases. They first introduced the definition of " aggressive angiomyxoma" to emphasize the peculiar tendency of this neoplasia to be a recurrent disease. To date, 29 cases of angiomyxoma of the vagina have been documented (1-6). Incidence is especially high in the third and fourth decade of life. This neoplasia is usually only locally invasive and slow growing but relapses are frequent and often bigger than the first incidence. No metastatic diffusion has ever been documented. This peculiar behaviour makes the diagnosis quite difficult. In the Fletcher case series eight out of ten cases   of angiomyofibroblastoma were first diagnosed as angiomyxomas. In the case we observed, a 49 years old woman was admitted in the Internal medicine department of Padua Hospital for abdominal pain. After colonoscopy for suspected colonopathy, the patient underwent gynaecologic examination, colpocytology, endometrial cytology and colposcopy which revealed a pedunculated mass on the right inferior third of the vaginal wall. The neoplasia was excised   with local anesthesia. The recovery was uneventful and the three month follow-up was negative for relapse. At the histological examination the angiomyxoma of the vagina presented as a polypoyd white-grey mass about 2,5 by 1,5 cm. The neoplastic stroma was characterized by thin-walled vessels; thicker vessels were frequent in the mixoid stroma while the back-up stroma was generally hypocellular with rare areas of higher cellularity. Some collagenous fibers were also present. We observed a strong positive reaction for estrogen receptors in 75% of the fusiform cells and in the pericytes surrounding the vasal wall which is consistent with the theory suggested by Rosai that this neoplasia may originate in the perineal mixoid vascular stromal cells producing estrogen receptors. A higher incidence during fertility and highly selective anathomic localization support this hypothesis.

Key-words: Vaginal cancer; Angiomixoma.

INTRODUCTION

Aggressive vaginal angiomyxoma is a rare neoplasia of the soft tissue which relapses but does not metastasize. In 1983 Stepper and Rosai published a study on 13 cases. They first introduced the definition of " aggressive angiomyxoma" to emphasize the peculiar tendency of this neoplasia to be a recurrent disease. To date, 29 cases of angiomyxoma of the vagina have been documented (1-6) with various histopathological diagnoses.

The Authors report on a case observed at the Institute of Gynaecology and Obstetrics of Padua University, describing the clinical and pathological aspects of this neoplasia and discussing its possible pathogenesis.

CLINICAL CASE

A.D., 49 years old, was admitted on 21 March 1994 at the III Department of Internal Medicine of Padua Hospital complaining abdominal pain. Serious obesity and a tractable abdomen were found by objective examination. Therapy with lactulose caused the symptoms to recede in the first days of hospitalization. Direct abdominal X-rays were negative whereas abdominal ecography showed a cholecystic calculus with no sign of cholecystopathy. A colonoscopy was performed for suspected colonopathy, which revealed the presence of diverticula of the sigma, discendens and transversus colon. Gynaecologic consultation was also required for amenorrhea probably of climateric origin. Obstetric-gynaecologic story was unremarkable: menarche at 10 years, regular cycles for rhythm, quantity and duration, Para 2002, eutocic deliveries, last cycle December 1993. β-HCG dosage was negative. The patient underwent gynaecologic examination colpocytology and colposcopy, endometrial cytology. Colposcopy revealed a pedunculated, greyish-white, well-capsulated mass on the right inferior third of the vaginal wall, measuring about 2.5 x 1.5 cm. Excision of the mass was performed under local anesthesia with a lozenge incision

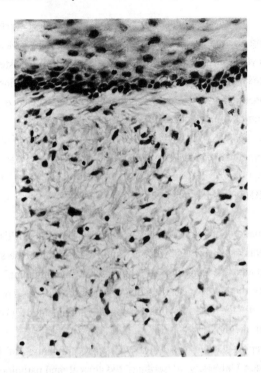

FIG.1 The pavimentous epithelium covers laxe stromal structure with a moderate cell component, represented by fibroblasts with big, thick nucleus, sometimes atypical with spindle-straped, cigar-like nuclei.

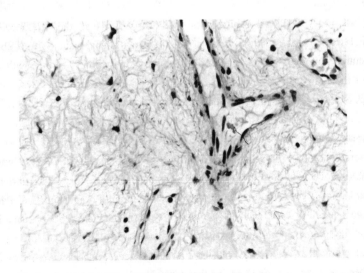

FIG.2 In the laxe stromal ambit are often observed vascular structures, sometimes ramificated, with evident endothelium.

- including the base of the mass and about 1 cm of disease free tissue - and with interrupted suture.

The neoformation was fixed in 10% buffered formaldehyde solution and embedded in paraffin except for a small quantity of material which was trasferred to glutaraldehyde for electron microscopic examination. Paraffin sections were obtained and afterwards stained with haematoxylin and eosin, van Gieson, PAS and Alcian Blue; these sections were also used for immunohistochemical examination. Histopathological findings. During operation it was revealed a polypoid mass of greyish-white colour 2.5 x1.5 cm located on the right vaginal wall. Microscopically the lesion appeared to be clearly marginated by a thin capsula. The neoplastic stroma was generally characterized by thin-walled vessels whereas some thick-walled vessels were immersed in mixoid stroma. The supporting stroma was mainly hypocellular with rare areas of high cellularity. Collagen fibers were also found. Occasionally the blood vessels had a plexiform appearance. Isolated or small groups of fusiform cells were present in the mixoid stroma. In fibrous areas, cells were clustered in aggregates. These cells had round and swollen nuclei with clear limits, finely granular chromatine, small and well- separated nucleoli while mitosis were very rare. In the stroma, mast cells, overflowing erythrocytes, rare lymphocytes and histocytes were also found. Special Alcian Blue staining for mucin showed a strong positive reaction in many histocytes but not in the tumoral acellular stroma which also resulted Pas-negative. Immunohystochemical staining with monoclonal antibodies for desmin, vimentine, collagen 4 and factor 8 was negative in the fusiform elements. Only endothelial cells stained with factor 8 were positive as were the vessel walls stained with collagen 4. We also used monoclonal antibodies for estrogen and progesterone and observed a strong estrogenic positive reaction in 75% of the fusiform cells and in the pericytes surrounding the vasal wall.

DISCUSSION

Aggressive angiomyxoma can be distinguished from other mixoid tumours by three main criteria: its occurrence has a peak in the third and fourth decade (range 18-63 years); it is locally invasive and slow-growing; histologically it is characterized by low cellularity and rare mitosis. The mixoid stroma shows fusiform or stellate cells, collagen fibrils and numerous vessels (1,9). Relapses are described as bigger than the first incidence and can often be multifocal and latent up to 14 years. Ten cases out of the 29 described in the literature relapsed (1,2,4,5,7,10). No metastases have ever been reported. In the case we observed there was no relapse in three months follow-up. A differential diagnosis can be useful with the angiomyofibroblastoma recently described by Fletcher (3). Fletcher reported on ten cases, eight of which were first considered angiomyxomas. No relapses were reported in a very long follow-up period of these cases (up to 14 years). Angiomyofibroblastoma is much smaller and better defined than angiomyxoma; thin-walled vessels are more frequent and no hemorrhages can be observed: the stroma is slightly hypercellular with polynucleal fusiform mast-cells gathering around the vessels. Another difference is immunohistochemical positive staining for desmine due to high myofibrillar differentiation which is characteristic of angiomyofibroblastoma.

Hormonal factors may play an important role in the pathogenesis of aggressive angiomyxoma. A higher incidence during fertility and highly selective anathomic localization support this hypothesis. Rosai suggested that aggressive angiomyxoma may originate in the perineal vascular stromal cells which produce estrogen (9). The pericytes and the stromal fusiform cells characteristic of this neoplasia react to estrogen stimulation thus supporting Rosai's theory. The rare incidence of this tumor makes the diagnosis difficult. In the past it has been often considered as a mixoid variety of benign and malignant soft tissue tumours (1,9).

CONCLUSIONS

Even if aggressive angiomyxoma has never shown metastatic potential it can be locally invasive and aggressive with a high relapse rate. The clinician and the pathologist must pay special attention to the equivocal behaviour of these neoplastic forms. Surgical removal must be radical and deep enough to avoid possible multinodal relapses which would cause more serious mutilations.

REFERENCES

1) Stepper T.A., Rosai J. (1983): Aggressive angiomixoma of the female pelvis and perineum. Am. J. Surg. Pathol. 7, 463.

2) Allen P.W., Dymock R.B., MacCorman L.B. (1988): Superficial angiomyxoma with and without epithelial components. Report of 30 tumors in 28 patients. Am. J. Surg. Pathol. 12, 519.

3) Flechter C., Tsang W.Y., Fischer C., Lee K.C., Chan J.K.C. (1992): Angiomyofibroblastoma of the vulva. Am. J. Surg. Pathol. 16 (4), 373.

4) Hilgers R.D., Pai R., Bartow S.A., Aisenbrey G., Bowling M.C. (1986): Aggressive angiomyxoma of the vulva. Obstet. Gynaecol. 68, 60s-62s.

5)Mandai K., Moriwaki S., Motoi M. (1990): Aggressive angiomyxoma of the vulva: report of a case. Acta Pathol. Jap., 40, 927.

6) Begin L.R., Clement P.B., Kirk M.E., Jothy S., McCaughey W.T.E., Ferenozy A. (1985): Aggressive angiomyxoma of pelvic soft parts. A clinicopathologic study of nine cases. Hum. Pathol. 16, 621.

7) Chen K.T.K., Hafez G.R., Gilbert E.F. (1980): Myxoid variant of epithelioid smooth muscle tumor. Am. J. Clin. Pathol. 74, 350.

8) Lovelady S.B., McDonald J.R., Waugh J.M. (1991): Benign tumors of vulva. Am. J. Obstet. Gynecol. 42, 309.

Serous papillary ovarian carcinoma: solitary uterine polyp metatstase

A. Azzena, R. Salmaso*, F. Vasoin, G. Cerri, S. Polonio and G. Altavilla*

Università degli Studi di Padova, Istituto di Ginecologia ed Ostetricia "G.B. Revoltella" and *Istituto di Anatomia Patologica, Padova, Italy

SUMMARY

A 64 year old woman affected by an ovarianserous papillary carcinoma presented an uterine metastase arised on a solitary endometrial fibroadenomatous polyp of the uterine fund, diagnosed after hysterectomy. This is the first report, to our knowledge, of a metastase of an ovarian carcinoma to an uterine polyp.

Key-words: Ovarian carcinoma; uterine metastase.

INTRODUCTION

Ovarian serous papillary carcinoma may metastase extensively, occasionally to unusual sites (1,2).

Caracteristically, the metastases to other gland forming tissues, can rise serious diagnostic problems.

The patient, examined in this report,incidentally at the time of the histhological examination, has presented an uterine metastase, arised on fibroadenomatous endometrial polyp. The polyp had a focal poorly differentiated neoplastic involvement, confined to the mucosa of its proximal part. Histologically, the adenocarcinoma in the polyp resembled the serous papillary ovarian carcinoma.

This is the first reported case of a metastase to an fibroadenomatous polyp of the uterus.

897

CASE REPORT

Patient I.Z., 64 years-old, menarche at 9 years old, PARA 3003, physiological menopause at 50 years old, in good health till march 1994 when, during a normal outpatient gynaecologic control, a left ovarian and an anterior vaginal-wall masses were diagnosed. Further ultrasound examination confirmed the presence of a cystic 8 cm diameter left ovarian mass. The patient was admitted to the Gynaecologic Clinic of Padua University and the 17th March 1994 underwent radical hysterectomy with bilateral oophorectomy, omentectomy, appendectomy and asportation of a paraurethral mass, the bladder trigon, bladder-vaginal septum and posterior trigonal tissue.

Frozen sections showed an infiltrating serous papillary adenocarcinoma of the left ovary.

Subsequent tissue examinations confirmed the frozen sections of serous papillary ovarian adenocarcinoma and demonstrated controlateral ovarian metastase and in an endometrial polyp without extension to the endometrium. Omental metastases were confirmed. Fibrous fatty tissue and muscle cells with adenocarcinomatous infiltration were found at trigonal and paraurethral level.

PATHOLOGICAL FINDINGS

Uterus ranged in size from 4x4x3,5 cm. The left ovarian mass (8x8x4 cm) was rubbery and firm with an attached fimbriated fallopian tube. The external surface was glistening and mattled yellow-pink to dark red-gray. The cut surface revealed encapsulated, apparently viable, soft, rubbery ton-white tumor with hemorrhagic areas. The right adnexa, less than 3 cm in diameter had a smooth external surface while cut surface revealed a tumor mass similar to the controlateral. In the uterine cavity, a single, peduncolated uterine polyp with fundal location was found. The polyp head (proximal part) measured 0,8 cm in greatest dimension; it was present an a 0,6 stalk.

Microscopic section of the ovarian mass revealed a poorly differentiated serous papillary carcinoma with cluster of psammoma bodies in the tumor capsula near islands of adenocarcinoma. Metastatic implant of papillary serous adenocarcinoma associated with psammoma bodies was present on the controlateral (right) ovary and in the head of the uterine fibroglandular polyp; metastatic implants were also found in the omentum, paraurethral tissue, bladder trigon, bladder-vaginal septum and posterior trigonal tissue.

Sections of the fibroglandular polyp showed a typical peduncolated fibro-adenoma, which head contained a focus of carcinoma. The stalk was delined by normal endometrium. The "muscolaris mucosae" of the polyp head was intact; there was no

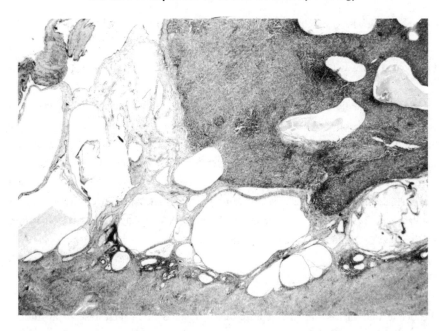

FIG.1 In the bottom of the figure is shown the uterine wall with endometrial atrophy, from which arises the polyp, at right represented by a fibroblandular structure while at left by the neoplastic portion (E-E 20X).

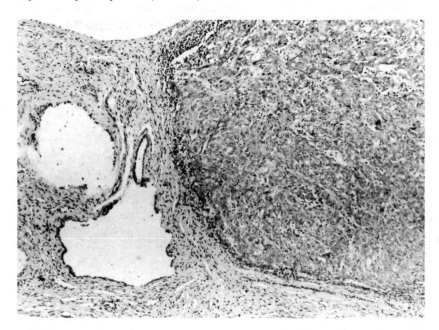

FIG.2 This particular points out the interface between neoplastic portion of the polyp and its fibroglandular structure (E-E60X).

evidence of invasive carcinoma into the submucosa but evidence of tumor in the lymphatics and veins of the polyp stalk was seen. The malignant neoplasm in the polyp was located halfway between the surface of the polyp and the muscolaris mucosae (Fig. 1).

Histologically, it did not resemble the usual carcinomas arising in adenomas, which generally progress through an orderly multistep neoplastic process (1). Rather it was surrounded by typical fibro-adenomatous gland without evidence of the cellular anaplasia characteristic of intraepitelial or intramucosal carcinoma. The neoplastic cells were extremely pleomorphic and atypical, with frequent mitoses (Fig. 2). The lesion was well delimited from the rest of the polyp, and there was no clean evidence of cellular transition from adenomatous to malignant tissue (Fig. 2). No other involvement of the endometrium was noted.

COMMENT

We belive that this is the first reported case of an ovarian metastase to an uterine fibroadenomatous polyp from an ovarian cancer. The evidence sostains the theory that the malignant neoplasm in the polyp is a metastase of the ovarian carcinoma. First the malignant neoplasm was confined to the mucosa of the polyp head, not involving the muscolaris mucosae. We know that malignant tumors arising in fibroglandular polyps must reach the level of the muscolaris mucosae (2). On the other hand, the polyp malignant cells were identical to those seen in the ovarian cancers. There is no evidence of displasia or other neoplastic foci at endometrial level. The proof that the polyp metastases reached this site throughout a venous diffusion-way is that few lymphatics were present at mucosal level.

REFERENCES

1) Ulbright T., Roth L. (1985): Metastatic and independent cancers of the endometrium and ovary. Hum. Pathol., 16, 28-34.
2) Silva E.G., Jenkins R. (1990): Serous carcinoma in endometrial polyp. Modern Pathology, 3, 2, 120-124.

Relationships between proliferative activity and oncogene expression in human breast cancer

M. Massobrio, L. Bianchi Malandrone*, A. Demurtas*, A. Durando, M. Geuna*, N. Ravarino**, M. Sberveglieri, B. Torchio** and G. Palestro*

Clinic of Gynecology and Obstetrics, *Department of Biomedical Sciences and Human Oncology, University of Turin and **Department of Pathology, Mauriziano Hospital, Turin, Italy

Background. Approximately 60 percent of patients with breast cancer have disease that is apparently confined to the breast, without axillary node involvement. The presence of tumor in axillary lymph nodes remains the strongest predictor of recurrence (1). If axillary lymph nodes are free from disease, prognosis is improved, nevertheless 30% of these patients have a recurrence at 10 years. Several recent studies have been focused on the identification of patients subsets with high risk of recurrence, even with negative nodes, using not conventional prognostic factors (2). In this view, some biological parameters have been identified and regarded as new independent prognostic factors consistent with the risk of relapse of the disease (3). These may be classified as a) proliferation markers, i.e. Ki67 (MIB-1), cyclins, PCNA, b) growth factors and receptors such as erbB-2/Neu, epidermal growth factor (EGF) receptor, insulin growth factor (IGF) receptor and transforming growth factor α (TGF-α), c) invasion markers such as cathepsin D, laminin receptors, plasminogen activator, collagenase IV, angiogenetic factors, d) tumor suppressor genes p53 and rb, e) others oncogenes such as nm23, ras, c-myc, Bcl-2, f) other factors such as chemoresistant protein gp 170 and pS2 protein.

Experimental evidence supports the role of oncogenes and tumor suppressor genes in regulating apoptotic cell death (4). The Bcl-2 proto-oncogene encodes an inner mitochondrial membrane protein responsible for specific prevention of apoptosis in several cell types.

The p53 suppressor gene encodes for a nuclear phosphoprotein able to regulate the cell cycle and also induce the apoptotic pathway (5). The p53 gene is the most commonly altered tumor suppressor gene in human malignancies and its alteration probably represents a relatively early event in cancer progression (3). About 30% of human breast cancers have mutations in p53 gene, and as many as 60% of tumors have p53 detectable by immunohistochemistry. The presence of mutant p53 in tumor cells is associated with poorer prognosis, but it remains uncertain whether p53 is an independent prognostic factor.

In this study we analyzed flow cytometric findings (DNA Index - DI and S phase fraction - SPF) in association with clinical and pathologic features and p53 and Bcl-2 protein expression in order to investigate the existence of correlations between oncogene expression, cytokinetic activity and conventional prognostic factors.

Methods and results. In 51 breast cancers we performed on fresh/frozen tumor fragments flow cytometric evaluation of DI (ploidy) by means of propidium iodine staining (Cycletest Plus, Becton Dickinson, San Josè, CA), on 43 (84%) of them we also could calculate SPF. Bcl-2 (MoAb 124, Dako, Glostrup, Denmark) and p53 (MoAb DO7, specific for both wild type and mutant protein, Medac, Germany) protein expression were evaluated on the same group of tumors using avidin–biotin complex (LSAB, Dako) immunohistochemical method on tissue section obtained from the same formalin fixed and paraffin embedded tissue block on wich breast cancer was diagnosed. The main features of the 51 breast cancers studied are reported in the table I, where the cases are divided on the basis of their pathologic characters (pT, pN and grading), hormone receptor status, cytokinetics parameters (DI and SPF) and protein Bcl-2 and p53 expression.

Table I. Distribution of pathologic and biologic features in 51 breast cancers ⊕.

	no. of cases	%
pT≤2cm	21	41.1
pT>2cm	30	58.9
pN=0	27	52.9
pN=1	24	47.1
G1	12	23.5
G2	21	41.2
G3	18	35.3
ER+	38	74.5
ER−	13	25.5
PR+	18	35.3
PR−	33	64.7
DI=1	13	25.4
DI≠1	38	74.6
SPF<7*	21	48.8
SPF≥7*	22	51.2
Bcl-2+•	38	74.5
Bcl-2−•	13	25.5
p53+#	23	45.1
p53−#	28	54.9

⊕ Bcl-2 vs p53: R=−0.44; p=0.001,
  Bcl-2 vs grading: R=−0.35; p=0.01,
  Bcl-2 vs SPF: R=−0.38; p=0.01,
  p53 vs SPF: R=0.4; p=0.007.
* SPF cut–off was decided on the basis of the median value. • Bcl-2 cut–off was <30% stained tumor cells = negative case and ≥30% stained tumor cells = positive case (6). #p53 cut–off was ≤ 5% stained tumor cells = negative case and >5% stained tumor cells = positive case (7).

Bcl-2 and p53 were inversely related (R=-0.44, p=0.001) as well as Bcl-2 and nuclear grading (R=-0.35, p=0.01). Moreover, Bcl-2 positive tumors were also significantly related to a lower proliferative activity, as detected by SPF (R=-0.38, p=0.01). By contrast, p53 expression was associated with a greater proliferation (R=0.4, p=0.007). No significant difference was found between tumor size, lymph node status, hormone receptor status, DI and both Bcl-2 and p53 protein expression.

Analyzing only node negative tumors (27 cases), another significant difference was found when comparing tumors progesterone-receptor positive with p53 expression: 18% of p53 positive tumors were PR+ and 69% of p53 negative tumors were PR+ (p=0.01).

Conclusive remarks. In this preliminary study, the analysis of Bcl-2 and p53 protein expression, investigated in a series of 51 invasive breast cancers may be summarized as follow. Bcl-2 expression was found in high percentage of breast cancer and was inversely related to proliferative activity. This result may suggest that Bcl-2 expression, besides protecting the cell from apoptosis, may also be involved in processes controlling (slowing down) cell proliferation. As a consequence, Bcl-2 positive tumors could be genetically more stable and with more favourable clinical course (6, 8). This hypotesis could also be supported by the well differentiated grading that we observed in Bcl-2 positive tumors.

By contrast, p53 expression seems to be correlated to a higher proliferative rate of tumor cells, and, at least in node negative tumors, to the absence of PR receptors. The last finding is in keeping with previous reports (9) wich suggested that mutations and consecutive accumulation of the mutant p53 protein will enhance clonal expansion of primary tumor cells, conferring selective growth advantage to p53-immunoreactive breast cancer.

The strong inverse correlation existing between Bcl-2 and p53 provides a further demonstration of the opposite roles that these two genes play in controlling cell growth. Moreover, recently it has been proposed an inhibitory activity of mutant p53 on Bcl-2 expression (10).

Silvestrini et al (6) have found a good correlation between Bcl-2 and pathological features (tumor size and oestrogen receptors) in a series of breast cancer patients. The difference between these and our results may be due to different criteria in patient selection: in the former series only cases without lymph node involvement were considered.

In our series the lack of correlation between p53 and tumor size, lymph node status and hormone receptor is in agreement with previous reports (9,11). However, an over-expression of p53 is thought to be an indipendent prognostic factor (7,11). Further studies are in course to better assessing the prognostic value of Bcl-2 and p53 expression and to understand the contribution of these genes to the biological and clinical behaviour of breast cancer.

References.

1) McGuire WL and Clark GM (1992) N Engl J Med 326:1756–61.

2) Gasparini G et al (1993) J Natl Cancer Inst 85:1206–19.

3) Shapiro CL and Henderson IC eds (1994) Hematol Oncol Clin North Am vol 8, no 1.

4) Oren M (1992) Metastasis Rev 11:141–8.

5) Lowe SW et al (1993) Cell 74:957–67.

6) Silvestrini R et al (1994) J Natl Cancer Inst 86:499–504.

7) Silvestrini R et al (1993) J Natl Cancer Inst 85:965–70.

8) Pezzella F et al (1993) New Engl J Med 690.

9) Caleffi M et al (1994) Cancer 73:2147–56.

10) Haldar S et al (1994) Cancer Res 54:2095–7.

11) Friedrichs K et al (1993) Cancer 72:3641–7.

Ornithine decarboxylase activity, P21 overexpression and P53 mutation in progestin treated endometrial adenocarcinoma

R. Bellino, A. Venuti, L. Leo, A. Re, M. Tessarolo, S. Colombatto*, L. Gubetta**, S. Cappia**, T. Wierdis and A. Lanza

*Department B of Gynecology and Obstetrics Institute, *Department of Experimental Medicine and Oncology, Biochemistry Section, University of Turin and **Department of Pathology, S. Luigi Hospital, Turin, Italy*

INTRODUCTION

Endometrial carcinoma is the most common gynecologic malignancy and approximately 30 % of women will have recurrences and die of disease.

The most important risk factors are grade of the tumours (   ), depth of myometrial invasion, cervical involvement, hystologic type, lymphonode metastases.

In recent years some data have been reported about growth - factors, oncogene mutation and oncogene products of normal and neoplastic endometrium: these efforts try to discover other independent risk - factors.

In other works (1, 2) we examined Ornithine Decarboxilase (ODC) activity and polyamines concentration in normal and neoplastic human endometrial tissue with and without progestin therapy according to our high dose schedule (medroxiprogesterone acetate, 1000 mg os daily).

It is known that the most activated cellular oncogenes are members of the ras family genes (3, 4, 5); H - ras, K - ras and N - ras encode p21 proteins that are related to the process of signal transduction which regulates cell growth and differentiation. K - ras mutation and overexpression are related to endometrial carcinogenesis.

In the same way more data are becoming available about the tumour suppressor p53 gene; the loss of wild - type p53 is associated with cell transformation (6, 7) as well as p53 overexpression.

In this works we studied the effect of high MPA dose on ras - p21 overexpression and p53 mutated protein in paraffin embedded specimens from human endometrial carcinoma, using an immunohistochemical method.

The results were related to ODC activity and to other clinico - pathological features.

MATERIAL AND METHODS

Thirty patients with uterine endometrial adenocarcinoma were included in this study. ODC activity was determinated in fresh tissue obtained at D & C before MPA treatment and at hysterectomy after the progestin therapy.

Progestin therapy consisted of administration of MPA 1000 mg / day orally for 30 days before the appropriate surgery.

The tissue was immediately frozen and homogenated with 19 volumes of 0.15 MHCl in an ultra turrax within 20 minutes.

Part of the homogenate was centrifuged at 12.000 x g for 10 minutes and the supernatant was used for measuring ODC activity.

It was measured according to Janne and William-Ashman method (8); CO2 formed from (1-14 C) D L-ornithine in 60 minutes incubation in a shaking incubator, was trapped in MCS contained in plastic center wells and counted in PPO-POPOP in toluene solution.

Expression of P53 mutation was studied in 19 of the same paraffin-embedded specimens where ODC activity was detected before MPA treatment and in 30 paraffin- embedded uteruses after progestin therapy.

P53 activity was detected by immunohistochemical technique according to Hsu et al method (Avidin - biotin Peroxidase complex (9). P 53 mutation was classified in 4 groups: in the group A the p53 mutation was not expressed, in the group B < 10 % of the nuclei were stained, in the group C 10 - 40 % of the nuclei were stained and the group D > 40 % of the nuclei were stained.

Similar technique was used to determine Estradiol (ER) and Progesterone (PR) receptors.

Tissue sections were deparaffinized and rehydrated, rinsed with Phosphate Buffered Saline 0.1 M, ph 7.4 (PBS).

Before immunohistochemical staining the sections were treated 4 times in microwave oven (750 W), immersed in citrate buffer 1.0mM ph 6.0 for 20 minutes at room temperature, and then immersed in PBS for 40 minutes to have again ph 7.4.

Endogenous peroxidase was inhibited by treatment with hydrogen peroxidase 3 % for 10 minutes at room temperature.

The sections, rinsed again many times with PBS, were incubated at room temperature with non immune horse serum (Protein Blocking Reagent)and then in wet room for 1 hour with primary monoclonal antibody anti-P53 (Clone DO 1 - Oncogene Science Inc.), primary monoclonal antibody anti - estrogen receptors (Primary Monoclonal Antibody or Mouse Estrogen Receptors Clone 1 D 5 DAKO SpA), or with primary monoclonal antibody anti - progesterone receptors (Primary Monoclonal Mouse Antibody Progesterone Receptors Clone 1 A 6 Novo CASTRA). After more rinses with PBS, the sections were incubated with antimouse antibodies conjugated with biotin (VECTOR) for 30 minutes in wet room.

Then the rinsed sections were incubated with the complex Avidin - Biotin peroxidase and then immunostained with 3-3'-diaminobenzidine (DAB Sigma) and hydrogen peroxidase.

The last step was the staining of nuclei with Mayer's hematoxylin and the mounting of the sections, cleared in xylene, in a non -acqueous mounting medium.

Positive and negative control slides were made to confirm our specimens; in the negative controls the primary antibody was not used and the positive slides should be prepared from tissue known to contain the antigen under study.

The intense, clear, and brown staining of the specimens was considered positive.

The immunohistochemical analysis of p21 protein was performed on paraffin embedded specimens which were deparaffinized and rehydrated. Endogenous peroxidase was inhibited by treatment with hydrogen peroxidase 3 % for 10 minutes at room temperature.

The section after numerous rinses were incubated at 37 °C on thermostat with protein K for 4 minutes (250 µ g / ml with PBS; stored at 20 ° C; before use than were diluted at 1:10 with PBS.

The technique used was the same as in p53, ER and PgR analysis.

We considered positive the sections that showed an evident cytoplasm staining. P 21 overexpression was searched in 23 cases before MPA and in 30 cases after MPA.

RESULTS

Among the 25 cases in which p21 overexpression was detected there were 13 G1 tumours, 9 G2 and 3 G3 tumours. Among the G1 tumours the negative cases (without p21 overexpression) were 31 % (4 / 13) and the positives were 69 % (9 / 13): a positive immunostaining in < 10 % of the cells was observed in 8 at of the 9 positive cases. In G2 tumours the negative cases were 33.5 % as well as in G3 tumours (Tab.1).

On the whole, before MPA treatment 68 %, of the cases overexpressed p21 and in 20 % (5 / 25) the immunostaining was present in > 10 % of the cells.

Among the 30 cases after MPA treatment (the 25 cases + 5 new cases) 74 % of G1 tumours, 55 % of G2 tumours and 35 % of G3 tumours did not overexpress p21. (Tab.2).

Among the 6 G3 tumours the overexpression was present in 4 / 6: in 3 cases out of the 4, the overexpression was present in > 10 % of the cells.

Table 1 Ras-p21 overexpression in 25 cases before MPA treatment accordy to grading subgrouping

	P21 -	P21 +	P21 ++
G1 (n = 13)	4 (31 %)	8 (62 %)	1 (7 %)
G2 (n = 9)	3 (33.5 %)	3 (33 %)	3 (33.5 %)
G3 (n = 3)	1 (33.5 %)	1 (33 %)	1 (33.5 %)

Legend:
  - : no immunostaining is showed
  +: immunostaining is present in < 10 % of the cells
  ++: immunostaining is present in > 10 % of the cells

Table 2 Ras-P21 overexpression in 30 cases after MPA treatment according to grading subgroupyng

	P (-)	P (+)	P (++)
G1 (n = 15)	11 (74 %)	3 (20 %)	1 (6 %)
G2 (n = 9)	5 (55 %)	4 (43 %)	0 (0 %)
G3 (n = 6)	2 (35 %)	1 (15 %)	3 (50 %)

Legend:
  -: no immunostaining is showed
  +: immunostaining is present in < 10 % of the cells
  ++: immunostaining is present in > 10 % of the cells

On the whole, after MPA treatment, 40 % overexpressed p21 and in 13 % the overexpression occurred in > 10 % of the cells.
The decrease of ras-p21 overexpression after MPA is statistically significative ($p = 0.003$).
As showed in Tab. 1, there were no differences of p21 overexpression by subgrouping according to grade of the tumour, before MPA. .
The MPA treated cases showed an increased p21 overexpression related to undifferentiation (p = n.s.).
Among the 30 patients there were six patients died of the disease: 16 out of the 24 NED cases did not overexpress p21, in 7 / 24 the overexpression occurred in < 10 % of the cells and 1 / 24 it occurred in > 10 % of the cells. Among the six patients who died, 3 / 6 overexpressed p21 in > 10 % of the cells and 1 / 6 in < 10 % of the cells.
Statistically, p21 overexpression is not related with poor prognosis. On the other hand, if we consider the relationship between poor prognosis and p21 overexpression when it is showed in > 10 % of the cells, significativity is high ($p = 0.003$).
Among the six patients who died there were 5 G3 tumours. All these cases had a high ODC activity after MPA treatment and 4 / 5 overexpressed p21. In 3 out of 4 the overexpression occurred in > 10 % of the cells.
The only G3 case who is alive did not express p21 and had high ODC activity after MPA.
Among the 30 patients after MPA treatment 4 cases overexpressed p21 in > 10 % of the cells: 3 of these 4 cases died, had high ODC activity and were G3.
The only patient alive with p21 overexpression in > 10 % of the cells was a G1 with low ODC activity.

Table 3 Expression of mutated P53 before treatment with MPA

Group	A	B	C	D
N° Cases	3 (15 %)	12 (65 %)	3 (15 %)	1 (5 %)

Group A = negative cases

    "   B = < 10 % of the cells are stained

    "   C = 10 - 40 % of the cells are stained

    "   D = > 40 % of the cells are stained

Table 4 After treatment with MPA

Group	A	B	C	D
N° Cases (30)	11 (37 %)	13 (43 %)	3 (10 %)	3 (10 %)

Table 5 Relationship between grading and P53 after MPA treatment

Grading	A (0 %)	B (< 10 %)	C (10 - 40 %)	D (> 40 %)	Total
G1	9	5	1	0	15
G2	2	6	1	0	9
G3	0	2	1	3	6
Total	11	13	3	3	30

Among the 19 cases before MPA treatment, p53 mutation was not expressed in 15 % of cancers, the expression was in less than 10 % of the cells in 20 % and it was present in > 10 % of the cells in 65 % (Tab.3).

On the whole, 85 % of the cases had p53 expression: there was not correlation between p53 and grade of the tumour in those patients.

Among the 30 MPA treated cases the 37 % did not express p53 mutation, in 43 % of the patients the immunostaining was present in less than 10 % of the cells in 65 % and in 20 % of the cases in > 10 % of the cells. (Tab.4).

In Tab. 5 we showed the relationship between grading and p53 and expression after treatment with MPA. We observed that 60 % of adenocarcinomas G1 did not express p53 while 22 % of G2 did not too.

There was an expression < 10 % of the cells in 33 % of G1 and in 66 % of G2. In 50 % of G3 there was an expression of p53 in > 10 % of the cells.

Neither G1 cases nor G2 ones belong to C and D groups; on the other hand there were no G3 neoplasms with no expression of p53.

A statistically significant difference exists between G1 / G2 and G3 adenocarcinomas in the expression of p53 after MPA treatment (Fisher's test $P < 0.004$).

In Tab. 6 ODC activity before and after hormonal therapy is demonstrated.

ODC activity is 119 ± 18 nmoles CO_2 g / h in G1 cancers, 143 ± 42 nmoles CO_2 g / h in G2, and 315 ± 25 nmoles CO_2 g / h in G3. There is a statistically significant difference in ODC activity between G1 / G2 and G3 groups.

ODC activity increased 30 times in G1 - G2 and 80 times in G3 adenocarcinomas compared with normal menopausal endometrium.

Table 6 Ornithine decarboxilase in neoplastic endometrium

DIAGNOSTIC CATEGORIES	N° of Cases	ODC nmoles CO_2 $g/h/37\,°C$
Grade 1 adenocarcinoma	10	119 ± 18
Post MPA	10	11.5 ± 4.9
Grade 2 adenocarcinoma	10	143 ± 42
Post MPA	8	67.5 ± 65
Grade 3 adenocarcinoma	5	315 ± 25
Post MPA	6	425 ± 418

Table 7. Correlation between ODC activity post MPA and survival

	ODC activity $< 20\ nmoles\ CO2/g/h$	ODC activity $> 20\ nmoles\ CO2/g/h$
NED	21	3
DOT	0	6

In G1 cancers MPA therapy induced a ODC activity decrease (10 times lover), lowering its value to that of advanced secretory endometrial phase.

We did not observe any change in ODC activity among G3 neoplasms while in G2 cases the reduction was not significative.

All the 6 patients who died of cancer had P53 expression: 4 patients belonged to C and D groups and 2 belonged to B group.

In 5 of those 6 cases the adenocarcinoma was indifferentiated and there was no change in ODC activity after MPA treatment.

The lack of ODC reduction produced by MPA was significatively related to survival. (Tab. 7).

Seven cases (24 %) did not show a decrease in ODC activity after hormonal therapy: all of them had p53 expression (4 medium-high) and 6 were G3.

Among the 24 cases before MPA therapy, in which we determined ER, 50 % did not show receptors, 20 % had a weak positivity, and the rest showed strong positivity.

Among the 12 ER- there were 7 G1, 2 G2, and 3 G3 while among the 12 ER+ there were 6 G1, 5 G2, and 1 G3.

In 21 of these 24 specimens we also determined PR. Positivity was found in 7 cases (66 %).

Six cases were negative for both ER and PR.

Among the 21 cases positivity for ER and for PR was seen in 9 of the 12 G1 tumors (75 %), 5 of the 7 G2 tumors (71 % 9, and 1 of the 2 G3.

After MPA therapy both ER and PR significantly decreased in G1 and G2 neoplasm as showed in Tab.8.

Table 8. Correelation between PgR positivity

pre and post MPA in G1 - G2

	PRE MPA	POST MPA
PgR +	14	2
PgR -	5	19

Table 9. Relationship between P53 ex and survival

	NED	DOT
P53 NEGATIVE	11	0
P53 POSITIVE	19	6

NED = not evident disease

DOT = death of tumour

DISCUSSION

The monoclonal antibody against p21 used in our study is able to recognize both the altered and normal proteins of the three members of the ras-gene family.

Differently from other antibodies there is immunostaining only when p21 overexpression occurres: infact normal endometrium is always negative by using this antibody. This is of great importance because it is not possible a comparison with other works (10) in which other monoclonal antibodies were used.

In our series, before MPA treatment, we showed a p21 overexpression in 68 % of the cases; this is in agreement with Long et al. (11) who demonstrated that 70 % of endometrial adenocarcinomas expressed high levels of p21 oncoprotein. In agrement with other reports (12, 13, 14) before MPA treatment we did not find any relationship between p21 overexpression and grade of the tumors.

It is known that K-ras mutation have been detected in 10 to 30 % of endometrial cancers (15, 16): in our work we found a positive immunostaining, in > 10 % of the cells, in 20 % of the cases. This rate did not significantly vary after MPA therapy (from 20 % to 13 %) while, on the whole, the decrease of p21 overexpression was statistically significant (from 68 % to 40 %). The significant modification occurred in the cases with a positive immunostaining in < 10 % of the cells: in these tumours the antiproliferative and anti DNA synthesis activity of MPA have caused the decrease of p21 overexpression.

It is interesting to note that 3 out of the 4 cases with a positive immunostaining in > 10 % of the cells, were G3 tumours on which MPA had no activity.

It has been shown that p21 overexpression may have a prognostic value in breast cancer (12) and in advanced stage of ovarian cancer (14). In our work if we assume as positives the cases with immunostaining in > 10 % of the cells, the overexpression of p21 is significantly related with poor prognosis. It is necessary to remember that 5 out of the six patients who died had G3 tumours and that the only patient who survived in spite of an overexpression of p21 in > 10 % of the cells, had a G1 tumour with low ODC activity. On the other hand the G3 surviving case, did not overexpress p21 despite the high ODC activity.

At the moment it is not possible to establish if p21 overexpression would be a prognostic factor indipendent from grading: it is necessary to study more G3 cases in order to express an absolut judgement.

In our study 85 % of endometrial adenocarcinomas showed a positive nuclear immunostaining for p53 before MPA treatment.

This incidence is higher than that found by other Authors (17, 18 , 19, 20, 21). It is interesting to observe that only 20 % of the cases showed a positive immunostaining in > 10 % of the nuclei in 10 HPF. The difference between our data and the Literature's could be explained by the different technique and the lower cut-off used in our series.

After MPA therapy, even though we had 11 more cases checked, the expression of p53 in > 10 % of the cells was still 20 % while a difference was observed in the negative cases (37 % Vs 15 %) and in the low expression ones (< 10 % of stained nuclei)(43 %).

This behaviour is similar to that of p21 overexpression in which MPA was able to modify the cases with positive immunostaining in < 10 % of the cells.

In agreement with Koshijama et al (17) we did not find any relationship between P53 expression and grade after tumour; after MPA treatment the relationship became significant which meant that p53 expression in G1 tumours was significantly less than that in G3 tumours.

There may be two explanations: the first is that the statistical power of the study before treatment was too low; the second is that MPA could differentiate and select the population.

In other words MPA antiproliferative and anti DNA synthesis activity occurring in G1 and in part of G2 tumours determined a decreased number of cells expressing p53 mutation. Another possibility is that the antiproliferative activity reduced the chances to have cellular clones which expressed the mutated p53.

ODC activity increased 30 and 80 times in G1-G2 and G3 tumours respectively in comparison to normal menopausal endometrium, MPA therapy decreased ODC activity almost 10 times in G1 tumours with values comparable to those of endometrial late secretory phase. In G2 cancers the decrease was not significance while in G3 we did not observe any change.

Because ODC is a key enzyme in cellular proliferation, the lack of MPA inhibition on its activity in G3 tumours explains the absence of antiproliferative action on indifferentiated neoplasms.

This results is in agreement with lacks or shortage of ER and PR in G3 tumours (22, 23, 24, 25) and the clinical data of G3 poor prognosis in spite of MPA treatment. (26).

Therefore we demonstrated a lot of MPA activities: in differentiated adenocarcinomas it was able to act through a reduction of ODC activity, a reduction of P21 overexpression and P53 mutated expression. The decreased ODC activity occurred in post- transcriptional level; infact, as demonstrated in new unpublished study of our laboratory, these is no relationship between ODC activity and mRNA levels in vitro coltures. At present it is not possible to establish the level of reduction of P21 overexpression and P53 expression. The hypotheses, which explain MPA activity on P53, may be good for P21 as well.

The correlation between ODC activity reduction after MPA and survival is statistically significant; 100 % of the 6 patients who died of cancer had a high ODC activity after MPA treatment while only 3 out of 24 NED patients (14 %) showed high ODC activity. Despite this datum we can not affirm that the lack of ODC reduction should be on indipendent risk factor; 5 out of the 6 death were G3 tumours. It is interesting to note that all the 6 cases had P53 expression and 4 out of the 6 overexpressed P21. Even though there was not a significative relationship between P53 expression after MPA and survival (p = 0.07) and the relationship for P21 overexpression is significant only for the cases with positive immunostaining in > 10 % of the cells, a link certainly exists among G3 tumours-high P53 expression- P21 overexpression- high ODC activity - lack of MPA activity - poor prognosis. The high ODC activity reflects a strong proliferative activity in G3 tumours. We can not say whether the high frequency of P53 mutated expression should be either the cause or the simple minor of biological aggressiveness, as well as P21 overexpression.

Koshijama et al (17) showed a relationship between p53 mutation and advanced stages; it may mean that the mutation of p53 gene is a late event in carcinogenesis. On the other hand it is possible that p53 mutation could develop a more malignant phenotype with a quick spread of disease.

The high p53 expression in G3 should confirm the letter hipotesys.

In our series G3 tumours showed an high p21 overexpression: their biological aggressiveness would carry out throught many mechanisms that should determine a chain reaction, able to increase cellular proliferative activity. The high p21 overexpression, p53 mutation, and high ODC activity would be the witnesses of it.

Acknowledgment: the authors thank Pharmacia / Farmitalia Carlo Erba

REFERENCES

1. Lanza, A., Colombatto, S., Bellino, R., Re, A., Tessarolo, M., Ferraris, G. (1990). Biochemical aspects of the hormonal therapy of endometrial adenocarcinoma. *Eur. J. Gynaecol. Oncol.* **XI**, 4.

2. Lanza, A., Colombatto, S., Re, A., Bellino, R., Tessarolo, M., Leo, L. (1991). Prognostic significance of ornithine decarboxylase (ODC) activity in endometrial adenocarcinoma. *The primate Endometrium. Annals of the New York Academy of Sciences*, **622**, 485.

3. Nishimura, S., and Sekiya, T.. (1987). Human cancer and cellular oncogenes. *Biochem. J.*, **243**,313-327.

4. Forrester, K., Almoguera, C., Jordano, J., Grizzle, W. E., and Perucho, M.. (1987).High incidence of c-K -ras oncogenes in human colon cancer detected by the RNAse a mismatch cleavage method. *J. Tumor Marker Oncol.*, **2**, 113-123.

5. Barbacid, M. (1987). Ras genes. *Annu. Rev. Biochem.*, **56**, 776-827.

6. Hollstein, M., Sidransky, D., Volgestein, B., Harris, C.C.. (1991). P53 mutations in human cancers. *Science*, **253**, 49-53.

7. Levine, A. J., Momand, J., Finlay, C. A.. (1991). The p53 tumours suppressor gene. *Nature*, **351**,453-456.

8. Janne, J., and William-Ashman (1971). On the purification of L- Ornithine decarboxilase from rat prostate and effects of thiol compounds on the enzyme. *Biol. Chem.*, **246**, 1725.

9. Hsu, S. M., Raine, L., and Fanger, H.. (1981). Use of Avidin- Biotin peroxidase complex (ABC) in immunoperoxidase techiniques: a comparison between ABC and unlabeled antibody (PAP) procedures. *J. Histochem. Cytochem.*, **29**, 577-580.

10. Scambia, G., Catozzi, L., Benedetti -Panici, P., Ferrandina, G., Battaglia, F., Giovannini, G., Distefano, M., Pellizzola, D., Piffanelli, A., and Mancuso, S.. (1993). Expression of ras p21 Oncoprotein in normal and neoplastic human endometrium. *Gynecologic Oncology*, **58**, 339-346.

11. Long, C. A., O'Brien, T. J., Sanders, M., Bard, D. S., and Quirk, J. G. Jr. (1988). Ras Oncogenes is expressed in adenocarcinoma of the endometrium. *Am. J. Obstet. Gynecol.*, **159**, 1512-1516.

12. Clair, T., Miller, W.R., and Cho-Chung, Y. S.. (1987). Prognostic significance of the expression of a ras protein with a molecular weight of 21,000 by human breast cancer. *Cancer Res.*, **47**, 5290-93.

13. Rodenburg, C. J., Koelma, I. A., Nap, M., and Fleuren, G. J.. (1988). Immunohistochemical detection of the ras oncogene product p21 in advanced ovarian cancer. *Arch. Pathol. Lab. Med.*, **112**, 151-154.

14. Scambia, G., Catozzi, L., Benedetti- Panici, P., Ferrandina, G., Coronetta, F., Barozzi, R., Baiocchi, G., Uccelli, L., Piffanelli, A., and Mancuso, S.. (1993). Expression of ras oncogene p21 protein in normal and neoplastic ovarian tissue: Correlation with histopathological features

and receptors for estrogen, progesterone, and epidermal growth factor. *Am. J. Obstet. Gynecol.,* **168/1**, 71-78

15. Ignar- Trowbridge, D., Risinger, J. I., Dent, G. A., Kohler, M., Berchuck, A., McLachlan, J. A., and Boyd, J.. (1992). Mutations of the Ki-ras oncogene in endometrial carcinoma. *Am. J. Obstet.Gynecol.,* **167**, 227-232.

16. Fujimoto, L., Shimizu, Y., Hiray, Y., Chen, J., Teshima, H., Hasumi, K., Masebuchi, K., and Takamashi, M.. (1993). Studies on ras oncogene activation in endometrial carcinoma. *Gynecol.Oncol.,* **48**, 196-202.

17. Koshiyama, I., Konishi, D., Wang, M., Mandai, T., Komatsu, S., Yamamoto, K., Nanbu, M. F.Naito, T. Mori. (1993). Immunohistochemical analysis of p53 protein over-expression in endometrialcarcinomas: inverse correlation with sex steroid receptors status. *Virchows Archiv. A Pathol. Anat.,* **423**, 265-271.

18. Okamoto. A., Sameshima, Y., Yamada, Y., Teshima, S., Terashima, Y., Terada, M., Yokota, J.. (1991). Allelic loss on chromosome 17 p and p53 mutations in human endometrial carcinoma of the uterus. *Cancer Res.,* **51**, 5632-5636

19. Kohler, M. F., Berchuck, A., Davidoff, A. M., Humphrey, P. A., Dodge, R. K., Iglehart, J. D., Soper, J. T., Clarke-Pearson, D. L., Bast, R. C., Marks, J. R.. (1992). Overexpression and mutation of p53 in endometrial carcinoma. *Cancer Res.,* **52**, 1622-1627

20. Enomoto, T., Fujita, M., Inoue, M., Rice, J.M., Nakajima, R., Tanizawa, O., Nomura, T. (1993). Alteration of the p53 tumor suppressor gene and its association with activation of the c-K-ras-2 protooncogene in premalignant and malignant lesions of the human uterine endometrium. *Cancer Res,* **53**, 1883-1888.

21. Honda, T., Kato, H., Imamura, T., Gima, T., Nishida, J., Sasaki, M., Hoshi, K., Sato, A., Wake, N. (1993). Involvement of p53 gene mutation in human endometrial carcinomas. *Int. J. Cancer,* **53**, 963-967.

22. Kauppila, A., Isotalo, H.E., Kivien, S.T., Viihko, R.K. (1986). Prediction of clinical outcome with estrogen and progestin receptor concentrations and their relationships of clinical and histopathological variables in endometrial cancer. *Cancer Res,* **46**, 5380-84.

23. Geisinger, K.R., Homesley, H.D., Morgan, T.M., Kute, T.E., Marchall, R.B. (1986). Endometrial carcinoma: a multiparameter clinicopathologic analysis including the DNA profile and the sex steroid hormone receptors. *Cancer,* **58**, 1518-25.

24. Creasman, W.T., Soter, J.T., McCarty, K.S. Sr., Hinshaw, W., Clarke-Pearson, D.L. (1985). Endometrial carcinoma. *Am. J. Obstet Gynecol.,* **151**, 922-32.

25. De Nardone, F.C., Benedifto, M.T., Rossiello, F., Bongiorno, M., Jacobelli, S., Mancuso, S., et al. (1989). Hormone receptor status in human endometrial adenocarcinoma. *Cancer,* **64**, 2572-78.

26. Friberg, L.G., Kullander, S. (1978). On receptors for estrogen (E2) and androgens (DMT) in human endometrial carcinoma and ovarian tumors. *Acta Obstet. Gynecol. Scand.,* **57**, 261-64.

Ovarian carcinoma metastases to the breast and axillary node: case report

M. Tessarolo, L. Leo, A. Re, R. Bellino, B. Ghiringhello*, A. Venuti, T. Wierdis, G. Visca and A. Lanza

Department B, Gynecology and Obstetrics Institute, University of Turin and *Department of Pathology, S. Anna Hospital, Turin, Italy

INTRODUCTION

Although primary malignant tumors of the breast are frequently seen, metastatic tumors to the breast are uncommon particularly from ovarian carcinoma, excluding breast involvement from terminal disseminated malignancies such as lymphoma, malignant melanoma, and leukemia.

Only 34 cases have been reported in English literature and the most were metastases which developed in patients with known ovarian neoplasms (1-23). Metastases to the breast from ovary signal widespread dissemination and generally lead to a rapid deterioration and death.

The recognition of the disease is important because the prognosis and treatment differ significantly from that of primary breast cancer.

We present a case of ovarian carcinoma with metastases to the breast and with axillary involvement and review the previous literature of this unusual entity.

CASE REPORT

A 55-year-old Caucasian woman, P2002, was admitted to Department B of the Insitute of Obstetrics and Gynecology, University of Torino, on September 12, 1989, after undergoing total abdominal hysterectomy, bilateral salpingo-oophorectomy, appendectomy, omentectomy and multiple diaphragmatic and peritoneal biopsies in another hospital. Microscopic examination of the 10.5 x 10 cm right ovarian mass revealed a moderately differentiated papillary serous cystadenocarcinoma with areas of endometrioid carcinoma with progesterone and estrogen receptors positivity . The disease was staged as FIGO stage IIIc and referred for chemotherapy. Three weeks after the surgical procedure and just before initiation of chemotherapy her serum CA125 level was under 35 IU/ml. Six courses of *cis*-platin, 20 mg/m/day Days 1 to 5, cyclophosphamide 500mg/m/day and epirubicin 50mg/m/day Day 1 were administred i.v. every four weeks.

After six cycles of chemotherapy, the patient was reassessed by clinical examination, a chest X ray, an ultrasound examination of the abdomen and pelvis and a CT. Second-look surgical reassessment with washing of the abdomen and pelvis,with pelvic and paraaortic lymphadenectomy and with multiple liver and random biopsies were performed. Thus the patient was considered in complete remission.

In May 1991 a CT and ultrasound examinations of the abdomen and pelvis revealed ascites and multiple nodules on the liver surface. The value of CA125 was 459 IU/ml (normal ≤ 35). The mammogram was normal. Six courses of carboplatin 400mg/m/day, i.v. every four weeks were performed. Two months later her serum CA125 level was 2,2 IU/ml.

In November 1991, at the end of chemotherapy, ultrasound examination of abdomen and pelvis did not find ascites and liver scan was negative. Follow-up, six and twelve months later, found the patient in generally well health. In May 1992 and 1993 bilateral mammograms and palpation of breasts were normal.

Eight months later the examination revealed a poorly definited, movable, non tender,oval shaped, 1.5 x 3.7-cm mass in the upper outer quadrant of the left breast near to the axilla. There was no nipple discharge or skin retraction and axillae and right breast were unremarkable. A mammogram showed an irregular, well defined mass in this area with no microcalcification. Serum CA125 was markedly elevated (480 IU/ml). Excisional breast biopsy was performed. The breast mass was found to be an extensive metastasis as well as the axillary nodes (16 / 26) of a papillary serous adenocarcinoma (Fig.1,2).

The patient was treated with taxol (135 mg/m^2 on day 1 every 4 weeks i.v.) and megestrol acetate (160 mg b.i.d.) (Megace, Bristol-Mayer). The patient died six months later.

DISCUSSION

Ovarian neoplasms are responsible for approximately 50% of the deaths due to malignancies of gynecologic tract. Since specific symptoms are not apparent in the early phase of the disease, ovarian carcinoma had already spread beyond the ovaries in about 70% of the cases by the time of diagnosis through the different ways of diffusion of the tumor (24).

The breast is a frequent site of primary neoplasms but it is an uncommon site of metastatic disease from extramammary tumors; the common malignancies metastasizing to the breast are those of hematologic origin, lung, stomach and malignant melanoma (1,5,10,21).

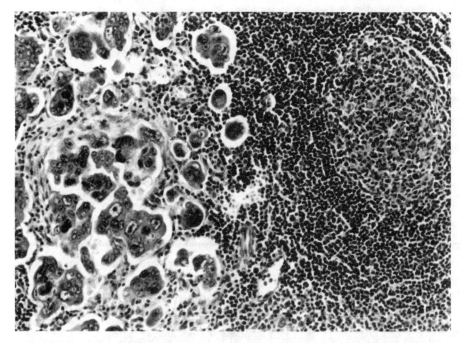

Figure 1   Axillary node metastasis on the left and germination node center on the right

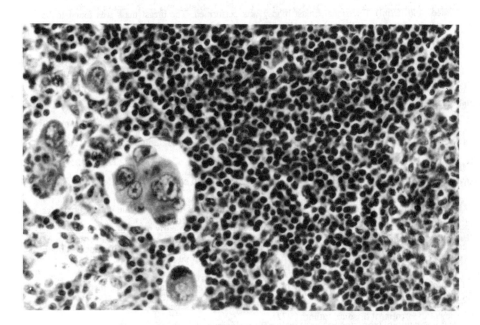

Figure 2 Higher magnification of the previous field enhancing the poor differentiation of the serous papillar adenocarcinoma

Table 1   Patients reported with ovarian cancers metastatic to the breast

Ref.	N° of cases	Age	Type of ovarian tumor	Survival after finding breast metastasis
1,4,5,6,7,9,11, 12,13,14,16,17, 18, 19, 22, current case	26	57,3 (mean)	Serous Papillary Adenocarcinoma	>2 months-3 years
2	1	56	Pseudomucinous Cystoadenocarcinoma	N.A
3	1	56	Lymphosarcoma	N.A
8	1	50	Granulose cell carcinoma	11 months
10	1	37	Cystoadenocarcinoma Mesonephric type	8 months
15	1	69	Choriocarcinoma	2 months
20	1	16	Dysgerminoma	> 16 months
23	1	52	Carcinoid	> 8 months
21	1	63	Endometriod	> 16 months
17	1	N.A	N.A	N.A

N.A. data not avaible

The few reported cases in English Literature indicate the rarity of metastatic mammary tumors from ovarian tumors and show the limited experience with this condition. The actual incidence is unknown.

The first case of ovarian cancer with breast metastasis was described by Sitzenfrey in 1907, who described a papillary serous cystoadenocarcinoma of the ovary metastases to one breast, the opposite ovary, the uterus, and intestine (25). Since then, in Literature, 34 cases of ovarian neoplasms metastatic to the breast have been reported (1-23) (table 1). Metastases have been reported as late as 10 years following the primary diagnosis (19). Breast metastases concurrent with an ovarian neoplasms are rare.

The epithelial ovarian neoplasm most often seen in breast metastatic lesion is the papillary serous cystoadenocarcinoma as our case and it is interesting to note that also the hystologic form with low malignant potential is able to metastasize outside of peritoneal cavity to the breast (21).

Breast metastases appear approximately 2.0 years after discovery of the primary lesion, most commonly as a solitary lesion appearing quite benign on both clinical and mammographic exams (13). The lesion tends to be superficially located in the upper outer quadrant of the breast, and axillary node involvement is frequently reported (7). On mammogram, the lump appears as a well demarcated, dense lesion ; microcalcifications in metastatic tumors are so uncommon than some authors think that the presence of tumor calcification virtually excludes metastatic disease to the breast (17).

It is important that metastases to the breast should be accurately differentiated from primary breast cancer because treatment and prognosis differ significantly. Immunohistochemical studies of tumor tissue can be useful to identify the site of origin of the neoplasms; the combination of tumor markers OC125 and OV632, DNA analysis and serum markers, as antigen CA-125 have been evaluated for the efficacy of the treatment by some authors (5,22).

Metastasis from ovarian cancer to the breast implies widespread tumor dissemination; in fact the average survival for these patients is less than one year after the discovery of breast metastases. Ron et al. reported an average survival of 8.1 months (21).

In the case reported the lump emerged in the upper outer quadrant of the left breast near to the axillary; however we cannot rule out the possibility that other metastatic sites are present in the breast when axillary node metastases are clinically recognized (19).

Many theories have been offered to explain the possible way of metastasis from the ovaries to the breast . It is suggested that this kind of metastasis affects first the axillary nodes and then the breast and it is caused by reverse lymph flow. Simple excisional biopsy and chemotherapeutic agents correctly chosen by the clinician for this tumor constitute the preferred choice of treatment and mastectomy may be recommended only for palliation in the case of a very large lesion.

Acknowledgment: the authors thank Pharmacia / Farmitalia Carlo Erba

REFERENCES

1. Abrams, H.L., Spiro, R. and Goldestein, N. (1950). Metastases in carcinoma: analysis of 1000 autopsied cases. *Cancer*, **3**, 74-85

2. Bohman, L.G.,Bassett,L.H. and Gold, R.H. (1982). Breast metastasis from extramammary malignancies. *Radiology*, **144**, 309-312

3. Brown, J.B. and O'Keefe, C.D. (1928). Sarcoma of the ovary with unusual oral metastasis. *Ann.Sur.*, **87**, 467-71

4. Charache, H. (1953). Metastatic tumors to the breast. *Surgery*, **33**, 385-390

5. Duda, R.B., August C.Z. and Schink, J.C. (1991). Ovarian carcinoma metastatic to the breast and axillary node. *Surgery*, **110**, 552-6

6. Frauenhoffer, E.E., Ro, J.Y., Silva, E.G. and El-Naggar, A. (1991). Well-differentiated serous ovarian carcinoma presenting as a breast mass: a case report and flow cytometric DNA study. *Int.J.Gynecol.Pathol.*, **10**, 79-87

7. Hajdu, S.I. and Urban, J.A. (1972). Cancers metastatic to the breast. Cancer, **29**, 1691-6

8. Harwood, T.R. (1971). Metastatic carcinoma to the breast. *JAMA*, **218**, 97

9. Hughes, J.D., Hynes, H.E. and Lin, J.J. (1983). Ovarian carcinoma metastatic to the breast. *South. Med. J.*, **76**, 667-9

10. Ibach, J.R. (1964). Carcinoma of the ovary metastatic to breast. *Arch.Surg.*, **88**, 410-4

11. Krishnan, E.U., Phillips, A.K., Randell, A., Taylor, B. and Grag, S.K. (1980). Bilateral metastatic inflammatory carcinoma in the breast from primary ovarian carcinoma.*Obstet.Gynecol.*,**55**(suppl), 94-6

12. Laifer, S., Bushema, J., Parmley, T.H. and Rosenshein, N.B. (1986). Ovarian carcinoma metastatic to the breast. *Gynecol.Oncol.*, 24, 97-102

13. Loredo, D.L., Powell, J.L., Reed, W.P. and Rosembaun, J.M. (1990). Ovarian carcinoma metastatic to the breast : a case report and review of literature. *Gynecol.Oncol.*, 37, 432-6

14. Matseoane, S.L. (1988). Ovarian carcinoma metastatic to the breast : a literature review and report of two cases. *Obstet.Gynecol.*, 43, 645-654

15. McIntosh, I.H., Hooper, A.A., Millis, R.R. and Greenberg, W.P. (1976). Metastatic carcinoma within the breast. *Clin. Oncol.*, 2, 393-401

16. Moncada, R., Cooper, R.A., Garces, M. and Badrinath, K. (1974). Calcified metastases from malignant ovarian neoplasm. *Radiology*, 113, 31-5

17. Paulus, D.D. and Libshitz, H.I. (1982). Metastasis to the breast. *Radiol. Clin. N. Am.*, 20, 561-8

18. Royen, P.M. and Ziter, F.M.H. (1974). Ovarian carcinoma metastatic to the breast. Br. J. Radiol., 47, 356-7

19. Scotto, V., Masci, P. and Sbiroli, C. (1985). Breast metastasis of ovarian cancer during cis-platinum therapy. *Eur. J. Gynecol. Oncol.*, 6, 62-5

20 .Kattan, J., Droz, J.P., Charpentier, P., Guy, M., Lhomme, C., Boutan-Laroze, A. and Prade, M. (1992). Ovarian dysgerminoma metastatic to the breast. *Gynecol. Oncol.*, 46, 104-6

21. Ron, I.G., Inbar, M., Halpern, M. and Chaitchik, S. (1992). Endometroid carcinoma of the ovary presenting as primary carcinoma of the breast. *Acta Obstet. Gynecol. Scand.*, 71, 81-3

22. Yamasaki, H., Saw, D., Zdanowitz, J. and Faltz, L.L. (1993). Ovarian carcinoma metastasis to the breast case report and review of the literature. *Am. J. Surg. Pathol.*, 17 (2), 193-7

23. Fishman, A., Kim, H.S., Girtanner, R.E. and Kaplan, A.L. (1994). Solitary breast metastasis as first manifestation of ovarian carcinoid tumor. *Gynecol.Oncol.*, 54(2), 222-6.

24. Twaalfhoven, F.C.M., Fleuren, G. J., Cornelisse, C.J., Peters, A.A.W., Trimbos, J.B. and Logendoorn, P.C.W. (1994). Metastasis of breast carcinoma to a primary mucinous cystadenocarcinoma of the ovary. *Gynecol. Oncol.*, 52, 80-6

25. Sitzenfrey, A. (1907). Mammakarzinom zwei jahre nach abdonimaler radikaloperation wegen doppelseitigen carcinoma ovarii. *Prag. Med. Woch.*, 32, 221-235

Author Index

Abós, M.D.   547
Abubakari, M.N.J.   469
Agosti, S.   541
Agostini, R.   293, 319
Aidala, V.   497, 577, 583, 649
Alba, E.   493, 609, 793
Alberico, S.   569
Albrecht, A.   225
Alfonso, R.   335
Aloi, J.A.   3
Altavilla, G.   897
Alviggi, C.   271
Ambrosini, A.   843
Ambrosini, G.   301, 315, 501
Ambrosio, D.R.   319
Angioni, S.   431
Anile, C.   169
Annicchiarico, C.   817
Ansaldi, C.   259
Anzivino, M.   665
Apa, R.   125
Ardita, F.V.   341, 661
Ardito, P.   453
Ardizzi, A.   141
Ardizzoja, M.   385
Arnone, P.   797
Artini, P.   53
Artini, P.G.   11, 47, 277, 325, 345, 441
Azzena, A.   363, 707, 891, 897

Bagella, M.P.   701, 843, 887
Baischer, W.   225
Balconi, G.   807
Balerna, M.   259
Ban, C.   319
Barbaro, L.   519
Barreca, A.   47
Barri, P.N.   233
Battaglia, C.   47, 277, 325, 345, 441
Baviera, G.   849, 863
Beleslin, B.Z.   163

Bellina, C.R.   821
Bellino, R.   217, 523, 529, 803, 869, 905, 915
Bellodi, P.   489, 507
Belloni, C.   671
Benagiano, G.   679
Benedetto, V.   307, 341, 511, 661
Benzi, L.   557
Bianchi Malandrone, L.   733, 901
Bianchi, A.   157
Bianchi, R.   811, 817, 821
Bianchi, S.   297
Bilezikjian, L.M.   5
Bili, H.   39
Blankenstein, M.A.   147
Boada, M.   233
Bocconcello, B.   351
Bogatti, P.   569
Bogdanskiene, G.   631
Bombelli, C.   541
Boni, G.   821
Bonuccelli, A.   811
Bori, S.   469
Borovský, M.   473
Boulet, M.   375
Bracco, G.L.   837
Britton, K.T.   9
Brot, M.D.   9
Brunetti, V.   707
Brus, L.   87
Brusati, M.   855
Burger, H.G.   27
Busacca, M.   297

Cadente Colucci, C.   271
Calò, G.   183
Canavese, A.   797
Candiani, M.   297
Cantarella, R.   497, 577, 583, 649
Cantù, M.G.   807
Capetta, P.   351

Capone, F. 613, 619
Cappia, S. 509
Carani, A. 193, 643
Carbonaro, A. 497, 577, 583, 649
Cardozo, L.D. 389
Carravetta, C. 271, 311
Carta, Q. 665
Caruso, A. 67, 125, 131, 285
Castaldo Tuccillo, A. 619
Castaldo, A. 613
Castellani, C. 817
Catinella, A. 671
Cela, V. 11, 47, 325
Celano, M.A. 637, 693
Celona, A. 519
Cerri, G. 363, 707, 891, 897
Cersosimo, L. 331, 797
Certo, M. 189
Cherchi, P.L. 315, 501, 701, 843, 887
Cianci, S. 371
Ciccarese, M. 671
Cicinelli, E. 175
Cirillo, D. 655, 827, 833
Coccia, M.E. 837
Coccollone, E. 501
Colacurci, N. 311
Colombatto, S. 905
Colombo, A. 193, 643
Comar, M. 683
Conte, G. 157, 169
Contu, G. 53
Corvetto, L. 493, 793
Costin, N. 211
Cotrozzi, N. 541
Cotta-Pereira, G. 787
Coviello, D. 541
Cozzolino, V. 613
Crea, E. 511
Criscuolo, M. 11
Crosignani, P.G. 17
Cucinelli, F. 67, 131
Curtiss, L.K. 9

D'Ambrogio, G. 47, 325
D'Amico, C. 169
D'Aniello, G. 613

D'Anna, R. 341
D'Auria, C. 613, 625
Dal Maso, J. 707
Dalkin, A.C. 3
Dalprà, L. 541
De Domenico, P. 469
De Luca, A.M. 131
De Luca, P. 619
De Luigi, G. 385
De Marinis, L. 157, 169, 189
De Medici, C. 183
De Placido, G. 271, 311
De Punzio, C. 637, 693
De Stefano, R. 357
De Vita, D. 589
de la Cueva, P. 393
de Micheroux, A.A. 11, 325
Decko, A. 793
Dei, M. 301, 315
Delli Carpini, R. 193, 489, 507
Demurtas, A. 733, 901
Depypere, H.T. 253
Desiderio, E. 613, 619, 625
Dessole, S. 301, 315, 501
Devroey, P. 265
Di Carlo, C. 73, 357
Di Cianni, G. 557
Di Giorgio, A. 797
Di Giulio, N. 697
Di Gregorio, A. 523
Dirsaite, I. 631
Drezgić, M. 163
Durando, A. 733, 901
Dyer, C.A. 9

Egozcue, J. 233
Ehrly, A.M. 463
El-Farra, K. 237
Esposito, F. 701, 843, 887

Fabrizi, M.L. 157
Facchini, V. 811, 817, 821
Fadda, G. 189
Faiman, C. 103
Falco, T. 175
Farina, M. 315

Fauser, B.C.J.M. 35
Fedele, L. 297
Fenocchio, M. 609, 793
Fenu, M.A. 431
Ferdeghini, M. 811, 817, 821
Ferrara, A. 363
Ferrara, P. 655, 827, 833
Ferraris, G. 875
Filippa, N. 671
Filosofi, M.T. 319
Fiorentino, G. 519
Fiozzi, R. 193, 643
Florio, P. 589
Fontanesi, M. 855
Franco, G.B. 843
Frigo, P. 457
Fujii, S. 715
Fulghesu, A.M. 67, 125, 131, 285

Gadducci, A. 811, 817, 821
Gagetti, O. 811
Gaiola, O. 733
Galli, P. 193, 489, 507, 643
Gallinelli, A. 589
Gallo, M. 385
Galossi, S. 293
Gandulfo, V.G. 687
Gardiman, M. 891
Gargiulo, A.R. 73
Garizio, M. 881
Ge, Q.-S. 153
Gelfand, M.M. 413
Genazzani, A.D. 21, 53, 441
Genazzani, A.R. 11, 47, 325, 589, 811,
    817, 821
Genta, F. 763
Geuna, M. 733, 901
Ghiringhello, B. 915
Giannone, E. 469, 697
Giovannetti, G. 693
Gordini, G. 523, 803
Gramellini, F. 541
Graziano, V. 827
Grieco, M. 625
Grosso, M. 821
Gruber, D.M. 457

Grudzinskas, J.G. 245, 535, 631
Grugni, G. 141, 183
Gu, C. 153
Guaschino, S. 569, 683
Guazzelli, G. 637, 693
Gubetta, L. 905
Guerzoni, G. 489, 507
Guidetti, R. 193, 643
Guido, M. 67, 125
Guo, Ai-Li 11
Guzzaloni, G. 183

Haisenleder, D.J. 3
Hartmann, B. 225
He, F. 153
Hegg, R. 727
Hergueta, J. 547, 777
Herold, J. 407
Hill, S. 389
Huang, S. 153
Huber, J. 225
Huber, J.C. 457

Ilardi, P. 541
Insler, V. 59

Jurado, A.R. 437

Kauppila, A. 423, 721
Kauppila, S. 721
Keckstein, J. 119
Kerrigan, J.R. 3
Khullar, V. 389
Kirchengast, S. 225
Kirk, S.E. 3
Knogler, W. 457
Kocijančič, A. 137
Koinig, G. 225
Komatsu, T. 715
Konishi, I. 715
Koob, G.F. 9
Koshiyama, M. 715
Kováč, G. 485
Krstić, N. 163

La Rusca, C. 271

Lambalk, C.B.   87
Langer, G.   225
Lanza, A.   217, 523, 529, 803, 869, 905, 915
Lanzone, A.   67, 125, 131
Lauricella, A.   869
Lauro, V.   469, 697
Leybaert, L.   253
Lecca, P.   701, 887
Legan, M.   137
Leo, L.   523, 529, 803, 869, 905, 915
Leonardi, J.   307, 341, 511, 661
Leonardi, R.   307, 341, 661
Leotta, A.   453
Lerro, R.   493, 609
Lio, S.G.   453
Liprandi, V.   351
Lollo, F.   613, 619, 625
Lombardo, M.   589
Lubrano, G.   613, 625
Lunenfeld, B.   59
Luoto, R.   515
Lyras, I.   787

Maccarini, U.   671
Macchia, E.   31
Macciò, A.   53
Maffei, S.   523, 529, 793
Maheux, R.   419
Maiorino, R.   175
Maira, G.   169
Manca, L.   701
Mancini, A.   131, 157, 169, 189
Mancuso, A.   341
Mancuso, S.   67, 125, 131
Mandai, M.   715
Mangiacasale, A.   371
Mangioni, C.   807
Markussis, V.   63
Marra, L.   189
Marshall, J.C.   3
Marzola, M.   807
Maso, G.   569
Masoni, S.   637, 693
Massobrio, M.   259, 385, 665, 733, 901
Mastrantonio, P.   357

Masturzo, B.   665
Mattei, A.M.   351
Matteo, G.   175
Matteucci, F.   821
Mauri, A.   605
Maxia, N,   53
Mehta, A.E.   103
Melpignano, M.   855
Menato, G.   665
Menendez, C.   437
Mercuri, N.   453
Merialdi, A.   855
Merisio, C.   855
Micalizzi, M.   307, 511
Milewicz, A.   113
Milluzzo, L.   371
Minocci, A.   141
Modotti, M.   259
Molaro, R.   613, 625
Mollo, A.   271, 311
Monaco, A.   881
Montaldo, C.   431
Montaldo, P.L.   431
Monti, P.   351
Montoneri, C.   281
Morabito, F.   141, 183
Morali, F.   807
Mori, T.   715
Moro, D.   141
Morollón, I.   393, 777
Moskovic, T.   479
Murgia, F.   125

Nanbu, K.   715
Nappi, C.   73, 203, 357, 655, 827, 833
Nappi, R.E.   11
Nardo, F.   281
Nassif, T.   787
Nauert, C.   463
Navalesi, R.   557
Neri, E.   637
Nocera, G.   541
Nuzzo, L.   493, 793
Nyman, T.   43

Orsini, P.   557

Osnengo, G. 523

Padula, L. 489, 507
Pagano, C. 613
Palacios, S. 437
Palestro, G. 733, 901
Palmara, V. 307, 511, 661
Palumbo, M.A. 11
Papa, M.C. 637, 693
Paradisi, G. 285
Parastie, S. 211
Parducci, R. 693
Parente, E. 655
Parri, C. 47, 325
Passannanti, G. 827, 833
Pavone, V. 125
Peg, V. 547
Pekonen, F. 43
Pellicano, M. 203, 357
Pellicer, A. 107
Penezić, Z. 163
Pereira, N.R. 633
Pérez Sanz, R. 393, 777
Pérez-López, F.R. 393, 547, 745, 777
Perotti, F. 671
Perrelli, M. 157
Perutelli, A. 817
Pesce, G. 293
Petraglia, F. 11, 21, 67, 589
Petrone, A. 203, 655, 827, 833
Petruzzelli, P. 665
Petruzzi, D. 175
Pezzella, P. 331
Piccione, E. 605
Pinchera, A. 31
Pinna Nossai, L. 701, 887
Pinotti, J.A. 727
Pinzano, R. 569
Piras, G. 701, 887
Piscopo, M. 613, 625
Pitanguy, I. 787
Pittau, G. 431
Platania, R. 577
Polatti, F. 671
Polonio, S. 897
Porcelli, A. 197

Powell, K.J. 535
Prato, B. 821
Prontera, C. 811
Puistola, U. 721
Pullè, C. 519, 849, 863
Purdy, R.H. 9
Putzolu, M. 887

Quinzi, A. 293, 319

Ragno, G. 175
Ragonesi, G. 493, 793
Ramella, A. 733
Rao, Ch. V. 715
Rapicano, C. 655
Rapti, P. 787
Raudaskoski, T. 423
Ravarino, A. 733, 901
Re, A. 523, 529, 803, 869, 905, 915
Regnani, G. 277
Reitano, S. 497, 577, 583, 649
Remohi, J. 107
Revelli, A. 259
Rigano, A. 849, 863
Rigano, M. 511, 661, 849, 863
Risteli, J. 721
Risteli, L. 721
Robbins, A. 93, 99
Robert, J. 547
Robertson, D.M. 27
Rohr, U.D. 463
Ronsini, S. 203, 833
Rosca, A. 211
Rossi, L. 189
Rossmanith, W.G. 119
Rosso, M. 803, 869
Rota, S. 807
Rowe, P. 679
Ruccia, C. 175
Ruiu, G. 843
Runic, S. 479
Rutanen, E.-M. 43, 515

Sagliocco, R. 311
Sajtos, B. 407
Salmaso, R. 363, 891, 897

Salvatori, M. 277, 345
Salvestroni, C. 589, 637, 693
Sammartano, L. 189
Sansebastiano, L. 855
Santala, M. 721
Santaló, J. 233
Santoro, T. 311
Sarpa, G. 523, 529
Sator, M.O. 457
Sbernardori, F. 843
Sberveglieri, M. 733, 901
Scapinelli, A. 301, 501, 701, 887
Scarcella, V. 453
Scarselli, G. 837
Scatena, E. 837
Schindler, A.E. 401, 407, 773
Schneider, H.P.G. 739
Schoemaker, J. 87
Schönauer, L.M. 175
Scida, P. 589
Scribanti, A. 881
Serrani, M. 351
Sgherzi, M.R. 277, 345, 441
Shoham, Z. 37
Silva, J.B. 633
Simón, C. 107
Simonelli, M. 589
Sismondi, P. 763
Sjöberg, N.-O. 595
Skret, A. 599
Slijepčević, D. 163
Smitz, J. 265
Soi, P. 431
Šoka, A. 485
Sole, E. 655, 827, 833
Soranna, L. 67
Spitz, I.M. 93, 99
Stenbäck, F. 721
Stjernquist, M. 595
Stojanović, M. 163
Sturlese, E. 849, 863
Surcel, I.V. 211
Surico, N. 197, 875
Šuška, P. 473, 485
Šuškova, E. 485
Suvanto-Luukkonen, E. 423

Taccani, C. 197
Tacconis, P. 259
Tarabusi, M. 325
Tarlatzis, B.C. 39
Tavernnari, D. 193, 489, 507
Tessarolo, M. 217, 523, 529, 803, 869, 905, 915
Thijssen, J.H.H. 147
Ticconi, C. 605
Tolino, A. 203, 655, 827, 833
Tolis, G. 63
Tomás, C. 721
Tonelli, E. 183
Torchio, B. 733, 901
Traficante, G. 293
Traversi, P. 277, 345, 441
Trentini, G.P. 11
Trojano, V. 335
Tronci, M. 431
Turnu, E. 53

Ubaldi, F. 265
Uherčík, D. 473
Ulrich, U. 119

Vadalà, P. 453
Vadora, E. 855
Vairo, G. 613, 619, 625
Vale, W.W. 5
Valle, D. 131, 157, 169, 189
Van Steirteghem, A. 265
Vargiu, N. 301, 501
Vasile, C. 363, 707
Vasoin, F. 363, 707, 891, 897
Vavalà, V. 881
Veiga, A. 233, 239
Veloce, N. 335
Venuti, A. 523, 529, 803, 869, 905, 915
Vescio, F. 453
Vezzani, M.A. 489, 507, 643
Vidal, F. 233
Vignali, M. 297
Villa, P. 125, 131
Villavieja, L. 393
Visca, G. 217, 523, 529, 609, 869, 915

Volpe, A.   21, 53, 345, 431, 441
Volpe, L.   557
Vujović, S.   163

Walker, S.M.   243
Wierdis, T.   523, 529, 803, 869, 905, 915
Winkler, U.H.   407, 447

Yamamoto, S.   715
Yasin, M.   3

Yeh, L.   153
Yip, A.   389
Ylikorkala, O.   427, 565
Yu, Q.   153

Zarbo, G.   281
Zen, T.   891
Zhu, G.-G.   721
Zona, G.   307, 341, 511, 661
Zullo, F.   357